ESSENTIALS
OF
PAIN MEDICINE
AND
REGIONAL ANESTHESIA

HONORIO T. BENZON, M.D.
PROFESSOR OF ANESTHESIOLOGY
Northwestern University
Medical School
Chief, Section of Pain Medicine
Northwestern Memorial Hospital
Chicago, Illinois

SRINIVASA N. RAJA, M.D.
PROFESSOR OF ANESTHESIOLOGY
Johns Hopkins University
School of Medicine
Baltimore, Maryland

DAVID BORSOOK, M.D, Ph.D.
ASSISTANT PROFESSOR OF NEUROLOGY
AND ANESTHESIOLOGY
Harvard Medical School
Director, Pain Management Center
Massachusetts General Hospital
Boston, Massachusetts

ROBERT E. MOLLOY, M.D.
ASSISTANT PROFESSOR OF ANESTHESIOLOGY
Northwestern University
Medical School
Chicago, Illinois

GARY STRICHARTZ, Ph.D.
PROFESSOR OF PHARMACOLOGY
AND ANESTHESIOLOGY
Harvard Medical School
Chairman of Anesthesia Research
Brigham and Women's Hospital
Boston, Massachusetts

CHURCHILL LIVINGSTONE

A Division of Harcourt Brace & Company
New York, Edinburgh, London, Philadelphia, San Francisco

CHURCHILL LIVINGSTONE
A Division of Harcourt Brace & Company

The Curtis Center
Independence Square West
Philadelphia, Pennsylvania 19106

Library of Congress Cataloging-in-Publication Data

Essentials of pain medicine and regional anesthesia / [edited by]
Honorio T. Benzon . . . [et al.].

p.   cm.

ISBN 0–443–06509–8

1. Conduction anesthesia. 2. Pain—Treatment. 3. Analgesia.
    I. Benzon, Honorio T.   [DNLM: 1. Pain. 2. Anesthesia,
    Conduction.   WL 704 E78 1999]

RD84.E87 1999   616′.0472—dc21

DNLM/DLC   98–24849

ESSENTIALS OF PAIN MEDICINE AND REGIONAL ANESTHESIA   ISBN 0-443-06509-8

Printed in the United States of America.

Last digit is the print number: 9   8   7   6   5   4   3   2   1

To our families.

To the Departments of Anesthesiology at Northwestern University Medical School, Johns Hopkins University School of Medicine, Massachusetts General Hospital, and Brigham and Women's Hospital.

To all our contributors.

Contributors

HONORIO T. BENZON, M.D.
Professor, Department of Anesthesiology, Northwestern University Medical School; Chief, Section of Pain Medicine, Northwestern Memorial Hospital, Chicago, Illinois.

Taxonomy: Definitions of Pain Terms and Chronic Pain Syndromes; Local Anesthetic Infusions for Pain Management; Patient-Controlled Analgesia; Epidural Opioid Infusion; Outcome Studies in Postoperative Pain Control; Spontaneous Intracranial Hypotension; Injection of Epidural Steroids; Facet Arthropathy and Facet Joint Injections; Facet Nerve Blocks and Rhizotomy; Anesthesiologic Treatment for Complex Regional Pain Syndrome; Phantom Pain; Sickle Cell Anemia; Celiac Plexus Block; Infraclavicular Brachial Plexus Block; Suprascapular Nerve Block; Lumbar Plexus, Femoral, Lateral Femoral Cutaneous, and Obturator Nerve Blocks; Sciatic Nerve Block in the Popliteal Fossa; Lumbar Paravertebral Sympathetic Block; Signs of Sympathetic Blockade: Correlation With Pain Relief

DINNA BILLOTE, M.D.
Clinical Instructor, Northwestern University–McGraw Medical School; Attending Anesthesiologist, Northwestern Memorial Hospital, Chicago, Illinois.

Interscalene Brachial Plexus Block

PATRICK K. BIRMINGHAM, M.D.
Assistant Professor, Northwestern University Medical School; Director, Acute Pain Management Service Co-director, Pain Management Service, Attending Physician, Department of Pediatric Anesthesia, Children's Memorial Hospital, Chicago, Illinois.

Pediatric Postoperative Pain

E. RICHARD BLONSKY, M.D.
Associate Professor of Clinical Neurology, Northwestern University Medical School; Director, Pain and Rehabilitation Clinic of Chicago, Chicago, Illinois.

Determination of Disability

DAVID BORSOOK, M.D., Ph.D.
Assistant Professor of Neurology and Anesthesiology; Harvard Medical School; Director, Pain Management Center, Massachusetts General Hospital, Boston, Massachusetts.

Opioids in Pain Management; Psychotropic Drugs Use-

ful in Pain Treatment; Membrane Stabilizers; Pharmacologic Treatment of Headache

ONASSIS A. CANERIS, M.D.
Assistant in Anesthesia (Neurology), Department of Anesthesia and Critical Care, Massachusetts General Hospital, Boston, Massachusetts.

Differential Diagnosis of Headache

KENNETH CHIOU, M.D.
Fellow, Section of Pain Medicine, Northwestern University Medical School, Chicago, Illinois.

Low Back Pain: Differential Diagnosis and Physical Examination

LUCY A. CHRISTOPHERSON, M.D.
Fellow, Department of Neuroradiology, Northwestern University Medical School, Chicago, Illinois.

Radiology of the Spine

MICHAEL R. CLARK, M.D., M.P.H.
Assistant Professor, Department of Psychiatry and Behavioral Sciences, Johns Hopkins University School of Medicine; Director, Chronic Pain Treatment Programs, Johns Hopkins Medical Institutions, Baltimore, Maryland.

Substance Use Disorders and Chronic Pain; Detoxification: Assessment and Methods

JAMES C. CREWS, M.D.
Associate Professor, Department of Anesthesiology, Wake Forest University School of Medicine; Director, Acute Pain Service, Pain Control Center, Department of Anesthesiology, Wake Forest University Baptist Medical Center, Winston-Salem, North Carolina.

Epidural Hematoma; Epidural Abscess

OSCAR A. de LEON-CASASOLA, M.D.
Assistant Professor, Department of Anesthesia, State University of New York at Buffalo, Buffalo, New York.

Superior Hypogastric Plexus Block Neurolysis for Cancer Pain; Ganglion Impar Block

KERRY GILL DeLUCA, M.D.
Resident, Physical Medicine and Rehabilitation, North-

western University Medical School; Resident, Rehabilitation Institute of Chicago, Chicago, Illinois.

Neurologic Assessment of the Pain Patient

CARMEN L. DOMINGUEZ, M.D.

Clinical Instructor, Department of Anesthesiology, Columbia Presbyterian Medical Center, New York, New York.

Trigeminal Neuralgia

PATRICK M. DOUGHERTY, Ph.D.

Departments of Neurosurgery and Neuroscience, Johns Hopkins University School of Medicine, Baltimore, Maryland.

Pain and the Neurophysiology of Somatosensory Processing; Pain and the Neurochemistry of Somatosensory Processing

FRANK D. FERRIS, M.D.

Lecturer, Department of Family and Community Medicine, University of Toronto; Coordinator, Inpatient and Research Services, Temmy Latner Centre for Palliative Care, Mount Sinai Hospital, Toronto, Ontario, Canada.

Approach to Management of Cancer Pain; Pharmacologic Management of Cancer Pain

MARC FISHMAN, M.D.

Assistant Professor, Department of Psychiatry and Behavioral Sciences Johns Hopkins University School of Medicine; Attending Physician, Motivated Behaviors Unit, Johns Hopkins Medical Institutions, Baltimore, Maryland.

Substance Use Disorders and Chronic Pain; Detoxification: Assessment and Methods

SCOTT M. FISHMAN, M.D.

Assistant Professor of Anesthesia, Assistant Professor of Psychiatry, Harvard Medical School; Medical Director, MGH Pain Center, Massachusetts General Hospital, Boston, Massachusetts.

Opioids in Pain Management; Psychotropic Drugs Useful in Pain Treatment

RICHARD V. GREGG, M.D.

Director, Pain Management Associates, Anesthesia Associates of Cincinnati; The Christ Hospital, Cincinnati Ohio.

Acute Herpes Zoster; Postherpetic Neuralgia

EDWARD P. GRIMES, M.D.

Instructor, Department of Anesthesiology, Northwestern University School of Medicine; Staff Anesthesiologist, Northwestern Memorial Hospital, Chicago, Illinois.

Supraclavicular Approaches to Brachial Plexus Block

ANTHONY GUARINO, M.D.

Director, Department of Pain Medicine, Barnes–Jewish West County Hospital, St. Louis, Missouri.

Terminology and Pathophysiology of Complex Re-

gional Pain Syndromes; Diagnosis of Complex Regional Pain Syndrome

ROBERT C. HAMILTON, M.B., B.Ch., F.R.C.P.C.

Clinical Professor, University of Calgary; Senior Anaesthesiologist, Gimbel Eye Centre, Calgary, Alberta, Canada.

Orbital Nerve Blocks

R. NORMAN HARDEN, M.D.

Assistant Professor of Physical Medicine and Rehabilitation, Northwestern University Medical School; Attending Physiatrist, Rehabilitation Institute of Chicago, Chicago, Illinois.

Tests of the Autonomic Nervous System

PATRICIA HARRISON, M.D.

Assistant Professor of Clinical Anesthesia, Director, USC Pain Management Center, Department of Anesthesiology, University of Southern California, Los Angeles, California.

Transdermal Fentanyl

JENNIFER A. HAYTHORNTHWAITE, Ph.D.

Associate Professor, Department of Psychiatry and Behavioral Sciences, Johns Hopkins University School of Medicine, Baltimore, Maryland.

Psychological Evaluation and Testing; Psychological Interventions for Chronic Pain

LESLIE J. HEINBERG, Ph.D.

Assistant Professor, Department of Psychiatry and Behavioral Sciences, Johns Hopkins University School of Medicine, Baltimore, Maryland.

Psychological Evaluation and Testing; Psychological Interventions for Chronic Pain

JACLYN HO, M.D.

Resident, Physical Medicine and Rehabilitation, Northwestern University Medical School; Resident, Rehabilitation Institute of Chicago, Chicago, Illinois.

Neurologic Assessment of the Pain Patient

SHERWIN E. HUA, M.D.

Resident, Department of Neurosurgery, Johns Hopkins University School of Medicine, Baltimore, Maryland.

Epidural Spinal Cord Stimulation for Chronic Pain Control; Spinal Cord Stimulation for Failed Back Surgery Syndrome

JOSEPH H. INTROCASO, M.D., D.M.D.

Director, Interventional Neuroradiology, Lutheran General Hospital, Park Ridge, Illinois.

Radiology of the Spine

JEFFREY A. KATZ, M.D.

Assistant Professor of Anesthesiology, Northwestern University Medical School; Director, Pain Management Clinic, Veterans Affairs Health Care System—Lakeside Division, Chicago, Illinois.

Diabetic and Other Neuropathies; Use of Nerve Stimulators for Peripheral Nerve Blocks

TOM C. KREJCIE, M.D.
Associate Professor of Anesthesiology, Northwestern University Medical School; Staff Anesthesiologist, Northwestern Memorial Hospital, Chicago, Illinois.
Cauda Equina Syndrome After Continuous Spinal Anesthesia

CHARLES E. LAURITO, M.D.
Medical Director, Center for Pain Management and Rehabilitation Medicine, University of Illinois at Chicago, Chicago, Illinois.
Caudal Anesthesia; Nerve Blocks at Elbow and Wrist

DAVID J. LEE, M.D.
Fellow in Pain Management, University of California at San Francisco, San Francisco, California.
Anesthesiologic Treatments for Complex Regional Pain Syndrome

MARK J. LEMA, M.D., Ph.D.
Associate Professor and Vice-Chairman of Anesthesiology, State University of New York at Buffalo, School of Medicine and Biomedical Sciences; Chairman of Anesthesiology and Pain Medicine, Roswell Park Cancer Institute, Buffalo, New York.
Ganglion Impar Block

ROBERT M. LEVY, M.D., Ph.D.
Associate Professor, Departments of Neurosurgery and Physiology, Director, Northwestern Comprehensive Pain Clinic, Northwestern University Medical School, Chicago, Illinois.
Implanted Drug Delivery Systems for Control of Chronic Pain; Neuroablative Procedures for the Treatment of Intractable Pain; Epidural Spinal Cord Stimulation for Chronic Pain Control; Spinal Cord Stimulation for Failed Back Surgery Syndrome

DWIGHT LIGHAM, M.D.
Clinical Fellow, Yale Center for Pain Management, Yale University School of Medicine, New Haven, Connecticut.
Sacroiliac Joint Dysfunction

HENRY M. LIU, M.D.
Chief Resident, Department of Anesthesiology, Northwestern University Medical School, Chicago, Illinois.
Acupuncture

SPENCER S. LIU, M.D.
Clinical Assistant Professor of Anesthesiology, University of Washington; Staff Anesthesiologist, Virginia Mason Medical Center, Seattle, Washington.
Local Anesthetics: Clinical Aspects

ONUR MELEN, M.D.
Assistant Professor of Neurology, Northwestern University Medical School; Attending Physician, Northwestern Memorial Hospital, Chicago, Illinois.
Muscle Relaxants

MICHAEL M. MINIEKA, M.D.
Assistant Professor of Neurology, Northwestern University Medical School; Attending Neurologist, Northwestern Memorial Hospital, Chicago, Illinois.
Role of Neurophysiologic Testing for Pain

VERONICA D. MITCHELL, M.D.
Instructor, Department of Anesthesia, Pain Management Center, Georgetown University Medical Center, Washington, D.C.
Preemptive Analgesia: Pathophysiology; Preemptive Analgesia: Clinical Studies

ROBERT E. MOLLOY, M.D.
Assistant Professor, Department of Anesthesiology, Director, Residency Program, Northwestern University Medical School; Anesthesiologist, Northwestern Memorial Hospital, Chicago, Illinois.
Diagnostic Nerve Blocks; Injection of Epidural Steroids; Myofascial Pain Syndrome; Fibromyalgia; Intrathecal and Epidural Neurolysis; Celiac Plexus Block; Agents Used for Neurolytic Block; Cervical Plexus Block; Occipital Nerve Block; Axillary Brachial Plexus Block; Intercostal Nerve Block; Sciatic Nerve Block; Ankle Block

RAJESHRI NAYAK, M.D.
Assistant Professor of Clinical Anesthesia, University of Cincinnati College of Medicine, Cincinnati, Ohio.
Maxillary, Mandibular, and Glossopharyngeal Nerve Blocks

RIMAS NEMICKAS, M.D.
Assistant Professor, Department of Anesthesiology, University of Texas Medical Branch at Galveston; Anesthesiologist, University of Texas Medical Branch at Galveston Hospital, Galveston, Texas.
Spontaneous Intracranial Hypotension

TAKASHI NISHIDA, M.D.
Assistant Professor of Neurology, Northwestern University Medical School; Attending Neurologist, Northwestern Memorial Hospital, Chicago, Illinois.
Role of Neurophysiologic Testing for Pain; Tests of the Autonomic Nervous System

KATHLEEN A. O'LEARY, M.D.
Assistant Professor of Clinical Anesthesiology, State University of New York at Buffalo School of Medicine and Biomedical Sciences; Chief of Surgical Anesthesia, Roswell Park Cancer Institute, Buffalo, New York.
Interpleural Analgesia

SAM PAGE, M.D.
Attending Anesthesiologist, St. John's Mercy Medical Center, St. Louis, Missouri.

Opioid Receptors; Epidural Morphine for Postoperative Pain; Paravertebral Somatic Nerve Block

UMESHRAYA T. PAI, M.D.
Professor of Clinical Anesthesia, Adjunct Professor of Anatomy, University of Cincinnati College of Medicine, Cincinnati, Ohio.

Maxillary, Mandibular, and Glossopharyngeal Nerve Blocks

SUNIL J. PANCHAL, M.D.
Assistant Professor of Anesthesiology and Critical Care Medicine, Johns Hopkins University School of Medicine; Co-director, Chronic Pain Service, Director, Pain Medicine Fellowship Program, Johns Hopkins Medical Institutions, Baltimore, Maryland.

Pelvic Pain

MARCO PAPPAGALLO, M.D.
Assistant Professor, Departments of Neurology, Neurosurgery and Anesthesia and Critical Care Medicine, Johns Hopkins University School of Medicine; Attending Physician, Johns Hopkins Hospital, Baltimore, Maryland.

Central Pain States; Entrapment Neuropathies

PAUL M. PARK, M.D.
Fellow, Section of Pain Medicine, Northwestern University Medical School, Chicago, Illinois.

Myofascial Pain Syndrome; Fibromyalgia; Phantom Pain

ARTI PATEL, M.D.
Assistant Professor of Anesthesiology, Northwestern University Medical School; Children's Memorial Hospital, Chicago, Illinois.

Post–Dural Puncture Headache

JAMES C. PHERO, D.M.D.
Professor of Clinical Anesthesia, Pediatrics, and Surgery, University of Cincinnati College of Medicine; Greater Cincinnati Pain Consortium Faculty, University of Cincinnati Medical Center, Cincinnati, Ohio.

Orofacial Pain

HEIDI PRATHER, D.O.
Instructor, Physical Medicine and Rehabilitation, Northwestern University, Chicago, Illinois.

Physical Medicine and Rehabilitation Approaches to Pain Management

JOEL M. PRESS, M.D.
Assistant Clinical Professor, Physical Medicine and Rehabilitation, Northwestern University Medical School; Medical Director, Center for Spine, Sports, and Occupational Rehabilitation, Rehabilitation Institute of Chicago, Chicago, Illinois.

Physical Medicine and Rehabilitation Approaches to Pain Management

SRINIVASA N. RAJA, M.D.
Professor, Department of Anesthesiology and Critical Care Medicine, Division of Pain Medicine, Johns Hopkins University School of Medicine, Baltimore, Maryland.

Pain and the Neurophysiology of Somatosensory Processing; Pain and the Neurochemistry of Somatosensory Processing; Preemptive Analgesia: Pathophysiology; Preemptive Analgesia: Clinical Studies; Terminology and Pathophysiology of Complex Regional Pain Syndrome; Diagnosis of Complex Regional Pain Syndrome; Phentolamine Infusion Test

JAMES P. RATHMELL, M.D.
Associate Professor, University of Vermont College of Medicine; Staff Anesthesiologist, Director, Pain Management Center, Fletcher Allen HealthCare, Burlington, Vermont.

Diabetic and Other Peripheral Neuropathies

GARY M. REISFIELD, M.D.
Medical Director, Pain Institute of Northeast Florida, Orange Park, Florida.

Pharmacologic Treatment of Headache

JACK M. ROZENTAL, M.D., Ph.D.
Associate Professor of Neurology, Northwestern University Medical School; Chief, Neurology Service, Chicago Veterans Affairs Health Care System—Lakeside Division, Chicago, Illinois.

Migraine Headache; Tension Headache; Cluster Headache

ERIC J. RUSSELL, M.D.
Professor of Radiology and Otolaryngology and Head and Neck Surgery, Northwestern University Medical School; Director of Neuroradiology, Northwestern Memorial Hospital, Chicago, Illinois.

Radiology of the Spine

LLOYD R. SABERSKI, M.D.
Associate Professor of Anesthesiology, Yale University School of Medicine; Medical Director, Yale Center for Pain Management, New Haven, Connecticut.

Sacroiliac Joint Dysfunction; Epidural Endoscopy

HARSHA V. SHARMA, M.D.
Assistant Professor, Director Fellowship Education, Department of Anesthesiology, University of Cincinnati, College of Medicine, Cincinnati, Ohio.

Postherpetic Neuralgia

NIGEL E. SHARROCK, M.B., Ch.B.
Assistant Clinical Professor of Anesthesiology, Cornell University Medical School; Attending Anesthesiologist, Hospital for Special Surgery, New York, New York.

Epidural Anesthesia

EDWARD R. SHERWOOD, M.D., Ph.D.
Assistant Professor, Department of Anesthesiology, University of Texas Medical Branch, Galveston, Texas.

Patient-Controlled Analgesia

CHARLES B. SISSON, M.D.
Fellow, Pain Medicine, Northwestern University Medical School, Chicago, Illinois.

Tramadol; Mexiletine

JAN SLEZAK, M.D.
Northeast Pain Consultants, Somersworth, New Hampshire.

Classification of Headache Disorders

ROM A. STEVENS, M.D.
Associate Professor of Anesthesiology, Mayo Medical School, Jacksonville, Florida; Associate Clinical Professor of Anesthesiology, Uniformed Services University of the Health Sciences, Bethesda, Maryland.

Spinal Anesthesia; Epidural Anesthesia

MILAN STOJANOVIC, M.D.
Director, Outpatient Center and Interventional Pain Program, Department of Anesthesia and Critical Care, Massachusetts General Hospital, Boston, Massachusetts.

Classification of Headache Disorders; Trigeminal Neuralgia

GARY STRICHARTZ, Ph.D.
Professor of Pharmacology and Anesthesiology, Harvard Medical School; Vice-Chairman for Research, Brigham and Women's Hospital, Boston, Massachusetts.

Physiology of the Nerve Impulse; Mechanisms of Local Anesthetic Action; Local Anesthetic Pharmacology; Complications

GURURAU SUDARSHAN, M.D., F.R.C.A.
Assistant Professor of Clinical Anesthesia, University of Cincinnati College of Medicine; Director, Greater Cincinnati Pain Consortium, University of Cincinnati Medical Center, Cincinnati, Ohio.

Orofacial Pain

RADHA SUKHANI, M.D.
Associate Professor, Loyola University Medical Center, Stritch School of Medicine; Associate Professor and Medical Director, Ambulatory Surgery Center, Loyola University Medical Center, Maywood, Illinois.

Spinal Anesthesia

SANTHANAM SURESH, M.D.
Assistant Professor of Anesthesiology, Northwestern University Medical School; Attending Anesthesiologist, Co-director, Pain Management Services, Children's Memorial Hospital, Chicago, Illinois.

Chronic Pain Management in Children

RAGHAVENDER THUNGA, M.D.
Clinical Instructor, Department of Anesthesiology, Medical College of Wisconsin, Milwaukee, Wisconsin; Director, Pain Management Center, Staff Anesthesiologist, Provena St. Therese Medical Center, Waukegan, Illinois.

Botulinum Toxin for Myofascial Pain Syndrome; Stellate Ganglion Block

WILLIAM F. URMEY, M.D.
Assistant Professor of Clinical Anesthesiology, Cornell University Medical College; Attending Anesthesiologist, Hospital for Special Surgery, New York, New York.

Combined Spinal-Epidural Technique

CHARLES F. VON GUNTEN, M.D., Ph.D.
Assistant Professor of Medicine, Division of Hematology/Oncology, Northwestern University Medical School; Director, Center for Palliative Medicine Education and Research, Northwestern Memorial Hospital, Chicago, Illinois.

Approach to Management of Cancer Pain; Pharmacologic Management of Cancer Pain

TO-NHU H. VU, M.D.
Clinical Assistant in Anesthesia, Department of Anesthesia and Critical Care, Massachusetts General Hospital, Boston, Massachusetts.

Membrane Stabilizers

DAVID R. WALEGA, M.D.
Fellow in Pain Medicine, Northwestern University Medical School, Chicago, Illinois.

Sickle Cell Anemia; Brachial Plexus Anatomy

VERNON B. WILLIAMS, M.D.
Fellow in Pain Medicine, Department of Anesthesia and Critical Care Medicine, Johns Hopkins University School of Medicine, Baltimore, Maryland.

Central Pain States; Entrapment Neuropathies

CYNTHIA A. WONG, M.D.
Assistant Professor, Northwestern University Medical School; Chief, Section of Obstetrical Anesthesiology, Northwestern Memorial Hospital, Chicago, Illinois.

Intrathecal Opioid Injections for Postoperative Pain; Unintentional Subdural Injections; Back Pain After Epidural Chloroprocaine Injection; Transient Radiculitis After Subarachnoid Lidocaine Injection

HAK YUI WONG, M.B.B.S.
Assistant Professor of Anesthesiology, Northwestern University Medical School; Attending Anesthesiologist, Northwestern Memorial Hospital Chicago, Illinois.

Nonsteroidal Anti-inflammatory Drugs; Epidural Opioid Infusion; Outcome Studies in Postoperative Pain Control

BING XUE, M.S.
Department of Anesthesiology, State University of New York at Buffalo, Buffalo, New York.

Ganglion Impar Block

JEFFREY L. YOUNG, M.D.
Associate Professor, Department of Physical Medicine and Rehabilitation, Albert Einstein College of Medicine of Yeshiva University; Associate Director, Spine and Sports Rehabilitation, Beth Israel Medical Center, New York, New York.

Physical Medicine and Rehabilitation Approaches to Pain Management

● P r e f a c e

This book was written to provide an up-to-date, concise, and authoritative discussion of the essential topics in pain medicine and regional anesthesia. The chapters are short; in some cases, single topics are divided into separate chapters. This was done to provide a quick reference and for easy reading. The format was adapted in consideration of the rigors of residency and fellowship training as well as of the time constraints imposed on busy clinical and academic practitioners. Hopefully, residents, fellows, and anesthesiologists will find this book a welcome and useful tool.

Honorio T. Benzon, M.D.
Srinivasa N. Raja, M.D.
David Borsook, M.D., Ph.D.
Robert E. Molloy, M.D.
Gary Strichartz, Ph.D.

Contents

SECTION ONE

Basic Considerations

Chapter 1

Pain and the Neurophysiology of Somatosensory Processing

Srinivasa N. Raja, M.D.,
and Patrick M. Dougherty, Ph.D.

Pain is the most common symptom that brings a patient to a physician's office. Pain is usually a physiologic consequence of tissue injury and serves a vital protective function. For example, clinical observations in patients with congenital insensitivity to pain and in patients with leprosy have clearly demonstrated that the absence of pain results in chronic disabilities. However, pain itself sometimes becomes the disease when it persists despite appropriate healing of injured tissue. Such a chronic pain state can often be incapacitating and have considerable impact on an individual's life.

The International Association for the Study of Pain defines pain as "an unpleasant sensory and emotional experience associated with actual or potential tissue damage, or described in terms of such damage." The definition recognizes that pain is not only a sensory experience, but it may be associated with affective and cognitive responses. The definition also indicates that the relationship between pain and tissue damage may not be constant. This chapter provides an understanding of the neurophysiologic mechanisms by which noxious and non-noxious stimuli are perceived, to equip the reader with the necessary background for an understanding of the chronic pain state.

SOMATOSENSATION, NOCICEPTION, AND PAIN

Somatosensation refers to the physiologic process by which sensory neurons are activated by physical stimuli, resulting in the perception of what we describe as, for example, touch, pressure, pain. *Nociception* refers to the physiologic process of activation of specialized neural pathways, specifically by tissue-damaging or potentially tissue-damaging stimuli. In experimental situations, a stimulus is considered to be nociceptive on the basis of a behavioral avoidance or escape response of an animal, or by observing the activity evoked by the stimulus in specialized groups of afferent fibers. Clinically, the degree of nociception is inferred by overt evidence of tissue damage. Pain, in contrast to nociception, is a conscious experience, and although the stimulus-induced activation of afferent neural pathways may play an important role, other factors may influence the overall perception of pain. These factors may include the alterations in somatosensory processing following injury to tissues and/or nerves as well as psychosocial factors. The experience of pain, particularly chronic pain, often results in suffering. Suffering results from a multitude of factors, including loss of physical function, social isolation, family distress, and a sense of inadequacy or spiritual loss. This chapter focuses on the neurophysiologic aspects of the neural pathways that respond to somatosensory stimuli, especially nociceptive stimuli, and emphasizes the plasticity in this system after an injury occurs. This knowledge is fundamental in the evaluation and subsequent management of patients with pain disorders.

The sequence of events by which a stimulus is perceived involves four processes: (1) transduction, (2) transmission, (3) modulation, and (4) perception. *Transduction* occurs in the peripheral terminals of primary afferent neurons, where different forms of energy (e.g., mechanical, heat or cold) are converted to electrical activity (action potentials). *Transmission* is the process by which electrical activity induced by a stimulus is conducted through the nervous system. The transmission system has three major components. The peripheral sensory cells in the dorsal root ganglia transmit impulses from the site of transduction at their peripheral terminal to the spinal cord, where the central terminals synapse with second-order neurons. The spinal neurons are the second component in the transmission network. These cells send projections to various brainstem and diencephalic structures. Finally, neurons of the brain stem and diencephalon form the third component of the transmission network as they project to various cortical sites. *Modulation* is the process whereby neural activity may be altered along the pain transmission pathway. The dorsal horn of the spinal cord is one major site at which modulation occurs involving a multitude of neurotransmitter systems. Activation of pain modulation systems usually results in less

2

activity in the pain transmission pathway following a noxious stimulus. Examples of activation of this process include stress-induced analgesia. However, in some circumstances modulation can also result in an enhancement of pain signaling. *Perception* is the final stage of the pain signaling process by which neural activity in the somatosensory transmission pathway results in a subjective sensation of pain. It is presumed that this process results from the concerted activation of primary and secondary somatosensory and limbic cortices.

PERIPHERAL MECHANISMS

There are three classes of primary afferent fibers in skin that may be activated by a given cutaneous stimulus. The fibers that are largest and have the fastest conduction velocity are the large-diameter myelinated (Aβ) fibers. These fibers, when activated, do not normally result in a sensation of pain, but rather of light touch, pressure, or hair movement. The axons of the nociceptive neurons are generally unmyelinated (C fibers) or thinly myelinated (Aδ fibers). Nociceptors have the capacity to respond to intense heat, cold, mechanical, and chemical stimuli. Information on the intensity of the stimulus is coded by the frequency of impulses in a population of nociceptive afferent fibers. There is usually a monotonic relationship between the stimulus intensity and the number of impulses generated by the noxious stimulus. The functional role of the A-fiber and C-fiber nociceptors may be different. The C fibers (0.3 to 3.0 μM) conduct at velocities of less than 2m/second and are the predominant type of afferent fiber (> 75%) in peripheral nerves. Recordings from C fibers in humans suggest that C-fiber activity is associated with a prolonged burning sensation. In contrast, activation of Aδ fibers evokes a sharp, intense, pricking sensation. Thus, the fast-conducting (5 to 20 m/second) Aδ fibers are thought to signal the first pain sensation, whereas the slower-conducting C fibers are thought to be responsible for the second pain sensation that follows brief, intense, heat stimulation to the skin. The pain signaling system encodes information on the intensity, location, and duration of the noxious stimulus.

Recent studies indicate that not all cutaneous nociceptors respond to mechanical stimuli. About half of the A-fiber nociceptors and 30% of the C-fiber nociceptors have either a very high mechanical threshold or fail to respond to mechanical stimuli. These nociceptors have been termed *mechanically insensitive nociceptors* (MIAs). Some of the MIAs respond to chemical stimuli, whereas others respond to intense heat or cold stimuli. MIAs have been shown to become sensitive to mechanical stimuli after inflammation and may play an important role in the mechanical hyperalgesia that develops following tissue injury.

SPINAL MECHANISMS

The first synapse in somatosensory signaling occurs either at the spinal dorsal horn or in the dorsal column nuclei at the spinal cord-brain stem junction. Evidence has accumulated to indicate that both nociceptive and non-nociceptive fibers provide input to both of these initial targets. However, under normal circumstances, the dorsal column nuclei can be considered to selectively process inputs from the large myelinated fiber classes related to light touch, whereas the spinal dorsal horn primarily processes inputs of the nociceptive primary afferent fibers. This separation of modalities in the somatosensory system is the basis for the localization of neural lesions based on quantitative sensory examination.

At the spinal level, nociceptive afferent fibers from the periphery terminate in a highly ordered way in the dorsal horn of the spinal cord on the same side of the body as the dorsal root ganglion (DRG), where the primary sensory neurons are located (Fig. 1-1). The dorsal horn is anatomically organized in the form of laminae (Rexed's). The unmyelinated C fibers terminate primarily in lamina I, whereas the thinly myelinated Aδ fibers end in lamina I and in laminae III to V. The collaterals of the large myelinated fibers (Aβ) that terminate in the dorsal horn do so in laminae III to V.

Two predominant types of second-order nociceptive spinal projection neurons have been identified in the spinal cord: wide dynamic range (WDR) neurons and nociceptive specific (NS) neurons. WDR cells are especially concentrated in the deeper laminae of the dorsal horn (laminae III to V) where they receive input from both low-threshold (Aβ) and nociceptive afferent fibers, and, hence, are activated by both innocuous and noxious stimuli. However, the responses of WDR cells to these stimuli are graded so that noxious stimuli evoke a greater response than non-noxious stimuli. For example,

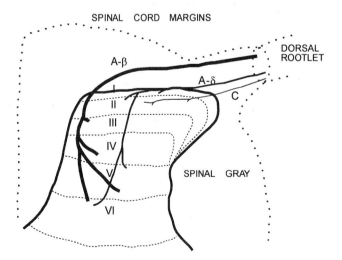

FIGURE 1–1. Schematic diagram of the terminations of the primary afferent fibers in the spinal dorsal horn. Rexed's laminae in the dorsal horn gray matter are indicated by the numerals I to VI. Representative patterns of the terminations of afferent fibers of different classes into the dorsal horn are also shown. The large myelinated (Aβ) fibers segregate in the dorsal aspect of the spinal rootlet, course medially in the dorsal horn, and terminate in laminae III to V. The small myelinated (Aδ) fibers and the C fibers that carry nociceptive information are located ventrally in the rootlets; they course laterally in the spinal dorsal horn and terminate in the more superficial layers (laminae I and II) of the dorsal horn.

WDR spinal projection neurons in monkeys have an average spontaneous discharge rate of approximately 11 Hz; average responses to innocuous cutaneous stimulation by a soft camel's hair brush, approximately 25 Hz; and average responses to noxious mechanical stimulation by a small arterial clip applied to the skin, approximately 50 Hz. WDR neurons may receive convergent input from skin, muscle, and visceral organs. This convergence of sensory input is considered to account for the *referred pain* from the viscera (e.g., angina).

In contrast to WDR cells, NS projection cells respond only to noxious stimuli under physiologic conditions. The majority of NS cells are found in the superficial laminae of the dorsal horn (I and outer II). These cells have a lower rate of spontaneous activity than WDR cells, averaging about 3 to 5 Hz. The discharge rates to the noxious stimuli of NS cells are comparable to those of WDR cells, averaging about 50 Hz. Figure 1–2 illustrates response characteristics of WDR and NS cells.

The axons of both WDR neurons and NS second-order neurons cross the midline near the spinal level of the cell body, gather into a bundle of ascending fibers in the contralateral anterolateral spinal region, and then ascend toward targets in the brain stem and diencephalon. The conduction velocity of the WDR cells is usually faster than that of the NS cells (approximately 30 m/second v. 12 m/second). Additionally, the axons of the NS cells, which largely arise from lamina I of the dorsal horn, and those of the WDR cells, which primarily arise from laminae III to V, tend to run in slightly different positions in the anterolateral spinal funiculus. In the anterolateral spinal column, the NS cell axons are found in the dorsal medial region, whereas axons of WDR cells are more concentrated in the ventrolateral region.

SPINAL MODULATION

The concept of modulation of noxious inputs at spinal levels was highlighted by the gate-control theory of Melzack and Wall. This theory suggested that input along low-threshold (Aβ) fibers inhibited the response of WDR cells to nociceptive input. The theory was offered as an explanation for the efficacy of transcutaneous electrical stimulation for pain relief. Subsequent studies have identified intrinsic spinal neurons that release several different neurotransmitters in the spinal cord, which play a role in the modulation of nociceptive impulses. Furthermore, a number of inputs to the dorsal horn from various brain-stem sites have been shown to also modulate peripheral inputs as well as outputs of intrinsic cells. Both types of modulation, that arising in the local network of cells at the spinal levels as well as that from the descending inputs, can result in either augmented or inhibited output from spinal cord pain-signaling neurons. It is the combined effects of spinal excitatory and inhibitory systems that determine what messages are delivered to the higher levels of the central nervous system.

A special type of spinal modulation that is observed under certain circumstances is known as *central sensitization*. In this phenomenon, the capacity for transmission in the nociceptive system is changed or shows *neuronal plasticity*. The result of this plasticity is that following a noxious stimulus of sufficient intensity and duration, such as a surgical incision, the coding of pain-signaling neurons for a given stimulus may be increased. One example of central plasticity is the phenomenon of *windup* whereby C-fiber stimulation repeated at intervals of 0.5 to 1.0 Hz results in a progressive increase in the number of discharges evoked by each volley. In addition to the increase in discharges evoked by a given stimulus, other characteristics of sensitization of spinal neurons include an expansion of receptive field size and an increase in spontaneous discharge rate. WDR cells tend to become sensitized more readily than do NS cells. However, in circumstances in which NS cells do show sensitization, they often acquire novel responsiveness to innocuous stimuli, and could therefore be recategorized as WDR neurons. Increases in the understanding of the pharmacology of this and other types

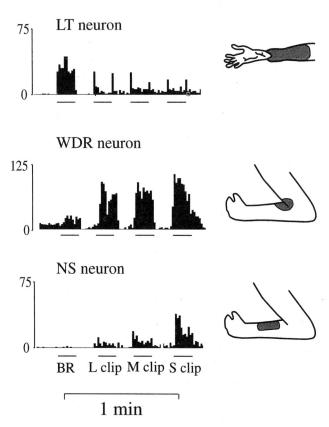

FIGURE 1–2. Rate histograms illustrate the response of low-threshold (LT) mechanoreceptor, wide dynamic range (WDR), and nociceptive-specific (NS) neurons, recorded from the thalamus, to cutaneous stimuli. Responses to innocuous brush (BR) stimuli and large (L), medium (M), and small (S) clips applied to the receptive field are shown. The times of application for all stimuli are indicated by the lines below each histogram set. The receptive fields are shown by the outlines on the limbs shown next to each histogram, and a 3-second sample of the raw signal is shown for each cell. Note that the LT neuron responds maximally to the low-threshold stimulus and minimally to the noxious stimuli. The WDR cell shows a graded response with increasing intensities of stimuli. Finally, the NS neuron shows minimal response to any stimuli except the most intense pinch. The response characteristics of the neurons in the dorsal horn are similar to those of the thalamic neurons shown here.

of plasticity will have profound consequences in the development of new analgesic pharmacotherapies.

BRAIN STEM, MIDBRAIN, AND DIENCEPHALIC MECHANISMS

There are two sets of somatosensory inputs to the brain stem and diencephalon (Fig. 1–3). First, many axons and axon collaterals of the spinal projection neurons that ascend in the anterolateral spinal quadrant depart this ascending tract to terminate in a number of nuclei of the brain stem and midbrain. These target sites include brain stem autonomic regulatory sites that influence cardiovascular and respiratory functions, whereas the midbrain contains multiple inputs to centers from which both descending and ascending (e.g., to thalamus) modulation of somatosensory processing is evoked. The remainder of the so-called anterolateral system fibers continue through the brain stem and midbrain to terminate in the hypothalamus and posterior regions of the lateral thalamus as well as in some medial thalamic regions.

The second set of somatosensory inputs to the brain stem include primary afferent fibers that ascend in the dorsal (posterior) columns of the spinal cord to form their first synapse at the dorsal column nuclei. These inputs are organized so that the fibers from the lower extremities are most medial in the nucleus gracilis, and inputs from the upper extremities are most lateral in the nucleus cuneatus. The trunk is represented in a region between these two nuclei. Finally, inputs from the most distal body regions are dorsal, and the more proximal body regions are ventral. The axons of the second-order cells in the dorsal column nuclei cross the midline and gather into the medial lemniscus on the contralateral side of the brain stem. The fibers then ascend through the brain stem and midbrain toward their site of termination in the so-called core of the ventral posterior lateral (VPL) nucleus of the thalamus.

Thalamic neurons, in turn, project to specific cortical regions. The cells in the core of the VPL that received inputs from the dorsal column–medial lemniscus fibers project to somatosensory cortical areas SI and SII. The neurons in the posterior region of the lateral thalamus receiving inputs from the anterolateral system project to SII and the retroinsular areas of cortex. Finally, the medial thalamic nuclei ultimately project to the anterior cingulate cortex.

SUPRASPINAL MODULATION OF NOCICEPTION

Several lines of research have clearly indicated that plasticity and modulation of somatosensory signaling occurs at brain stem, midbrain, and diencephalic levels. Examples of plasticity of responses of dorsal column neurons following intradermal injection of the irritant capsaicin have been documented in the rat and monkey. Similarly, with the development of acute inflammation and following deafferentation, neurons of the thalamus alter their patterns of spontaneous discharge, and a large increase in bursting of these cells is observed. Ascending modulation from the brain-stem dorsal raphe nucleus also influences signaling of thalamic neurons. However, our understanding of these processes at the higher levels of the somatosensory system, unlike our

FIGURE 1–3. Schematic diagram of nociceptive pathways in the CNS. The boxes represent the anatomic sites at which nociceptive signals are processed and/or registered. The lines indicate the nerve tracts interconnecting the anatomic sites.

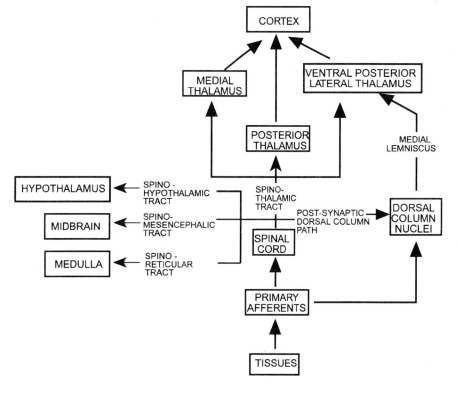

knowledge of spinal-level activity, is not as fully developed.

SUMMARY

Four different processes—transduction, transmission, modulation, and perception—are involved in the sequence of events that results in the sensation of pain from a noxious external stimulus. A subset of primary afferent nerve fibers, nociceptors, are excited only by noxious stimuli under physiologic circumstances. Signals in nociceptors are conducted toward the spinal cord, where they synapse with WDR and NS neurons. Spinal neurons that signal pain are dynamic, and their output is modulated by segmental and descending control mechanisms. The somatosensory system is composed of two main signaling channels. The anterolateral (spinothalamic) system is the primary pain-signaling channel. In contrast, the dorsal column–medial lemniscal system is primarily a high-speed, very discrete signaling channel for innocuous stimuli. The two channels tend to project to slightly different but somewhat overlapping brain regions. Derangements can occur in both of these signaling systems at any and all levels, and may result in the generation of chronic pain states.

BIBLIOGRAPHY

Benson JM, Chaouch A: Peripheral and spinal mechanisms of nociception. Physiol Rev 67:67–186, 1987.

Dougherty PM, Lenz FA: Plasticity of the somatosensory system following neural injury. *In* Boivie J, Hansson P, Lindblom U (eds): Touch, Temperature, and Pain in Health and Disease: Progress in Pain Research and Management, vol 3. Seattle, IASP Press, 1994.

Dubner R, Basbaum AI: Spinal dorsal horn plasticity following tissue or nerve injury. *In* Wall PD, Melzack R (eds): Textbook of Pain, ed 3. Edinburgh, Churchill Livingstone, 1994, pp 225–241.

Fields HL, Basbaum AI: Central nervous system mechanisms of pain modulation. *In* Wall PD, Melzack R (eds): Textbook of Pain, ed 3. Edinburgh, Churchill Livingstone, 1994, pp 243–260.

McMahon SB, Lewin GR, Wall PD: Central hyperexcitability triggered by noxious inputs. Curr Opin Neurobiol 3:602–610, 1993.

Pockett S: Spinal cord synaptic plasticity and chronic pain. Anesth Analg 80:173–179, 1995.

Treede RD, Meyer RA, Raja SN, et al: Peripheral and central mechanisms of cutaneous hyperalgesia. Prog Neurobiol 38:397–421, 1992.

Willis WD Jr: Central plastic responses to pain. *In* Gebhart GF, Hammond DL, Jensen TS (eds): Proceedings of the 7th World Congress on Pain: Progress in Pain Research and Management, vol 2. Seattle, IASP Press, 1994, pp 301–324.

Willis WD Jr: Mechanical allodynia: A role for sensitized nociceptive tract cells with convergent input from mechanoreceptors and nociceptors? APS Journal 2:23–33, 1993.

Woolf CJ: Evidence for a central component of post-injury pain hypersensitivity. Nature 306:686–688, 1983.

Chapter 2

Pain and the Neurochemistry of Somatosensory Processing

Patrick M. Dougherty, Ph.D.,
and Srinivasa N. Raja, M.D.

The neurochemistry, unlike the neurophysiology, of somatosensory processing in both the anterolateral and dorsal column–medial lemniscal systems (see Chapter 1) is very similar. Both systems involve three classes of transmitter compounds: excitatory neurotransmitters, inhibitory neurotransmitters, and neuropeptides that are found in three anatomic compartments (sensory afferent terminals, local circuit terminals, and descending [or ascending] modulatory circuit terminals). In this chapter, the role of each type of transmitter is addressed.

EXCITATORY NEUROTRANSMITTERS

The main excitatory neurotransmitters in the somatosensory system are the amino acids, glutamate and aspartate. These excitatory amino acids appear to mediate the transmission at each of the afferent connections in the somatosensory system, including the synaptic connection between primary afferent fibers and spinal neurons, from spinal neurons to thalamic neurons, etc. There are four receptor types for glutamate and aspartate in the somatosensory system. These receptors are named for the synthetic agonists by which they are best activated. Thus, one class of receptors best activated by *N*-methyl-D-aspartate (NMDA) is termed the *NMDA glutamate receptor*. A second class of receptors not activated by NMDA (non-NMDA receptors) includes three subtypes: a *kainate* receptor, an *AMPA* (R,S)-α-amino-3-hydroxy-5-methylisoxazole-4-propionic acid) receptor, and an *ACPD* (trans-(±)-1-amino-cyclopentane-1,3-decarboxylate) receptor. The AMPA and kainate receptors are linked to sodium channels and are considered to mediate the majority of the fast synaptic afferent signaling in this system, for all modalities and intensities of stimuli. The NMDA receptor is usually considered as recruited only by intense and/or prolonged somatosensory stimuli. This characteristic is due to the NMDA receptor's well-known magnesium block, which is only relieved by prolonged depolarization of the cell membrane. The NMDA receptor is linked to a calcium iono-

phore that, when activated, results in many long-term changes in excitability of sensory neurons (*sensitization*). The AMPA/kainate and NMDA receptors are also frequently considered to mediate monosynaptic and polysynaptic contacts of primary afferent fibers to dorsal horn neurons (Fig. 2–1). Finally, the ACPD site, often termed the *metabotropic glutamate receptor*, is a G-protein–linked site that, when activated, results in liberation of the second messenger, inositol phosphate, which in turn results in the release of cytosolic calcium. The role of the ACPD receptor in somatosensory signaling is unclear.

A second type of excitatory substance that may have a transmitter role in the somatosensory system is adenosine triphosphate (ATP). ATP excited some dorsal horn neurons in an in vitro preparation. Excitation by ATP in vivo was found to be rather specific for cells receiving only low-threshold mechanoreceptive inputs in spinal laminae II and III.

INHIBITORY NEUROTRANSMITTERS

The primary inhibitory neurotransmitters of the somatosensory system include the amino acids glycine and γ-aminobutyric acid (*GABA*). *Glycine* is particularly important at spinal levels, whereas GABA is the predominant inhibitory transmitter at higher levels. Glycine has two receptor sites. (1) a chloride-linked strychnine-sensitive inhibitory receptor and (2) a strychnine-insensitive modulatory site on the NMDA glutamate receptor complex. GABA also has two receptor sites. The GABA-A receptor is a chloride-linked ionophore that is also the site of action for barbiturates and benzodiazepines. GABA-B receptors are part of the seven transmembrane-spanning protein receptor superfamily that activates G proteins.

Alterations in the functions of the inhibitory neurotransmitters may be particularly important with the induction of hyperalgesia and following the development of neuropathic pain. For example, a GABA-A mediated link between large myelinated fibers and C-fiber noci-

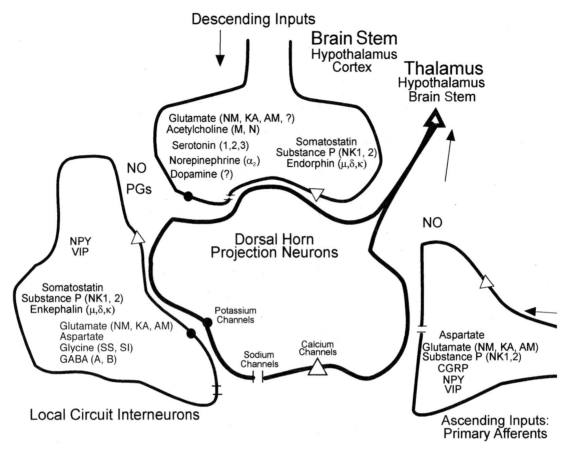

FIGURE 2–1. Neurochemistry of nociception. The complex neurochemical mechanisms in the spinal dorsal horn are shown schematically. The terminals of primary afferent fibers release excitatory amino acids and peptides. Other neurotransmitters, released by either local circuit interneurons or from descending inputs from the brain stem, that have a modulatory role on the dorsal horn projection neurons are also shown. Abbreviation in parentheses indicate the receptors at which the neurotransmitters interact. NM, NMDA; KA, kainate; AM, AMPA; NK, neurokinin; SS, strychnine-sensitive; SI, strychnine-insensitive; PGs, prostaglandins; CGRP, calcitonin-gene–related peptide; NPY, neuropeptide Y; VIP, vasoactive intestinal peptide; NO, nitric oxide.

ceptors has been proposed as a mechanism for the development of allodynia following intradermal injection of the irritant capsaicin. Additionally, a selective loss of inhibitory interneurons at both spinal and thalamic levels has been suggested as contributing to some neuropathic pain conditions.

Norepinephrine is an important inhibitory neurotransmitter in descending brainstem projections to the dorsal horn. The adrenergic receptors include two broad classes, termed the α- and β-receptors, each of which in turn has several subtypes. The α2-adrenergic receptor is the primary form found in the spinal dorsal horn and has an inhibitory role on the processing of sensory information. However, it should be noted that in some circumstances the function of norepinephrine following injury to the nervous systems might become reversed from an inhibitory, analgesic role to one of promoting and/or sustaining an ongoing chronic pain state.

Serotonin has historically been considered an important inhibitory transmitter in descending projections to the spinal dorsal horn from the midbrain raphe nuclei. There are multiple serotonin (5-hydroxytryptamine, or 5-HT) receptor subtypes, including 5-HT-1, -2, and -3 receptors; each of these major types also has several

subtypes. Controversy remains concerning which of these subtypes mediates the analgesic properties of serotonin. In part, this controversy may be due to the fact that some serotonin receptor subtypes in fact promote nociception, whereas others are inhibitory. If more selective tools are developed to help dissect the pharmacology of serotonin, potentially useful clinical targets may emerge.

Another important secondary inhibitory neurotransmitter at spinal levels is the purine *adenosine*. There are at least two types of adenosine receptors, termed the A1 and A2 sites. Occupation of these sites by adenosine results in G-protein–mediated alterations of cyclic adenosine monophosphate (cAMP) levels in target cells. However, both increases and decreases in cAMP formation have been reported in various conditions. Adenosine may mediate a portion of the analgesia produced by brain stem norepinephrine projections to the spinal cord, and it appears to have especially robust analgesic properties in neuropathic pain conditions.

Acetylcholine is yet another neurotransmitter that appears to mediate anti-nociception at the level of the spinal dorsal horn. The anti-nociceptive effects appear to be mediated predominantly by the muscarinic rather than by the nicotinic acetylcholine receptor subtypes.

NEUROPEPTIDES

There are multiple neuropeptides that contribute to signaling of somatosensory information. Some of these could be classified as excitatory compounds and others as inhibitory. However, instead of considering these compounds together with the excitatory and inhibitory neurotransmitters mentioned above, they are discussed separately because of the distinct profile of action of these compounds as opposed to that of the neurotransmitters. Unlike the very rapid onset and termination of action of the transmitters, neuropeptides tend to have more gradual onset of effects as well as much more prolonged duration of action once released.

The excitatory neuropeptides in the somatosensory system include *substance P* and *neurokinin A*. These peptides are especially concentrated in primary afferent fibers, but they also may be present in intrinsic neurons of the spinal dorsal horn and thalamus. The receptors for these peptides include the neurokinin-1 and -2 sites, each of which has been associated with elevation of intracellular calcium levels, perhaps through liberation of inositol phosphate. At the spinal level these peptides are only released following application of noxious stimuli that are sufficient to produce sustained discharges in C-fiber nociceptive afferents, although some small myelinated (Aδ) fibers may also contain substance P. These peptides do not appear to signal as synaptic transmitters, but rather as transsynaptic transmitters. Thus, once released, the peptides are not confined to a site of action on the immediate postsynaptic membrane, but instead tend to spread throughout the dorsal horn, potentially acting on multiple synapses at some distance from their point of release. It has been suggested that stimuli of particular modalities (e.g., mechanical vs. thermal) are associated with selective release of one peptide vs. another; however, this suggestion has not been corroborated. It is agreed that activation of neurokinin-1 and/or -2 receptors by substance P and/or neurokinin A are key steps necessary for the induction of sensitization and, hence, the expression of hyperalgesia following cutaneous injury. It has been further proposed that the mechanism of neurokinin receptor involvement in the expression of sensitization is through facilitation of the synaptic actions of the excitatory amino acid neurotransmitters.

The inhibitory neuropeptides at spinal levels include *somatostatin*, the *enkephalins*, and possibly *dynorphin*. These peptides are contained in both intrinsic neurons of the dorsal horn and in the fibers descending to the dorsal horn from various brain-stem nuclei. At thalamic levels, the inhibitory neuropeptides also include the *endorphins*, which are contained in ascending anti-nociceptive pathways. The receptor types for the opioid peptides include the μ, δ, and κ receptor subtypes at all levels of the somatosensory system. These receptors are associated with modulation of both intracellular cAMP and potassium levels. There is also an important cooperative functional link between μ opioid and α_2-adrenergic receptors that has yet to be fully exploited for clinical applications.

Finally, a number of neuropeptides are present in the somatosensory system whose function is yet to be clearly identified; at present these need to be considered as a third category. These peptides include, calcitonin gene-related peptide (CGRP), vasoactive intestinal peptide (VIP), neuropeptide Y (NPY), and cholecystokinin (CCK), among others. Future studies will no doubt have more to say about the role of these peptides in the neurochemistry of synaptic transmission in the somatosensory system.

SUMMARY

The sensation of pain involves a complex interaction of excitatory and inhibitory neurotransmitter mechanisms. Both classical neurotransmitters, such as glutamate and aspartate, and peptides, such as substance P, are released from primary afferents. Both local circuit interneurons and descending inputs from the brain stem release a number of neurochemicals, such as GABA, glycine, norepinephrine, serotonin, and acetylcholine, that play an important role in spinal modulation of nociceptive signals.

BIBILIOGRAPHY

Bloom FE: Neuropeptides and other mediators in the central nervous system. J Immunol 135:743s–745s, 1985.

Coderre TJ: The role of excitatory amino acid receptors and intracellular messengers in persistent nociception after tissue injury in rats. Mol Neurobiol 7:229–246, 1993.

Dougherty PM, Mittman S, Sorkin LS: Hyperalgesia and amino acids: Receptor selectivity based on stimulus intensity and a role for peptides. APS Journal 3:240–248, 1994.

Dray A, Urban L, Dickenson A: Pharmacology of chronic pain. Trends Pharmacol Sci 15:190–197, 1994.

Levine JD, Fields HL, Basbaum AI: Peptides and the primary afferent nociceptor. J Neurosci 13:2273–2286, 1993.

Salt TE, Eaton SA: Functions of inotropic and metabotropic glutamate receptor in sensory transmission in the mammalian thalamus. Prog Neurobiol 48:55–72, 1996.

Yaksh TL, Malmberg AB: Central pharmacology of nociceptive transmission. *In* Wall P, Melzack R (eds): Textbook of Pain, ed 3. Edinburgh, Churchill Livingstone, 1994, pp 165–200.

Yaksh TL, Chaplan SR: Physiology and pharmacology of neuropathic pain. Anesthesiol Clin North Am 15:335–352, 1997.

Chapter 3

Taxonomy: Definitions of Pain Terms and Chronic Pain Syndromes

Honorio T. Benzon, M.D.

Allodynia — Pain from stimulus that does not normally provoke pain.

Analgesia — Absence of pain in response to a stimulus that is normally painful.

Anesthesia — Absence of all sensory modalities.

Anesthesia dolorosa — Pain in an area or region that is anesthetic.

Central pain — Regional pain caused by a primary lesion or dysfunction in the central nervous system (CNS), usually associated with abnormal sensibility to temperature and to noxious stimulation.

Complex regional pain syndrome (CRPS) — A term describing a variety of painful conditions following injury, which appear regionally and have a distal predominance of abnormal findings. The conditions exceed the expected clinical course of the inciting event in both magnitude and duration, often resulting in significant impairment of motor function and showing variable progression over time. CRPS is a new term for disorders previously called *reflex sympathetic dystrophy* (RSD).

Type I CRPS (RSD)

1. Type I CRPS is a syndrome that develops after an initiating noxious event.

2. Spontaneous pain or allodynia/hyperalgesia occurs, is not limited to the territory of a single peripheral nerve, and is disproportionate to the inciting event.

3. There is or has been evidence of edema, skin blood flow abnormality, or abnormal sudomotor activity in the region of the pain since the inciting event.

4. This diagnosis is excluded by the existence of conditions that would otherwise account for the degree of pain and dysfunction.

Type II CRPS (Causalgia)

1. Type II CRPS is a syndrome that develops after a nerve injury. Spontaneous pain or allodynia/hyperalgesia occurs and is not necessarily limited to the territory of the injured nerve.

2. There is or has been evidence of edema, skin blood flow abnormality, or abnormal sudomotor activity in the region of the pain since the inciting event.

3. This diagnosis is excluded by the existence of conditions that would otherwise account for the degree of pain and dysfunction.

Chronic pain — Pain that (1) persists beyond either the course of an acute disease or a reasonable time for an injury to heal; (2) is associated with a chronic pathologic process that causes continuous pain; or (3) recurs at intervals of months or years. Some investigators use a duration of 6 months or more to designate pain as being chronic.

Deafferentation pain — Pain resulting from loss of sensory input into the CNS. This may occur with lesions of peripheral nerves, such as avulsion of the brachial plexus or with pathologic lesions of the CNS.

Dysesthesia — An unpleasant, abnormal sensation, spontaneous or evoked.

Fibromyalgia — Diffuse musculoskeletal aching and pain with multiple, predictable tender points.

Hyperalgesia — An increased response to a stimulus that is normally painful.

Hyperesthesia — Increased sensitivity to stimulation; this excludes the special senses.

Hyperpathia — A painful syndrome characterized by increased reaction to a stimulus, especially a repetitive stimulus, and an increased threshold.

Hypoalgesia — Diminished sensitivity to noxious stimulation.

Hypoesthesia — Diminished sensitivity to stimulation; this excludes the special senses.

Lateral epicondylitis (tennis elbow) — Pain in the lateral epicondylar region of the elbow due to strain or partial tear of the extensor tendon of the wrist.

Neuralgia — Pain along the distribution of a nerve or nerves.

Neuritis — Inflammation of a nerve or nerves. (Not to be used unless inflammation is thought to be present.)

Neurogenic pain — Pain initiated or caused by a primary lesion, dysfunction, or transitory perturbation in the peripheral or CNS.

Neuropathic pain — Pain initiated or caused by a primary lesion or dysfunction in the CNS.

Neuropathy — A disturbance of function or pathologic change in a nerve. This may involve one nerve (mononeuropathy) or several nerves (mononeuropathy multiplex), or it may be bilateral or symmetrical (polyneuropathy).

Nociceptor — A receptor preferentially sensitive to a noxious stimulus or to a stimulus that would become noxious if prolonged.

Noxious stimulus — A stimulus that is actually or potentially damaging to body tissue.

Pain — An unpleasant sensory and emotional experience associated with actual or potential tissue damage, or described in terms of damage.

Pain of psychological origin — Pain attributed by the patient to a specific delusional cause (delusional or hallucinatory) or pain specifically attributable to the thought process, emotional state, or personality of the patient in the absence of an organic or delusional cause or tension mechanism (hysterical, conversion, or hypochondriacal).

Pain threshold — The least experience of pain that a subject can recognize.

Pain tolerance level — The greatest level of pain that a subject is prepared to tolerate.

Paresthesia — An abnormal sensation, spontaneous or evoked. (Note: Paresthesia is an abnormal sensation that is not unpleasant, whereas dysesthesia is an abnormal sensation that is considered unpleasant. Dysesthesia does not include all abnormal sensations, but only those that are unpleasant.)

Peripheral neuropathy — Constant or intermittent burning, aching, or lancinating limb pain due to generalized or focal diseases of peripheral nerves.

Phantom pain — Pain referred to a surgically removed limb or a portion thereof.

Piriformis syndrome — Pain in the buttock and posterior thigh due to myofascial injury of the piriformis muscle itself, or dysfunction of the sacroiliac joint, or pain in the posterior leg and foot, groin, and perineum due to entrapment of the sciatic or other nerves by the piriformis muscle within the greater sciatic foramen, or a combination of these causes.

Radicular pain — Pain perceived as arising in a limb or the trunk wall, caused by ectopic activation of nociceptive afferent fibers in a spinal nerve or its roots or by other neuropathic mechanisms.

Radiculopathy — Objective loss of sensory and/or motor function as a result of conduction block in axons of a spinal nerve or its roots. (Note: Radicular pain and radiculopathy are not synonymous. The former is a symptom caused by ectopic impulse generation. The latter relates to objective neurologic signs resulting from conduction block. The two conditions may coexist and may be caused by the same lesion.)

Raynaud's disease — Episodic attacks of aching, burning pain associated with vasoconstriction of the arteries of the extremities in response to cold or emotional stimuli.

Raynaud's phenomenon — Attacks similar to those of Raynaud's disease but related to one or more other disease processes. Systemic and vascular diseases, such as collagen disease, arteriosclerosis obliterans, nerve injuries, and occupational trauma, may all contribute to the development of Raynaud's phenomenon.

Referred pain — Pain perceived as occurring in a region of the body topographically distinct from the region in which the actual source of pain is located.

Somatic — Derived from the Greek word for body (*sōmatikos*). Although somatosensory input refers to sensory signals from all tissues of the body, including skin, viscera, muscles, and joints, it usually signifies input from body tissue other than the viscera.

Stump pain — Pain at the site of an extremity amputation.

Suffering — A state of severe distress associated with events that threaten the intactness of the person; this may or may not be associated with pain.

Stylohyoid process syndrome (eagle syndrome) — Pain following trauma in the region of a calcified stylohyoid ligament.

Thoracic outlet syndrome — Pain in the root of the neck, head, or shoulder that radiates down the arm into the hand, owing to compression of the brachial plexus by hypertrophied muscle, congenital bands, post-traumatic fibrosis, cervical rib or band, or a malformed first thoracic rib.

BIBLIOGRAPHY

Bonica JJ: The Management of Pain, ed 2. Philadelphia, Lea & Febiger, 1990, pp 18–27.

Mersky H, Bogduk N: International Association for the Study of Pain (IASP) Classification of Chronic Pain, ed 2. Seattle, IASP Press, 1994.

Stanton-Hicks M, Janig W, Hassenbuch S, et al: Reflex sympathetic dystrophy: Changing concepts and taxonomy. Pain 63:127–133, 1995.

Clinical Evaluation and Diagnostic Examinations

Chapter 4

Neurologic Assessment of the Pain Patient

Jaclyn Ho, M.D., and Kerry Gill DeLuca, M.D.

A thorough history and physical examination are essential in the evaluation of any patient. In the assessment of the patient with chronic or acute pain, additional emphasis is placed on the neurologic examination. This includes a careful analysis of both the central nervous system (CNS) (brain and spinal cord) and peripheral nervous system to determine, if possible, the location of the lesion. The physical examination should be well planned and orderly, and the patient should be informed about the impending process. Areas to be examined include mental status, cranial nerve function, sensation, motor, reflexes, coordination, and gait. Finally, provocative tests are performed in the presence of specific conditions.

MENTAL STATUS

Although mental status can be largely assessed by the quality and nature of the history given by the patient, a more detailed evaluation may sometimes be required. In such an instance, a more formal assessment should be made, and the level of alertness and cooperation should be noted. The following should be assessed:

Orientation to person and place, date repetition
Ability to name objects (e.g., pen, watch)
Memory (immediate, at 1 minute, and at 5 minutes)
Ability to calculate serial 7s (if patient refuses, the examiner may have patient spell the word "world" backward)
Signs of cognitive deficits, aphasia

CRANIAL NERVES

A screening assessment of the cranial nerves can be completed within a few minutes. A summary of cranial nerve functions and tests is listed in Table 4–1.

SENSATION

When assessing the pain patient, the examiner may use the various parts of the sensory examination to focus on which fibers may be affected as well as on where the lesion is located along the sensory pathway.

Peripheral nociceptors, which respond selectively to damaging stimuli, are connected to the CNS via axons belonging to Aδ and C fibers. There are three main types of nociceptors: *mechanical nociceptors* are activated by pin-prick or pinch; *heat nociceptors* respond when the field is heated to greater that 45°C; *polymodal nociceptors* respond equally to many types of noxious stimuli—mechanical, heat, and chemical.

Two distinct types of pain may be sensed, reflecting the two types of pain fibers. *Fast pain* is carried by well-localized myelinated Aδ fibers and is sometimes characterized by shooting or sharp sensation. *Slow pain*, which is carried by unmyelinated C fibers, is often described as being poorly localized, dull, or burning in nature.

Ideally, sensory stimuli should be applied to all four limbs, the face, and the trunk. If an area of abnormal sensation has been identified by the patient's history, test the area of normal sensation first. The patient is to report if the stimulus feels normal or abnormal. Abnormal sensations are subcategorized in Figure 4–1.

Hyperesthesia is a general term for sensation that is out of proportion to the stimulus applied. Specific types of hyperesthesia include hyperalgesia (severe pain in response to mild noxious stimulus, such as pin-prick) and allodynia (pain perceived after non-noxious stimulation, such as light stroking of the skin).

Sensory innervation may be described in terms of dermatomes, reflecting sequential nerve roots, or in terms of the distribution of peripheral nerves. Both patterns are illustrated in Figures 4–2 and 4–3. Easy landmarks to remember include C4 distribution over the shoulders, T4 dermatome at the nipple line, and T10 at the umbilicus. More landmarks are listed in Table 4–2.

Specific tests of sensation include temperature, pain, light touch, vibration, position, and cortical interpretation.

Temperature (Thermal Perception) (C Fibers)

Traditionally, a cold tuning fork has been used for the temperature test. It may be more appropriate, especially

TABLE 4–1. SUMMARY OF CRANIAL NERVE FUNCTIONS AND TESTS

Cranial Nerve	Function	Test
I. Olfactory	Smell	Use coffee, mint, etc., held to each nostril separately; consider basal frontal tumor in unilateral dysfunction
II. Optic	Vision	Assess optic disc, visual acuity; name number of fingers in central and peripheral quadrants; direct and consensual pupil reflex; note Marcus-Gunn pupil (paradoxically dilating pupil)
III, IV, and VI. Oculomotor, trochlear, and abducens	Extraocular muscles	Pupil size; visually track objects in 8 cardinal directions, note diplopia (greatest on side of lesion); accommodation; note Horner's pupil (miosis, ptosis, anhydrosis)
V. Trigeminal: motor, sensory	Facial sensation, muscles of mastication	Cotton-tipped swab/pin-prick to all 3 branches; recall bilateral forehead innervation (peripheral lesion spares forehead, central lesion affects forehead); note atrophy, jaw deviation to side of lesion
VII. Facial	Muscles of facial expression	Wrinkle forehead, close eyes tightly, smile, purse lips, puff cheeks; corneal reflex
VIII. Vestibulocochlear (acoustic)	Hearing, equilibrium	Use tuning fork, compare side-side; Rinne's test for air vs. bone conduction (BC>AC); Weber's test for sensorineural hearing
IX. Glossopharyngeal	Palate elevation, taste to posterior third of tongue, sensation to posterior tongue, pharynx, middle ear, and dura	Palate elevates away from the lesion; check gag reflex
X. Vagus	Muscles of pharynx, larynx	Check for vocal cord paralysis, hoarse or nasal voice
XI. Accessory	Muscles of larynx, sternocleidomastoid, trapezius	Shoulder shrug, sternocleidomastoid strength
XII. Hypoglossal	Intrinsic tongue muscles	Protrusion of tongue; deviates toward lesion

in patients with sensory complaints, to test with a glass tube containing warm water alternating with a tube containing cool water.

Pain (C Fibers, Aδ Fibers)

Pain is usually assessed by pin-prick, using a clean pin or the sharp edge of a broken tongue blade that will not puncture the skin. The patient is to report if the stimulus is "prickly" or "sharp." Sensory dissociation, in which a patient reports a sharp sensation to a pin in an area with no temperature or pain sense, may be found in lesions in which fibers crossing the spinal cord are interrupted, such as a syrinx (progressive myelopathy, which presents as central high cervical cord syndrome with sensory loss in "cape" or "shawl" distribution and muscle wasting of the neck, shoulders, and arms).

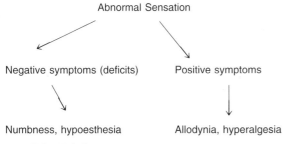

FIGURE 4–1. Subcategories of abnormal sensation.

Light Touch (Aδ and Aβ Fibers)

Light touch is assessed by stroking the skin with a cotton-tipped swab or tissue. One should compare proximal vs. distal and side-side and upper extremity vs. lower extremity sensation.

Vibration (Aβ Fibers)

Vibration is usually assessed using a 128-Hz tuning fork in all extremities. The examiner may be used as the normal control if deficits are found. Isolated decreased vibratory sense may be an early sign of large-fiber neuropathy. This should be tested in conjunction with position sense. If both are absent, one should suspect posterior column disease and/or peripheral nerve involvement.

Position (Conscious Joint Position Sense) (Aβ Fibers)

Conscious joint position sense is tested by moving the distal phalanx in the direction of the joint. Hold the phalanx on the sides to avoid tactile cues. Test all four limbs. If the patient is unable to perceive movement at the digit, test the next largest joint. Parietal lobe dysfunction or peripheral nerve involvement should be considered in position sense loss.

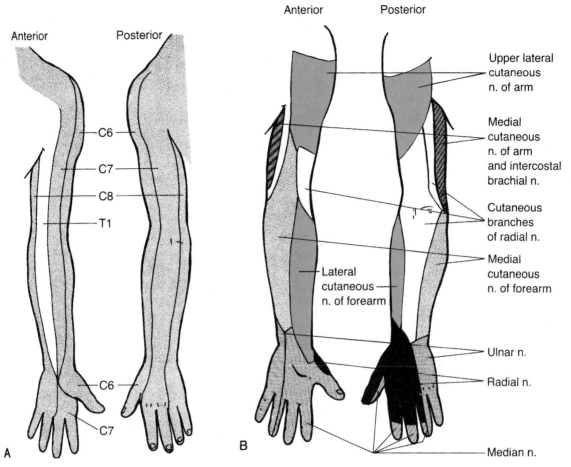

FIGURE 4–2. *A,* Cutaneous distribution of the cervical roots. *B,* Cutaneous distribution of the peripheral nerves. (From Wedel DJ: Nerve blocks. *In* Miller RD (ed): Anesthesia, ed 4. New York, Churchill Livingstone, 1994, p 1537.)

Cortical Function of the Sensory System

1. Two-point discrimination: This is tested by applying two stimuli at increasingly small distances apart. Ask the patient if he or she feels one or two stimuli. This test is usually reserved for evaluating areas of abnormal sensation.

2. Graphesthesia: The examiner draws numbers in the patient's palm or on the patient's calf, and the patient must tell the examiner which number has been drawn. The number of correct and incorrect trials are recorded. This is a useful assessment of posterior column function.

MOTOR EXAMINATION

In addition to observing for atrophy or wasting of any muscle groups, tone and muscle power should be thoroughly and completely evaluated.

Tone is defined as the sensation of resistance felt as one manipulates a joint through a range of motion while the patient attempts to relax.

Hypotonia, a decrease in the normal muscular resistance to palpation or passive manipulation, is thought to be secondary to depression of α or γ motor unit activity. Hypotonia may be seen in extrapyramidal or cerebellar motor disorders, polyneuropathy, myopathy, or spinal cord injury.

Hypertonia, a condition of increased tone, is a broad term used to describe both spasticity and rigidity. *Spasticity* is a velocity-dependent increase in tone that is elicited by movement about a joint. Spasticity may result from either increased excitation at the level of the spinal reflex arc or from loss of descending inhibitory control (e.g., reticulospinal or rubrospinal tracts) and is commonly seen with multiple sclerosis, brain injury, or spinal cord injury or after stroke. *Rigidity* is a condition of increased tone that usually involves all muscle groups. It is a prominent feature of many extrapyramidal diseases and is caused by lesions of the nigrostriatal system.

Muscle Power Test

Testing of muscle power is usually done in a proximal-to-distal and cephalad-to-caudal manner. The examiner must immobilize the muscle in order to test only one group at a time. In addition, the examiner must try to isolate the intended muscle as much as possible (e.g., the biceps is optimally tested with the elbow flexed and the forearm in full supination).

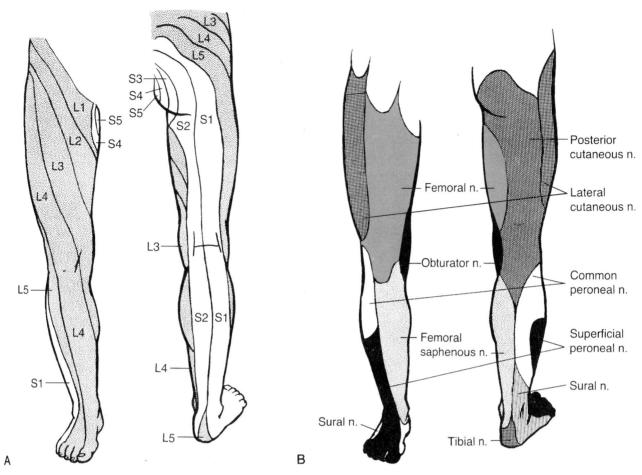

FIGURE 4–3. *A,* Cutaneous distribution of the lumbosacral nerves. *B,* Cutaneous distribution of the peripheral nerves of the lower extremity. (From Wedel DJ: Nerve blocks. *In* Miller RD (ed): Anesthesia, ed 4. New York, Churchill Livingstone, 1994, p 1547.)

Weakness that affects proximal more than distal musculature may reflect myopathy, whereas weakness affecting distal more than proximal musculature may represent polyneuropathy. Single nerve damage may be manifested by weakness in the distribution of that nerve.

Manual muscle testing is graded as follows:

0   No movement
1   Trace movement
2   Movement through the full range with gravity eliminated
3   Movement through the full range against gravity
4   Movement through the full range against gravity and with partial resistance
5   Movement through the full range against gravity and full resistance

Key muscle root levels are noted in Table 4–3.

REFLEXES

Referred to as *deep tendon reflexes* or *muscle stretch reflexes*, these are elicited by a brisk tap to the tendon of the muscle being tested. To test reflexes, place the joint in a physiologic position, usually flexed at ninety degrees. In patients in whom muscle stretch reflexes are hypoactive, techniques such as Jendrassik's maneuver (facilitation of underactive reflexes by voluntary contraction of other muscles) may be necessary to elicit accurate information.

TABLE 4–2. SENSORY INNERVATION LANDMARKS BY DERMATOME

Dermatome	Landmark
C4	Shoulder
C5	Lateral aspect of the elbow
C6	Thumb
C7	Middle finger
C8	Little finger
T1	Medial aspect of the elbow
T2	Axilla
T3–11	Corresponding intercostal space; T4, nipple line; T10, umbilicus
T12	Inguinal ligament at midline
L1	Halfway between T12 and L2
L2	Mid-anterior thigh
L3	Medial femoral condyle
L4	Medial malleolus
L5	Dorsum of foot
S1	Lateral heel
S2	Popliteal fossa at the midline
S3	Ischial tuberosity
S4–5	Perianal area

TABLE 4–3. KEY MUSCLE NERVE ROOT LEVELS

Root Level	Nerve	Muscle(s) tested	Position	Action
C4	Dorsal scapular	Levator scapulae	Sitting	Shoulder shrug
C5	Musculocutaneous (C5-6)	Biceps	Forearm fully supinated, elbow flexed 90 degrees	Patient attempts further flexion against resistance
C6	Radial (C5-6)	Extensor carpi radialis, longus, and brevis	Elbow flexed at 45 degrees, wrist extended	Maintain extension against resistance
C7	Radial (C6-8)	Triceps	Shoulder slightly abducted, elbow slightly flexed	Extend forearm against gravity
C8	Anterior interosseous (median) (C7-8)	Flexor digitorum profundus		Finger flexion of middle finger
T1	Ulnar, deep branch (C8-T1)	Dorsal interossei	Patient extends and spreads all fingers	Examiner pushes patient's fingers together, patient resists
L2	Femoral (L2-4)	Psoas, iliacus	Hip and knee flexed at 90 degrees	Flex hip further against resistance
L3	Femoral (L2-4)	Quadriceps femoris	Supine, hip flexed, knee flexed at 90 degrees	Extend knee against resistance
L4	Deep peroneal (L4-5)	Tibialis anterior	Ankle dorsiflexed	Maintain dorsiflexion against resistance
L5	Deep peroneal (L4-5)	Extensor hallucis longus	Great toe extended	Maintain extension against resistance
	Superficial peroneal	Peroneus longus and brevis	Foot everted	Maintain eversion against resistance
S1	Sciatic (L5-S2)	Hamstrings	Prone, knee flexed	Maintain flexion against resistance

Reflexes are graded as absent, neutral, or hyperactive (causing brisk excursion of the distal limb), and are usually quantified along a scale from 0 (no reflex elicited) to 4 (significant hyperreflexia and clonus). *Clonus* is the phenomenon in which sudden and sustained stretch of muscles causes rhythmic, uniphasic contractions, which may signify upper motor neuron disease.

When testing reflexes, the examiner must know which muscles and nerves are being tested. One technique for remembering the innervation for common reflexes is to count from 1 to 8 while proceeding from the Achilles reflex to the triceps reflex as follows:

1-2 (S1-2)   Achilles reflex
3-4 (L3-4)   Patellar reflex
5-6 (C5-6)   Biceps reflex
7-8 (C7-8)   Triceps reflex

Additional reflexes that may be tested are medial hamstrings (L5) and brachioradialis (C5-6).

Plantar or Babinski's reflex is tested by scratching along the lateral aspect and metatarsal heads on the plantar aspect of the foot, using a key or another similar object. A positive response is elicited when the great toe moves upward and/or the toes fan outward; this signifies upper motor neuron disease.

COORDINATION AND GAIT

Examination of cerebellar function traditionally includes finger-nose-finger and heel-knee-shin tests. Testing rapidly alternating movements (touching fingertips together, flipping hands, tapping feet) is a sensitive way to test cerebellar function as well as to assess sensory, motor, and extrapyramidal centers and pathways.

Gait represents a complex neurologic function; testing gait gives the examiner clues to disturbances and diseases of the entire nervous system. The examiner should first have the patient walk normally, then walk on the toes and, finally, on the heels (to observe lower extremity strength and how the system operates under stress). Testing tandem gait, in which the patient walks heel to toe along an imaginary line on the floor, is a sensitive test for coordination and equilibrium.

Pain secondary to an injury of the hip, knee, ankle, or foot can lead to an antalgic gait. The patient decreases the stance phase of gait on the affected side to remove the weight, and he or she may also support the affected area with one hand and use the other hand as a counterbalance.

Testing of postural reflexes (Romberg's test) also tests equilibrium. The patient stands with the feet together, arms outstretched, and eyes closed. The examiner then pushes the patient gently, while simultaneously preventing the patient from falling. The patient without equilibrium dysfunction is able to recover easily and to maintain balance.

PROVOCATIVE TESTS

In addition to the previous tests of neurologic function, other tests performed in the presence of specific neurologic conditions are called *provocative tests*. Although such tests for myofascial nerve root and orthopedic conditions are covered elsewhere, those for meningitis and neuroma are worth noting here. Tinel's sign is a provocative sensory test in which percussion is applied to an area innervated by the sensory nerve in question. Reproduction of the patient's characteristic symptoms with percussion over the nerve is a positive result. This test is particularly useful in conditions of possible nerve entrapment (e.g., carpal tunnel) or in neuralgic pain in a dermatomal distribution (e.g., postherpetic neuralgia). It also serves to identify the presence of a superficial neuroma, such as might exist following a limb amputation.

In the evaluation of a patient with headache or neck pain, especially in the setting of increased somnolence and/or confusion, maneuvers to elicit signs of meningeal irritation are helpful. Kernig's test is performed with the patient supine, hip flexed at 90 degrees, and knee flexed. The examiner attempts to straighten the patient's knee; inability to straighten the knee is considered a positive finding, but it should be present bilaterally. Hamstring pain and tightness may prevent completion of the test. Brudzinski's test is also performed with the patient supine. The examiner flexes the patient's neck; the test is considered positive if the patient's hips and knees flex automatically.

Throughout the examination of the nervous system, the examiner must keep in mind which part of the nervous system is being examined, to help localize the lesion. The neurologic examination should be performed consistently and methodically by the examining physician in all patients. A thorough examination can be done efficiently, allowing time for more detailed examination of the affected region.

BIBLIOGRAPHY

Adams RD, Victor M: Principles of Neurology, ed 5. New York, McGraw-Hill, 1993.

American Spinal Injury Association/International Medical Society of Paraplegia: International Standards for Neurological and Functional Classification of Spinal Cord Injury (revised 1992). Chicago, ASIA, 1994.

Backonja M: Introduction to the Neurological Examination. Madison, University of Wisconsin Board of Regents, 1992.

Bates B: A Guide to Physical Examination and History Taking. Philadelphia, JB Lippincott, 1987.

Borenstein DG, Wiesel SW: Low Back Pain: Medical Diagnosis and Comprehensive Management. Philadelphia, WB Saunders, 1989.

Camic PM, Brown FD (eds): Assessing Chronic Pain: A Multidisciplinary Clinic Handbook. New York, Springer-Verlag, 1989.

Devinsky O, Feldman E: Examination of the Cranial and Peripheral Nerves. New York, Churchill Livingstone, 1988.

Kandel E, Schwartz J (eds): Principles of Neural Science, ed 2. New York, Elsevier Science, 1985.

Magee DJ: Orthopedic Physical Assessment. Philadelphia, WB Saunders, 1992.

Chapter 5

Radiology of the Spine

Joseph H. Introcaso, M.D., D.M.D.,
Lucy A. Christopherson, M.D.,
and Eric J. Russell, M.D.

ANATOMY

The morphology of the spinal vertebrae is quite consistent throughout, with a few exceptions. These exceptions are the first two cervical segments, the sacrum, and the coccyx. The typical vertebra consists of a body, pedicles, transverse processes, articular processes, laminae, and a spinous process (Fig. 5-1).

In the cervical region, the vertebral arteries pass through foramina in the transverse processes as they ascend to the skull base. This usually begins at the C6 level, but may also begin at C7. Uncinate processes are also found in the lower five cervical vertebrae. These form synovial articulations with the vertebrae above. Occasionally, cervical ribs may be present at the C7 level, which may result in thoracic outlet syndrome.

The superior and inferior aspects of the articular processes are covered with articular cartilage and form the facet joints. These synovial joints are enclosed by loose capsular ligaments. Orientation of the facet joints varies, depending on the region of the spine. These factors allow for the variable degrees of motion required.

Ligaments of the spine provide stability while allowing flexion, extension, and rotation. The anterior and posterior longitudinal ligaments run along their respective aspects of the vertebral bodies. The liga-

mentum flavum courses along the deep surface of each of the laminae. Interspinous ligaments connect the spinous processes and the supraspinous ligament courses over the superficial surface of the spinous processes.

Intervertebral discs separate the vertebral bodies and contribute a significant proportion (20% to 35%) of the height of the spinal column. Discs consist of a dense outer fibrous covering (annulus fibrosus), which surrounds the nucleus pulposus. The nucleus pulposus is a much softer, hydrated material, which can act as a shock absorber.

The first (atlas) and second (axis) cervical vertebrae (C1 and C2) differ significantly in their morphology from other vertebrae. C1 is a ring comprising anterior and posterior arches separated by articular processes (lateral masses). There is no body to C1; therefore no intervertebral disc is present at the C1-2 level. C2 has a body with an odontoid process extending superiorly and articulating with the anterior arch of C1. This articulation is stabilized by the transverse ligament.

Nerve roots exit through the intervertebral foramina at each level. In the cervical spine, eight nerve roots are present, with the first exiting the spinal canal between the skull base and C1. Therefore, in the cervical spine, the number of the nerve root passing through the foramen is one greater than the number of the pedicle that it passes beneath. For example, the nerve root passing through the foramen at C3-4 is the C4 nerve root. Innervation of the synovial membrane of the facet joints and the joint capsule has contributions from the nerve roots above and below. The spinal cord terminates in the conus medullaris, normally located at the L1 level. The level of the conus medullaris may vary, being as high as T12 or as low as L3. The nerve roots arising from the conus medullaris are referred to as the *cauda equina.*

PROJECTION RADIOGRAPHY (CONVENTIONAL RADIOGRAPHS)

Plain radiographic projections should always be the initial imaging study of the spine. These images provide

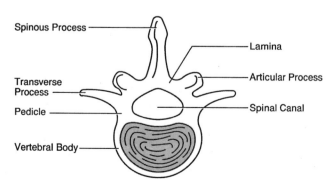

FIGURE 5-1. Axial diagram of a vertebral body.

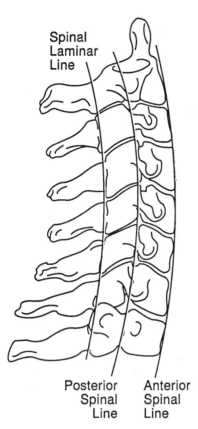

Spinal
Laminar
Line

Posterior   Anterior
Spinal   Spinal
Line   Line

FIGURE 5–2. Lateral diagram of the cervical spine demonstrating the spinal laminar, posterior spinal, and anterior spinal lines.

important information about both structure and alignment. Standard frontal (including odontoid view) and lateral projections are the minimum required for adequate evaluation. Often in the cervical and lumbar regions, oblique projections are helpful in evaluating the facet joints, articular processes, and neural foramina. When spondylolithesis or spondylolysis is present, flexion and extension views aid in demonstration of abnormal motion. Flexion and extension views may be supplemented by direct real-time observation using fluoroscopy. On occasion, evaluation of the odontoid process of C2 may be improved by the use of complex motion tomograms in the sagittal and coronal planes. However, this type of equipment is rapidly becoming extinct and may be replaced with digital multiplanar reconstructions of thin-section helical computed tomographic (CT) images.

Projection radiographs can provide excellent information through depiction of the "big picture." This is often important in the diagnosis of systemic diseases and metabolic disorders. Paraspinal soft tissue abnormalities may also be more apparent on projection radiographs than on planar imaging studies, such as CT and magnetic resonance imaging (MRI).

Diagnosis of compression fracture is often most easily performed on projection radiographs. Fractures of the odontoid process of C2 and of the spinous processes are also usually better demonstrated by projection radiography. Demonstration of these types of fractures by

planar imaging modalities (CT and MRI) is often less than satisfactory.

Conventional radiography is the easiest and most cost-effective method of assessing alignment of the spine. On lateral projection, three longitudinal curves may be used to evaluate alignment of the vertebrae (Fig. 5–2). The anterior and posterior spinal lines trace the course of the anterior and posterior longitudinal ligaments, respectively. The spinal laminar line traces the course of the ligamentum flavum along the deep surface of the laminae. On frontal projection, a vertical line drawn through the tips of the spinous processes serves as a reference for evaluation of lateral curvature. The relationship of this line and the pedicles will demonstrate rotational malalignment (Fig. 5–3).

MYELOGRAPHY

Myelography is the radiographic technique utilized to evaluate the contents of the spinal canal by the introduction of an iodinated contrast material into the spinal subarachnoid space. This contrast material outlines the spinal cord and nerve roots, which appear as filling defects in the contrast column on projection radiographs. Oil-based contrast materials used previously have been replaced by non-ionic water-soluble materials. Myelography should always be followed by a postmyelography CT scan to provide better definition of anatomic relationships of the contents of the spinal canal to the surrounding structures. The indications for myelography have declined in recent years due to improvements in MRI techniques. The risks associated with the intrathecal administration of contrast material (e.g., severe headache, seizures, infection) have limited its use in recent years to those patients with contraindications to MRI examination.

COMPUTED TOMOGRAPHY

Advantages of CT over conventional projection radiography (Fig. 5–4) are based in the inherent properties of a tomographic examination and the greater contrast resolution of the technique. CT provides the best possi-

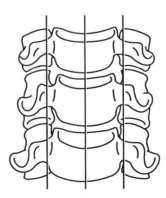

FIGURE 5–3. Frontal diagram of the cervical spine showing normal alignment of the spinous processes.

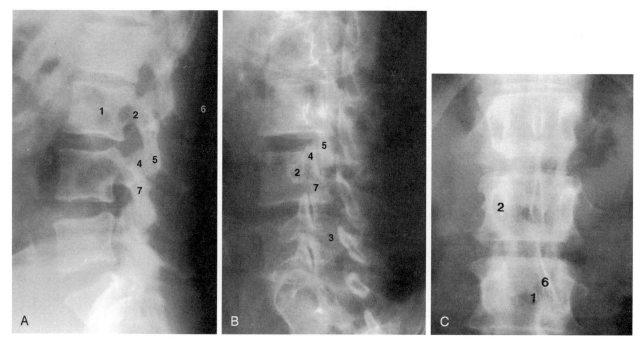

FIGURE 5–4. Plain radiographs of the lumbar spine showing the normal structures. Lateral *(A)*, oblique *(B)*, and AP *(C)* views of the lumbar spine: L3 vertebral body *(1)*, pedicle *(2)*, lamina *(3)*, superior articular process of L4 *(4)*, inferior articular of process L3 *(5)*, spinous process of L2 *(6)*, and pars interarticularis *(7)*. Note that the spinous process of L2 overlies the L3 vertebra on the AP view.

ble definition of osseous structures. Differences in radiographic density of ligament, disc material, and cerebrospinal fluid make identification of disk herniations and ligamentous disorders possible using CT (Fig. 5–5). Windowing techniques used in the display of CT images allow optimal viewing of image data, depending on the tissue type of interest (i.e., bone or soft tissue). The administration of intravenous iodinated contrast material may be valuable in certain circumstances to highlight vascular structures, such as the epidural venous plexus or adjacent arteries.

CT examinations of the spine are performed utilizing slice thicknesses ranging from 1 to 3 mm, depending on the region being examined and the abnormality being investigated. Limitations imposed by the heat capacity of the x-ray tube, as well as other technical factors, require that CT examinations be targeted to specific regions of the spine. These regions of interest may be identified by clinical examination, conventional radiography, or MRI. Recent developments in helical CT data acquisition have made possible high-resolution multiplanar reconstruction of CT images (Fig. 5–6). This has largely supplanted the need for complex motion tomography. Artifacts from metallic surgical implants, such as spinal rods, transpedicular screws, and ligature wires, can severely limit the diagnostic value of CT images. In these cases, projection radiography and myelography may prove to be the best diagnostic imaging modalities.

MAGNETIC RESONANCE IMAGING

The superb soft tissue contrast resolution afforded by MRI combined with its multiplanar tomographic capability make it the most versatile diagnostic imaging mod-

ality for spinal disorders. It provides a wide field of view with excellent definition of tissue types, such as bone marrow, muscle, ligament, disc material, and nerve roots (Fig. 5–7). MRI allows precise definition of extradural, intradural, extramedullary, and intramedullary pathology. Evaluation of medullary bone with MRI is excellent, having the ability to demonstrate edema or metastatic disease within the marrow. However, demonstration of dense cortical bone and osteophytes by MRI is less precise than by CT.

Standard MRI imaging protocols for degenerative disc pathology include sagittal spin echo-images with T1, proton density, and T2 weighting (Fig. 5–8). When evaluating scoliosis, coronal T1- or T2-weighted imaging may be added. In the cervical and thoracic spine, thin-section axial two- or three-dimensional gradient-echo images are utilized to further evaluate spinal and neural foraminal stenosis. The degree of stenosis produced by osteophytes tends to be exaggerated on gradient-echo sequences. Proton density and T2-weighted axial images are utilized in the lumbar region. Gradient-echo and T2-weighted images provide a "myelographic" effect by making the cerebrospinal fluid within the thecal sac appear white. When evaluating for infection, multiple sclerosis, intramedullary neoplasm, metastatic disease, or post-operative scarring, sagittal and axial T1-weighted images prior to and following the intravenous administration of gadolinium contrast material are indicated. This will increase diagnostic sensitivity in cases of epidural abscess, meningitis, leptomeningeal carcinomatosis, and perineural scarring.

Unfortunately, some patients cannot be examined using MRI. The most common problem encountered is claustrophobia. Although this is a relative contraindication which can usually be overcome using appropriate

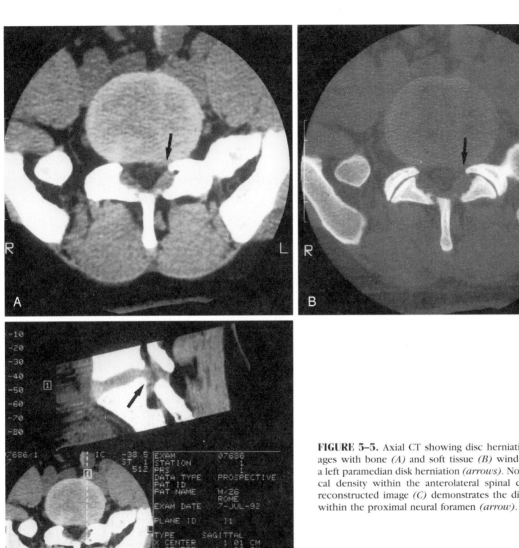

FIGURE 5–5. Axial CT showing disc herniation. Axial images with bone *(A)* and soft tissue *(B)* windows showing a left paramedian disk herniation *(arrows)*. Note asymmetrical density within the anterolateral spinal canal. Sagittal reconstructed image *(C)* demonstrates the disk herniation within the proximal neural foramen *(arrow)*.

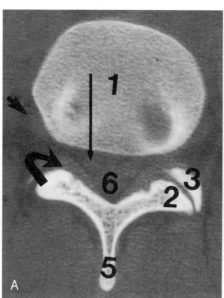

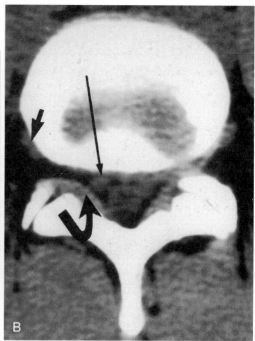

FIGURE 5–6. Axial CT image of a lumbar vertebra. Axial CT image with bone *(A)* and soft tissue *(B)* windows. L4 vertebral body *(1)*, inferior articular process of L4 *(2)*, superior articular process of L5 *(3)*, L4 spinous process *(5)*, ligamentum flavum *(curved arrows)*, thecal sac *(6)*, traversing L5 nerve roots *(long arrows)*, and exiting L4 nerve root *(short arrows)*. Note preservation of the fat plane around the exiting nerve root.

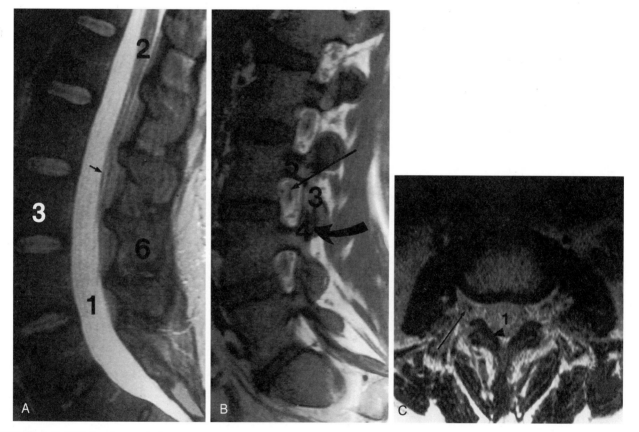

FIGURE 5–7. MRI showing normal anatomy of the lumbar spine. T2-weighted midline sagittal *(A)*, T1-weighted lateral sagittal *(B)*, and T2-weighted axial *(C)* MR images: thecal sac *(1)*, conus medullaris *(2)*, nerve roots of the cauda equina *(small arrow)*, inferior articular process of L3 *(3)*, superior articular process of L4 *(4)*, facet joint at L3–4 *(curved arrow)*, exiting L3 nerve root within the foramen *(long arrow)*, pedicle *(5)*, spinous process *(6)*, and ligamentum flavum *(arrowhead)*. Note the "myelographic effect" of the hyperintense CSF within the thecal sac on the T2-weighted images.

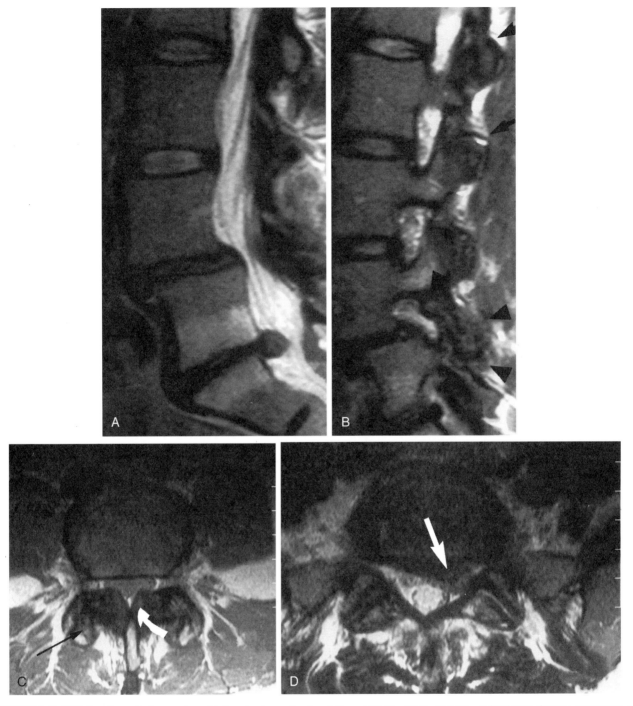

FIGURE 5-8. MRI showing spinal stenosis at L4-5 and a large disc herniation at L5-S1. *(A)* Sagittal T2-weighted MRI showing narrowing of spinal canal at L4-5 secondary to severe facet arthritis and disc height loss resulting in anterolisthesis of L4 on L5. Note abnormal low signal in the L4-5 and L5-S1 discs and the large disc herniation at L5-S1. Hyperintense signal within vertebral endplates adjacent to the L5-S1 discs represents reactive degenerative change. *(B)* Sagittal T2-weighted MRI (more lateral) showing severe facet arthritic changes at L4-5 *(arrowheads)* narrowing the superior aspect of the neural foramen. Note the more normal appearance of the facets at L1-2 and L2-3 *(short arrows)*. *(C)* Axial proton density-weighted MRI at the L4-5 disc level showing severe concentric spinal canal stenosis. Bilateral facet hypertropy *(long arrow)*, ligamentous thickening *(curved arrow)*, and degenerative anterolisthesis of L4 on L5 all contribute to the narrowing of the central canal at this level. *(D)* Axial T2-weighted MRI at L5-S1 showing the left paramedian disc herniation compressing the left S1 nerve root *(arrow)*.

oral and intravenous sedation, certain patients may require general anesthesia. "Open"-magnet MRI systems also help to reduce this problem.

Strict contraindications for MRI relate to the very strong magnetic field required for imaging. Patients with cardiac pacemakers, metallic foreign bodies, and specific metallic surgical implants cannot be examined using MRI. Cardiac pacemakers may be disabled or reprogrammed or their leads repositioned by the magnetic field. Metallic foreign bodies or surgical implants, such as cerebral aneurysm clips or heart valves, may be displaced by the magnetic field with catastrophic consequences. Comprehensive references are available to determine which implants are safe to be placed into the magnetic field. In certain cases metallic spinal implants will be safe to examine with MRI, but artifact created by these metallic devices may distort the images significantly, rendering them nondiagnostic.

BIBLIOGRAPHY

Atlas SW: Magnetic Resonance Imaging of the Brain and Spine. New York, Raven Press, 1996.

Clemente CD: Anatomy: A Regional Atlas of the Human Body. Philadelphia, Lea & Febiger, 1975.

Dalinka MK, Dixon L, Verstandig, A: Spinal Trauma Radiology: Diagnosis, Imaging, Intervention. Philadelphia, JB Lippincott, 1989.

Modic MT, Masaryk TJ, Ross JS (eds): Magnetic Resonance Imaging of the Spine. Chicago, Year Book Medical Publishers, 1989.

Netter FH: The CIBA Collection of Medical Illustration, vol 1, part 1. West Caldwell, NJ, CIBA Pharmaceutical Company, 1983.

Osborn AG: Diagnostic Neuroradiology. St Louis, Mosby–Year Book, 1994.

Chapter 6

Role of Neurophysiologic Testing for Pain

Takashi Nishida, M.D.,
and Michael M. Minieka, M.D.

Electrophysiologic testing, when properly applied, is a useful tool for the evaluation of patients with pain. Understanding the indications and limitations of each test is absolutely essential for appropriate diagnosis and subsequent treatment.

Electrophysiologic studies are a very sensitive indicator of central and peripheral nervous system involvement but do not indicate underlying disease. For example, testing can diagnose radiculopathy but cannot determine if it is caused by osteophytes, a herniated disc, or diabetes. This chapter describes conventional electrophysiologic tests, such as electromyography (EMG) and short-latency somatosensory evoked potentials (SSEPs), as well as newer techniques, including quantitative sensory testing (QST) and laser evoked potentials (LEPs).

ELECTROMYOGRAPHY

When strictly defined, EMG indicates only a needle examination of muscles. However EMG is often used to include both needle studies and nerve conduction studies. Nerve conduction studies are often referred to by the letters NCV, with "V" standing for velocity, although nerve conduction studies measure more than velocity. For clarity, we use EMG/NCV to indicate the combination of needle electromyography and nerve conduction studies.

EMG/NCV is extremely useful in the evaluation of the peripheral nervous system. Indeed, the three most common diagnoses in EMG laboratories—peripheral neuropathy, carpal tunnel syndrome, and lumbosacral radiculopathy—all cause pain. EMG/NCV can identify the anatomic site of injury (anterior horn cell, root, plexus, nerve, neuromuscular junction, or muscle), the type of neurons or fibers involved (motor, sensory, or mixed), the nature of pathologic alteration (demyelination, axonal degeneration, or both), time course (acute, subacute, or chronic), and severity of injury.

By stimulating peripheral nerve with supramaximal intensity, compound muscle action potential (CMAP) for motor nerve and sensory nerve action potential (SNAP) for sensory nerve are recorded. Amplitude of action potentials as well as the time from stimulation to response are recorded. Latency is the interval between the onset of a stimulus and the onset of a response, expressed in milliseconds. Conduction velocity is obtained by dividing the distance between two stimulation points (in millimeters) of the same nerve by the difference between proximal and distal latencies (in milliseconds). This calculated velocity, expressed in meters per second, represents the conduction velocity of the fastest nerve fibers between two points of stimulation. It is important to note that studies may be normal if a disorder is limited to small nerve fibers, such as Aδ and C fibers.

The amplitude of CMAP is measured from baseline to negative peak in millivolts, and the amplitude of SNAP is measured from the first positive peak to negative peak in microvolts. Most laboratories have their own normal values for major motor and sensory nerves, with minor differences occurring among laboratories. A lower temperature will prolong distal latencies, reduce conduction velocities, and increase the amplitude of CMAP and SNAP. Age also affects NCVs. Adult values are not attained until 4 years of age, and they decline after age 60 years at a rate of 1 to 2 meters/second per decade. The amplitude of a response should be similar when the same nerve is stimulated proximally and distally. A greater than 20% reduction between distal and proximal stimulation of a motor nerve suggests an abnormal block in conduction between two stimulation points. Many laboratories are now computerized, and the area under an action potential curve can be calculated. Greater than 40% reduction in area also suggests conduction block. A significant reduction in amplitude from proximal to distal stimulation sites without a reduction in area under the response curve and a significant increase in duration (15%) suggest temporal dispersion resulting from a relative desynchronization of the components of an action potential, which is due to different rates of conduction of each nerve fiber. This also suggests a nerve pathology between the proximal and distal stimulation sites (Fig. 6-1).

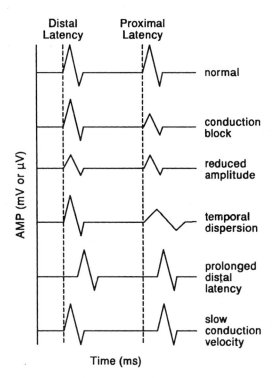

FIGURE 6–1. Schematic representation of normal and pathologic findings obtained from an NCV study.

The H reflex is the electrophysiologic equivalent of a muscle stretch reflex. A sensory nerve is stimulated with submaximal intensity, and a late motor response is recorded owing to reflex activation of motor neurons. In adults, H reflexes are easily obtained from soleus muscles, and less easily from flexor carpi radialis muscles, following the stimulation of tibial and median nerves, respectively. The tibial H reflex is useful in identifying S1 radiculopathy.

F waves are a late response recorded from muscle after supramaximal stimulation of a motor nerve. F waves represent a response to a stimulus that travels first to and then from the cord via motor pathways; thus, F waves are useful in studying the proximal portion of motor nerves (Fig. 6–2). Unfortunately there is no consensus as to methodology for obtaining responses and to the patterns of abnormality to be identified.

Repetitive nerve stimulation (RNS) studies are used primarily for evaluation of neuromuscular junction disorders, such as myasthenia gravis. As such they are not usually useful in the evaluation of pain, and therefore they will not be discussed further.

The electrical activity in a muscle can be measured using disposable needle electrodes. Needle examination is performed in proper steps. An examiner observes activity on insertion of a needle (insertion activity), activity when the needle is maintained in a relaxed muscle (spontaneous activity), and activity during varying degrees of voluntary muscle contraction. The electrical activity is evaluated by sight and sound, as specific activities have specific wave forms and characteristic sounds. Observations are made by the electromyographer during the study; therefore, the results of a needle

examination are dependent on the experience of the examiner.

Insertion activity, also referred to as injury potential, is caused by movement of the needle electrode, resulting in mechanical damage to the muscle fibers. Increased insertion activity consists of unsustained fibrillation potentials and positive sharp waves. A muscle at rest should be electrically silent. Spontaneous activity in a resting muscle usually suggests a pathologic condition. The type and significance of various spontaneous activities are summarized in Table 6–1, and some examples are shown in Figure 6–3.

As a muscle contracts, motor unit action potentials (MUAPs) are observed. MUAP represents the summation of muscle fiber action potentials of a given motor unit. With increasing voluntary muscle contraction, individual motor units fire more frequently, and more motor units are recruited to fire. The term *onset frequency* is used to describe the firing rate of a single MUAP maintained at the lowest voluntary muscle contraction (normally less than 10 Hz). Recruitment frequency is defined as the frequency of first MUAP when second MUAP is recruited (normally less than 15 Hz). Reduced recruitment (high recruitment frequency) can be seen in neuropathic processes. Rapid recruitment (low recruitment frequency), however, can be seen in myopathic disorder or defect of neuromuscular junction. During maximum contraction, a full interference pattern, consisting of overlapping motor units, is seen. MUAPs are analyzed in terms of amplitude, duration, number of phases, and stability. The morphology of the MUAPs is affected by the type of needle electrode used, location of the needle within the motor unit territory, age, temperature, and specific muscle being examined. Large, long-duration, polyphasic units suggest denervation and reinnervation. Short-duration, small polyphasic units can be seen in myopathic processes. EMG findings in neuropathic and myopathic disorders are summarized in Table 6–2.

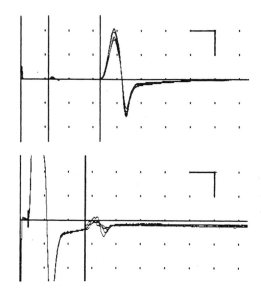

FIGURE 6–2. H reflex with tibial nerve stimulation *(top)*; time marker, 10 ms; amplitude marker, 5 mV. F response with median nerve stimulation *(bottom)*; time marker, 10 ms; amplitude marker, 1 mV.

TABLE 6–1. POTENTIALS RECORDED IN THE MUSCLE AT REST

Spontaneous Activity	Firing Pattern	Frequency (Hz)	Wave Form	Amplitude	Duration (ms)	Significance
Complex repetitive discharge	Regular, abrupt onset and cessation	5–100	Polyphasic or serrated, MFAP	100 μV–1 mV		Neurogenic (chronic), myopathic (dystrophy)
Cramp discharge	Increase and subside gradually	1. <150 2. 4–15	MUAP			1. Ischemic, ↑Na 2. ↓Ca, ↓Mg, ↑K
Endplate noise	Dense and steady, "sea shell" sound	>150	Monophasic (negative), MEPP	10–20 μV	0.5–1	Normal
Endplate spike	Irregular short bursts	50–100	Biphasic (negative-positive), MFAP	100–300 μV	2–4	Decrease in denervated muscle, increase in reinnervated muscle
Fasciculation potential	Spontaneous, sporadic	0.1–10	MUAP			Normal, neurogenic (motor neuronopathy), myopathic
Fibrillation potential	Regular, "rain on a tin roof" sound	1–50	Biphasic (positive-negative), MFAP	<1 mV	<5	Neurogenic, NMJ defect, myopathic
Myokymic discharge	Semi-regular	1. 2–60 brief 2. 1–5 continuous	MUAP			Normal, neurogenic (chronic, radiation) Face (MS, brain-stem tumor, Bell's palsy)
Myotonic discharge	Wax and wane, "dive bomber" sound	20–80	1. Biphasic (positive-negative) 2. Positive	<1 mV <1 mV	<5 5–20	Myopathic (myotonic syndromes)
Neuromyotonic discharge	Start and stop abruptly, wane, "pinging" sound	150–300	MUAP			Isaac's syndrome, stiff-man syndrome, tetany
Positive sharp wave	Regular	1–50	Biphasic (positive-negative), MFAP	<1 mV	10–100	Same as fibrillation

MFAP, muscle fiber action potential; MUAP, motor unit action potential; MEPP, miniature endplate potential; NMJ, neuromuscular junction.

While performing an EMG/NCV study, several questions, specified in the following text, must be answered by the examiner.

Where Is the Lesion? (Localization)

EMG/NCV is very useful in localizing the specific anatomic site of a lesion that is causing pain. For example, a complaint of burning feet can be caused by a diffuse peripheral neuropathy (as in diabetes), by a plexus injury after surgery, or by lumbosacral radiculopathy due to spinal stenosis. Each of these has different findings and can be localized by EMG/NCV. In general, changes in conduction, either a prolonged distal latency or a slow velocity, suggest a pathologic lesion between the site of stimulation and the recording site. An abnormally small amplitude, however, can occur from an injury anywhere along the nerve. A sampling on needle examination of muscles representing different nerves and roots can further localize the site of injury. Using the example of burning feet, let us examine the differential diagnosis and its EMG/NCV findings. In radiculopathy, motor conduction velocity would be normal, and CMAP amplitude would be reduced if there were axonal degeneration from nerve root compromise. SNAP would be normal because the lesion is proximal to the dorsal root ganglion. (Please note that most radiculopathies occur within the spinal canal. The dorsal root ganglion, which is sensory, is located in the neuroforamina distal to most radicular pathologic lesions. The dorsal root ganglion is a bipolar neuron with one axon extending distally to the limb and one extending proximally to the spinal cord.) EMG abnormalities first appear in appropriate paraspinal muscles, because of their proximity to the injury site. Abnormalities are next seen in proximal and then distal muscles within the specific myotomal distribution of the injured nerve root. In a plexus injury, both CMAP and SNAP amplitudes would

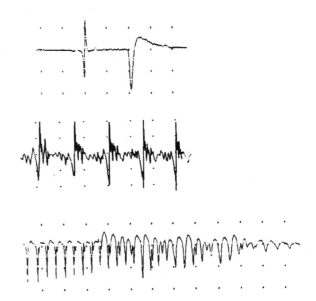

FIGURE 6–3. Spontaneous activities. Fibrillation potential and positive wave *(top panel).* Complex repetitive discharges *(middle panel);* time marker, 10 ms; amplitude marker, 100 μV. Myotonic discharges *(bottom panel);* time marker, 20 ms; amplitude marker, 200 μV.

TABLE 6–2. EMG FINDINGS IN NEUROGENIC AND MYOPATHIC DISORDERS

EMG	Normal	Neurogenic (Axonal)	NMJ Defect	Myopathic
Insertional activity	N	↑	↑	↑
Spontaneous activity	—	+	+	+
MUAP				
Amplitude (mV)	0.1–5	↑	↓	↓
Duration (ms)	3–15	↑	↓	↓
Phase	<5	↑	N	↑
Stability	N	N	Variable	N
Recruitment	N	↓	N	↑

MUAP, motor unit action potential; NMJ, neuromuscular junction; N, normal.

be decreased if axons were injured. NCV is usually normal, unless stimulation is applied proximal to the lesion. Paraspinal muscles are spared because posterior rami innervate these muscles, while the plexus is in the anterior rami distribution. Combined motor and sensory NCV abnormalities are characteristic of most peripheral neuropathies. Needle findings would depend on the severity of motor nerve involvement, and they are usually normal unless the neuropathy is severe. Anatomic localization based on EMG/NCV is summarized in Table 6–3.

Is the Lesion Axonal or Demyelinating? (Pathophysiology)

Based on the EMG/NCV findings, the distinction can be made with relative ease. If an injury occurs at the cell body or axon, axonal degeneration results. If an injury is directed against the myelin, demyelination ensues. In the majority of cases of peripheral neuropathy, both demyelination and axonal injury occur; however, characterizing the primary pathologic process is important to establish an etiology and to assess the extent of injury. Demyelinating neuropathies can be further divided into segmental (acquired) and uniform (hereditary) types. In the former, non-uniform slowing in individual myelinated nerve fibers results in conduction block and temporal dispersion. In the latter, prolonged latency and slowing of conduction predominate as a result of uniform involvement of all myelinated fibers. Table 6–4 summarizes the EMG/NCV characteristics of demyelinating and axonal injuries.

Is the Lesion Motor, Sensory, Mixed, or Autonomic? (Fiber Type Specificity)

NCVs test motor and sensory components separately. Many peripheral nervous system diseases affect both motor and sensory nerves. In a case of distal sensory or motor neuropathy, amplitudes as well as velocities are abnormal. With a dorsal root ganglion lesion or anterior horn cell disease, NCV studies show small-amplitude SNAP or CMAP, respectively, and, as a rule, normal velocities. Routine EMG/NCV studies do not test the autonomic nervous system. Autonomic nervous system tests are discussed in Chapter 7.

Is the Lesion Focal, Multifocal, or Diffuse?

By determining the distribution of abnormalities, neuropathy, for example, can be further divided into mononeuropathy, multifocal neuropathy, and polyneuropathy. A focal lesion such as carpal tunnel syndrome will result in abnormalities limited to the distal segment of a median nerve. If the same nerve is affected disproportionately in the opposite limb, or one nerve is affected more than the other in the same limb, a multifocal disorder is suggested. In a fully developed polyneuropathy, motor and sensory nerves in both upper and lower extremities are affected in equal and symmetrical fashion; in milder cases, however, the abnormalities will be more significant in distal sensory nerves of the lower extremities.

How Old Is the Injury? (Chronicity)

Following an axonal injury, the nerve distal to the lesion undergoes wallerian degeneration. For the first 2

TABLE 6–3. ANATOMIC LOCALIZATION BASED ON THE EMG AND NCV STUDIES

Lesion	Motor Nerve Conduction	Sensory Nerve Conduction	RNS	EMG
Dorsal root ganglion (sensory neuronopathy)	N	N, ↓ amp	N	N
Anterior horn cell (motor neuronopathy)	N, ↓ amp	N	N/Abn	Abn
Root (radiculopathy)	N, ↓ amp	N	N	Abn
Plexus (plexopathy)	N, ↓ amp	N, ↓ amp	N	Abn
Nerve (neuropathy)	Abn	Abn	N	Abn
NMJ defect	N, ↓ amp	N	Abn	Abn
Muscle (myopathy)	N, ↓ amp	N	N/Abn	Abn

RNS, repetitive nerve stimulation; NMJ, neuromuscular junction; N, normal; Abn, abnormal; amp, amplitude.

TABLE 6–4. NCV AND EMG CHARACTERISTICS OF THE DEMYELINATING AND AXONAL INJURIES

	NCV	EMG
Demyelination	1. Prolonged latency, more than 13% of normal 2. Slow NCV, less than 70% of normal 3. Conduction block 4. Temporal dispersion	1. Normal insertional activity, no spontaneous activity 2. Reduced recruitment with conduction block 3. Normal MUAP morphology
Axonal injury	1. Normal latency 2. Slow NCV, more than 70% of normal 3. Small CMAP/SNAP amplitude	1. Increased insertional activity, spontaneous activity 2. Reduced recruitment 3. Large-amplitude, long-duration polyphasic with reinnervation 4. Satellite potential

CMAP, compound muscle action potential; SNAP, sensory nerve action potential; MUAP, motor unit action potential.

to 3 days, motor conduction distal to a lesion is normal. Then CMAP amplitude drops progressively, reaching a nadir at about 7 days. SNAP amplitudes distal to a lesion are unaffected for 5 to 6 days, but by day 10 to 11, the nadir is reached. After an axonal motor nerve injury, needle findings change slowly. Initially, insertional activity is increased. Positive sharp waves and fibrillation potentials may not occur for 2 to 3 weeks following a nerve injury, depending on the length between site of nerve injury and corresponding muscles. The abnormal spontaneous activities can resolve in 3 to 6 months. Therefore, needle studies performed less than 2 to 3 weeks after injury, or later than 3 to 6 months after injury, may be normal. Large-amplitude, long-duration polyphasic MUAPs seen in denervation and reinnervation develop 3 to 6 months after an injury. Table 6–5 summarizes the chronology of EMG/NCV findings after axonal injury.

How Bad Is the Injury? (Severity and Prognosis)

The severity of an injury can be determined if EMG/NCV is done in a timely manner. The amplitude difference between the same nerves on affected and unaffected sides gives an idea of extent of injury and potential recovery if they are determined sequentially. A paucity of spontaneous activity in affected muscles 3 weeks after injury indicates an excellent outcome for the return of muscle function. Markedly reduced recruitment of MUAPs indicates a severe lesion, except for

TABLE 6–5. CHRONOLOGY OF THE NCV AND EMG FINDINGS FOLLOWING AXONAL INJURY

Time After Injury	NCV	EMG
0–1 wk	↓ Amp, proximal	↓ Recruitment
1–2 wk	↓ Amp, proximal and distal	↓ Recruitment ↑ Insertional activity
2–3 wk	↓ Amp, proximal and distal	↓ Recruitment ↑ Fibrillation potentials
1–3 mo	↑ Amp	↓ Fibrillation potentials ↓ Amp, ↑ duration, ↑ phase
3–6 mo	↑ Amp	↑ Recruitment ↑ Amp, ↑ duration, ↑ phase

Amp, amplitude.

neurapraxia. In general, axonal injury has a worse prognosis than demyelinating disorders.

QUANTITATIVE SENSORY TESTING

The test provides a quantitative measure to detect large- and small-fiber dysfunction. Various stimuli at varying intensities are applied to the skin, and a patient is asked to indicate when he or she begins to feel the stimulus. The recent consensus report defines "sensory detection threshold" as "the smallest stimulus that can be detected at least 50% of the time." By increasing and decreasing stimulus intensity from the predetermined level, "appearance" and "disappearance" thresholds can be determined. Sensory modalities commonly used are vibration and thermal senses—warm, cold, heat pain, and cold pain (Fig. 6–4). Vibration threshold measures large myelinated fiber function, whereas warm, heat pain, and cold pain thresholds reflect the function of unmyelinated C fibers. Cold threshold measures small myelinated Aδ-fiber function.

QST measures not only peripheral nerve fiber function but also central pathway function. Vibratory sense is carried by the dorsal columns and thermal senses via the spinothalamic tract. Normal values depend on methodology, sensory modality tested, and site of test. Sensory detection threshold increases with age; therefore, results should be compared with the age-matched reference values.

QST can be used to detect subtle sensory changes that may be missed by NCV study. Increased or decreased thermal detection threshold (hypoesthesia or hyperesthesia) and thermal pain threshold (hypalgesia or hyperalgesia) have been reported in many painful neuropathies. Cold or heat hyperalgesia is a feature of reflex sympathetic dystrophy. Heat hyperalgesia is common in erythromelalgia, and *angry backfiring C* nociceptor (or ABC) syndrome. Cold hypoesthesia, cold hyperalgesia, and cold limb are features of the CCC syndrome, whereas thermal hypoesthesia and hyperalgesia (anesthesia dolorosa) are typical manifestations of postherpetic neuralgia.

QST allows early detection of disease. Sequential testing can be used to monitor disease progression and therapeutic efficacy. However, QST is not objective and relies on patient cooperation. QST does not localize a

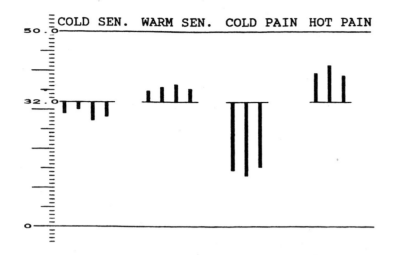

FIGURE 6–4. Example of a thermal QST in a normal subject. Temperature, in degrees centigrade, on vertical scale. *Solid bar* represents each trial. Sen., sensation.

lesion, as it tests the integrity of the entire sensory pathway from nerve ending to cortex.

SHORT-LATENCY SOMATOSENSORY EVOKED POTENTIALS

Conventional sensory NCV studies assess a lesion distal to the dorsal root ganglion. SSEPs provide a quantitative measure to study the entire sensory pathway. Typically, a mixed nerve, such as the median nerve at the wrist or tibial nerve at the ankle, is repeatedly stimulated, and responses are recorded along the sensory pathway. These responses are then averaged to improve the signal-to-noise ratio. Stimulations of skin within a dermatome or cutaneous nerve, such as superficial radial or sural nerve, have more limited value because of the low-amplitude response. Submaximal intensity and longer duration of stimulus are required to elicit an optimal response.

Stimulations are mediated by group Ia and II sensory afferents, dorsal root ganglion (neuron I), dorsal columns, gracilis and cuneatus nuclei (neuron II), contralateral medial lemniscus, ventroposterolateral nucleus of the thalamus (neuron III), and sensory cortex. Clinically, touch-pressure, position-movement senses are affected with the injury to the dorsal column pathway in both the central and peripheral nervous system. Each identifiable component is labeled according to its polarity (negative or positive) and its mean peak latency (in milliseconds) following stimulation. Useful obligate potentials after median nerve stimulation include EP (Erb's potential), N13 (dorsal column of the cervical cord), P14 (caudal medial lemniscus), N18 (thalamus), and N20 (sensory cortex). Identifiable potentials after tibial nerve stimulation are PF (popliteal fossa), LP (lumbar potential), P31 (caudal medial lemniscus), N34 (thalamus), and P37 (sensory cortex) (Fig. 6–5). Knowledge of the generator source of these peaks allows us to localize lesions to parts of the pathway. Age, tempera-

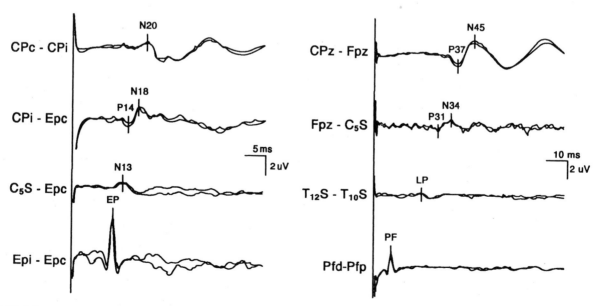

FIGURE 6–5. Median *(left)* and tibial *(right)* SSEPs in a normal subject. CPc, contralateral central-parietal; CPi, ipsilateral central-parietal; Epc, contralateral Erb's point; Epi, ipsilateral Erb's point; CPz, midline central-parietal; Fpz, midline frontopolar; Pfd, popliteal fossa, distal; Pfp, popliteal fossa, proximal; EP, Erb's potential; LP, lumbar potential; PF, popliteal fossa potential.

TABLE 6–6. TYPICAL SSEP FINDINGS AND RESULTING LOCALIZATION

SSEPs	Abnormality	Lesion
Median nerve	1. Absent EP	Median nerve–brachial plexus
	P14	Above plexus
	N20	Above medulla
	2. Prolonged EP–P14	Brachial plexus–medulla
	P14–N20	Medulla–sensory cortex
Tibial nerve	1. Absent LP	Tibial nerve–cauda equina
	P37	Above lumbar spinal cord
	2. Prolonged LP–P37	Spinal cord–sensory cortex

EP, Erb's potential; LP, lumbar potential.

ture, limb length, medications, level of attention, and sleep may alter latency and amplitude. Therefore, every laboratory has its own normal values. Adult norms are reached at about 8 years of age. Criteria for abnormality includes absence of any obligate waves and prolongation of interpeak intervals. For example, absence of N18 or N20 or a prolonged P14–N20 interval suggests a lesion between the medulla and sensory cortex. Table 6-6 summarizes some typical SSEP findings and resulting localization. Absolute latency is a less reliable indicator of abnormality because it varies with limb length. A side-to-side amplitude ratio less than half is considered abnormal by some. Application of SSEPs for a patient with pain is limited to the identification of a potential structural or compressive lesion involving peripheral or central sensory pathway.

LASER EVOKED POTENTIALS

A carbon dioxide laser can also be used to generate pain-related cerebral potentials. Laser stimulation produces heat quickly and activates $A\delta$ and C fibers. Late component, which occurs at approximately 500 ms following stimulation of the hand, corresponds to $A\delta$-fiber conduction, and ultra-late component at 1500 ms corresponds to C fiber; both components are maximum in amplitude at the vertex (CZ). LEP is a noninvasive test, and no tissue damage has been reported. LEPs provide an objective measure to assess the function of pain pathway in patients with neuropathic pain. LEP is not yet available in most electrophysiology laboratories.

BIBLIOGRAPHY

AAEE glossary of terms in clinical electromyography. Muscle Nerve 10(suppl):G1–G60, 1987.

Carmon A, Mor J, Goldberg J: Evoked cerebral responses to noxious thermal stimuli in humans. Exp Brain Res 25:103–107, 1976.

Dawson GD: Cerebral responses to electrical stimulation of peripheral nerve in man. J Neurol Neurosurg Psychiatry 10:137–140, 1947.

Guidelines in electrodiagnostic medicine. Muscle Nerve 15:229–253, 1992.

Guidelines on evoked potentials. J Clin Neurophysiol 11:40–73, 1994.

Quantitative sensory testing: A consensus report from the Peripheral Neuropathy Association. Neurology 43:1050–1052, 1993.

Yarnitsky D: Quantitative sensory testing. Muscle Nerve 20:198–204, 1997.

Chapter 7

Tests of the Autonomic Nervous System

Takashi Nishida, M.D.,
and R. Norman Harden, M.D.

In diseases of the central or peripheral nervous system, autonomic dysfunction results in alteration of vascular tone, skin temperature, and sweat secretion. The role of the sympathetic nervous system in the production of pain is complex and controversial; nonetheless, testing of autonomic function is important for evaluation of pain complaints because it gives an objective measure of autonomic nervous system involvement as well as evidence of the effectiveness of therapeutic interventions, such as sympathetic nerve blocks. The most frequent referrals to the autonomic testing laboratory are patients with painful peripheral neuropathy, such as diabetic polyneuropathy, and so-called complex regional pain syndrome/reflex sympathetic dystrophy (CRPS/RSD). Autonomic testing that is available for the assessment of pain is basically for the vasomotor and sudomotor functions. For the former, thermography is performed, and for the latter, numerous tests with different stimulation and recording modes are available. Based on accuracy, reproducibility, and ease of performance, two quantitative methods (sympathetic skin response and quantitative sudomotor axon reflex test) are discussed here.

THERMOGRAPHY

Thermography is a noninvasive, safe, and sensitive technique for measuring body surface temperature. It measures emitted heat from a surface, reflecting the temperature of the distal 6 mm of skin in the human. It is a direct measure of cutaneous vascular flow and an indirect measure of sympathetic vasomotor activity. The function of the intact sympathetic nervous system in the cutaneous layer is to regulate (and, when activated, to decrease) superficial blood flow rates, which has the effect of decreasing the emitted infrared radiation. Therefore, thermography measures the functional condition of the vascular beds as regulated by sympathetic efferent neurons. In certain pathologic conditions, an apparently asymmetrical sympathetic efferent dysfunction occurs (such as in CRPS/RSD), and thermography

is useful in detecting and measuring these asymmetries. The device can detect very small differences in emitted heat (down to 0.05°C) with a resolution of 1 mm² or less. Side-to-side differences in humans are usually less than 0.5°C, and a difference of greater than 1°C is defined as abnormal.[1, 2] Thermographic asymmetry can occur not only in the traditional dermatomes[3] but also, more importantly, in "thermatomes" that probably reflect the distribution of functional sympathetic efferent groups. Thermography is best at detecting regional patterns of asymmetry (e.g., in a distal extremity), but it can also be used to detect abnormalities in specific somatic efferent patterns (e.g., specific dermatomes). Thermography does not measure "pain," and like many other physiologic tests, it lacks a high degree of specificity.[4-8] However, interobserver reliability is good.[8]

Many factors influence cutaneous temperature (e.g., humidity, evaporation, ambient and core temperature, chemical and mechanical stimuli), and the skilled thermographer must control these effects as much as possible and interpret the results in the context of a careful clinical examination to make best use of the test. Thermography is therefore a very useful adjunctive test, but it should never be used in isolation.

The great amount of controversy recently generated about thermography stems primarily from arguments based on the test's solitary use, and they often reflect emotional bias rather than actual deficiencies in the test. The fact of the matter is that thermography is a very sensitive (although not particularly specific) test that is enormously useful in the complete clinical context.[4-8]

There are two basic types of thermography: the newer electronic infrared telethermography and the older liquid crystal contact thermography. The former translates emitted infrared temperatures into discrete color bands, which can be arbitrarily adjusted to represent a temperature range (e.g., 0.5°C per band). Homuncular mapping of these bands is then displayed using arbitrary colors to represent each temperature band, usually on a television screen which can either be photographed or digitally transcribed for hard-copy storage.

For more qualitative information, a black-and-white picture can also be generated, which represents the continuum of temperatures over the surface being studied. Various provocative techniques are often employed, such as immersing an unaffected limb in ice water, which causes activation of the sympathetic nervous system. There are rigorous, specific guidelines available for the thermographic technique, and it is essential that these be closely adhered to in order to obtain the maximum diagnostic information from the test.[1, 3]

Thermography is particularly useful in the documentation of baseline temperature patterns in diseases associated with autonomic dysregulation, such as CRPS/RSD.[9] Although temperature asymmetry is easily documented at the bedside, displays of specific thermographic patterns and regional dysregulation are important to completely understand the degree and extent of disease. CRPS/RSD can be manifested either by increased temperature in the affected limb in the early phases or by a very cold limb, which is the more common chronic picture. If thermography is used to document a baseline temperature, then it can also be useful to document the impact of relevant therapeutic measures. As a dynamic test, it can be used in the regional anesthesiology suite to document the effect of procedures such as sympathetic blocks. Although the effect of these blocks is easily seen in the clinical context (e.g., development of Horner's syndrome), thermography documents the complete field of the effect of the sympathoplegia, and it can also be used to demonstrate duration of effect. Some of the devices are portable and can easily be moved from the procedure suite to the bedside for whatever documentation of dynamic surface temperature changes is needed. Thermography is also useful for demonstrating specific nerve root irritation, and it commonly shows a "heat stripe" in the relevant dermatomes.[3] Again, it is important that the test be taken in the context of other relevant tests (such as electromyography [EMG]), especially an astute clinical examination.

Thermography has been examined in a variety of other conditions that involve vasomotor asymmetry, such as the mammographic cold spots associated with tumors, and as a rapid screening device for such problems as carpal tunnel syndrome in the industrial medicine setting. Essentially, any disease that involves disturbance of the cutaneous vasomotor beds can theoretically be demonstrated, documented, and diagnosed using thermography.

SYMPATHETIC SKIN RESPONSE

The first report of the galvanic skin response was by Tarchanoff in 1890.[10] Since then, various terminology has been introduced on the basis of different stimulating and recording methods (e.g., electrodermal activity,[11] sympathetic skin response,[12] peripheral autonomic surface potential,[13] and psychogalvanic reflex[14]). A standard method of obtaining sympathetic skin response (SSR) is to place a recording electrode (9-mm silver/silver chloride electrode) on the palmar surface, which is referenced to phalanx, and on the plantar surface, also referenced to phalanx, because these recording sites yield higher amplitudes. A bipolar stimulator is placed on either the median or the tibial nerve of the opposite limb, and the stimulus is given randomly at a rate of less than one per minute, with a stimulus duration of 0.1 to 0.3 ms, and a stimulus intensity of 80 mA, which is sufficient to cause mild pain. Amplifier settings for two-channel simultaneous recording from hand and foot are high-frequency filter at 100 Hz; low-frequency filter, 0.1 Hz; sweep velocity, 1 second/cm; and sensitivity, 1 mV/cm (for hand) and 0.2 mV/cm (for foot). A minimum of five to ten responses should be recorded, and SSR responses are obtainable 60% to 100% of the time in normal subjects. Wave forms are usually triphasic, with an initial small negativity followed by a large positive wave and a subsequent prolonged negative wave (Fig. 7-1). Wave forms can also be monophasic or diphasic, with an initial negative or positive peak. Maximal peak-to-peak amplitudes and mean latencies are measured. Amplitude and latency variability can be minimized by reducing stimulus frequency, increasing stimulus intensity, and/or changing stimulus site or mode. Low skin temperature, low level of attention, medication (especially anticholinergics), age, and habituation will also attenuate the response. Normal amplitude is more than 1 mV for hand and more than 0.2 mV for foot. Mean palmar latency is 1.4 ± 0.1 second, and plantar latency is 1.9 ± 0.1 second. SSR measures change of epidermal resistance due to sweat gland activity. The somatic afferent limb depends on the stimulus type (electrical shock, loud noise, visual threat, deep breathing); with the electrical stimulation, the afferent limb occurs via large myelinated fibers. The efferent limb is a sympathetic pathway originating in the posterior hypothalamus, descending through the spinal cord to the intermediolateral cell column (T1 to L2) and paravertebral ganglia and then to the sweat gland via small unmyelinated fibers. Therefore, it is important to note that neuropathy affecting large myelinated fibers exhibits abnormal SSR when electrical stimulation is used.

Low-amplitude or absent response indicates abnormal

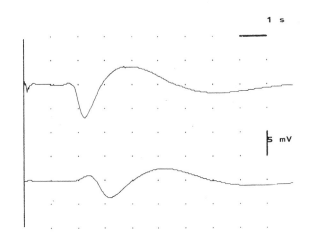

FIGURE 7-1. Normal sympathetic skin response (SSR) recorded simultaneously from the palm of the hand *(top)* and sole of the foot *(bottom)* by electrical stimulation.

sympathetic reflex arc, and the lesion can be central or peripheral, preganglionic or postganglionic. A side-to-side amplitude difference of more than 50% is considered to be abnormal by some. In studies of diabetic, uremic, and amyloid neuropathies, the result of SSR correlated well with autonomic symptoms. As a rule, SSR is abnormal in axonal neuropathies.[12] An exception is a demyelinating neuropathy with prominent autonomic features, such as Guillain-Barré syndrome. Some studies have reported abnormal SSR test results in patients with CRPS/RSD, and others have not.[15] Immediately following the sympathetic nerve block or sympathectomy, SSR is absent or reduced in amplitude. The SSR is usually normal in entrapment neuropathy and radiculopathy.

SSR evoked by magnetic stimulation in the neck bypasses the afferent limb and directly stimulates postganglionic fibers. This method has less propensity to habituate, and therefore less fluctuation of amplitude and latency occurs.[16]

QUANTITATIVE SUDOMOTOR AXON REFLEX TEST AND RESTING SWEAT OUTPUT TEST

This is a sensitive, reproducible, and quantitative method to test sudomotor function. A multicompartment plastic "sweat cell" is tightly secured to the skin. The outer compartment is filled with 10% acetylcholine solution via a cannula, and a constant-current stimulator is attached to a wire inside the compartment. Nitrogen gas flows constantly at the rate of about 100 mL/minute to an inner compartment through an instrument that measures the change in humidity (sudorometer). The middle compartment serves as a barrier between the inner and outer compartments. A 2 mA direct current is applied for 5 minutes, and the water content in the inner compartment is continuously measured before, during, and after the stimulus (Fig. 7-2). The basis of the test is that the axon terminal of the sweat gland under the outer compartment is activated by acetylcholine iontophoresis; the impulse travels centripetally to a branch point and then distally to the axon terminal

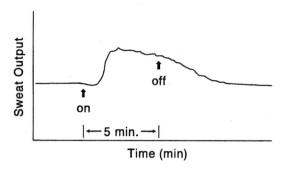

FIGURE 7–3. Example of a normal quantitative sudomotor axon reflex test (QSART). On, off, stimulator on and off.

under the inner compartment, where acetylcholine is released and a sweating response results. Use of the term "axon reflex" should be discouraged, because only the postganglionic sympathetic sudomotor axon is considered to be involved in this setup. With a latency of 1 to 2 minutes after the induction of the stimulus, sweat output increases rapidly while stimulation continues; then the stimulator is turned off, and sweat output returns to its prestimulus baseline within 5 minutes (Fig. 7-3). The area under the curve represents the total amount of sweat output expressed in microliters per square centimeter, and the normal value varies depending on the site of testing and sex and age of the subject. Distal limbs, male subjects, and younger subjects tend to sweat more. Reduced or absent response indicates postganglionic disorder. Normal response does not rule out preganglionic involvement. Excessive and persistent sweating is also considered abnormal. Comparison is made between the two limbs, and an asymmetry of more than 25% is considered to be abnormal. The resting sweat output (RSO) test is basically similar to the quantitative sudomotor axon reflex test (QSART): a capsule with one chamber is attached to the skin, and the rate of water evaporation is continuously monitored for 5 minutes. The presence of RSO indicates that the sweat gland is spontaneously activated by the sympathetic fibers.

In a patient with painful diabetic neuropathy, RSO studies show the presence of increased sweat activity, and QSART exhibits short-latency, excessive, and persis-

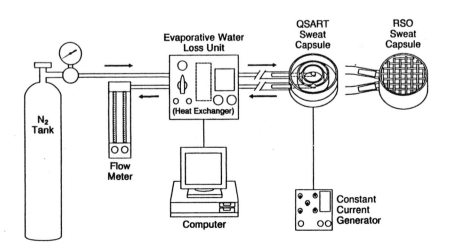

FIGURE 7–2. Physiologic setup for the quantitative sudomotor axon reflex test (QSART). *Arrow* indicates direction of gas flow. (Figure is not drawn to scale.) RSO, resting sweat output.

tent sweat patterns, which is evidence of sympathetic overactivity.[17] A most recent study seems to indicate that sweat test abnormalities correlate well with the symptoms of CRPS/RSD-related pain,[18] for which the pathophysiologic mechanism is uncertain; perhaps a lower firing threshold or an increased firing frequency due to denervation hypersensitivity of the sudomotor axons may produce excitation of the sweat glands.

REFERENCES

1. Wexler CE: Thermographic evaluation of trauma (spine). Acta Thermogr 5:3-10, 1980.
2. Uematsu S, Jankel WR, Edwin DH, et al: Quantification of thermal asymmetry: I. Normal values and reproducibility. J Neurosurg 69:552-555, 1988.
3. Standards for neuromuscular thermography of the Academy of Neuromuscular Thermography: Clinical thermography. J Acad Neuromusc Thermogr, Aug:1-18, 1989.
4. Chafetz N, Wexler CE, Kaiser JA: Neuromuscular thermography of the lumbar spine with CT correlation. Spine 13:922-925, 1988.
5. Uematsu S, Jankel WR, Edwin DH, et al: Quantification of thermal asymmetry: II. Application in low back pain and sciatica. J Neurosurg 69:556-561, 1988.
6. Uricchio J, Walbroel C: Blinded reading of electronic thermography. Postgrad Med (special ed):47-53, 1986.
7. Cabot W, Bothe B: A multidisciplinary treatment program for back and neck injuries utilizing computerized electronic thermography as a diagnostic tool. Clin Thermogr Aug:145-150, 1989.
8. Wiesel SW, Tsourmas N, Feffer HL, et al: A study of computer assisted tomography: The incidence of positive CAT scans in an asymptomatic group of patients. Spine 9:549-551, 1984.
9. Uematsu S, Hendler U, Hungerford, et al: Thermography and electromyography in the differential diagnosis of chronic pain syndromes and reflex sympathetic dystrophy. Electromyogr Clin Neurophysiol 21:165-182, 1981.
10. Tarchanoff G: Über die galvanischen Erscheinungen an der Haut des Menschen bei Reizung der Sinnesorgane und bei vershiedenen Formen der physische Tätigkeit. Pflugers Arch 46:46-55, 1890.
11. Christie MJ: Electrodermal activity in the 1980s: A review. J R Soc Med 74:616-622, 1981.
12. Shahani BT, Halperin JJ, Boulu P, et al: Sympathetic skin response: A method of assessing unmyelinated axon dysfunction in peripheral neuropathies. J Neurol Neurosurg Psychiatry 47:536-542, 1984.
13. Knezevic W, Bajada S: Peripheral autonomic surface potential: A quantitative technique for recording sympathetic conduction in man. J Neurol Sci 67:239-251, 1985.
14. Lader MH, Montagu JD: The psycho-galvanic reflex: A pharmacologic study of the peripheral mechanism. J Neurol Neurosurg Psychiatry 25:126-133, 1962.
15. Rommel O, Tegenthoff M, Peru U, et al: Sympathetic skin response in patients with reflex sympathetic dystrophy. Clin Auton Res 5:205-210, 1995.
16. Uozumi T, Nakano S, Matsunaga K, et al: Sudomotor potential evoked by magnetic stimulation of the neck. Neurology 43:1397-1400, 1993.
17. Low PA, Caskey PE, Tuck RR, et al: Quantitative sudomotor axon reflex test in normal and neuropathic subjects. Ann Neurol 14:573-580, 1983.
18. Chelimsky TC, Low PA, Naessens JM, et al: Value of autonomic testing in reflex sympathetic dystrophy. Mayo Clin Proc 70:1029-1040, 1995.

Chapter 8

Psychological Evaluation and Testing

Leslie J. Heinberg, Ph.D.,
and Jennifer A. Haythornthwaite, Ph.D.

The experience of pain is a private, subjective phenomenon. There is no simple instrument, such as a thermometer, that can accurately assess an individual's pain experience. As a result, numerous instruments have been offered to measure multiple domains of pain. Voluminous research data have demonstrated that a psychological perspective is helpful in conceptualizing, evaluating, and treating chronic pain. This chapter focuses on evaluation and assessment of chronic pain from a psychological perspective. The components of a psychological evaluation for chronic pain are reviewed and the psychological assessment of pain is examined in the domains of pain severity, disability/impairment, negative affect, and coping. Multidimensional instruments and measures of more global psychopathology are outlined, followed by a discussion of specialized assessment.

PSYCHOLOGICAL EVALUATION

A comprehensive evaluation of individuals with chronic pain must include assessment of psychological, social, and behavioral factors associated with their experience of pain. This is best accomplished by combining interview techniques with the administration of one or more standardized questionnaires. Psychological evaluation should not only include an examination of psychological aspects of the pain experience but also a more comprehensive psychiatric interview to diagnose current or past psychiatric disorders, particularly depression.

Although structured clinical interviews for pain have been developed, the majority of practitioners choose to conduct semi-structured interviews. Because patients with chronic pain complaints may be reticent to undergo psychological evaluation, it is recommended that a history of the pain complaint be taken first. This assessment will focus on the intensity, frequency, and affective and sensory quality of pain as well as the efficacy of previous treatment interventions. It is important to identify events that act as precipitants to pain

exacerbations; to assess daily activities, disability, and perceived interference; to evaluate familial and/or social factors; and to identify any psychiatric disorders. Because of the high co-prevalence of chronic pain and major depression, it is recommended that all depressive symptoms be carefully assessed. In addition, practitioners generally assess symptoms of anxiety disorders, alcohol and substance abuse and dependence, personality disorders, and any relevant family psychiatric history.

PSYCHOLOGICAL ASSESSMENT/TESTING

Pain Severity

Pain and suffering are internal, subjective events that cannot be directly observed by clinicians. Assessment of pain severity is therefore reliant on self-report measures. Such measures of pain severity provide a quantitative estimate of the intensity of the pain experience. Patients' self-report can also be used to compare their reported experience to norms of large pain populations. The majority of these measures are brief and unidimensional. For instance, a *verbal rating scale* consists of a list of adjectives describing increasing levels of pain intensity. The extremes of the scale are anchored by a description of "no pain" and some description reflecting the "worst pain." Verbal rating scales are generally scored by assigning increasing numbers as a function of rank. Verbal rating scales are brief, easily administered and scored, and comprehended by patients. They have been shown to correlate with more detailed measures of pain severity and are sensitive to treatment interventions.[1] However, it is not clear, because of its unidimensional quality, whether the intervals between the descriptors are equal, and it is not recommended that these scales be chosen as the sole measure of pain severity.

A *visual analogue scale* (VAS) consists of a 100-mm line whose ends are labeled as the extremes of pain (e.g., "no pain" and "worst pain imaginable"). VASs generally assess sensory and affective components of pain intensity. Patients are asked to indicate which point along the line best represents their pain experience. The distance from the left end of the line is measured in millimeters and yields a pain intensity score. Like verbal rating scales, VASs correlate well with other measures of pain intensity and are sensitive to treatment effects. Although VASs are easy to administer, the scoring is more time-consuming than that for a verbal rating scale. Further, patients often have difficulty understanding how to complete the VAS correctly.

One of the most comprehensive measures of pain intensity is the *McGill Pain Questionnaire*,[2] which assesses sensory, affective, and evaluative aspects of pain intensity. Adjectives are categorized to describe the sensory quality of the experience (e.g., thermal) and are arranged in increasing intensity (e.g., hot, burning, scalding, and searing). Similarly, adjectives are selected that describe increasingly intense affective qualities of pain (e.g., fearful, frightful, terrifying). In addition to the list of pain descriptions, the questionnaire contains line drawings of the body to show the spatial distribution of the pain experience as well as a single five-item verbal rating scale for the present pain intensity. The McGill Pain Questionnaire has acceptable psychometric properties and has been translated into a dozen languages. The McGill Pain Questionnaire has been criticized for lacking a consistent scoring technique, and administration can be time-consuming. More recently, a short form of the McGill Pain Questionnaire (SF-MPQ)[3] has been developed that correlates highly with the longer version.

Disability/Impairment

Individuals with chronic pain describe significant variability in the degree of interference, impairment, and disability due to their pain complaints. As a result, a number of measures have been offered to assess perceived disability. One of the most widely used is the *Sickness Impact Profile* (SIP).[4] The SIP assesses a number of daily activities and assumes that changes in related behavior are sensitive to changes in health status. The SIP has been comprehensively tested and revised, and norms have been established for a number of medical populations, including individuals with chronic pain. The 136 items of the SIP are separated into 12 scales: (1) sleep and rest, (2) eating, (3) work, (4) home management, (5) recreation and pastimes, (6) ambulation, (7) mobility, (8) body care and movement, (9) social interaction, (10) alertness behavior, (11) emotional behavior, and (12) communication. Often, investigators use only the scales of interest, because this is a lengthy questionnaire.

The *Pain Disability Index* (PDI)[5] is a brief self-report measure of pain-related disability. It consists of seven questions assessing functioning in the following domains: (1) family/home, (2) recreation, (3) social activities, (4) occupation, (5) sexual behavior, (6) self-care, and (7) life support activities. This measure is often favored due to its brevity and practicality, but, it has been criticized for its face-validity (i.e., informants are aware of what it is attempting to measure).

Negative Affect

Because depression and other types of negative affect often result from chronic pain and unduly influence its experience, it is important to determine whether the patient has experienced any change in mood or affect.[6] One of the most frequently utilized measures is the *Beck Depression Inventory* (BDI).[7] The BDI is a 21-item, multiple-choice measure that requires individuals to endorse one of a series of four statements that best describes his or her subjective experience. The four statements reflect progressively more severe symptoms. The BDI was developed to measure symptoms of depression or distress as operationally defined by alterations in mood, a negative self-concept associated with self-devaluation and self-blame, self-punitive wishes, vegetative symptoms, and alterations in activity level.[7] The BDI is frequently used in psychiatric and general medical populations. Although it is brief and easy to score and interpret, the BDI may overestimate the degree of depression among chronic pain patients because of its focus on a number of somatic and vegetative symptoms.

Another frequently used measure of depression is the *Center for Epidemiological Studies Depression Scale* (CES-D).[8] The CES-D was originally developed for use in large epidemiologic studies involving the general population and has been shown to be quite reliable and valid. Patients are asked to report the frequency with which they have experienced each of 20 symptoms during the past week on a four-point scale. Like the BDI, the CES-D is brief and has excellent psychometric properties. However, because of the overlap in somatic symptoms of depression and symptoms of chronic pain, it also has been criticized for possibly overestimating the prevalence and severity of depression among pain populations. Comparative analysis suggests that the CES-D and BDI are relatively comparable, with the CES-D demonstrating greater sensitivity and the BDI exhibiting better specificity.[9]

Coping

Coping is a term that includes techniques that people utilize to attempt to control or tolerate stressors, including the experience of pain. The use of some pain-specific coping strategies has been found to differentially relate to outcome among chronic pain patients.[10] Because of the interest in reducing maladaptive and increasing adaptive coping techniques, a number of measures of coping in chronic pain patients have been developed. The *Coping Strategies Questionnaire* (CSQ)[11] is a 50-item measure that assesses six cognitive and two behavioral coping strategies, including (1) diverting attention, (2) reinterpreting pain sensations, (3) use of coping self-statements, (4) ignoring pain sensations, (5) praying and hoping, (6) catastrophizing, (7) increasing behavioral activity, and (8) increasing pain behaviors. Catastrophizing (e.g., "I feel I can't stand it anymore") has been consistently identified as a maladaptive coping strategy. Despite the inclusion of cognitive strategies in psychological interventions for pain management (e.g., coping self-statements), these strategies have not been consistently demonstrated to be adaptive.[10]

The *Vanderbilt Pain Management Inventory* (VPMI)[12] is a 19-item scale that differentiates between active and passive coping strategies. That is, patients may be differentiated on the basis of the amount of effort put forward as compared with their tendency to rely on others. Passive coping has been shown to be associated with increased depressive symptoms during periods of increased pain.[13]

More recently, a more behaviorally oriented measure of coping in chronic pain patients has been developed in the *Chronic Pain Coping Inventory* (CPCI).[14] The scale was designed to include strategies that are encouraged, as well as discouraged, in multidisciplinary pain treatment, which have not been assessed with other measures of coping. This 65-item scale has 12 subscales, including (1) guarding, (2) resting, (3) asking for assistance, (4) employing relaxation techniques, (5) task persistence, (6) exercising/stretching, (7) seeking social support, (8) using coping self-statements, and (9) using medication. Guarding, resting, asking for assistance, and task persistence are closely associated with measures of functioning.

Multidimensional Instruments

Rather than administering large batteries of assessments to patients to measure the various domains of interest, multidimensional instruments have been developed. One of the most frequently used and widely studied is the *Multidimensional Pain Inventory* (MPI).[15] This 56-item measure is comprised of three sections and examines multiple pain domains including pain severity; interference of pain with daily activities, work, family relationships, and social activities; pain-specific support from spouse or significant other; perceived life control; and negative affect. Patients' responses may be compared against normative data from other chronic pain patients. In addition, validity studies[16] demonstrate that MPI profile patterns, labeled "dysfunctional," "interpersonally distressed," and "adaptive coper," can be readily identified and interpreted. This measure is valuable in its ability to assess multiple dimensions of pain within a relatively short period and its demonstrated sensitivity to treatment.

The *Short Form 36 Health Survey* (SF-36)[17] is a 36-item self-report measure of health-related quality of life yielding eight subscales. The scale was developed for diverse applications, and factor analysis yields two major factors: physical health and mental health. An advantage of the SF-36 is the opportunity to compare different diagnostic groups, as this instrument has been widely used.

Measures of Psychopathology

In addition to assessing the presence of psychopathology during a psychiatric interview, psychologists often administer self-report instruments of psychopathology to patients with chronic pain. Unlike interview data, these measures provide standardized, reliable, and valid assessments of psychopathology that may influence the experience of pain. The *Minnesota Multiphasic Personality Inventory* (MMPI) is the psychological instrument most commonly used to evaluate the psychological status of patients with chronic pain. A revised version, the MMPI-2,[18] has been introduced; like the original MMPI, it includes ten clinical scales that assess psychopathology and three validity scales. The MMPI has been shown to differentiate samples of rheumatoid arthritis and low back pain. However, it has been criticized for its length (566 items), large number of items relating to physical symptoms, and lack of predictive validity among populations with chronic pain.[19]

Shorter inventories, such as the 90-item *Symptom Checklist-90-Revised* (SCL-90-R),[20] have been utilized to assess psychopathology among chronic pain patients. The SCL-90-R assesses nine different types of psychological disturbance and yields three global measures of distress. Although often favored for its briefer length and, because of its focus on symptoms, less patient resistance, it also has not demonstrated predictive validity with regard to treatment outcome.

SPECIALIZED ASSESSMENT
Presurgical Evaluations

Psychological evaluation is often recommended prior to undertaking a number of pain-related surgical interventions. Such evaluations have numerous goals, including screening for major psychopathology, retardation, dementia, or delirium, which could impede the patient's ability to provide informed consent. In addition, it has been suggested that active psychosis, suicidality and/or homicidality, untreated major depression, somatization disorder, alcohol or drug dependency, and lack of social support should in some cases be considered exclusionary criteria.[21] Independent of depression, most patients with chronic pain will not evidence these conditions. As such, presurgical evaluation focuses on screening for, and potentially intervening in, psychological factors that may impede optimal outcome (e.g., a high degree of disability); helps educate the patient as part of preparation for informed consent, and guides both the patient and physician in identifying the individual's strengths and weaknesses. Presurgical evaluations generally include psychological testing, a psychiatric interview, and an educational component. Such evaluations are often recommended prior to the implantation of an intrathecal pump or a spinal cord stimulator or undertaking more extensive orthopedic and/or neurologic surgery. It is important to note that both physical and psychological criteria for patient selection for surgery are somewhat imprecise, and the predictive ability of psychological measures is relatively mixed.[21]

Chronic Opioid Therapy

Patients are often referred for evaluation to a clinical psychologist who specializes in chronic pain before chronic opioid therapy is initiated. This evaluation provides a baseline assessment of the patient's pain intensity, affective state, disability, and quality of life prior to initiation of chronic opioid therapy. In addition, potential behavioral and/or psychological contraindications for chronic opioid use can be identified, such as current alcohol abuse or dependence, illicit or prescription drug abuse or dependence, severe major depression, or antisocial or borderline personality disorder. Other psychological factors that may require closer supervision either by the physician or psychiatric care can also be assessed.

Psychological evaluation is frequently helpful for patients who are concerned about the effects of opioid treatment on cognitive functioning, particularly if they continue to work. Brief screening of intellectual functioning, memory, psychomotor speed, and attention, both before initiation of chronic opioid therapy and after titration to therapeutic doses, can demonstrate to patients (and often to employers) the lack of significant cognitive effects of opioid medications. If such an evaluation is considered, it is important that the baseline testing occur when the patient has not taken any opioid therapy for at least 1 week and has not taken other medications (e.g., benzodiazepines) that may impair cognitive functioning.

SUMMARY

Assessment of chronic pain requires careful multidisciplinary assessment to arrive at an optimally helpful treatment plan. A physical examination is generally not sufficient to capture the number of psychological and behavioral factors that should be considered. Psychological assessment and clinical interviewing can be helpful adjuncts to physicians' evaluations. However, it is important that the assessment be multidimensional and utilize instruments that are reliable and valid. The preceding discussion of instruments should provide a starting place for the selection of appropriate instruments.

REFERENCES

1. Jensen MP, Karoly P: Self-report scales and procedures for assessing pain in adults. *In* Turk DC, Melzack R (eds): Handbook of Pain Assessment. New York, Guilford Press, 1992 (p 135.)
2. Melack R: The McGill Pain Questionnaire: Major properties and scoring methods. Pain 1:277, 1975.
3. Melzack R: The short-form McGill Pain Questionnaire. Pain 30:191, 1987.
4. Bergner M, Bobbitt RA, Carter WB, et al: The Sickness Impact Profile: Development and final revision of a health status measure. Med Care 19:787, 1981.
5. Pollard CA: Preliminary validity study of the Pain Disability Index. Percept Mot Skills 59:974, 1984.
6. Fishbain DA, Cutler R, Rosomoff HL, et al: Chronic pain-associated depression: Antecedent of consequence of chronic pain? A review. Clin J Pain 13:116, 1997.
7. Beck AT, Rush AJ, Shaw BF, et al: Cognitive therapy for depression. New York, Guilford Press, 1979.
8. Radloff L: The CES-D scale: A self-report depression scale for research in the general population. Appl Psychol Meas 1:385, 1977.
9. Geisser ME, Roth RS, Robinson ME: Assessing depression among persons with chronic pain using the Center for Epidemiological Studies–Depression Scale and the Beck Depression Inventory: A comparative analysis. Clin J Pain 13:163, 1997.
10. Jensen MD, Turner JA, Romano JM, et al: Coping with chronic pain: A critical review of the literature. Pain 47:249, 1991.
11. Rosensteil AK, Keefe FJ: The use of coping strategies in low-back pain patients: Relationship to patient characteristics and current adjustment. Pain 17:33, 1983.
12. Brown GK, Nicassio PM: The development of a questionnaire for the assessment of active and passive coping strategies in chronic pain patients. Pain 31:53, 1987.
13. Zautra AJ, Manne SL: Coping with rheumatoid arthritis: A review of a decade of research. Ann Behav Med 14:31, 1992.
14. Jensen MP, Turner JA, Romano JM, et al: The Chronic Pain Coping Inventory: Development and preliminary validation. Pain 60:203, 1995.
15. Kerns RD, Turk DC, Rudy TE: The West Haven-Yale Multidimensional Pain Inventory (WHYMPI). Pain 23:345, 1985.
16. Turk DC, Rudy TE: The robustness of an empirically derived taxonomy of chronic pain patients. Pain 43:27, 1990.
17. Ware JE, Snow KK, Kosinski M, et al: SF-36 Health Survey: Manual and Interpretation Guide. Boston, Nimrod Press, 1993.
18. Hathaway SR, McKinley JC, Butcher JN, et al: Minnesota Multiphasic Personality Inventory–2: Manual for Administration. Minneapolis, University of Minnesota Press, 1989.
19. Main CJ, Spanswick CC: Personality assessment and the Minnesota Multiphasic Personality Inventory 50 years on: Do we still need our security blanket? Pain Forum 4:90, 1995.
20. Derogatis L: The SCL-90R Manual–II: Administration, Scoring and Procedures. Baltimore, Clinical Psychometric Research, 1983.
21. Nelson DV, Kennington M, Novy DM, et al: Psychological selection criteria for implantable spinal cord stimulators. Pain Forum 5:93, 1996.

Determination of Disability

E. Richard Blonsky, M.D.

Disability is defined as the inability of an individual to perform various activities of daily living based on the physical and/or cognitive requirements of the tasks relevant to the individual's impairments. Impairment is an alteration of an individual's health status and includes the loss of, or loss of use of, a physical, cognitive, or psychological part or function.

Physicians are trained to determine impairment, but the majority do not evaluate patients from a functional perspective unless specifically requested to do so. The goal of most physicians is to establish a diagnosis and determine a course of treatment as quickly and accurately as possible. Acute disorders are most easily dealt with. Chronic illness and impairment are more difficult matters because of the demands made on the physician to look beyond the medical model.

The American Medical Association's *Guides to Evaluation of Permanent Impairment*[1] enables the examiner to assess an individual and to accurately establish the nature and degree of each impairment displayed. Every organ system is considered in this book, as are chapters on psychiatric disturbances and pain. All but these two chapters assign a value for a particular impairment (e.g., loss of the part due to injury or disease; loss of use due to immobility [ankylosis], injury, or disease; diminished function of a part or system).

The determination of disability is administrative, not medical, although the question is regularly asked of treating and examining physicians. To establish disability status it is necessary (1) to fully identify all pertinent impairments exhibited by an individual, (2) to determine what restrictions are imposed on performance by the impairments, (3) to understand the complete requirements of the tasks or job to be completed, and (4) to be aware of possible accommodations that would enable the impaired individual to perform the requisite tasks.

DETERMINATION OF IMPAIRMENT

The *Guides to Evaluation of Permanent Impairment* integrate the effects of injury, disease, and disuse in an evaluation process that assesses disturbance in functional use of the affected part or system. The first two chapters of the fourth edition provide the philosophy and methodology of the work. Inherent in the impairment ratings are associated phenomena such as pain and sensory changes. For example, a surgically treated disc lesion with residual medically documented pain receives a higher rating than a similar lesion with no residual symptoms. This is a well-recognized situation, and an additional rating for pain is not warranted.

Each affected part, organ, or system must be individually evaluated and documented. Impairment, however, affects the whole person, and the *Guides to Evaluation of Permanent Impairment* are structured according to this principle. Impairment of a finger relates to a percentage of the hand, which is a proportion of the upper extremity, which is a percentage of the whole person (Tables 9-1 and 9-2). If multiple parts and/or systems are affected, each impairment percentage is determined and the cumulative impairment is established, based on the grid located at the end of the book that facilitates this process. The concept behind use of the *Guides to Evaluation of Permanent Impairment* is that any competent physician who utilizes the methods described should arrive at a determination of impairment consistently comparable to that determined by another evaluator. Another essential concept is that the condition being evaluated is stable and permanent. No attempt to determine impairment should be made until complete resolution has occurred. If additional treatment can be expected to improve function, it should be recommended; if the treatment is carried out, reevaluation should be performed subsequently.

The chapter on pain discusses how residual pain interferes with performance of activities of daily living. It utilizes a grid arrangement (Table 9-3) whereby an individual's symptoms are classified in terms of intensity vs. frequency, and an impairment rating is assigned on the basis of the examiner's perception of the problem.

There is no way to objectify pain. This assessment is entirely dependent on the patient's statements regarding pain characteristics (location and distribution, quality,

TABLE 9–1. RELATIONSHIP OF IMPAIRMENT OF THE DIGITS TO IMPAIRMENT OF THE HAND*

% Impairment		% Impairment		% Impairment	
Thumb	Hand	Index or Middle Finger	Hand	Ring or Little Finger	Hand
0–1 =	0	0–2 =	0	0–4 =	0
2–3 =	1	3–7 =	1	5–14 =	1
4–6 =	2	8–12 =	2	15–24 =	2
7–8 =	3	13–17 =	3	25–34 =	3
9–11 =	4	18–22 =	4	35–44 =	4
12–13 =	5	23–27 =	5	45–54 =	5
				55–64 =	6
				65–74 =	7
				75–84 =	8
				85–94 =	9
49–51 =	20			95–100 =	10
52–53 =	21				
54–56 =	22	73–77 =	15		
57–58 =	23	78–82 =	16		
59–61 =	24	83–87 =	17		
62–63 =	25	88–92 =	18		
64–66 =	26	93–97 =	19		
		98–100 =	20		
87–88 =	35				
89–91 =	36				
92–93 =	37				
94–96 =	38				
92–93 =	37				
97–98 =	39				
99–100 =	40				

*The table is illustrative only. Material has been deliberately deleted for brevity. Deletions indicated by dotted lines.

Modified from Guides to the Evaluation of Permanent Impairment, ed 4. Chicago, American Medical Association, 1993.

TABLE 9±2. RELATIONSHIP OF IMPAIRMENT OF THE HAND TO IMPAIRMENT OF THE UPPER EXTREMITY*

% Impairment		% Impairment		% Impairment	
Hand	Upper Extremity	Hand	Upper Extremity	Hand	Upper Extremity
0 =	0	53 =	48	88 =	79
1 =	1	54 =	49	89 =	80
2 =	2				
3 =	3	55 =	50	90 =	81
4 =	4	56 =	50	91 =	82
		57 =	51	92 =	83
5 =	5	58 =	52	93 =	84
6 =	5	59 =	53	94 =	85
7 =	6				
8 =	7				
9 =	8	60 =	54	95 =	86
		61 =	55	96 =	86
10 =	9	62 =	56	97 =	87
11 =	10	63 =	57	98 =	88
12 =	11	64 =	58	99 =	89
13 =	12				
14 =	13	65 =	59	100 =	90
		66 =	59		
15 =	14	67 =	60		
16 =	14	68 =	61		
17 =	15	69 =	62		

*The table is illustrative only. Material has been deliberately deleted for brevity. Deletions indicated by dotted lines.

ModiÆed from Guides to the Evaluation of Permanent Impairment, ed 4. Chicago, American Medical Association, 1993.

intensity, duration, frequency of occurrence, and precipitating and relieving factors) and on the examiner's experience with similar conditions (either personally or through training), his or her belief in the patient's description, and personal bias.

Impairment for psychiatric reasons is based on an individual's inability to perform in society because of his mental and emotional disturbances. The chapter "Mental and Behavioral Disorders" requires determination of a diagnosis based on specific criteria as set forth in the fourth edition of the *Diagnostic and Statistical Manual of Mental Disorders (DSM-IV)*. This mandates obtaining a detailed history from the patient regarding onset, precipitating causes, duration, periodicity, and interference in functional state caused by the disorder. A person with a mental disorder is often least qualified to provide an accurate statement concerning these issues. Other observers (e.g., family, friends, previous treaters) need to be interviewed or their records and/or reports reviewed to determine the chronologic and longitudinal aspects of a mental disorder; this is a time-consuming process that is rarely carried out. A clever, tutored person could easily say the appropriate things to establish the presence of a major emotional disturbance if he or she were trying to gain a disability rating.

Unlike physical impairments, those relating to pain and psychiatric issues are almost entirely dependent on the clinician's judgment. There are projective tests (e.g., Rorschach test, Thematic Apperception Test) that provide some measurable data regarding mental impairment and thought disorders and are useful in confirming such a diagnosis. The Minnesota Multiphasic Personality Interview (revised version) (MMPI-2) is a well-established means of determining a person's self-perception and likely behavioral response to situations. The validity measures can be utilized effectively to determine whether responses meet criteria for credibility or represent the subject's attempt to make himself appear more or less impaired than he is.

TABLE 9–3. PAIN INTENSITY-FREQUENCY GRID

		Frequency			
		Intermittent	Occasional	Frequent	Constant
Intensity	Minimal				
	Slight				
	Moderate				
	Marked				

From Guides to the Evaluation of Permanent Impairment, ed 4. Chicago, American Medical Association, 1993.

RESTRICTIONS

The limitations imposed on a person based on a specific set of impairments is usually related to the training and experience of the evaluator. A student adopts principles and practices espoused by a respected mentor, but, ideally, modifies them on the basis of subsequent personal experiences. Lifting, carrying, walking, sitting—the numerous and varied activities of daily living—may be restricted in the subject because of the nature of the original problem, the effects of surgical and other techniques employed to correct it, and potential problems in the future if restriction were not imposed.

Examiner bias also plays a role, unfortunately. When setting limits for a personal patient the physician tends to be more lenient regarding duration of recovery time and restrictions following return to work or other activities. When evaluating a person as an independent medical examiner the physician tends to be more rigorous and expectant of higher levels of performance than if the patient had been referred for a consultative opinion by the treating physician. Realistically, financial issues (continued referrals) or legal considerations (concern about legal action if the person is judged to be fit and claims reinjury on return to work) may cloud the objectivity of the evaluation process.

In an attempt to objectify this process, many physicians and insurance companies rely on the findings of a functional capacity assessment (FCA) and/or work capacity assessment (WCA). Several standardized protocols have been established, but all require that a person perform a set number of different tasks over a measured period of time in various positions. Validity measures are built in, and some incorporate the Waddell criteria[2] as measures of symptom magnification. Because all of these protocols allow the person to discontinue an activity on the basis of pain or fatigue, for example, similar activities presented in a different format (for distraction) allow the evaluator to confirm the disparity or reproducibility of performance. Motivation on the part of the examinee also is crucial. A person who makes no attempt to perform at maximal effort will, predictably, have a poor outcome, and the performance would be unreliable as an indicator of the person's potential.

A functional capacity assessment (FCA) looks at the maximum physical performance of a person and determines limits that should allow for regular, consistent performance. If the maximum lift is 50 lb, the person would not be expected to perform at that level continuously. Reducing the lift by 20% would allow a 40-lb lift occasionally, and reducing it by 30% would justify a 35-lb lift on a regular basis. Tolerances for sitting, standing, walking, and climbing, for example, can be determined in a similar fashion, by direct observation for a given session and extrapolation for longer periods. For this reason, an FCA should be carried out over at least 5 to 6 hours over a span of 2 days to establish a confident analysis.

A work capacity assessment (WCA) gauges an individual's ability to carry out all of the numerous physical tasks required in the performance of a specific job. Availability of heavy tools, special equipment, mock-up vehicles, for example, are necessary for this evaluation, and only specialized centers are equipped to properly perform these assessments. Sedentary and light-level jobs can be simulated more easily, and a determination of ability to perform them can be made in the regular physical and occupational therapy department settings.

It is acceptable for a physician to rely on the results of such testing to specify restrictions for an individual only if the results are valid and are based on maximal effort and motivation; less effort on the part of the subject would produce a flawed outcome and results would be unreliable.

JOB REQUIREMENTS

The physician must have an accurate and complete job description for the individual in question. This must include not only the purpose of the job (what should be accomplished as a result of its performance) but also its physical and cognitive requirements. Regarding the former, the physician must be aware of how much actual time is spent sitting, standing, walking, pushing, pulling, lifting, and carrying; the weights of items lifted, carried, pushed, or pulled; how often the task is performed in an hour or a day; what positions are required for the head and neck, upper limbs, trunk, and legs; and how often various movements are performed by the fingers, hands, wrists, forearms, elbows, upper arms, and shoulders, for example.

From a cognitive perspective, the physician must understand the amount of decision-making required by the patient vs. performance of simple repetitive activities; the amount of interaction with co-workers, supervisors, and outsiders; and the level of stress produced by production quotas. Knowledge of these and other issues is essential for the physician to provide a realistic and reasonable statement regarding the patient's capabilities. It is not enough to rely on a written job description provided by the patient's company if it is several years old, particularly when it is at great variance with the description given by the patient.

ACCOMMODATIONS

It is reasonable to suggest simple accommodations at work to enable an impaired, handicapped worker to perform his or her job, or another job, as mandated by the Americans With Disabilities Act. The vast majority of accommodations or work-site modifications cost less than $300. These recommendations may emanate from the evaluator's own clinical experience with other patients with similar problems or may reflect observations and statements contained in the FCA/WCA reports. The optimal vocational outcome would be for the injured person to return to the previous job for the previous employer. An uncooperative employer creates major problems in getting an injured person back to work.

SUMMARY

The evaluating physician has an obligation to the injured person, the employer and/or insurance carrier, and society to perform a scrupulous examination of the injured person and to provide as honest, unbiased, and realistic a report as possible—to truly be an independent expert. Although reasonable minds might differ to some extent regarding physical capability, those differences should be slight and explicable. There should be no disagreement between examiners about the degree of impairment. For that reason, a claims adjuster or other administrator should realistically be able to determine disability on the basis of the information provided by the physician.

REFERENCES

1. Guides to the Evaluation of Permanent Impairment, ed 4. American Medical Association, Chicago, 1993.
2. Waddell G, McCullock JA, Kummel E, et al: Nonorganic physical signs in low-back pain. Spine 5:117, 1980.

FURTHER READING

Dusik LA, Menard MR, Cooke C, et al: Concurrent validity of the ERGOS work simulator versus conventional functional capacity evaluation techniques in a workers' compensation population. J Occup Med 35:759, 1993.
Isernhagen SJ: Role of functional capacities assessment after rehabilitation. In Bullock MI (ed): Ergonomics: The Physiotherapist in the Workplace. New York, Churchill Livingstone, 1990, p 259.
Matheson LN: Functional capacity evaluation. In Demeter SL, Andersson GBJ, Smith GM (eds): Disability Evaluation. St Louis, Mosby-Year Book, 1996, p 168.
Ogden-Niemeyer L: Procedure for the WEST Standard Evaluation. Long Beach, Calif, Work Evaluation Systems Technology (WEST), 1989.

Pharmacology and Pharmacologic Modalities

Chapter 10

Opioid Receptors

Sam Page, M.D.

Opioids continue to provide the gold standard for analgesia. Historically, opioids were thought to provide analgesia through central and spinal mechanisms; however, evidence for a peripheral site of action is emerging.

In general, opioid receptors are coupled to the regulation of response to mechanical, thermal, or chemical stimuli. Net effect is activation of inhibition. Injections of μ, δ, and κ agonists produce analgesia that is naloxone sensitive. Stereospecific opioid receptors are found in the central nervous system (CNS) and other tissues, showing stereoselectivity for levorotatory isomers. These receptors are activated by endogenous ligands called *endorphins*, with analgesia mediated through a complex interaction of μ, δ, and κ receptors. Affinity for binding parallels potency. The term "opiate" is used for drugs derived from the poppy plant and other semisynthetic derivatives, including morphine, methylmorphine (codeine), and diacetylmorphine (heroin). The term "opioid" is used generally to describe all natural and synthetic substances that bind to opioid receptors.

The five subtypes of opioid receptors are μ, κ, δ, σ, and ε receptors.

The μ (morphine) receptors are responsible for generalized analgesia. They are divided into two subtypes, based on two affinity states. The $μ_1$ receptors have the same affinity for all opioid peptides. Receptors in this affinity state are responsible for supraspinal analgesia, euphoria, miosis, nausea, vomiting, urinary retention, and pruritus. The $μ_2$ opioid receptors have a greater selectivity for morphine. This receptor subtype is responsible for ventilatory depression, sedation, bradycardia, and ileus.

The κ receptors have specific ligands: ketocyclazine and dynorphin A. These receptors are responsible for spinal analgesia and sedation. There are three subdivisions: $κ_1$ and $κ_3$ have selective ligands, whereas $κ_2$ has no selective ligand. $κ_2$ is the only receptor to which β-endorphin does not bind (Table 10–1).

The specific ligand for δ receptors is leu-enkephalin. Although this receptor has selective agonist and antagonist receptors that are distinct from μ receptors, it

may be coupled with a μ receptor. It is thought to be responsible for the modulation of μ-receptor activity, such as physical dependence.

The σ receptor is no longer considered an opioid receptor. It does not mediate analgesia, and it is not antagonized by naloxone. There are two σ-receptor subtypes: $σ_1$ is stimulated by dextro(+)-pentazocine and dextromethorphan; $σ_2$ is stimulated by levo(−)-pentazocine and many antipsychotic drugs. The $σ_2$ receptor is associated with psychomimetic symptoms such as dysphoria, hypertonia, mydriasis, hypertension, and tachycardia. The ε-receptor subtype is now thought to be the second κ subtype. It mediates the stress response.

SIGNAL MECHANISMS

Most opioid receptors rely on the G-protein receptor superfamily. G_i, the inhibitory form of the G protein, inhibits adenylate cyclase, which is the most common second messenger. Binding results in inhibition of adenylate cyclase, hyperpolarization of the neuron, and suppression of spontaneous discharge and evoked responses. μ and δ receptors are associated with the opening of potassium channels, and κ receptors are associated with the closing of calcium channels. Stimulation produces a primary inhibitory effect on the neuron (hyperpolarization of the nerve terminal), and a reduction of calcium influx and transmitter release. If the inhibited cell is inhibitory, then the next cell in line is released from inhibition.

Tolerance is defined as a decreased receptor response to a given concentration of agonist. Receptor uncoupling from the intracellular second messenger is the primary mechanism. Downregulation, or a decreased number of available receptor sites, also contributes to the development of tolerance.

Independent supraspinal κ activity is unconfirmed. κ- and δ-receptor agonists produce less dependence. Prolonged production of enkephalins by protease inhibitors has no dependence liability.

TABLE 10-1. OPIOID RECEPTORS AND THEIR LIGANDS

	Receptor		
	μ	δ	κ
Endogenous ligands	β-endorphin	Met-enkephalin	Dynorphins
	Dermorphin	Leu-enkephalin	
	Metorphamide		
Exogenous ligands	Morphine	DPDPE	Butorphanol
	Fentanyl, sufentanil	DTLET	Bremazocine
	Methadone	DSTBULET	Spiradoline
	Meperidine		Pentazocine
Antagonists	Naloxone (low-dose)	Naloxone (medium-dose)	Naloxone (high-dose)
	β-funaltrexamine	Naltrindole	Norbinaltorphimine
	Naltrexone		

Data from Yaksh TL, Malmberg AB: Central pharmacology of nociceptive transmission. *In* Wall PD, Melzak R: Textbook of Pain, ed 3. New York, Churchill Livingstone, 1994, p 165; and Yaksh TL: Pharmacology and mechanisms of opioid analgesic activity. Acta Anaesthesiol Scand 41:1, 1997.

ANATOMIC LOCATION

Supraspinal

There are several sites of action of opioid receptors, including the medial brain-stem nucleus raphae magnus and mesencephalic periaqueductal and periventricular gray matter. In addition, receptors are situated at thalamic levels and in the sensory cortex. The solitary tract (visceral afferents of cranial nerves IX and X) contains large numbers of opioid receptors. These are associated with respiratory effects, cough suppression, and nausea and vomiting. The locus ceruleus and ventral trigeminal area are associated with reward processes and dependence.

Opioid peptides need to cross the blood-brain barrier to effect supraspinal analgesia. Rather than activating nociceptive neurons, the opioid peptides act by reducing the contrast, or intensity, of the pain signal, which blurs the perception of pain and the emotional response to pain. Morphine enhances descending inhibitory control, which decreases cephalad transmission of pain signals and increases the release of norepinephrine and serotonin.

Spinal

The μ receptors are close to C terminals in laminae I and II in the dorsal horn of the spinal cord. Small doses of μ agonists enhance C-fiber activity, whereas larger doses have analgesic activity. μ and δ agonists may precipitate a synergistic action through a presynaptic event, which may prevent release of primary afferent neurotransmitters. In the spinal cord, μ receptors dominate, but no endogenous opioid μ agonist is present in spinal cord. The division of receptors types is as follows: μ, 70%; δ, 24%; and κ, 6%; with a notable difference among species. Activation of opioid receptors blocks the spinal transmission of pain, both sensory and affective responses. Opioid peptides may also spread to supraspinal sites. Some opioids have local anesthetic activity.

Analgesic effect of κ agonists at the spinal level is controversial, because κ agonists can antagonize μ-receptor-mediated analgesia in the spinal cord. Spinal (epidural and subarachnoid) doses 50- to 100-fold less than systemic doses may cause itching, ileus, and urinary retention. The mechanism of epidural analgesia is thought to be local spread to the dorsal horn and rostral flow in CSF to brain-stem receptors. In addition, venous absorption and systemic delivery to supraspinal sites may play a role, depending on lipophilicity, volume, and location.

Peripheral Effects

Opioid receptors are absent in undamaged tissue, but they appear in damaged tissue within minutes to hours. All three receptors (μ, δ, and κ) are active. They have been proven to be stereospecific and antagonized by naloxone. C-fiber neurons mediate the peripheral antinociceptive effects of morphine. Inflammatory mediators, such as prostaglandin E_2, activate adenylate cyclase via stimulatory G protein, causing nociceptor sensitization. Activation of μ receptors switches off this process via G_i protein and prevents sensitization.

The anti-nociceptive and anti-inflammatory effects may also work through δ and κ agonists, by preventing bradykinin-induced sensitization. Bradykinin stimulates the release of nociceptor-sensitizing agents from the postganglionic sympathetic nerves. This discovery led to the use of intra-articular morphine for analgesia after knee arthroscopy.

Inflammation enhances the peripherally directed axonal transport of opioid receptors. Endogenous opioids have been detected in immune cells in inflamed tissue. They are synthesized in these cells. The exact method of opioid secretion is unknown; they may be released by cytokines. Low doses of naloxone may elicit analgesia, suggesting the presence of presynaptic opioid receptors that control the release of endogenous opioids.

The perineural application of opioid peptides is less effective than nerve terminal (intra-articular) application. It may be difficult to elicit response to intra-articular opioids in patients with spinal or epidural anesthesia, because preemptive analgesia may prevent the induction of peripheral opioid receptors, and development could lead to the avoidance of centrally mediated side effects. Non-analgesic peripheral effects remain a problem. These include inhibition of intestinal motility, urinary retention, pruritus, and increased tone of pancreatic, biliary, and rectal sphincters.

Other Neurotransmitters That Interact With Opioid Receptors

Amino Acids. Excitatory amino acids glutamate and aspartate combine with N-methyl-D-aspartate (NMDA) receptors. NMDA and glutamate produce analgesia when injected into the periaqueductal gray matter; this response is not naloxone sensitive. NMDA receptors can amplify and extend nociceptive inputs. Morphine may disinhibit neurons containing NMDA receptors and prevent hyperresponsiveness when given preemptively.

Monoamines. The α_2 agonists have sedative and analgesic activity and reduce the requirements for opioid and inhalation analgesics. The κ agonists, but not morphine, activate noradrenergic and serotoninergic pathways in mice. The μ and α_2 receptors regulate the same potassium conductance. Histamine is involved in the anti-nociceptive activity of morphine.

Cholecystokinin. CCK-B receptors mediate opioid activity. Cholecystokinin acutely enhances opioid activity, but chronically antagonizes endogenous opioids.

Organ System Effects of Opioids

Cardiovascular Effects. Cardiovascular effects include decreased sympathetic nervous system tone to peripheral veins, resulting in orthostatic hypotension. This may be a direct effect on smooth muscle. Bradycardia may occur from stimulation of vagal nucleus in medulla, enhancing parasympathetic tone.

Ventilation. Responsiveness to the stimulatory effects of carbon dioxide is decreased, and the ventilatory response to hypoxia is blunted. The respiratory rate is decreased, and the tidal volume is increased. There is also a direct depressant effect on the cough center in the medulla. Muscle rigidity may make ventilation difficult.

CNS. Opioids do not reliably produce unconsciousness. Normeperidine, a meperidine metabolite, may cause seizures. Most are cerebral vasoconstrictors, decreasing cerebral blood flow and intracranial pressure (ICP). Fentanyl and sufentanil can increase ICP in patients with trauma. Miosis, nausea, and vomiting may be due to stimulation of dopaminergic receptors in the chemotactic trigger zone of the medulla.

Skeletal and Smooth Muscle Spasm. This is mediated by μ receptors. Chest wall rigidity may interfere with ventilation. Spasm of the sphincter of Oddi may make the interpretation of intraoperative cholangiograms difficult.

Histamine Release. This leads to hypotension, tachycardia, and decreased systemic venous resistance. Morphine sulfate and meperidine present more drug to mast cells, causing more histamine release.

Gastrointestinal. The μ receptors are located on neuronal, smooth muscle, and mucosal cells throughout the gastrointestinal (GI) tract. Smooth muscle contraction (central and peripheral) leads to hypertonicity and decreased rhythm and propulsive activity.

Hormonal. Opioids act on the hypothalamus, decreasing nociceptive input and blunting the stress response, by decreasing the release of gonadotropin-releasing factor and adrenocorticotropic hormone–releasing factor.

SUMMARY

Synthesis of non-μ opioids, peptidase inhibitors, opioids with only peripheral actions, and adjuvants that would reduce anti-opioid systems may lead to alternative therapy. This would allow avoidance of central-acting opioid side effects, such as respiratory depression, sedation, nausea, vomiting, pruritus, dysphoria, and dependence. The presence of endogenous opioids in immune cells within inflamed tissue needs more investigation.

FURTHER READING

Cousins MJ, Bridenbaugh PO: Acute and chronic pain: Use of spinal opioids. *In* Cousins MJ, Cherry DA, Gourlay GK (eds): Neural Blockade in Clinical Anesthesia and Management of Pain, ed 2. Philadelphia, JB Lippincott, 1988, p 955.

Dickenson AH: Mechanisms of analgesic actions of opiates and opioids. Br Med Bull 47:690, 1991.

Murkin JM: Central analgesic mechanisms: A review of opioid receptor physiopharmacology and related antinociceptive systems. J Cardiothorac Vasc Anesth 5:268, 1991.

Pleuvry BJ: Opioid receptors and their relevance to anaesthesia. Br J Anaesth 71:119, 1993.

Stein C, Schafer M, Hassan A: Peripheral opioid receptors. Ann Med 27:219, 1995.

Yaksh TL: Opioid receptor systems and the endorphins: A review of their spinal organization. J Neurosurg 67:157, 1987.

Yaksh TL: Pharmacology and mechanisms of opioid analgesic activity. Acta Anaesthesiol Scand 41:94, 1997.

Yaksh TL, Malmberg AB: Central pharmacology of nociceptive transmission. *In* Wall PD, Melzak R (eds): Textbook of Pain, ed 3. Edinburgh: Churchill Livingstone, 1994, p 165.

Chapter 1 1

Opioids in Pain Management

Scott M. Fishman, M.D.,
and David Borsook, M.D., Ph.D.

OPIOID ANALGESICS

Opioid analgesics remain the gold standard for treating severe or unremitting pain. Traditionally, physicians have been tentative about prescribing them because of high abuse potential and fear of adverse effects, tolerance, and dependence. Use of opioids for terminally ill patients is less encumbered by social, legal, and professional taboos. Opioids may be the only effective analgesic for some cases of severe cancer pain, even when visceral or neuropathic pain is prominent. Extensive documented experience in treating cancer pain with opioids has broadened the understanding of this important area of drug therapy that has long been characterized by stigma and apprehensive application.

With an informed and cautious approach, opioids are safe and effective for treating severe pain of both malignant and nonmalignant origin. Because all limitations of opioid therapy cannot be prevented, close follow-up must be maintained to monitor for toxic effects and addictive tendencies. Patients with substance abuse histories and severe pain present a particularly challenging dilemma. Portenoy[1] proposes that a history of substance abuse indicates a relative contraindication to opioid administration for nonmalignant pain. For patients with substance abuse histories and pain that has proved resistant to all other therapeutic options, or pain associated with terminal illness, the relative nature of this contraindication must yield to compassionate use of narcotics.

Individual opioids vary in potency and degree of adverse effects. Their mechanism of action involves binding to opioid receptors, either centrally or peripherally. Subtypes of opioid receptors have been identified, which explains the varying effects of opioids (see later). Acutely, severe pain is well treated with opioids, because they produce reliable analgesia, and their adverse effects, such as respiratory suppression, sedation, constipation, and nausea and vomiting, are either reversible or manageable. Mild to moderate complications can either be anticipated and avoided or treated with complementary medications. Severe complications can usually be reversed by naloxone, a narcotic antagonist that blocks the effect of morphine at its receptor. Another class of narcotic analgesics consists of the mixed agonist-antagonist agents: butorphanol (Stadol), nalbuphine (Nubain), and pentazocine (Talwin). They have both stimulatory and inhibitory actions at opioid receptors (agonism at one receptor subtype and antagonism at another). The agonist-antagonist agents have found a role in treatment of severe acute pain in selected opioid-naive patients in the postoperative setting, or for pain related to biliary or pancreatic dysfunction, when strong analgesia is necessary but morphine-related spasm of the sphincter of Oddi must be avoided. Use of agonist-antagonist drugs in opioid-sensitized patients is contraindicated owing to the potential to induce withdrawal and, at elevated dosages, psychotomimetic effects.

Morphine sulfate is the prototypical opioid drug. Morphine and morphine-related compounds are the most commonly used opioids in treating severe pain, either acute or chronic. The bioavailability of oral morphine is between 35% and 75%, and its half-life is only 2 to 3 hours. Morphine's duration of analgesia is slightly shorter than its plasma half-life, which limits the risk of toxic accumulation. Its favorable linear pharmacokinetics with repeated doses offer reliable dosing and ease of use. In 1982, the World Health Organization (WHO) declared oral morphine its drug of choice in treating cancer pain and requested that it be part of the essential drug list and be made available throughout the world. Other opioid choices include hydromorphone (Dilaudid) and levorphanol (Levo-Dromoran), both congeners of morphine. Hydromorphone has a half-life comparable to that of morphine, but it offers greater solubility than morphine or even heroin. Levorphanol offers analgesic potency with a longer half-life. Its clinical profile is similar to that of methadone, requiring close monitoring for potential accumulation.

Controversy has surrounded the oral preparation of morphine because it can be readily converted to heroin in the laboratory. Heroin is a pro-drug: its effect requires metabolic conversion to 6-acetylmorphine and morphine. Heroin and morphine have comparable analgesic profiles and adverse effects. Heroin is a legal drug within the Canadian medical system and has been viewed by some to be a unique analgesic agent that has been indiscriminately withheld from needy patients in the American health system. No study has shown that heroin has any advantage over morphine or other similarly available opioid analgesics. In a non–drug-oriented society without substantial abuse problems, heroin might be considered a reasonable analgesic option for severe pain management. However, because serious social and legal implications are associated with its use, and because many other equally efficacious preparations are available, its use will likely not become favored. Methadone (Dolophine) is also a stigmatized drug that is associated with drug abuse, despite its use in rehabilitative efforts. Methadone is the least expensive oral opioid preparation. It is commonly used for maintenance treatment of heroin addiction, but it is also an effective analgesic. The bioavailability of oral methadone is approximately 85%, although its half-life may range from 13 to 50 hours in contrast to a duration of analgesic effect of 4 to 8 hours. Because the analgesic half-life of methadone is a fraction of its plasma half-life, the drug is ideal as a once-per-day maintenance agent. However, in multiple doses for analgesia, it poses some risk of metabolic accumulation and requires careful monitoring. For this reason, it is usually not a first-line opioid analgesic option. Methadone is often reserved for patients who have become tolerant to morphine or for those in whom an inexpensive opioid with a long half-life is required.

Meperidine (Demerol) is a commonly used analgesic, particularly by the intramuscular (IM) route. However, its use is problematic because of its tendency, with repeated doses, to lead to accumulation of the toxic metabolite normeperidine. The half-life of normeperidine is 12 to 16 hours, and it is well documented to produce central nervous system (CNS) hyperactivity and ultimately seizures. This metabolite is excreted by the kidneys, and its adverse effects are most commonly, though not exclusively, seen in patients with renal failure. These adverse effects manifest initially as subtle mood alteration, and may progress to tremors, myoclonus, and seizures. Because the hyperexcitabilty of normeperidine can occur in patients with normal renal function, repeated dosages of meperidine are not recommended.

Administration

The goal of effective opioid administration is to provide constant, sustained analgesia over regular intervals. This requires consideration of multiple factors. Some have been discussed earlier, such as half-life in relation to duration of analgesia to prevent toxic accumulation. Changing from one opioid to another requires knowledge of equianalgesic dosages. Because cross-tolerance between opioids may be incomplete, a patient who has become tolerant to one opioid drug can respond with effective analgesia to another opioid of less-than-equianalgesic dose. Tolerance occurs when increasing opioid dosage is required over time to maintain a stable

level of analgesia, or when analgesia decreases while opioid dosage remains fixed. Pain in the tolerant patient can be a challenge, because typical dosages for the opioid-naive patient do not apply. In these cases, careful titration is required.

Whether fixed dosing is better than PRN (*pro re nata*, "as-needed") dosing is controversial, with each method having advantages for different situations. Fixed dosing allows consistent delivery for reaching the steady state and avoiding the high-peak-and-low-trough effect associated with on-demand dosing. It also prevents delays in delivery, which often occur in on-demand schedules. However, opioids with longer half-lives may accumulate in fixed doses, and patients receiving their first exposure to opioids may require test dosing that is most safely given on demand. Morphine and hydromorphone may take less than 24 hours to reach a steady state, whereas levorphanol or methadone can take up to a week. Employing conservative fixed dosing combined with PRN "rescue" dosing can be effective, particularly when there is a need to assess analgesia threshold.

Analgesic therapy with long-acting opioids offers convenient dose intervals that reach safe, effective steady-state levels. Various controlled-release opioids are now available, including morphine (MS Contin, Oramorph), oxycodone (OxyContin), and fentanyl (Duragesic transdermal patch). Long-acting and immediate-release narcotics have made the oral route a practical option. Many cancer patients, however, are unable to tolerate oral ingestion. Intravenous or subcutaneous infusion is commonly used in these cases, often with continuous dosing for constant effect. Infusion eliminates the first-pass effect and can be supplemented by "rescue" bolus doses. The subcutaneous route has several advantages: faster onset of analgesia compared with most oral preparations (although slower than IV), access that is usually uncomplicated (e.g., use in patients without IV access), and safer administration compared with the IM route in patients with bleeding disorders or reduced muscle mass.

Various means of opioid administration are advantageous for patients with cancer as well as for patients undergoing surgery or other invasive or chemical therapies. Rectal suppositories are an alternative in patients unable to receive parenteral or oral preparations. Suppositories containing morphine, hydromorphone, and oxymorphone are available. Sublingual, buccal, intranasal, and transdermal administration of opioids is also possible. Fentanyl, an opioid with many times the potency of morphine, has become available by transdermal patch, with dosing every 3 days. It has the advantage of easy application in almost all patients with chronic severe pain, but it may be limited by skin sensitivity to the adhesive patch. Epidural and intrathecal routes of opioid administration are also available, presumably making opioids available to CNS regions densely populated with opioid receptors. This form of selective analgesia has the advantage of requiring small quantities of narcotics, which predisposes patients to significantly fewer central and autonomic nervous system complications. This route is widely used in postoperative and obstetric settings as well as for cancer patients.

Patient-controlled analgesia (PCA) consists of delivery of intravenous or subcutaneous doses of analgesic when the patient pushes a button. Ceilings can be placed on frequency and maximal dosage, and records of usage are easily maintained. Essentially, the patient titrates his or her own dosage, delivered at individualized intervals according to the parameters set by the physician. PCA is widely used for treating postoperative pain and is finding broader use in cancer patients.

Adverse Effects

Adverse effects of opioids can significantly undermine therapy. Which patients will experience which set of side effects and which narcotics will produce them is not predictable. When using opioids, it is wise to expect side effects and to take preventive action before they manifest. Opioids most commonly produce constipation, nausea, vomiting, sedation, confusion, and respiratory depression. Anticipation of and preventive measures against these complications is the best approach to management.

Constipation is the most commonly encountered side effect of narcotics. Tolerance to this effect develops slowly or not at all. Thus, constipation should be expected throughout the entire course of opioid administration. It should be prevented with laxatives rather than with passive agents, such as stool softeners or bulking agents. Respiratory depression is a potentially serious complication of opioid administration. Tolerance to this effect occurs early in chronic therapy. Significant respiratory depression can be managed with the opioid receptor antagonist naloxone. Rapid administration of naloxone can precipitate severe withdrawal in the patient with prolonged exposure to opioids.

Severe nausea and vomiting due solely to opioids is rare. These symptoms are usually mild and may be adequately managed with antiemetics. Patients rapidly become tolerant to this opioid side effect, at which time antiemetic therapy should be discontinued. If nausea or vomiting persist, changing to a different narcotic may reduce emetic side effects. For this reason, only patients with prior histories of gastrointestinal symptoms should be given prophylaxis with antiemetic medications prior to starting a regimen of narcotics. It is not clear why one opioid produces nausea and vomiting while another does not. Sedation is also a common problem with opioids, but it is typically temporary, resolving as patients accommodate to the new drug. In those with persistent sedation, the opioid dose should be reduced to the minimal level required for adequate analgesia. Consideration should be given to whether the medication may be accumulating and, if so, adjustments should be made to either increase the dose interval or change to a shorter-acting agent. For unremitting sedation, stimulants such as dextroamphetamine or caffeine reduce sedation until accommodation occurs.

Endogenous Opioids and Opioid Receptors

The endogenous opioids represent an extensively studied group of analgesic peptides. Areas of greatest opioid concentration include the periaqueductal gray matter (gray matter around the aqueduct connecting the third and fourth ventricles) and the nucleus raphae magnus (within the rostral ventromedial medulla). All regions associated with descending pain control contain endogenous opioids.

All known endogenous opioids begin with the same sequence of four amino acids (Tyr-Gly-Gly-Phe). It is the sequence of the remaining amino acids that confers differing properties to different endogenous opioids. There are three major families of endogenous opioids, termed *endorphins*, *enkephalins*, and *dynorphins*. Each of these is synthesized from a larger precursor molecule. Precursor molecules possess no intrinsic biologic activity. However, when enzymatically cleaved, precursors yield fragments with potent opioid properties. Pro-opiomelanocortin (POMC) contains 265 amino acids and may be cleaved to produce β-endorphin. It also contains the biologically active peptide sequences for adrenocorticotropin (ACTH) and melanocyte-stimulating hormone (MSH). Pro-dynorphin, a 256–amino acid precursor, produces the high-potency peptide dynorphin. Met-enkephalin and leu-enkephalin are pentapeptides, identical in the first four amino acids, with the fifth and last amino acid being either methionine or leucine (as the name indicates). The enkephalins were the first endogenous opioids to be purified and named enkephalins (from the Greek *enkephalos*, or "in the head"). They arise from pro-enkephalin, a 263–amino acid prohormone containing four copies of the sequence for met-enkephalin and one sequence for leu-enkephalin.

The three families of endogenous opioids are paralleled by three major classes of opioid receptors: μ, δ, and κ. These pharmacologically distinct receptor types are found in varying proportions throughout the CNS. The anatomic mapping of receptor types and subtypes shows surprisingly little correlation with the receptor specificity of each endogenous ligand. Like morphine, β-endorphin and met-enkephalin show high in vitro affinity for the μ receptor. Unlike morphine, the δ receptor is preferentially activated in vitro by enkephalins. Dynorphin has the highest affinity for the κ receptor. Naloxone, the clinically useful opioid antagonist, is considered predominantly responsible for blocking μ receptors. However, in higher doses, naloxone also blocks δ and κ receptors. The variety of opioid receptor types and subtypes makes it possible to develop clinically useful drugs that are receptor selective. "Mixed agonist-antagonist" drugs such as nalbuphine, pentazocine, and butorphanol activate one receptor subtype while antagonizing another. As noted earlier, the initial four amino acids are the same for all known endogenous opioids, leaving the remaining sequence to confer characteristics such as receptor binding preference. Manipulating the peptide structure within or beyond the initial four amino acids offers the opportunity to develop opioids with new properties and clinical advantages. For example, although leu-enkephalin has a predilection for the δ receptor, adding extra amino acids beyond the first five can change its preference to the κ receptor. The complexity of receptor preference is illustrated by the discovery of two subtypes of the μ receptor. The high-affinity μ receptor (μ_1) is thought to mediate analgesia, whereas the low-affinity μ receptor (μ_2) is thought to mediate respiratory depression and withdrawal symptoms. This may explain why small doses of naloxone may improve respiratory rate or relieve opioid-induced pruritus while having, perhaps, little effect on analgesia. Future agents may be able to selectively activate only the μ_1 receptor to produce analgesia or block the μ_2 receptor to antagonize some of the opioid-related side effects.

REFERENCE

1. Portenoy RK: Chronic opioid therapy in nonmalignant pain. J Pain Symptom Manage 5:546–562, 1990.

Chapter 12

Transdermal Fentanyl

Patricia Harrison, M.D.

BACKGROUND

Since its introduction in the late 1980s, the transdermal fentanyl system has gained widespread popularity for the treatment of chronic cancer pain. It is a noninvasive, convenient method for delivering an opioid analgesic on a continuous basis and is of particular benefit to patients who are unable to take oral medication.

PHYSICOCHEMICAL PROPERTIES

The chemical name of the fentanyl base is *N*-phenyl-*N*(1-2-phenylethyl-4-piperidyl)propanamide. Fentanyl has a molecular weight of 336.5 kd and is one of a number of compounds with a molecular weight of less than 1000 kd that have been associated with relatively high skin permeability. It is also highly lipophilic and lipid soluble, making it suitable for transdermal administration.[1] As an opioid analgesic it has similar effects to morphine, but it is approximately 75 times more potent and produces less histamine release.

TRANSDERMAL SYSTEM

The fentanyl transdermal system or fentanyl patch (Fig. 12-1) holds the fentanyl and a small amount of alcohol as a gel with hydroxyethyl cellulose in a drug reservoir. Between the reservoir and the skin is the rate-controlling or release membrane, which regulates the amount of drug that is delivered to the skin surface. The adhesive layer, which is in contact with the skin,

prevents the patch from being dislodged while allowing the fentanyl that has passed through the release membrane to reach the skin. The small amount of alcohol in the gel increases the rate of diffusion through the membrane. The occlusive backing is a polyester film that is heat sealed around the perimeter of the rate-controlling membrane, which protects the system and prevents the loss of fentanyl to the outside. The protective layer is removed prior to use. When the patch is applied to the skin, fentanyl diffuses through the rate-controlling membrane and the adhesive to the skin surface. It is then concentrated in the upper layer of the skin as a depot, from where it is gradually absorbed into the systemic circulation, which explains the delay of at least an hour before measurable amounts of fentanyl are detected in the serum. Therapeutic serum concentrations are not reached until at least 6 hours, and constant blood levels are not observed before 12 to 24 hours.[2] This applies to the placement of a patch for the first time only. Subsequently, when the system is changed, medication from the depot under the initial patch will be released while a depot forms under the new patch. In one study,[3] plasma levels in patients with the 100 µg/hour system were compared to those in a group given a continuous intravenous infusion of fentanyl, and levels were found to be similar in both groups at 24 hours.

Dosing Options

The patches are currently available in doses of 25, 50, 75, and 100 µg/hour, which correlate with their surface area; they are supplied in boxes of five. They are de-

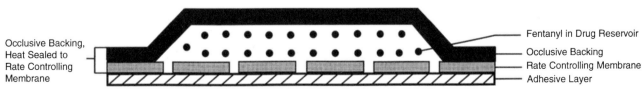

FIGURE 12-1. Diagram of cross-section of transdermal fentanyl system or patch.

Occlusive Backing, Heat Sealed to Rate Controlling Membrane

Fentanyl in Drug Reservoir
Occlusive Backing
Rate Controlling Membrane
Adhesive Layer

signed to release fentanyl for 72 hours, although in some patients more frequent changes are required. Multiple patches may be worn at any one time, which increases dosing options, because the dose of each patch is additive.

VARIABILITY

Certain factors affect the rate of absorption and the serum concentrations. Although it is recommended to apply the patch to an area of the upper body, the efficacy does not appear to be altered when comparing application to the chest, back, or upper arm.

Temperature

Drug-input rates have been found to vary with changes in temperature. Serum concentrations may increase by as much as 25% for every 3°C increase in body temperature,[4] and patients who develop a fever should be monitored for increased side effects. External heat sources, such as heating blankets or sun lamps, should not be applied close to the patch, as this may also increase absorption.

Skin Thickness

The absorption of fentanyl varies according to skin thickness. When applied to thicker skin, a slower rate of rise and a lower maximum serum concentration are noted.[4] Conversely, serum levels can reach five times normal when applied to broken skin.

Metabolism and Clearance

Fentanyl is metabolized primarily in the liver with no evidence of metabolism in the skin when given transdermally. It is then excreted, predominantly in the urine, with a small proportion excreted in the feces. There is significant variability in the clearance of fentanyl. Serum concentrations were measured at various intervals during multiple applications of a 100 μg/hour patch. Steady-state was said to have been reached at day 13, when the range was determined to be due to individual variation in skin permeability and fentanyl clearance. When the patch was removed at day 16, the serum concentration gradually declined to reach 50% between 13 and 22 hours (mean, 17 hours), but after 3 days, significant levels were still measured in some patients. This variability reflects different clearance rates between individuals and necessitates that enough time be allowed between dose changes for equilibration. It also illustrates the importance of dose titration to clinical effect.

USES AND INDICATIONS

Although many of the initial studies were done in the acute pain setting, the fentanyl patch is now recommended for use only in patients with chronic pain. This prescribing change follows a 20% incidence, reported in several studies, of hypoventilation in postoperative patients, many of whom were narcotic naive.[5]

In the cancer population, both patient acceptance and compliance are high. Desirable features of therapy in this situation include the control of continuous pain by the most convenient method without the need for expensive invasive techniques. Transdermal fentanyl fulfills this need and can be used for long periods of time. Simmonds and colleagues[6] described excellent acceptance and compliance in patients who were maintained for an average of 84 days (5 to 365 days) with a mean dose of 150 μg/hour (25 to 600 μg/hour).[6] The 72-hour duration of the patch is an advantage when compared with the sustained-release oral products, which only have an 8- to 12-hour duration, and many patients enjoy the ability to achieve pain control without the need to take frequent pills. Dose titration is facilitated by the four available sizes, and there is no upper limit to the number of patches that can be worn if the patient requires larger doses. When the oral route is unavailable because of nausea and vomiting or an inability to swallow, this system is a good alternative to parenteral therapy for providing analgesia.

Certain basic guidelines should be followed when treating chronic pain with fentanyl, which applies to any opioid analgesic. These include (1) continual assessment of the patient; (2) dose titration to achieve pain relief with minimal side effects; (3) the use of adjuvant analgesics to enhance the opioid effect; and (4) the anticipation and early treatment of side effects such as nausea, constipation, and sedation.

Rescue or breakthrough medication should be available at all times, particularly after the initial patch is applied or following dose changes, when there will be a delay in achieving a steady-state concentration. In some instances, initial pain control may be titrated with a rapidly acting opioid. The previous 24-hour opioid requirement is then calculated, and the fentanyl dose is selected by using a conversion chart similar to that shown in Table 12-1. This table gives many of the commonly used opioid analgesics for cancer pain and the equivalent fentanyl patch sizes. However, it appears that when using this chart, the conversion factors may be conservative, because as many as 50% of patients may require a dose increase after the initial application. It is also recommended that doses of greater than 25 μg/hour not be used for the initiation of therapy in non–opioid-tolerant patients. The morphine dose equivalent to this patch is between 45 and 134 mg/day, given orally, which is an adequate starting dose for the majority of opioid-intolerant patients, although they may be experiencing moderate to severe pain. The consequences of overdose are likely to be avoided, and rescue medication of short duration can still be available.

The fentanyl patch should be applied to nonirritated and nonirradiated skin over a flat surface of the upper body. Where no hairless site is available, the hair should be clipped, not shaved, and the skin cleansed with water and dried. At the time of a patch change, a new site should be selected and the initial patch removed

TABLE 12–1. TRANSDERMAL FENTANYL DOSAGE CONVERSION

Fentanyl (µg/hr)	Morphine (mg/Day)		Hydromorphone (mg/Day)		Oxycodone (mg/Day)	Levorphanol (mg/Day)		Codeine (mg/Day)	
	Oral	IM/IV	Oral	IM/IV	Oral	Oral	IM/IV	Oral	IM/IV
25	45–134	8–22	5.6–17	1.2–3.4	22.5–67	3–8.9	1.6–4.4	150–447	104–286
50	135–224	23–37	17.1–28	3.5–5.6	67.5–112	9–14.9	4.5–7.4	448–747	287–481
75	225–314	38–52	28.1–39	5.7–7.9	112.5–157	15–20.9	7.5–10.4	748–1047	482–676
100	315–404	53–67	39.1–51	8–10	157.5–202	21–26.9	10.5–13.4	1048–1347	677–871
125	405–494	68–82	51.1–62	10.1–12	202.5–247	27–32.9	13.5–16.4	1348–1647	872–1066
150	495–584	83–97	62.1–73	12.1–15	247.5–292	33–38.9	16.5–19.4	1648–1947	1067–1261
175	585–674	98–112	73.1–84	15.1–17	292.5–337	39–44.9	19.5–22.4	1948–2247	1262–1456
200	675–764	113–127	84.1–96	17.1–19	337.5–382	45–50.9	22.5–25.4	2248–2547	1457–1651
225	765–854	128–142	96.1–107	19.1–21	382.5–427	51–56.9	25.5–28.4	2548–2847	1652–1846
250	855–944	143–157	107.1–118	21.1–24	427.5–472	57–62.9	28.5–31.4	2848–3147	1847–2041
275	945–1034	158–172	118.1–129	24.1–26	472.5–517	63–68.9	31.5–34.4	3148–3447	2042–2236
300	1035–1124	173–187	129.1–141	26.1–28	517.5–562	69–74.9	34.5–37.4	3448–3747	2237–2431

Adapted from Duragesic Fentanyl Transdermal System: Clinical Monograph. Piscataway, NJ, Janssen Pharmaceutical, 1991.

and disposed of in a safe manner, as unused medication may still be contained within the patch.

Although there are no well-controlled studies of this therapy in children, reports[7] and anecdotal experience suggest that there is a place for its use in this population. Children who are opioid tolerant are the most likely to benefit from this convenient form of therapy, but current recommendations are that it be used only in a research setting.

DISADVANTAGES AND SIDE EFFECTS

The potential side effects of transdermal fentanyl are those that occur with any opioid drug as well as those that are specifically related to fentanyl in this vehicle. Table 12–2 lists the adverse events that were experienced by 153 cancer patients receiving long-term fentanyl therapy as well as events severe enough to cause discontinuation of therapy.[8] Hypoventilation, defined as a respiratory rate of less than 8 breaths/minute, had an incidence of only 2%, but was the most serious side effect. If hypoventilation does occur, the patient should

TABLE 12–2. ADVERSE EVENTS AND INCIDENCE OF DISCONTINUATION OF TRANSDERMAL FENTANYL

Adverse Event	Incidence (%)	Incidence of Discontinuation (%)
Nausea	23	6
Vomiting	22	3
Somnolence	17	2
Constipation	14	0
Sweating	14	0
Dry mouth	13	0
Confusion	13	1
Asthenia	12	0
Anorexia	8	1
Dizziness	7	0
Restlessness	6	0
Skin reactions	4	<1
Hypoventilation	2	2

Adapted from Duragesic Fentanyl Transdermal System: Clinical Monograph. Piscataway, NJ, Janssen Pharmaceutical, 1991.

be monitored closely and consideration given to removing the patch. With severe hypoventilation, an opioid antagonist, such as naloxone, will reverse the effect, but as significant amounts of fentanyl are detected for many hours after the patch is removed, monitoring should continue and naloxone repeated if necessary.

In the same series, somnolence occurred in 17% of patients, and although the incidence of nausea (23%) and vomiting (22%) were higher, only a small percentage of patients discontinued the patch as a result of these side effects (see Table 12–2). Many of the patients were also undergoing radiation and chemotherapy, which are known to cause nausea and vomiting and may have contributed to the incidence of these side effects. Other adverse effects that were severe enough for the patients to change to another form of therapy included confusion and anorexia.

A small number of skin reactions to the adhesive have occurred, and therapy should be discontinued in this situation. There is also a potential for the patch to become unknowingly removed or for the adhesive to lift off the skin. In the latter situation, the edges of the patch may be secured with adhesive tape to maintain contact with the skin. As already discussed, serum concentrations may increase at body temperatures of 40°C, necessitating close monitoring in patients who develop fever. Bradycardia, although occasionally seen with fentanyl given intravenously, has not been a feature of the transdermal route.

There is little evidence of teratogenicity when transdermal fentanyl is administered during pregnancy. However, it is recommended that it be used in this situation only if the potential benefit justifies the potential risk to the fetus. Similarly, it is not recommended for use in nursing mothers due to the excretion in breast milk.

The main disadvantages of transdermal fentanyl when compared with oral opioid therapy are the slower onset and elimination and the difficulty in rapid dose titration. Reversal of serious side effects, such as hypoventilation, may necessitate repeated doses of naloxone to offset the prolonged duration of action. It has a relatively higher cost than immediate-release morphine, but is comparable to some of the sustained-release oral preparations. However, with close monitoring and titration to clinical effect, many of the adverse effects can be minimized without resorting to termination of therapy.

SUMMARY

The properties of fentanyl make it suitable for use via the transdermal route. The patch in which it is contained provides a simple and convenient method of delivery of a continuous dose of this opioid analgesic. At the same time, the more expensive and labor-intensive invasive methods can be avoided. Transdermal administration minimizes the peaks and troughs of serum levels that occur when oral medications are given, which is an advantage in the treatment of the constant pain that is often associated with cancer. However, rescue medication must be available at all times. Transdermal fentanyl has a high patient acceptance and is of particular benefit when the oral route is unavailable. Due to the delay in achieving therapeutic effects, initial pain control may be titrated with more rapidly acting drugs, and the dose of fentanyl can then be selected using a dose-equivalency table. Side effects can be minimized with close monitoring and dose titration.

The success of transdermal fentanyl in the control of chronic pain has paved the way for the development of other drugs that may be given in this form.

REFERENCES

1. Caplan RA, Southam M: Transdermal drug delivery and its application to pain control. *In* Benedetti C (ed): Advances in Pain Research and Therapy. New York, Raven Press, 1990, p 233.
2. Plezie PM, Kramer JH, Lintard J, et al: Transdermal fentanyl: Pharmacokinetics and preliminary clinical evaluation. Pharmacotherapy 9:2, 1989.
3. Duthie DJR, Rowbotham DJ, Wyld R, et al: Plasma fentanyl concentrations during transdermal delivery of fentanyl to surgical patients. Br J Anaesth 60:614, 1988.
4. Gupta SK, Southam M, Gale R: System functionality and physicochemical model of fentanyl transdermal system. J Pain Symptom Manage 7:517, 1992.
5. Sandler A: Transdermal fentanyl: Acute analgesic clinical studies. J Pain Symptom Manage 7:527, 1992.
6. Simmonds MA, Payne R, Rickenbacher J, et al: TTS (fentanyl) in the management of pain in patients with cancer. Proc ASCO 8:324, 1989.
7. Patt RB, Lustik S, Litman RS: The use of transdermal fentanyl in a 6-year-old patient with neuroblastoma and diffuse abdominal pain: Case report. Anesth Analg 8:317, 1993.
8. Duragesic Fentanyl Transdermal System: Clinical Monograph. Piscataway, NJ, Janssen Pharmaceutical, 1991.

FURTHER READING

Miser AW, Narang PK, Dothage JA, et al: Transdermal fentanyl for pain control in patients with cancer pain. Pain 37:15, 1989.
The role of the fentanyl series for pain management: Novel delivery system. J Pain Symptom Manage 7:35, 1992.

Chapter 13

Tramadol

Charles B. Sisson, M.D.

Tramadol hydrochloride (1RS, 2RS)-2-[(dimethylamino)methyl]-1-(3-methoxyphenyl)-cyclohexanol HCl) is an orally and parenterally active, clinically effective, centrally acting binary analgesic with opioid and non-opioid analgesic mechanisms. In the United States, tramadol HCl (Ultram, Ortho-McNeil) has FDA approval for the management of moderate to moderately severe pain. It has a low abuse potential and is not classified as a controlled substance. In the United States, tramadol is currently only available in an oral form for clinical use.

STRUCTURE

There are similarities between the chemical structures of tramadol and opioid derivatives. In common with codeine, tramadol has a methyl group substitution on the phenolic moiety, which contributes to its weak affinity for opioid receptors (Fig. 13–1).

MECHANISM OF ACTION

Preclinical pharmacology studies found that tramadol-induced anti-nociception is mediated via opioid mechanisms.[1] Tramadol binds with modest activity to the μ-receptors and has a weaker affinity for the σ- and κ-receptors. Therefore, it acts in this manner like any other opioid by blocking pain impulse transmission. It binds to the μ-receptor approximately 6000-fold less than morphine. The mono-*O*-desmethyl metabolite of tramadol (M1) has a greater affinity for the opioid receptors than the parent compound and is thought to also contribute to the drug's analgesic effects.[2]

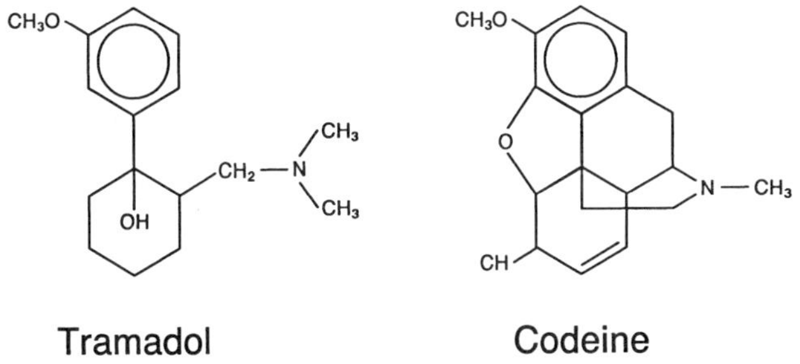

Clinical studies demonstrated that, unlike typical opioid analgesics, the therapeutic use of tramadol has not been associated with clinically significant side effects such as respiratory depression, constipation, or sedation.[3] In addition, analgesic tolerance has not been a clinically significant problem.[4] Tramadol does not work well as a substitute medication in methadone-dependent patients.[5] Tramadol did not produce morphine-like effects and did not produce withdrawal symptoms in methadone-maintained volunteers.[6]

Tramadol also inhibits the uptake of norepinephrine and serotonin. The (+) enantiomer mainly binds the μ-receptor and is responsible for inhibition of serotonin reuptake. The (−) enantiomer is more active in inhibiting norepinephrine reuptake. These findings suggest tramadol anti-nociception is mediated by both opioid (primarily μ-receptor) and non-opioid (inhibition of monoamine uptake) mechanisms. This dual mechanism of action affords tramadol a unique place among opioids. The opioid and non-opioid components interact in a synergistic fashion to relieve pain.[7, 8]

PHARMACOKINETICS

Onset

After an oral dose of 100 mg in healthy volunteers, tramadol was rapidly absorbed, and peak blood concentration (250 μg/L) was reached in 2 hours. Mean bioavailability is 68%. After repeated administration of 100-mg doses, four times daily, the steady-state plasma concentration doubled to twofold the desired therapeutic concentration. Therefore, in long-term administration the dose of tramadol should be reduced to 50 mg. Tramadol appears in the plasma 15 to 45 minutes after a single 100-mg oral dose, with a peak plasma concentration of 308 ± 68 ng/mL of racemic tramadol in 1.6

FIGURE 13–1. Chemical structure of tramadol and codeine.

to 2 hours. The mean plasma concentration for the M1 metabolite is 55 ± 20 ng/mL and occurs in 3 hours after a single 100-mg oral dose.[9]

Dose

In the acute postsurgical setting for obstetric patients, 100 mg of tramadol was equipotent to a single dose of aspirin, 650 mg, plus 60 mg of codeine.[10] Tramadol may be given in a 100-mg dose every 4 to 6 hours. The recommended dose is 50 to 100 mg as needed every 4 to 6 hours, with the total dose not to exceed 400 mg/day. According to the manufacturer, the 50-mg dose should be adequate for moderate pain. More severe pain may require the 100-mg dose. The dosage does not need to be adjusted for elderly patients. For patients with creatinine clearance less than 30 mL/minute, the dose interval should be increased to 12 hours and the maximum daily dose should be limited to 200 mg. In long-term treatment, the recommended dose is 50 to 100 mg, given orally two or three times daily, not to exceed 300 mg/day. Patients receiving dialysis can take a normal dose, because dialysis removes only 7% of the drug from the blood. For patients with hepatic cirrhosis, the recommended dose is 50 mg every 12 hours.[11]

Metabolism

Tramadol is metabolized extensively by the liver. Thirty percent of a single oral dose is excreted unchanged in the urine and 60% is excreted as metabolites.[11] Tramadol is metabolized to M1 by isoenzyme CYP2D6 of cytochrome P-450.[12] Plasma protein binding is 20%. Following multiple oral doses of tramadol, 100 mg four times daily for 1 week, oral bioavailability increases by 90% to 100%, possibly due to saturation of the first-pass hepatic metabolism.[13, 14] Tramadol crosses the placenta, with serum concentration in the umbilical veins being 80% of those in the maternal veins.[15] The elimination kinetics of tramadol are consistent with a two-compartment model, with a reported elimination half-life of 5.1 hours (SD, 0.8) after a single oral dose in young, healthy volunteers.[13] The elimination of the M1 metabolite was longer at approximately 9 hours. Within 48 hours of commencing a regimen of tramadol, 100 mg four times daily, tramadol and the M1 metabolite had accumulated twofold. In patients with severe renal or hepatic impairment the $t_{1/2\beta}$ of tramadol increases to twofold or threefold, respectively.[16]

TOLERABILITY AND SAFETY

The most frequently reported side effects are dose-related dizziness, nausea, constipation, anorexia, insomnia, vomiting, sedation, dry mouth, and headache.[17, 18] A cumulative analysis of the adverse effects found that tramadol was not associated with severe adverse effects including respiratory depression, addiction, or allergy. Overdose of tramadol can result in respiratory depression, dysphoria, and constipation. In children the effects of overdosage may result in significant respiratory de-

pression and concomitant symptoms of central nervous system (CNS) excitation, such as convulsions. Tramadol may increase the risk of seizure in patients taking monoamine oxidase (MAO) inhibitors, neuroleptics, and other drugs that reduce the seizure threshold. It should be used with caution in patients with epilepsy. Tramadol should also be used with caution and in reduced doses in patients taking CNS depressants. Tramadol has additive anti-nociceptive effects with nonsteroidal anti-inflammatory drugs (NSAIDs). Drugs that depress CNS function may enhance the sedative and other central effects of tramadol.[19] Tramadol should be used with caution in patients taking MAO inhibitors and in those with respiratory distress, increased intracranial pressure or head injury, and renal or hepatic disease.[20]

ABUSE AND TOLERANCE

The development of tolerance or dependence during long-term tramadol use is uncommon. In cancer patients the analgesic requirements do not escalate with time.[4, 20] Addictive potential of tramadol is minimal in studies of its euphoria-inducing effects and abuse potential.[5, 20]

SYSTEMIC EFFECTS

In Europe, tramadol is safely used in acute myocardial infarction. Cardiovascular effects of tramadol after intravenous tramadol are minimal.[21] In therapeutic doses the respiratory effects of oral tramadol are negligible in adults. Tramadol can cause CNS excitation in overdose. Tramadol does not appear to affect sphincteric muscle; therefore, it does not cause urinary retention or exacerbation of biliary and pancreatic disorders. Constipation is a common side effect.[22]

DRUG INTERACTIONS

Due to its low protein binding, tramadol does not interfere with the serum levels of anticoagulants or oral hypoglycemic agents. There are no restrictions on combining tramadol with other peripheral analgesics or NSAIDs.[23]

THERAPEUTIC USE

Acute Postoperative Setting

In acute therapeutic use, tramadol has analgesic efficacy and potency comparable to that of codeine, pentazocine, or propoxyphene. A review of single-dose studies found that tramadol is an effective oral analgesic for treating acute pain and that a dose of 100 mg provides optimal analgesia. A single 50-mg dose of tramadol provides relief similar to that of 60 mg of codeine in mild postoperative pain. The onset of analgesia with tramadol was rapid and paralleled its plasma concentration in patients with postoperative pain.[11, 24, 25] In 161 patients following cesarean section, tramadol, 75 mg given orally, was roughly comparable to a combination of acetaminophen-propoxyphene.[26, 27] In a double-blind randomized study of 144 total hip replacement patients, tramadol efficacy was inferior to that of acetaminophen and codeine and comparable to placebo for a single oral dose of 50 or 100 mg.[28] However, multiple doses of tramadol reduce the total requirements of patient-controlled administration of morphine in postoperative surgery patients.[29] In obstetric patients, intramuscular tramadol did not impair labor and had less analgesic efficacy than demerol, but it also had less respiratory depression in the neonates.[30, 31]

Chronic Pain Condition

Malignant Pain States

Morphine sulfate was shown to be superior to tramadol in analgesic efficacy for cancer patients with moderate to severe pain. Tramadol, however, was the drug of choice due to its better ratio of analgesic efficacy and side effects profile when compared to morphine.[20] Tramadol is effective in providing relief in patients with bone metastases and visceral pain.[32] The drug is ineffective in patients with pain due to nerve lesions.[33]

Nonmalignant Pain States

In patients older than 65 years, efficacy and safety for a variety of nonmalignant chronic pain states, including joint conditions and low-back neuropathic and orthopedic pain, were comparable to those of acetaminophen and codeine.[34] Adverse experiences led to discontinuation in a higher percentage (18% vs. 9%) of the tramadol group.[35] Patients older than 75 years should not receive more than 300 mg/day.[36] Tramadol is therapeutically useful for patients who are not receiving adequate relief from acetaminophen, in patients at risk for adverse affects from NSAIDs, or in patients who cannot tolerate narcotic analgesics. In another study, tramadol was more effective than propoxyphene in decreasing pain during daily activities, walking, and sleeping.[37]

SUMMARY

Tramadol is a safe and effective analgesic in adult patients who suffer from mild to moderately severe chronic pain. Data from two double-blind long-term clinical trials demonstrate a comparable overall cumulative incidence rate of adverse effects among tramadol, aspirin with codeine, and acetaminophen with codeine. The most common adverse effects with tramadol are dizziness, nausea, and constipation. These adverse effects occur at rates similar to or less than those seen with comparable agents. In addition, tramadol causes less dyspepsia. Physical dependence, withdrawal tolerance, and abuse potential are minimal with tramadol therapy.[36, 38]

REFERENCES

1. Hennies HH, Friderichs E, Wilsman K, et al: Effect of the opioid analgesic tramadol on inactivation of norepinephrine and serotonin. Biochem Pharmacol 31:1654, 1982.
2. Raffa RB, Friderichs E, Reimann W: Opioid and nonopioid components independently contribute to the mechanism of action of tramadol, an 'atypical' opioid analgesic. J Pharmacol Exp Ther 260:275, 1992.
3. Arend I, von Arnin B, Nijssen J, et al: Tramadol and pentazocine in a double blind crossover comparison. Arzneimittelforschung 28:199, 1978.
4. Flohe L, Arend I, Cogel A, et al: Clinical study on the development of dependency after long-term treatment with tramadol. Arzneimittelforschung 28:213, 1978.
5. Richter W, Barth H, Flohe L, et al: Clinical investigation on the development of dependence during oral therapy with tramadol. Arzneimittelforschung 35:1742, 1985.
6. Cami J, Lamas X, Farre M: Acute effects of tramadol in methadone-maintained volunteers. Drugs 47(suppl 1):39, 1994.
7. Raffa RB, Friderichs E, Reimann W, et al: Complementary and synergistic antinociceptive interaction between the enantiomers of tramadol. J Pharmacol Exp Ther 267:331, 1993.
8. Friderichs E, Reimann W, Selve N: Contribution of both enantiomers to antinociception activity in mice (abstract 36). Naunyn Schmiedebergs Arch Pharmacol 343 (suppl):9, 1991.
9. Lintz W, Barth H, Osterloh G, et al: Bioavailability of enteral tramadol formulations—first communication capsules. Arzneimittelforschung 36:1278, 1986.
10. Brown J, Jackson A, Wan Wagoner D, et al: Tramadol HCl: Dose response in pain following cesarean section. Clin Pharmacol Ther 51:121, 1992.
11. Lee R, McTavish D, Sorkin S: Tramadol: A preliminary review of its pharmacodynamic and pharmacokinetic properties, and therapeutic potential in acute and chronic pain states. Drugs 46:313, 1993.
12. Lintz W, Uragg H: Quantitative determination of tramadol in human serum by gas chromatography-mass spectrometry. J Chromatogr 341:65, 1985.
13. Liao S, Hill JF, Nayak RK: Pharmacokinetics of tramadol following single and multiple doses in man (abstract PPDM 8206). Pharm Res 9 (suppl):308, 1992.
14. Lintz W, Erlacin S, Frankus E, et al: Biotransformation of tramadol in man and animal (in German). Arzneimittelforschung 31:1278, 1986.
15. Husslein P, Kubista E, Egarter C: Obstetric analgesia with tramadol: Results of a prospective randomized comparison with pethidine. Z Geburtshilfe Perinatol 191: 234, 1987.
16. Dayer P, Collart L, Desmeules J: The pharmacology of tramadol. Drugs 47 (suppl):3, 1994.
17. Grond S, Zech D, Lynch J, et al: Tramadol: A weak opioid for relief of cancer pain. Pain Clin 5:241, 1992.
18. Cossmann M, Wilsmann KM: Behandlung langer andauernder Schmerzsyndrome: Beurteilung der Wirkung und Vertraglichkeit von Tramadol (Tramal) bei mehrmaliger Gabe. Muench Med Wochenschr 129:851, 1987.
19. Riedel F, von Stockhausen H-B: Severe cerebral depression after intoxication with tramadol in a 6-month-old infant. Eur J Clin Pharmacol 26:631, 1984.
20. Osipova NA, Novikov GA, Beresnev VA, et al: Analgesic effect of tramadol in cancer patients with chronic pain: A comparison with prolonged action morphine sulfate. Curr Ther Res 50:812, 1991.
21. Huber HP: Examination of psychic effects of a new analgesic agent of the cyclohexanol series (in German). Arzneimittelforschung 28:189, 1978.
22. Preston KL, Jasninski DR, Testa M: Abuse potential and pharmacological comparison of tramadol and morphine. Drug Alcohol Depend 27:7, 1991.
23. Radbruch L, Grond S, Lehmann K: A risk-benefit assessment of tramadol in the management of pain. Drug Safety 15:8, 1996.
24. Grond S, Meuser T, Zech D, et al: Analgesic efficacy and safety of tramadol enantiomers in comparison with the racemate: A randomised, double-blind study with gynaecological patients using intravenous patient-controlled analgesia. Pain 62:313, 1995.
25. Ilias W, Jansen M: Pain control after hysterectomy: An observer-

blind, randomised trial of lornoxicam versus tramadol. Br J Clin Pract 50:197, 1996.

26. Lehmann K: Tramadol for the management of acute pain. Drugs 47 (suppl 1):19, 1994.

27. Brown P, Mehlisch DR, Minn F: Tramadol hydrochloride: Efficacy compared to codeine sulfate, acetaminophen with dextropropoxyphene and placebo in dental extraction pain: Eleventh International Congress of Pharmacology, Amsterdam, the Netherlands, July 1990. Eur J Pharmacol 193:1441, 1990.

28. Sunshine A, Olson NZ, Zighelboim I, et al: Analgesic oral efficacy of tramadol hydrochloride in postoperative pain. Clin Pharmacol Ther 57:740, 1992.

29. Stubhaug A, Grimstad J, Breivik H: Lack of analgesic effect of 50 and 100 mg oral tramadol after orthopaedic surgery: A randomized, double-blind, placebo and standard active drug comparison. Pain 62:111, 1995.

30. Vickers MD, Paravicini D: Comparison of tramadol with morphine for post-operative pain following abdominal surgery. Eur J Anaesth 12:265, 1995.

31. Suvonnakote T, Thitadilok W, Atisook R: Pain relief during labor. J Med Assoc Thai 69:566, 1986.

32. Budd K: Chronic pain. Challenge and response. Drugs 47(suppl 1):33, 1994.

33. Barkin RL: Focus on tramadol: A centrally acting analgesic for moderate to moderately severe pain. Formulary 30:321, 1995.

34. Rodrigues N, Pereira ER: Tramadol in cancer pain. Curr Ther Res 46:1142, 1989.

35. Rauck R, Ruoff G, McMillen J: Comparison of tramadol and acetaminophen with codeine for long-term pain management in elderly patients. Curr Ther Res 55:1417, 1994.

36. Jensen EM, Ginsberg F: Tramadol versus dextropropoxyphene in the treatment of osteoarthritis. Drug Geriatr Invest 8:211, 1994.

37. Enck RE: Pain control in the ambulatory elderly. Geriatrics 46:49, 1991.

38. Dalgin PH: Use of tramadol in chronic pain. Clin Geriatr 3:17, 1995.

Chapter 14

Psychotropic Drugs Useful in Pain Treatment

*David Borsook, M.D., Ph.D., and
Scott M. Fishman, M.D.*

It is probably not a coincidence that a large proportion of drugs used to treat pain overlap with those used to treat psychiatric disorders. Because pain usually consists of both nociceptive and non-nociceptive features, the inability to treat all facets of pain may result in incomplete analgesia. Thus, adjuvant psychotropic medications are useful in both acute and chronic pain states. Patients in acute pain may experience anxiety, depression, agitation, sedation, fearfulness, or insomnia. In these cases, the use of agents such as benzodiazepines (e.g. Ativan), antidepressants, phenothiazines (e.g., Haldol), stimulants, or sedatives may be very beneficial. In chronic pain conditions, the issues are more complicated because psychotropic agents may be used for treatment of the pain itself (e.g., antidepressants have been shown to have local anesthetic effects on damaged nerve fibers) or for the treatment of associated mood disorders, such as depression or anxiety. Each of the different classes discussed herein contains numerous psychotropic agents. However, we have provided a short list of psychotropic agents that are useful in the treatment of pain and discuss their use and side effects.

ANTIDEPRESSANTS

Of the antidepressants, the tricyclic antidepressants (TCAs) have been the most widely used as analgesics. Although clearly documented as effective antidepressants and anxiolytics, most of the other antidepressant agents, including atypical antidepressants (e.g., trazodone), monoamine oxidase inhibitors (MAOIs), and the selective serotonin reuptake inhibitors (SSRIs) (e.g., fluoxetine, sertraline), have not undergone the same scientific scrutiny as the TCAs and have more limited use in pain therapy. Some reports have suggested that SSRIs benefit patients with chronic pain states, such as headache, although other anecdotal reports find that these agents may induce headaches.

TCAs potentiate the actions of biogenic amines by blockade of reuptake at the nerve terminals. The effects for each drug differ for blockade of reuptake of norepi-

nephrine, serotonin, and dopamine, and these profiles are thought to have an impact on antidepressant selectivity and efficacy. The agents also have inhibitory activity in the cholinergic, histaminergic, and adrenergic systems, and hence have significant side effect profiles that may limit therapy. As possible mechanisms in pain relief, TCAs inhibit noradrenergic neuronal firing, which perhaps underlies the early onset of analgesia seen in some patients.

Although used mainly for major depression, antidepressants have been shown to be useful in controlled clinical trials for chronic pain. These agents have little use in acute pain. Analgesic effects may be seen prior to the therapeutic effect for depressive symptoms, although efficacy may require passage of several weeks and dosages in the antidepressant range. TCAs should be carefully selected, depending on the patient's age and side effect profile. It is our practice to start patients at low doses (10 to 50 mg) and to choose agents based on the basis of the side effect profile of each drug (e.g., selecting agents that might have beneficial effects, such as somnolence, or avoiding others with bothersome side effects, such as constipation or dry mouth). Side effects include cardiovascular effects, which result from both the anti-α-adrenergic and local quinidine-like antiarrhythmic properties (e.g., tachycardia, orthostatic hypotension, heart block); anticholinergic effects that are particularly bothersome for patients (e.g., dry mouth, decreased tear flow, blurred vision, constipation, urinary retention); and antihistaminic effects (e.g., sedation, weight gain). Secondary amine TCAs, such as amitriptyline or imipramine, metabolize to the tertiary compounds nortriptyline and desipramine, respectively. Nortriptyline and desipramine have much fewer anticholinergic side effects than their parent compounds and are often preferable first-line analgesic antidepressants. Finally, the clinician should be aware of the potentially lethal signs and symptoms of TCA overdose. These include electrocardiographic (ECG) changes (e.g., PR widening, which is associated with the TCA plasma level; QRS and QT widening), tachycardia, delirium, hypotension, and respiratory depression. Care should

TABLE 14–1. USEFUL TRICYCLIC ANTIDEPRESSANTS

| Drug | Trade Name | Starting Dose (mg) (Range) | Side Effect Profile | | | $t_{1/2}$ (hr) |
			Sedative	Anticholinergic	Orthostatic	
Amitriptyline	Elavil	25–75 (75–300)	+ + +	+ + +	+ + + +	24
Desipramine	Norpramin	50–100 (75–300)	+	+	+ + + +	—
Doxepin	Sinequan	10–50 (75–300)	+ + +	+ + +	+ +	—
Imipramine	Tofranil	25–50 (75–300)	+ +	+ +	+ + + +	30
Nortriptyline	Pamelor	10–50 (30–150)	+	+	+ +	26
Clomipramine	Anafranil	25–50 (150–200)	+ + + + +	+ + + +	+ + + +	—

be taken not to give these drugs to patients with cardiac conduction disorders or to those receiving concurrent medications with the same side effect potential (e.g., mexiletine). Potentially serious side effects may be seen if these drugs are used with norepinephrine/epinephrine or the phenothiazines. Table 14–1 lists useful TCAs and their side effect profiles.

BENZODIAZEPINES

The efficacy of benzodiazepines is thought to result from pharmacologic effects on increasing γ-aminobutyric acid (GABA) levels in the spinal cord and brain following binding of these agents at the benzodiazepine receptor, an allosteric site within the GABA-A receptor complex. GABA produces inhibitory interneural effects. Benzodiazepines have minimal effects on cardiac and respiratory systems, and this accounts for a large margin of safety. Benzodiazepines increase sleep time and decrease sleep latency. They are potent muscle relaxants.

Benzodiazepines are useful in the treatment of acute anxiety that is sometimes seen in the postoperative period and can be mistaken for uncontrolled pain, especially in children. We find that lorazepam and clonazepam are particularly useful agents. These agents may also be helpful muscle relaxants in acute pain states (e.g., inhibition of muscle spasms sometimes seen in the postoperative period, particularly in postamputation states) or chronic pain states.

Benzodiazepines also may be useful in the treatment of chronic pain conditions (Table 14–2). Benzodiazepines such as clonazepam have been reported to be helpful with shooting pain conditions, although no controlled trials have been reported.

TABLE 14–2. USEFUL BENZODIAZEPINES

Drug	Trade Name	Dose (mg)	Onset of Effect	$t_{1/2}$ (hr)
Alprazolam	Xanax	0.5	Fast/intermediate	6–20
Clonazepam	Klonopin	0.25–0.5	Intermediate	20–40
Diazepam	Valium	5.0	Fast	30–100
Lorazepam	Ativan	1.0	Intermediate	10–20

Side effect profiles of benzodiazepines may be uncomfortable for the patient and also potentially serious and lethal. Withdrawal symptoms include the potential for seizures and may appear as late as 7 to 10 days after discontinuation due to the long half-life of the agents. Other side effects of benzodiazepines include hostility, disinhibition, and irritability; confusional states, particularly in the elderly; and sedation, which effect is additive with those of other CNS depressants, including alcohol. The literature does report that benzodiazepines are drugs of potential abuse or addiction when prescribed, and the Drug Enforcement Agency (DEA) informs us that these agents are among the most abused drugs.

NEUROLEPTICS

Neuroleptic drugs act mainly by their anti-dopaminergic actions. Anecdotal reports have suggested that neuroleptic drugs may be useful as primary analgesic agents or as adjuvant agents. We have found haloperidol, which is a butyrophenone, very useful in the treatment of delirium, agitation, and fearfulness, or in emergent situations in which benzodiazepines are contraindicated. The use of neuroleptics in chronic pain conditions is limited by potential serious side effects, such as dystonia and tardive dyskinesia (Table 14–3). They may also be used in controlling hiccups in the postoperative period, which can aggravate pain, particularly in patients undergoing chest-related surgery. Most neuroleptics are greater than 90% protein bound, and conditions that alter protein levels will alter the bioavailability of the drug. Most neuroleptic agents have endocrine effects, including increases in prolactin and decreases in luteinizing hormone and follicle-stimulating hormone. Potential serious side effects of all the neuroleptic drugs are predominantly neurologic in nature, including acute dystonia (spasm of muscles of face and tongue), akathisia (motor restlessness), parkinsonism, neuroleptic malignant syndrome (catatonia, stupor, fever), and tardive dyskinesia. The latter is usually only seen months or years after treatment. Other side effects include faintness, anticholinergic side effects, palpitations, drowsiness, and orthostatic hypotension.

TABLE 14-3. USEFUL NEUROLEPTIC AGENTS

| Drug | Trade Name | Dose (mg) | Side Effect Profile | | | $t_{1/2}$ |
			Sedative	*Extrapyramidal*	*Hypotensive*	
Droperidol	Inapsine	5-10	+	+ +	+ +	Unknown
Haloperidol	Haldol	1-20	+ +	+ + +	+ +	Unknown

SUMMARY

The complete pain clinician must be able to harness psychotropic medications for both nociceptive and non-nociceptive features of pain. These drugs can be important components in effective analgesia. It is suggested that the clinician have experience with a few agents in each class and understand their indications, dosages, and potential side effects. For a more extensive review of the use of these agents in pain treatment, the reader is referred to the references that follow.

FURTHER READING

Ardid D, Guilbaud G: Anti-nociceptive effects of acute and 'chronic' injections of tricyclic antidepressant drugs in a new model of mononeuropathy in rats. Pain 49:279-287, 1992.

Cameron LB: Neuropsychotropic drugs as adjuncts in the treatment of cancer pain. Oncology 6:65-72, 77-80, 1992.

Eija K, Tiina T, Pertti NJ: Amitriptyline effectively relieves neuropathic pain following treatment of breast cancer. Pain 64:293-302, 1996.

Gordon NC, Heller PH, Gear RW, et al: Temporal factors in the enhancement of morphine analgesia by desipramine. Pain 53:273-276, 1993.

Kerrick JM, Fine PG, Lipman AG, et al: Low-dose amitriptyline as an adjunct to opioids for postoperative orthopedic pain: A placebo-controlled trial. Pain 52:325-330, 1993.

Max MB, Zeigler D, Shoaf SE, et al: Effects of a single oral dose of desipramine on postoperative morphine analgesia. J Pain Symptom Manage 7:454-462, 1992.

Max MB: Treatment of post-herpetic neuralgia: Antidepressants. Ann Neurol 35(suppl):S50-S53, 1994.

Onghena P, Van Houdenhove B: Antidepressant-induced analgesia in chronic nonmalignant pain: A meta-analysis of 39 placebo-controlled studies. Pain 49:205-219, 1992.

Panerai AE, Bianchi M, Sacerdote P, et al: Antidepressants in cancer pain. J Palliat Care 7:42-44, 1991.

Rainov NO, Gutjahr T, Burkert W: Intra-operative epidural morphine, fentanyl, and droperidol for control of pain after spinal surgery: A prospective, randomized, placebo controlled, and double-blind trial. Acta Neurochir 138:33-39, 1996.

Reddy S, Patt RB: The benzodiazepines as adjuvant analgesics. J Pain Symptom Manage 9:510-514, 1994.

Tura B, Tura SM: The analgesic effect of tricyclic antidepressants. Brain Res 518:19-22, 1990.

Volmink J, Lancaster T, Gray S, et al: Treatments for postherpetic neuralgia—a systematic review of randomized controlled trials. Fam Pract 13:84-91, 1996.

Chapter 15

Membrane Stabilizers

To-Nhu H. Vu, M.D., and
David Borsook, M.D., Ph.D.

Unfortunately, no universal pain medication exists that provides pain relief without side effects. Recently, a large contribution has been made to the therapeutic armamentarium from a growing group of new membrane-stabilization agents. This chapter reviews the use of sodium- and calcium-channel blockers in the treatment of chronic neuropathic pain. The indications for and pharmacologic profiles of anticonvulsants and local anesthetics are discussed, as is the possible clinical application of calcium-channel blockers used in experimental animal models.

Chronic pain conditions may result from damage to the integrity of the axons of peripheral primary sensory neurons. Following an injury, an increase in membrane excitability occurs, which may be due to a number of processes, including the upregulation and accumulation of ion channels near the site of injury. Because of this increased excitability, abnormal or ectopic impulses are generated. These discharges may be perceived as pain, and they can lead to central hyperexcitability or sensitization. Membrane stabilizers that block sodium and calcium channels decrease the ectopic firings. Anticonvulsants, local anesthetics, and antiarrhythmics are some of the agents that exert their effects by sodium-channel blockade. Drugs that act at calcium channels include gabapentin, calcium-channel blockers, and a new class of agents, ω-conopeptides.

Clinical studies support the role of sodium- and calcium-channel blockers in pain management. In 1992, Devor and colleagues reported a reduction in the ectopic discharges from neuromas and dorsal root ganglia following the administration of lidocaine (a sodium-channel blocker) in rats. Controlled trials in humans also demonstrated the effectiveness of sodium-channel blockers over placebo in the treatment of neuropathic pain. Although less extensively studied than sodium-channel blockers, calcium-channel blockers have been shown to decrease ectopic discharges and reduce hyperalgesia and allodynia in animal models of nerve injury.

SODIUM-CHANNEL BLOCKING AGENTS

Anticonvulsant Agents

Anticonvulsant drugs, as a class, depress abnormal neuronal discharges and raise the threshold for nerve activation. They are thought to be effective in neuropathic pain, which typically is associated with sharp, shooting, electric shock–like sensations. Indeed, for more than five decades, phenytoin and carbamazepine have been used to treat trigeminal neuralgia, a condition characterized by episodic attacks of sharp, lancinating pain. Phenytoin, carbamazepine, and newer anticonvulsant agents, such as lamotrigine and topiramate, are used as either first-line or adjunctive therapy for postherpetic neuralgia, diabetic neuropathy, mononeuropathies and polyneuropathies, radiculopathy, complex regional pain syndrome, central pain syndrome, phantom limb pain, and cranial neuralgia. All anticonvulsants can cause cognitive impairment and sedation, which necessitates careful titration. Newer anticonvulsants, including lamotrigine, topiramate, and gabapentin, are relatively well tolerated when administered appropriately and do not require rigorous monitoring for hematologic and hepatic toxic effects (Table 15-1).

Phenytoin (Dilantin)

Phenytoin was the first anticonvulsant used for pain. It is a second-line agent for the treatment of trigeminal neuralgia. Two controlled studies have shown that phenytoin is statistically more efficacious than placebo in the treatment of diabetic neuropathy. Phenytoin may interact with other pain medications, and it decreases the effects of carbamazepine, lamotrigine, haloperidol, methadone, mexiletine, and meperidine. Tricyclic antidepressants and valproic acid may increase phenytoin levels. The most common side effects include nystagmus, ataxia, slurred speech, and mental confusion. Cos-

TABLE 15–1. MEMBRANE STABILIZERS

Drug	Trade Name/Formulation (mg)	Starting Dose	Side Effects/Drawbacks
Sodium-Channel Blocking Agents			
Anticonvulsants			
Phenytoin	Dilantin/30, 50, 100	100 mg b.i.d.–t.i.d.	CNS, cosmetic effects, drug interactions
Carbamazepine	Tegretol/100, 200	100 mg b.i.d.	Sedation, aplastic anemia, agranulocytosis
Lamotrigine	Lamictal/25, 100, 150, 200	25–50 mg (300–500 mg/day b.i.d.)	Rash, drug interactions with other anticonvulsants
Topiramate	Topamax/25, 100, 200	50 mg q.h.s. (200 mg b.i.d.)	Sedation
Local anesthetics			
Lidocaine	Xylocaine/1%, 2%	1–5 mg/kg	CNS and cardiovascular effects
Mexiletine	Mexitil/150, 200, 250	150 mg b.i.d. (1200 mg/day t.i.d.)	GI distress and CNS effects
Calcium-Channel Blocking Agent			
Gabapentin	Neurontin/100, 300, 400	300 mg q.h.s. (3600 mg/day t.i.d.–q.i.d.)	Sedation, frequent dosing

metic side effects include gingival hyperplasia and coarsening of the facial features. The initial dose for phenytoin is 100 mg, two or three times daily.

Carbamazepine (Tegretol)

Carbamazepine is chemically related to the tricyclic antidepressants. It is the drug of choice for trigeminal neuralgia. Controlled studies have also shown that carbamazepine is effective in diabetic neuropathy, migraine prophylaxis, central pain after stroke, and postherpetic neuralgia. The most frequent side effects include dizziness, drowsiness, nausea, and vomiting. With this drug, aplastic anemia and agranulocytosis occur at a rate five to eight times higher than that in the general population. Therefore, a complete blood cell count (CBC) should be obtained at the initiation of therapy and at 3 and 6 months' follow-up. The initial dose is 100 mg, given twice daily, to be increased at weekly intervals to a desirable effect. Slow titration appears to minimize the gastrointestinal side effects of this medication.

Lamotrigine (Lamictal)

In addition to blocking the voltage-gated sodium channels, lamotrigine also inhibits the release of glutamate. Lamotrigine has been shown to reduce pain behavior in induced acute and chronic hyperalgesia conditions in rats. One recent controlled study in humans showed that lamotrigine was more effective than placebo in the treatment of trigeminal neuralgia. In general, lamotrigine is well tolerated. The most common side effect is rash, seen in 5% to 10% of patients taking this medication. Factors that increase the risk for the development of rash include age, as demonstrated by occurrence in 1 in 50 or 100 pediatric patients; co-administration of valproic acid, which decreases the metabolism of lamotrigine twofold; and rapid initial dose titration. Lamotrigine also interacts with the other anticonvulsants: lamotrigine levels are decreased by 40% to 50% by

carbamazepine and phenytoin. The initial dose is 25 to 50 mg, taken at bedtime, which is gradually increased to 300 to 500 mg/day in two divided doses.

Topiramate (Topamax)

Topiramate is thought to have three distinct mechanisms of action. It blocks sodium channels, potentiates the action of the inhibitory neurotransmitter γ-aminobutyric acid (GABA), and antagonizes the kainate–α-amino-3-hydroxy-5-methylisoxazole-4-propionic acid (AMPA) subtype of the glutamate receptor. Controlled trials have not been done to examine the effectiveness of topiramate in neuropathic pain conditions. In general, topiramate is well tolerated. The most common side effects are somnolence, fatigue, and psychomotor slowing. There is a 1.5% incidence of kidney stones, a side effect associated with topiramate's weak carbonic anhydrase inhibitor activity. The usual starting dose is 50 mg, taken at bedtime, which is titrated up to 200 mg, twice daily.

LOCAL ANESTHETICS

Membrane-stabilizing agents such as lidocaine, tocainide, and mexiletine are also classified as class IB antiarrhythmic agents. In the management of neuropathic pain, systemically administered local anesthetics selectively block ectopic discharges and do not affect normal nerve conduction. The site of action is thought to be both central and peripheral. In both animal and human double-blind, randomized, placebo-controlled studies, these agents have been shown to be effective in neuropathic pain states such as radiculopathy, peripheral neuropathy, and trigeminal neuralgia. The routes of administration include intravenous (lidocaine), topical (lidocaine and prilocaine), and oral (mexiletine and tocainide) (see Table 15–1).

Lidocaine is an amide that is metabolized by the liver. The serum half-life is 1.6 hours; however, the analgesic effects last from several days to a month. Side effects mainly involve the central nervous and cardiovascular systems; they include lightheadedness and/or dizziness, drowsiness, tinnitus, blurred vision, seizures, hypotension, and bradycardia. Caution should be taken in patients with heart block. We usually obtain a preprocedural electrocardiogram (ECG). Blood pressure, heart rate, and ECG should be monitored during the administration of lidocaine. The usual dose is 1 to 5 mg/kg, given intravenously over 5 to 30 minutes.

Topical preparations of local anesthetics include lidocaine and a combination of lidocaine and prilocaine in EMLA cream. In clinical trials, topical 5% lidocaine was effective in relieving postherpetic neuralgia. EMLA cream has been used to prevent nociceptive pain from intravenous cannula placement and minor skin procedures. The eutectic mixture of local anesthetics provides 80% of active drug at the skin site. EMLA cream must be applied at least 1 hour prior to an elective procedure.

Structurally similar to lidocaine, tocainide and mexiletine are effective orally. Tocanide has been shown to be efficacious in treating trigeminal neuralgia. However, tocainide causes life-threatening complications, such as blood dyscrasias and pulmonary fibrosis. Therefore, it should not be used routinely for the treatment of pain. (Mexiletene is discussed separately in Chapter 16.) In one study, lidocaine infusion was shown to predict the response to mexiletine in patients with neuropathic pain.

CALCIUM-CHANNEL BLOCKING AGENTS

Several calcium-channel subtypes have been identified on the basis of their electrophysiologic profiles and binding affinity to calcium-channel blockers. The N- and L-type calcium channels are of great interest in the treatment of pain. ω-Conopeptides selectively block the N-type calcium channels. Dihydropyridines (nifedipine and nimodipine) have a higher affinity for the L-type calcium channels. Recently, gabapentin was also found to have binding site at the $\alpha_2\delta$-subunit of the L-type calcium channels.

Like sodium channels, the upregulation of calcium channels has been implicated in the generation of ectopic discharges in damaged nerve. However, calcium channels are also involved in the release of neurotransmitters and the modulation of opioid and N-methyl-D-aspartate (NMDA) receptors. Calcium-channel blockers are not selective for the sensory nerves. Their application in the treatment of pain is limited by their action at other sites, such as the heart.

Gabapentin (Neurontin)

Gabapentin is discussed here because it is the first drug found to have a binding site at the $\alpha_2\delta$-subunit at the L-type calcium channel in pig brain. Although gabapentin is structurally similar to the GABA analogue, it does not have GABAergic receptor activity. As an anticonvulsant, gabapentin possibly stabilizes the membrane by modulating the calcium channels. By reducing the abnormal firing in damaged nerve, it prevents central sensitization, which may result in allodynia and hyperesthesia. Gabapentin has been reported to be effective in complex regional pain syndrome and neuropathic pain conditions, although larger controlled studies are needed to validate the results. The most common side effects are somnolence, dizziness, ataxia, and fatigue. Unlike the other anticonvulsants, such as phenytoin and carbamazepine, gabapentin has few drug interactions. The starting dose is usually 100 to 300 mg, taken at bedtime, with doses being increased gradually every 3 days to a maximal dose of 2400 to 3600 mg/day. Because gabapentin has a short serum half-life, the dose should be given three to four times daily.

ω-Conopeptides

ω-Conopeptides were originally extracted from the venom of marine snails. They are potent blockers of the N-type calcium channels. In rats, the perineural administration of conotoxin reduces mechanoallodynia and heat hyperalgesia. The mechanism of action is likely due to a reduction in ectopic discharges leading to a decrease in central hyperexcitability. The N-type calcium-channel blocker is devoid of cardiovascular effects, unlike agents that act at the L-type calcium channels. Therefore, it can be used in the treatment of neuropathic pain. Selective perineural administration of conopeptide can provide pain relief without conduction or sensory blockade, like lidocaine with the similar route of administration. Conopeptide also effects sympathetic blockade and may be effective in sympathetically maintained pain. The side effects of conotoxin are hypotension, tremor, and histamine release.

Other Calcium-Channel Blockers

Calcium-channel blockers with unproven use in pain include nifedipine, nimodipine, and verapamil. They are primarily used in the treatment of migraine headache. Recently, these agents have been used to decrease the development of tolerance and to enhance the effect of opioids. The injection of nifedipine, nimodipine, or verapamil in the rat produces an antinociceptive effect on formalin and writhing tests. The mechanism of action is thought to be a decrease in central sensitization. In a small clinical study that involved 23 patients with cancer who received long-term morphine therapy, nimodipine was shown to decrease the development of tolerance. Larger controlled, randomized studies are needed to validate these results.

SUMMARY

Aside from sodium, other ions such as calcium are also involved in the generation of ectopic discharges that lead to chronic neuropathic pain. Currently, sodium-channel blockers such as anticonvulsants and local anesthetics are used in the treatment of chronic neuropathic pain. Future directions include targeting the different subtypes of calcium channels by using agents such as conopeptides or targeting specific sodium-channel blockers unique to pain fibers. These agents may provide more specific analgesia without significant side effects.

FURTHER READING

General References

Devor M, Wall PD, Catalan N: Systemic lidocaine silences ectopic neuroma and DRG discharge without blocking nerve conduction. Pain 48:261–268, 1992.

Dray A: Agonists and antagonists of nociception. *In* Proceedings of the 8th World Congress on Pain. Seattle, IASP Press, 1996, pp 279–292.

Elliott JR: Slow sodium channel inactivation and bursting discharge in a simple model axon: Implications for neuropathic pain. Brain Res 754:221–226, 1997.

Matzner O, Devor M: Sodium conductance and the threshold for repetitive neuronal firing. Brain Res 597:92–98, 1992.

Miller RJ: Multiple calcium channels and neuronal function. Science 235:46–52, 1987.

Sodium-Channel Blocking Agents
Anticonvulsant Agents

Brodie MJ: Lamotrigine versus other antiepileptic drugs: A star rating system is born. Epilepsia 35(suppl 5):S41–S46, 1994.

Hunter JC, Gogas KR, Hedley LR, et al: The effect of novel anti-epileptic drugs in rat experimental models of acute and chronic pain. Eur J Pharmacol 324:153–160, 1997.

Leach MJ, Marden CM, Miller AA: Pharmacological studies on lamotrigine, a novel potential antiepileptic drug: Neurochemical studies on the mechanism of action. Epilepsia 27:490–497, 1986.

McQuay H, Carroll D, Jadad AR, et al: Anticonvulsant drugs for management of pain: A systemic review. Br Med J 311:1047–1052, 1995.

Nakamura-Craig M, Follenfant RL: Effect of lamotrigine in the acute and chronic hyperalgesia induced by PGE$_2$ and in the chronic hyperalgesia in rats with streptozotocin-induced diabetes. Pain 63:33–37, 1995.

Shorvon SD: Safety of topiramate: Adverse events and relationships to dosing. Epilepsia 37(suppl 2):S18–S22, 1996.

Zakrzewska JM, Chaudhry Z, Nurmikko TJ, et al: Lamotrigine (Lamictal) in refractory trigeminal neuralgia: Results from a double-blind placebo controlled crossover trial. Pain 73:223–230, 1997.

Local Anesthetics

Abram SE, Yaksh TL: Systemic lidocaine blocks nerve injury–induced hyperalgesia and nociceptor-driven spinal sensitization in the rat. Anesthesiology 80:383–391, 1994.

Chabal C, Russell LS, Burchiel KJ: The effect of intravenous lidocaine, tocainide, and mexiletine on spontaneously active fibers originating in rat sciatic neuromas. Pain 38:333–338, 1989.

Ehrenstrom Reiz GME, Reiz SLA: EMLA: A eutectic mixture of local anaesthetics for topical anaesthesia. Acta Anaesthesiol Scand 26:596–598, 1982.

Glazer S, AB, Portenoy RK: Systemic local anesthetics in pain control. J Pain Symptom Manage 6:30–39, 1991.

Kastrup J, Petersen P, Dejgard A, et al: Intravenous lidocaine infusion: A new treatment of chronic painful diabetic neuropathy? Pain 28:69–75, 1987.

Lindstrom P, Lindblom U: The analgesic effect of tocainide in trigeminal neuralgia. Pain 28:45–50, 1987.

Calcium-Channel Blocking Agents

Basilico L, Parolaro D, Rubino T, et al: Influence of ω-conotoxin on morphine analgesia and withdrawal syndrome in rats. Eur J Pharmacol 218:75–81, 1992.

Bernstein MA, Welch SP: Alterations in L-type calcium channels in the brain and spinal cord of acutely treated and morphine-tolerant mice. Brain Res 696:83–88, 1995.

Chaplan SR, Pogrel JW, Yaksh TL: Role of voltage-dependent calcium channel subtypes in experimental tactile allodynia. J Pharmacol Exp Ther 269:1117–1123, 1994.

Coderre TJ, Melzack R: The role of NMDA receptor-operated calcium channels in persistent nociception after formalin-induced tissue injury. J Neurosci 12:3671–3675, 1992.

Gee NS, Brown JP, Dissanayake VUK, et al: The novel anticonvulsant drug, gabapentin (Neurontin), binds to the I2J subunit of a calcium channel. J Biol Chem 271:5768–5776, 1996.

Miranda HF, Bustamante D, Kramer V, et al: Antinociceptive effects of calcium channel blockers. Eur J Pharmacol 217:137–141, 1992.

Santillan R, Maestre JM, Hurle MA, et al: Enhancement of opiate analgesia by nimodipine in cancer patients chronically treated with morphine: A preliminary report. Pain 58:129–132, 1994.

Sluka KA: Blockade of calcium channels can prevent the onset of secondary hyperalgesia and allodynia induced by intradermal injection of capsaicin in rats. Pain 71:157–164, 1997.

Taylor CP: Emerging perspectives on the mechanism of action of gabapentin. Neurology 44(suppl 2):S18–S22, 1996.

Xiao WH, Bennett GJ: Synthetic ω-conopeptides applied to the site of nerve injury suppress neuropathic pains in rats. J Pharmacol Exp Ther 274:666–672, 1995.

Chapter 16

● Mexiletine

Charles B. Sisson, M.D.

Mexiletine (Mexitil) is an orally active lidocaine congener that is resistant to first-pass hepatic metabolism. It is a class IB antiarrhthymic agent that is used for the treatment of ventricular arrhythmia. In pain management it has been used for the treatment of dysesthetic pain secondary to peripheral vascular disease, diabetes mellitus, and central pain syndromes.

PHARMACOKINETICS

Mexiletine is rapidly absorbed (90%) after an oral dose. Peak plasma concentrations are reached in 2 to 3 hours, with a half-life of 10 to 12 hours. Mexiletine crosses the blood-brain barrier and has central effects. This is particularly true with serum levels greater than 2 μg/mL. Fine hand tremor, ataxia, dizziness, light-headedness, nystagmus, paresthesias, blurred vision, diplopia, confusion, drowsiness, seizures, and psychosis have been reported with mexiletine.[1]

There is marked individual patient variation in the pharmacokinetics of mexiletine. This is thought to be due to multiple factors, including urinary pH and genetic differences in hepatic metabolism.[2]

In healthy volunteers, a 200-mg dose of racemic mexiletine produced a peak plasma concentration of 217 ± 69 ng/mL for R(−)-mexiletine and 197 ± 56 ng/mL for S(+)-mexiletine. Mexiletine displays pH-dependent stereoselective binding to serum proteins. Mexiletine is highly metabolized, and only 3.68 ± 3.94% for S(+)-mexiletine appears in the urine unchanged.[3]

MECHANISM OF ACTION

Like lidocaine, mexiletine inhibits the inward sodium current and thus reduces the rate of rise of the action potential, phase 0. Mexiletine acts at the Na^+/K^+ channels in the peripheral nerve and dorsal root ganglion preparations.[4]

Mexiletine significantly inhibits the intensity of somatostatin and substance P-induced nociceptive effect in diabetic mice. Furthermore, mexiletine significantly inhibits the K^+-evoked release of substance P from slices of spinal cord of diabetic mice.[5] This suggests that the reduction of the release of substance P from the nociceptive afferent terminal in the spinal cord is involved in the mechanisms of mexiletine analgesia in diabetic mice.[6]

Other experimental studies in diabetic and nondiabetic mice suggest that a δ_1-opioid receptor–mediated mechanism may be involved in the antinociceptive effect of mexiletine.[7] In rat models, involving central sensitization using noxious chemical stimuli, mexiletine (10 to 100 mg/kg given subcutaneously) significantly attenuated hyperalgesia in formalin-treated (60 and 100 mg/kg) rats as well as tactile allodynia in neuropathic rat models (100 mg/kg).[8]

Stereoselective binding of mexiletine has been shown in skeletal tissue preparation of frogs, supporting potential usefulness of low doses of R(−)-mexiletine in the treatment of abnormal hyperexcitability of myotonic muscles.[9]

DOSAGE

Patients taking mexiletine for cardiac arrhythmia may take up to 900 mg/day; however, a significant number of these patients experience intolerable side effects. More commonly, for the treatment of neuropathic pain, if a patient fails to respond to doses less than 450 mg/day, increasing the dose yields more side effects than benefits. A reasonable approach to treatment is to start therapy with 150 mg/day and gradually increase the dose to therapeutic effect or to a target range of 300 to 450 mg/day in divided doses.[10]

ONSET

Intravenous lidocaine infusion (2 to 5 mg/kg) has been significantly correlated with oral mexiletine and may be predictive for response to mexiletine therapy.[11]

One study showed efficacy in the treatment of diabetic neuropathy with mexiletine at a dosage of 10 mg/kg.[12] A single dose of 200 mg in healthy males produced a peak plasma level of 300 ng/mL 3.5 to 4.0 hours after administration. Plasma half-life was 7.75 hours.[13]

TOLERABILITY AND SAFETY

In the treatment of neuropathic pain, some authors feel that mexiletine is safer and has fewer side effects than alternative drugs, such as phenytoin or tocainide.[14] However, ongoing studies with gabapentin may eventually prove it to be better tolerated and more efficacious than mexiletine.

ABUSE AND TOLERANCE

Mexiletine has little or no abuse potential. If a patient responds to mexiletine, tolerance rarely develops.[15]

SYSTEMIC EFFECTS AND SIDE EFFECTS

Contraindications to the use of mexiletine include preexisting second- or third-degree AV block, chronic hypotension, congestive heart failure, and hepatic injury. Patients should be periodically monitored for elevations of serum glutamic oxaloacetic transaminase and blood dyscrasias, which occur in approximately 0.1% of patients. Side effects are dose dependent, centrally mediated, and predominantly neurologic, including tremor, blurred vision, and lethargy. Nausea is also a common side effect.[15]

DRUG INTERACTIONS

Mexiletine increases serum levels of theophylline. In one controlled study, plasma theophylline levels increased by a mean of 72% by the second day of mexiletine therapy.[15]

THERAPEUTIC USE

The use of mexiletine for the treatment of chronic neuropathic pain is an off-label use of the drug. Mexiletine has been used for myotonia, chronic painful diabetic neuropathy, and spasticity.[14, 16] Several studies report the use of mexiletine and lidocaine for the treatment of painful diabetic neuropathy that is refractory to standard therapy.[17, 18] Mexiletine has a favorable effect on neuropathic pain in patients with diabetic neuropathy as assessed by the PRIT index of the McGill Pain Questionnaire, in doses of 350 to 450 mg/day, whereas at the dose of 675 mg/day, side effects limited patient tolerance. Mexiletine has also been used for the treatment of painful alcoholic neuropathy.[19]

Mexiletine effectively relieves allodynia-like symptoms at doses of 15 and 30 mg/kg in rats after ischemic spinal cord injury.[20] Mexiletine has been shown to provide protection from anoxia and/or ischemic injury in optic nerve preparations and hippocampal slices from the rat. These findings may support a role for mexiletine use to maximize clinical recovery of white matter tracts from injury due to stroke or spinal cord injury.[21] In humans, however, mexiletine has been shown to be ineffective in the treatment of spinal cord injury–related dysesthetic pain.[22] In non-spinal cord injury–patients, studies show that the use of intravenous lidocaine is effective in the treatment of pain in the acute postoperative state as well as in neuropathic conditions.[22]

Research supports the use of mexiletine in neuropathic pain involving peripheral nerve injury. A double-blind placebo-controlled study found that mexiletine produced a statistically significant reduction in reported pain when compared to baseline or placebo in patients with a history of peripheral nerve injury and neuropathic pain.[23]

Mexiletine has been used for the treatment of spasticity due to neurologic disorders that are unresponsive to trials of antispasticity drugs, such as dantrolene and baclofen. Takahiro and Yoshiro[24] reported that oral mexiletine, initially given at 25 mg/day with a gradual titration to 150 to 300 mg/day, abolished muscle cramps, reduced ankle clonus, and diminished spasticity in all limbs. They found that 7 of 12 patients had a reduction of muscle tone leading to improved functional status, such as the ability to walk.[25]

Finally, mexiletine has been used to treat pain in patients after stroke. In thalamic pain syndrome, a rare sequela of cerebrovascular accident, mexiletine has been used successfully.[25]

TOXICITY

In one case report of fatal overdose, the blood concentration of mexiletine was 44.8 µg/mL.[26] Toxicity from mexiletine occurs within a wide range of plasma levels and may occur within the therapeutic range. The incidence of central nervous system toxic effects, as evidenced by seizures, occurs in 2 in 1000 patients.[27, 28]

SUMMARY

Mexiletine is a viable therapeutic agent for use in central pain syndromes and peripheral neuropathies. Response to intravenous lidocaine infusions is predictive of the analgesic response to mexiletine therapy. The dose should be titrated to effect. For patients receiving long-term therapy, blood cell counts and liver function tests should be monitored at 6- to 12-month intervals.

REFERENCES

1. Lathers C, O'Rourke D: Antiarrhythmic agents. In Smith C, Reynard A (eds): Textbook of Pharmacology. Philadelphia, WB Saunders, 1992, pp 1, 539.

2. Lledo P, Abrams S, Johnston A: Influence of debrisoquine hydroxylation phenotype on the pharmacokinetics of mexiletine. Eur J Clin Pharmacol 44:63, 1993.
3. Kwok D, Kerr C, McErlane K: Pharmacokinetics of mexiletine enantiomers in healthy human subjects: A study of the in vivo serum protein binding, salivary excretion, and red blood cell distribution of the enantiomers. Xenobiotica 25:1127, 1995.
4. Zhang X, Wang T: Protection of mexiletine against hypoxic damage of synaptic function in hippocampal slices. Acta Pharmacol Sin 14:426, 1993.
5. Kamei J, Hitosugi H, Kasuya Y: Effects of mexiletine on formalin induced nociceptive responses in mice. Res Commun Chem Pathol Pharmacol 80:153-162, 1993.
6. Kamei, Hitosugi H, Kawashima N, et al. Antinociceptive effect of mexiletine in diabetic mice. Res Comm Chem Pathol Pharmacol 77:245-248, 1992.
7. Kamei J, Saitoh A, Kasuya Y: Involvement of delta 1-opioid receptors in the antinociceptive effects of mexiletine in mice. Neurosci Lett 196:169-172, 1995.
8. Jett MF, McGuirk J, Waligora D, et al: The effects of mexiletine, desipramine and fluoxetine in rat models involving central sensitization. Pain 69:161-169, 1997.
9. DeLuca A, Natuzzi F, Lentini G, et al: Stereoselective effects of mexiletine enantiomers on sodium currents and excitability characteristic of adult skeletal muscle fibers. Naunyn Schmiedebergs Arch Pharmacol 352:653, 1995.
10. Cambell N, Pantridge J, Adgey A: Long term oral antiarrhythmic therapy with mexiletine. Br Heart J 40:796, 1978.
11. Galer BS, Harle J, Rowbotham MC: Response to intravenous lidocaine infusion predicts subsequent response to oral mexiletine: A prospective study. J Pain Symptom Manage 12:161, 1996.
12. Tanelian D, Brose W: Neuropathic pain can be relieved by drugs that are use-dependent sodium channel blockers: Lidocaine, carbamazepine, and mexiletine. Anesthesiology 74:949, 1991.
13. Hutt V, Pabst G, Salama Z, et al. The pharmacokinetics and bioavailability of a new mexiletine preparation in healthy volunteers. Arzneimittelforschung 45:254, 1995.
14. Pouget J, Serratice G: Myotonia with muscular weakness corrected by exercise: Therapeutic effect of mexiletine. Rev Neurol 139:669 1983.
15. Physicians' Desk Reference, ed 50. Montvale, NJ, Medical Economics, 1995, p 640.
16. Dejard A, Petersen P, Kastrup J: Mexiletine for treatment of chronic diabetic neuropathy. Lancet 9:9, 1988.
17. Ackerman W 3rd, Colclough G, Juneja M, et al: The management of oral mexiletine and intravenous lidocaine to treat chronic painful symmetrical distal diabetic neuropathy. J Kentucky Med Assn 89:500, 1991.
18. Kubota K, Joshita Y, Tamura J, et al: Relief of severe diabetic truncal pain with mexiletine. J Med 22:307, 1991.
19. Nishiyama K, Sakuta M: Mexiletine for painful alcoholic neuropathy. Intern Med 34:577, 1995.
20. Xu X, Hao I, Seiger A, et al: Systemic mexiletine relieves chronic allodynia like symptoms in rats with ischemic spinal cord injury. Anesth Analg 74:649-652, 1992.
21. Stys P, Lesiuk H: Correlation between electrophysiological effects of mexiletine and ischemic protection in central nervous system white matter. Neuroscience 71:27-36, 1996.
22. Chiou-Tan F, Tuel S, Johnson J, et al: Effect of mexiletine on spinal cord injury dysesthetic pain. Am J Phys Med Rehabil 75:84-87, 1996.
23. Chabal C, Jacobson L, Mariano A, et al: The use of oral mexiletine for the treatment of pain after peripheral nerve injury. Anesthesiology 76:513, 1992.
24. Takahiro J, Yoshihiro W: Mexiletine for treatment of spasticity due to neurological disorders. Muscle Nerve. 10:885, 1993.
25. Awerbuch G, Sandyk R: Mexiletine for thalamic pain syndrome. Int J Neurosci 55:129, 1990.
26. Rorhrig T, Harty L: Postmortem distribution of mexiletine in a fatal overdose. J Anal Toxicol 18:354, 1994.
27. Denaro C, Benowitz N: Poisoning due to class IB antiarrhythmic drugs: Lignocaine, mexiletine, and tocainide. Med Toxicol Adverse Drug Exp 4:412, 1989.
28. Christie J, Valdes C, Markowsky S: Neurotoxicity of lidocaine combined with mexiletine. Anesth Analg 77:1291, 1993.

Chapter 17

Nonsteroidal Anti-inflammatory Drugs

Hak Yui Wong, M.B.B.S.

The nonsteroidal anti-inflammatory drugs (NSAIDs) include a diverse group of chemicals, excluding corticosteroids, that share the common primary property of possessing anti-inflammatory action. The analgesic effect is secondary and is related to interference with the chemical mechanisms of pain.

CHEMICAL MECHANISM OF PAIN

The phenomenon of pain is complex, incorporating biological factors as well as sociological, cultural, and psychological influences. After initial transmission of sharp first pain by fast-conducting myelinated Aδ fibers from the afferent nerve endings, a complex myriad of changes then occurs, both in the periphery as well as in the central nervous system, resulting in slow dull pain as well as other phenomena, including primary and secondary hyperalgesia, allodynia, sensitization, windup, expansion of receptor field, and enhancement of flexor reflex.

Many of these changes are brought about by chemical mediators that either act directly on neuronal cell membranes (e.g., H^+ ions, adenosine triphosphate, and serotonin), or react with membrane receptors to invoke intracellular second messengers. Examples of these receptor-binding mediators include bradykinin reacting with β_1- and β_2-receptors; tachykinins, such as substance P, with NK receptors; histamine with H_1-receptors; serotonin with $5\text{-}HT_1$-receptors; glutamate and aspartate with NMDA receptors, nitric oxide, cytokines, and eicosanoids. Platelet-activating factor (PAF), which mediates vasodilation, may also be involved.

THE ALGOGENIC ROLE OF EICOSANOIDS

Eicosanoids are products of metabolism of arachidonic acid released from membrane phospholipid (in response to tissue damage) by phospholipase A_2. The cyclooxygenase (COX) and lipoxygenase pathways lead to formation of cyclic prostaglandins and leukotrienes, respectively (Fig. 17–1).

Prostaglandins are algogenic by several mechanisms: (1) acting on prostaglandin receptors and second messengers to sensitize sensory neurons; (2) directly increasing the activity of nociceptors; and (3) stimulating the release of substance P from sensory neurons. The release, level, and activity of prostaglandins are enhanced by other algogenic substances released during inflammation, such as bradykinins and cytokines.

In visceral pain in which the mechanisms of pain include peritoneal inflammation, visceral distention, and exaggerated smooth muscle motility, prostaglandins may enhance pain by promoting biliary fluid production and gallbladder contraction, increasing renal blood flow and ureteric motility, inhibiting antidiuretic hormone (ADH), and increasing inflammation at the site of calculic ureteric obstruction.

At least two forms of cyclooxygenase are now recognized. COX-1 is the constitutive, ubiquitous form that provides prostaglandins for physiologic functions, such as maintenance of renal blood flow and gastric mucosal covering. COX-2 is the inducible form that expresses in endothelial cells, macrophages, fibroblasts, and mast cells and produces prostaglandin during inflammation. The level and activity of COX-2 are influenced by multiple factors, such as lipopolysaccharides, bacterial toxins, and an inducible form of nitric oxide synthetase.

The products of lipoxygenase activity, hydroxyeicosatetraenoic acid (HETE), and leukotrienes, have chemotactic activity for leukocytes. Leukotriene B_4 also stimulates the release of HETE from leukocytes, which produces hyperalgesia directly by decreasing the mechanical and thermal thresholds of C fibers.

CHEMICAL AND PHARMACOKINETIC FEATURES

Most NSAIDs are derivatives of carboxylic acid or enolic acid and are weakly acidic, with a pKa of 3 to 5, dissociating readily in acidic gastric environment and

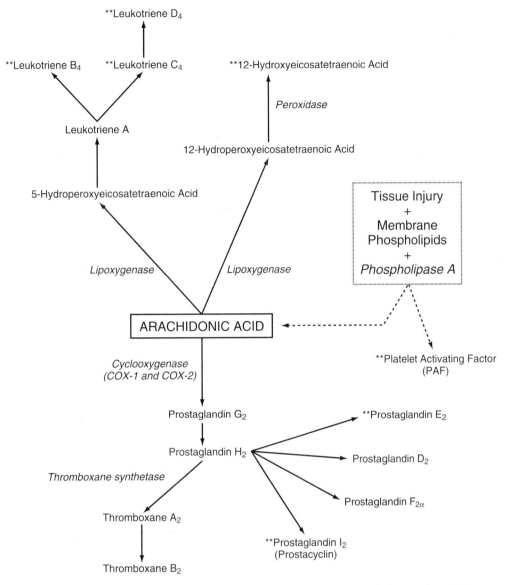

FIGURE 17-1. Algogenic compounds (indicated by *double asterisks*) from arachidonic acid metabolism.

allowing rapid absorption after oral intake and trapping in gastric mucosa. They are highly protein-bound, with a small volume of distribution and low hepatic clearance. Hepatic metabolism is extensive, whereas renal elimination of unchanged drug accounts for a very small percentage of the administered dose. In renal failure, enterohepatic recirculation of metabolites may lead to increased drug level.

Elimination half-life varies greatly, ranging from short (diclofenac, 1 hour) to intermediate (ketorolac, 5 hours) to long (piroxicam, 50 hours).

Two pro-drugs are available. Sulindac is metabolized in the liver to active sulindac sulfide, which is directly eliminated in the feces. Nabumetone is absorbed in the duodenum and metabolized in the liver to an active form, which does not undergo enterohepatic circulation and thus has little effect on the stomach.

Among this large group of drugs, parenteral formulations are only available for indomethacin, diclofenac, and ketorolac, thus greatly limiting the choice when oral intake may not be possible or desired (Table 17-1).

THE ANALGESIC ACTION OF NSAIDs

Analgesia by NSAIDs has been attributed primarily to peripheral inhibition of COX and decreased level of prostaglandins. The inhibition can be reversible (e.g., by ibuprofen) or irreversible (e.g., by aspirin). Future selective COX-2 inhibitors may permit a lower incidence of renal and gastrointestinal complications. Inhibition of lipoxygenase and leukotriene production also contribute to peripheral analgesia. NSAIDs may also directly uncouple membrane receptor and G-protein–mediated signal transduction. Finally, there may be central antinociceptive action by a decrease in central prostaglandin synthesis, an opioid-like effect, a decrease in central

TABLE 17–1. COMMONLY AVAILABLE NSAIDs

Chemical Group	Chemical Name	Sample Trade Names
Carboxylic acids		
Salicylic acids and esters	Aspirin	(Various)
	Diflunisal	Dolobid
Acetic acids		
Phenylacetic acid	Diclofenac	Voltaren
	Bromfenac	Duract
Carbocyclic and	Indomethacin	Indocin
heterocyclic acetic	Sulindac	Clinoril
acids	Tolmetin	Tolectin
	Ketorolac	Toradol
	Etodolac	Lodine
Propionic acids	Ibuprofen	Motrin, Advil
	Flurbiprofen	Ansaid
	Naproxen	Naprosyn
	Ketoprofen	Orudis
	Fenoprofen	Nalfon
	Oxaprozin	Daypro
Fenamic acids	Mefenamic	Ponstel
	Meclofenamic	Meclomen
Enolic acids		
Pyrazolidines	Phenylbutazone	Butazolidin
Oxicams	Piroxicam	Feldene
Nonacidic	Nabumetone	Relafen
Phenols	Acetaminophen	Tylenol

serotoninergic mechanism, and a decrease in spinal *N*-methyl-D-aspartate excitatory mechanism.

The analgesic effect of NSAIDs bears no direct relationship to the anti-inflammatory potency. For example, acetaminophen has little peripheral anti-inflammatory effect, but it is an effective analgesic and antipyretic. Ketorolac is designed primarily as a potent analgesic for short-term treatment.

CLINICAL ANALGESIC EFFECTS

The absence of significant depressant effect on respiration, cardiac function, and sensorium is the major advantage of NSAIDs over opioid analgesics in treatment of acute pain. For mild to moderate acute pain, such as minor musculoskeletal trauma, soft tissue inflammation, and pain after dental procedures, superficial surgery, and minor gynecologic procedures, NSAIDs are efficacious and comparable to opioid analgesics, although the onset is typically delayed by 15 to 30 minutes. NSAIDs are also effective against ureteric colic, including that after extracorporeal shock wave lithotripsy.

NSAIDs appear to exhibit a "ceiling effect" in analgesic efficacy and are clearly less effective than opioid analgesics for patients who have undergone major surgical procedures. Even so, they may reduce both visual analogue pain scores and postoperative opioid requirements and permit a more rapid return of bowel function.

The usefulness of NSAIDs (such as ketorolac) as the sole analgesic agent during balanced anesthesia is hampered by the delayed onset of action, lack of parenteral formulation, and variable potencies. Administering NSAIDs prior to or during surgery may, however, compensate for the delayed onset of analgesia postopera-

tively, and takes advantage of the opioid-sparing effect, which reduces adverse effects such as respiratory depression and nausea. NSAIDs can significantly improve analgesia in the early postoperative period, especially for ambulatory surgery patients. The efficacy of the NSAID depends on the timing, route of administration, and type of surgical procedure.

Because regional anesthesia results in profound analgesia, the peripheral anti-nociceptive action of NSAIDs provides negligible additional pain relief in the presence of local anesthetic-induced analgesia. However, when administration of local anesthetics results in less than profound analgesia (or if the local anesthetic effects are resolving), the use of NSAIDs may provide additional pain relief. NSAIDs have also been used as adjuvants to epidural and intrathecal opioid analgesia and morphine patient-controlled analgesia (PCA) to lower pain scores and reduce postoperative opioid requirement.

ADVERSE EFFECTS OF NSAIDs

Nonselective inhibition of ubiquitous COX has widespread consequences. Clinical data on adverse effects are usually derived from long-term use of NSAIDs, and direct applicability to short-term use in acute pain situations is unproved.

Renal Function

Prostaglandins are closely involved in the maintenance of renal blood flow, glomerular filtration, renin and aldosterone release, and sodium and potassium homeostasis. When renal perfusion is threatened by plasma volume depletion and/or increased circulating neurohumoral vasoconstrictors, COX inhibition may lead to acute deterioration of renal function. Hyporeninemic hyperkalemia, water retention, and hyponatremia are also seen. The effect of concomitant diuretics may be antagonized. Other adverse effects seen with more chronic use of NSAIDs include interstitial nephritis, papillary necrosis, and chronic renal failure.

Hemostasis

Reversible or irreversible inhibition of platelet COX decreases thromboxane A_2 synthesis. Platelet aggregability and hemostatic function are impaired, which may manifest as elevated bleeding time. The duration of such abnormality depends on the NSAID used. For reversible inhibitors, the duration ranges from 30 hours (ketorolac) to 12 days (piroxicam). For irreversible inhibitors of platelet COX (such as aspirin), return to normal hemostatic function would depend on the replacement of existing platelets by newly formed platelets. In the perioperative period, surgical hemostasis, safety of central neuraxial block, and the superimposed threat of gastric erosion are of concern. Except for increased bleeding after tonsillectomy in children who received ketorolac, data demonstrating increased surgical bleeding are scarce.

Presence of abnormal platelet function due to prior

intake of NSAIDs would contraindicate central neuraxial blockade. The safety of administering NSAIDs after a regional block has been established is still controversial.

Gastrointestinal Effect

Gastrointestinal symptoms constitute the most frequent complications of NSAID treatment. Chronic NSAID treatment is associated with de novo gastroduodenal ulceration as well as exacerbation of peptic ulcer disease (preventable by misoprostol, a prostaglandin analogue) and increase in ulcer complication, such as perforation and hemorrhage. The risk of ulceration and hemorrhage during a short course of treatment in the acute pain setting is unknown. Cumulative uncontrolled data suggest that in the absence of preexisting peptic ulcer disease, the risk is minimal.

Other Effects

Prostaglandins counteract the bronchoconstrictive effect of leukotrienes. NSAIDs have the potential to trigger acute attacks in asthmatics, and there is cross-sensitivity in patients who have aspirin intolerance or the aspirin triad: aspirin intolerance, asthma, and nasal polyps.

During long-term use, NSAIDs can exacerbate systemic hypertension or interfere with antihypertensive treatment. The effect during a short course of treatment is probably small.

By interfering with synthesis of connective tissue, cartilage, and bone, NSAIDs have the potential to interfere with wound healing and healing of bony fractures and prostheses.

CONTRAINDICATIONS TO NSAIDs

1. Known allergy to aspirin and/or other NSAIDs
2. Active erosive gastrointestinal disease: peptic ulcer and inflammatory bowel disease
3. Concomitant anticoagulation
4. Intrinsic renal disease and insufficiency
5. Contracted intravascular volume with high renal vascular tone: uncontrolled hypertension, severe congestive heart failure, cirrhosis with ascites, hypovolemia
6. Asthma and nasal polyps, chronic urticaria

SPECIAL CIRCUMSTANCES
Pregnant and Lactating Women

Due to the importance of prostaglandins in gestation, fetal development, and fetal circulation, NSAIDs are contraindicated during pregnancy as analgesics. In addition, prenatal exposure to NSAIDs has been linked to development of renal failure in neonates.

NSAIDs are excreted in human milk in minimal but variable amounts. NSAIDs with shorter half-lives and that form no active metabolites (e.g., ibuprofen and diclofenac) are preferable for the lactating patient.

Children

Acetaminophen, aspirin, and ibuprofen are the most commonly used. The analgesic profile of parenteral ketorolac, in a dosage of 0.5 mg/kg, is similar to that seen in adults. Currently, ketorolac is not recommended for use in children.

The Elderly

Significant decrease in clearance and increased plasma half-life is seen with many NSAIDs. With long-term use, the risk of complications (especially gastrointestinal and renal) is increased in the elderly. The risk (vs. the benefit of opioid-sparing effect) of short-term use in acute pain is unclear.

BIBLIOGRAPHY

Bennett WM, Henrich WL, Stoff JS: The renal effects of nonsteroidal anti-inflammatory drugs: Summary and recommendations. Am J Kidney Dis 28(suppl 1):S63–S70, 1996.

Cashman JN: The mechanisms of action of NSAIDs in analgesia. Drugs 52:(suppl 5):13–23, 1996.

Code W: NSAIDs and balanced analgesia (editorial). Can J Anaesth 40:401–405, 1993.

Coderre TJ, Melzack R: The contribution of excitatory aminoacids to central sensitization and persistent nociception after formalin-induced tissue injury. J Neurosci 12:3665–670, 1992.

Dahl JB, Kehlet H: Non-steroidal anti-inflammatory drugs: Rationale for use in severe postoperative pain. Br J Anaesth 66:703–712, 1991.

Gillis JC, Brogden RN: Ketorolac: A reappraisal of its pharmacodynamic and pharmacokinetic properties and therapeutic use in pain management. Drugs 53:139–188, 1997.

Kehlet H, Dahl JB: The value of "multimodal" or "balanced analgesia" in postoperative pain treatment. Anesth Analg 77:1048–1056, 1993.

McCormack K, Brune K: Dissociation between the antinociceptive and anti-inflammatory effects of the non-steroidal anti-inflammatory drugs. Drugs 41:533–547, 1991.

Souter AJ, Fredman B, White PF: Controversies in the perioperative use of nonsteroidal antiinflammatory drugs. Anesth Analg 79:1178–1190, 1994.

Woolf CJ: Recent advances in the pathophysiology of acute pain. Br J Anaesth 63:139–146, 1989.

Chapter 18

Muscle Relaxants

Onur Melen, M.D.

Muscle relaxants are a pharmacologically diverse group of agents that are used for various medical purposes. They may be classified into the three following broad categories:

1. Neuromuscular blocking agents, which are used as an adjunct to general anesthesia to facilitate endotracheal intubation and muscle relaxation during surgery and mechanical ventilation
2. Antispasticity drugs, which are indicated for treatment of spasticity and associated, sometimes painful, flexor and extensor spasms due to disorders of the central nervous system (CNS)
3. Drugs that are useful in short-term relief of pain and muscle spasm associated with acute musculoskeletal conditions.

This chapter discusses the drugs in the second and third categories.

ANTISPASTICITY DRUGS

Spasticity is an involuntary increase in muscle tone that occurs during muscle stretch. It is defined as a motor disorder characterized by an increase in tonic stretch reflexes, exaggerated tendon jerks, cutaneous nociceptive and flexor withdrawal reflexes, Babinski's response, and contractures. Its pathophysiology is not entirely clear. Spasticity is mediated peripherally by muscle spindle primary Ia fibers, which mediate monosynaptic reflex arc, and centrally through reticulospinal and vestibulospinal pathways. Accumulating evidence suggests that spasticity is primarily caused by long-term reduction in inhibition rather than in increase in excitation of α motor neurons. Current hypotheses suggest that decreased presynaptic inhibition of primary Ia afferent terminals, decreased reciprocal inhibition of antagonist motor neurons, and decreased nonreciprocal inhibition and dysfunction of Ia inhibitory interneurons are causes of spasticity. Presynaptic inhibition is mediated by synapses activated by γ-aminobutyric acid (GABA), a major inhibitory neurotransmitter in CNS. GABA re-

duces the amount of neurotransmitter released by Ia fiber terminals and inhibits sensory signals from muscle spindles. Glycine is a neurotransmitter released by inhibitory interneurons and is found to be reduced in spastic experimental animals.

Drugs that reduce spasticity act either centrally to enhance inhibitory neurotransmission (e.g., benzodiazepines, baclofen, tizanidine) or peripherally on contractile elements of the skeletal muscle (e.g., dantrolene).

Benzodiazepines

Benzodiazepines have unique pharmacodynamic and pharmacokinetic properties that allow their use for various therapeutic purposes. They are administered as sedatives, anxiolytics, hypnotics, anticonvulsants, and muscle relaxants. Only diazepam (Valium) and, to a much lesser extent, clonazepam (Klonopin) are used as muscle relaxants.

Mechanism of Action

The effects of benzodiazepines virtually all result from their action on the CNS. They exert their antispastic function by enhancing presynaptic inhibition in the spinal cord. Their targets are inhibitory neurotransmitter receptors that are directly activated by GABA. Experiments have demonstrated that benzodiazepines act presynaptically to facilitate the release of GABA and its binding to a subtype GABA receptor, GABA-A, which forms an integral part of multiple units of ligand-gated chloride channels. Most of the rapid inhibitory transmission in CNS is believed to be mediated by these chloride channels.[1, 2] Benzodiazepines are considered to be indirect GABA-ergic agents. They increase the gain of inhibitory transmission mediated by GABA-A receptors.[3, 4] As a result, the chloride channels open within the receptor-chloride channel complex, and chloride ion currents are magnified and inhibition of neurotransmission achieved. Benzodiazepines require normally functioning synapses to exert their action, which can be blocked by the GABA-A receptor antagonist bicuculline.

Diazepam is the only benzodiazepine to have found widespread use as a muscle relaxant. It can be administered alone or in combination with other muscle relaxants. It is most effective in patients with spinal cord disease and injury, but less so in those with cerebral palsy and spastic hemiplegia due to stroke. Painful, persistent, and disabling muscle spasms seem to respond to diazepam better than do periodic flexor spasms. In addition, diazepam is valuable in the treatment of tetanus, stiff-man syndrome, and occasionally in alleviating local muscle spasm and pain due to trauma, inflammatory joint disease, and radiculopathy. Diazepam induces hypotonia without interfering with locomotion, but it often produces loss of muscle strength. This side effect, along with its potential to cause somnolence, dizziness, and excessive sedation, makes nonambulatory patients better candidates for treatment with diazepam.

Pharmacokinetics, Dose, and Toxicity

Diazepam is absorbed from the gastrointestinal system, reaching the effective blood level in 30 minutes and the peak level within 3 hours. The half-life of a single dose is about 8 hours. It is detoxified by the liver and excreted in urine and feces. It crosses the placenta and is found in breast milk.

The usual starting dose of oral diazepam is 2 mg, twice daily. Depending on the patient's sensitivity and tolerance, the dose can be raised by increments of 2 to 4 mg/week to a maximum total daily dose of 20 to 30 mg. Smaller doses are often not very effective in reducing the muscle tone, but most patients do not show good tolerance of doses higher than 15 to 20 mg, no matter how slowly the dose is raised. Limiting side effects are dizziness, somnolence, lassitude, confusion, increased reaction time, memory loss, ataxia, and digestive disturbance. Sometimes adverse psychological effects are encountered, such as anxiety, irritability, euphoria, hypomania, depression, paranoia, and suicidal ideation. Concomitant use of CNS-acting drugs, such as baclofen, anticonvulsants, barbiturates, and narcotics, potentiate the side effects. Long-term use of diazepam carries the risk of dependence. Incidence of allergic and hematologic reactions and hepatotoxicity is low. Abrupt termination of diazepam therapy may lead to serious withdrawal symptoms, including delirium and seizures.[5, 6] Parenterally administered diazepam has little role in the long-term treatment of spasticity, but it is valuable in tetanus.

Baclofen (Lioresal)

Mechanism of Action

Baclofen (4-amino-3-[4-chlorophenyl]-butanoic acid) is structurally similar to GABA. It is a GABA-B receptor agonist. Baclofen is an overall powerful neuronal depressant that exerts its action by binding to presynaptic GABA-B receptors in the dorsal horn of the spinal cord and the brain stem and at other CNS sites. The site of its antispastic action is the spinal cord. By binding to GABA-B receptors, it suppresses the release of excita-tory neurotransmitters and inhibits excitatory afferent terminals that are involved in monosynaptic and poly-synaptic reflex activity at the spinal level.[7-9] In high concentrations, baclofen may block the postsynaptic action of excitatory neurotransmitters.[10] In addition, baclofen appears to have an inhibitory effect on the release of excitatory neurotransmitters from nociceptive afferent nerve endings that originate in the skin.[11]

Baclofen is indicated and is particularly useful in the treatment of spasticity of spinal cord origin. Patients with cord injury and multiple sclerosis are prime candidates. The efficacy of baclofen in the treatment of spastic hemiplegia due to various cerebral lesions is far less certain. Some patients with generalized or cervical dystonia, upper motor neuron disease, and stiff-man syndrome may partially benefit from baclofen. It provides long-term reduction in spasticity and decreases the frequency of flexor spasms in addition to alleviating the pain associated with them. Reduction of flexor spasms at night allows patients to enjoy uninterrupted sleep. Bladder and bowel function may benefit from baclofen. Release of adductor and flexor contractions facilitates nursing care. Modest muscle weakness is observed in some patients, but baclofen has little overall effect on locomotion.

Antispastic effects of baclofen and diazepam are similar. Baclofen is preferred over diazepam because it causes less sedation, which allows its use at maximum effective doses.

Pharmacokinetics, Dose, and Toxicity

Baclofen is available in 10-mg tablets. Usual starting dose is 5 mg, three times a day. The dose can be doubled every 3 to 4 days to a maximum daily dose of 80 mg, if needed and tolerated.

In a single dose, baclofen is rapidly absorbed. The serum half-life is about 4 hours. About 30% is bound to serum proteins and deaminated in the liver. The remainder is excreted unchanged in the urine and feces. Only a small fraction crosses the blood-brain barrier.

Baclofen is a safe drug and is tolerated well even in large doses. Somnolence and dizziness are the most frequent side effects, and with larger doses, confusion, ataxia, and even hallucinations may appear, especially in patients with cerebral lesions. Rarely does baclofen trigger seizure activity in epileptic patients. Abrupt withdrawal should be avoided because of the risk of increased flexor spasms, hallucinations, and seizures.

Because of low lipid solubility, baclofen does not cross the blood-brain barrier in sufficient amount to reach high concentrations in cerebrospinal fluid (CSF), even when given in large oral doses. Devices have been developed to deliver baclofen directly to the target sites in the spinal cord. Administering baclofen intrathecally offers the advantage of achieving rapid and sustainable effective CSF levels and reaching the receptor sites in the spinal cord without risking systemic side effects.

Intrathecal baclofen is delivered using an infusion system that consists of an implantable pump, an intrathecal catheter, and an external programmer with a programmer head. The pump is implanted into the abdominal wall, and the catheter is inserted into the lumbar intrathecal space. Communication with the pump is accomplished via a radiotelemetric link between the external programmer and the pump. Dosage titration can be selected with the programmer. Before placement of the pump, a trial dose is given, and the patient is observed for several hours. If decreased spasticity is observed, the patient is selected for pump placement.

Intrathecal baclofen is effective in reducing spasticity in patients with spinal cord injury and multiple sclerosis.[12, 13] Its usefulness in cerebral palsy, spastic hemiplegia due to stroke or cerebral injury, upper motor neuron disease, and dystonia has not yet been fully established.

Although intrathecal baclofen often eliminates the need for other antispasticity medications, it can still be used in conjunction with others in selected patients. Rare complications of intrathecal baclofen therapy include drowsiness, orthostatic hypotension, and pump-related complications such as malfunction, kinking, dislodgment, disconnection, breakage, and wound infections.

Dantrolene (Dantrium)

Mechanism of Action

Dantrolene is structurally an imidazoline derivative and is classified as a direct-acting muscle relaxant. Its primary action is on contractile elements of the muscle. Although some of its side effects, such as mental depression, confusion, and dizziness, suggest CNS effect, the central antispastic property of dantrolene has not been identified.

In resting muscle, calcium is stored in sarcoplasmic reticulum. For muscle contraction to take place, calcium has to be released from sarcoplasmic reticulum to activate myosin adenosine triphosphatase (ATPase) and excitation-contraction coupling. Dantrolene blocks the release of calcium and dissociates excitation-contraction coupling, leading to hypotonia and muscle weakness.[14] Heightened reflex activity and clonus are also reduced. Unless it is given in very large doses, the effect of dantrolene on myocardium and smooth muscle is negligible.

Dantrolene is primarily used to treat spasticity. It is indicated in patients with spinal cord injury, multiple sclerosis, cerebral palsy, and stroke. It is of particular benefit to patients who are nonambulatory and have prolonged muscle contractions due to chronic spasticity. Relief of spasticity and fixed contractions aids nursing care, enhances physical rehabilitation, and restores residual function. Ambulatory patients benefit less from dantrolene, because the induced muscle weakness interferes with the patient's ability to ambulate. Dantrolene is not indicated in the treatment of skeletal muscle spasm and pain resulting from rheumatologic disorders.

Pharmacokinetics, Dose, and Toxicity

Oral dantrolene is absorbed slowly and incompletely. It is metabolized by the liver to hydroxyl and amino derivatives and excreted in the urine. Risk of physical dependence and tolerance is low.

Standard oral starting dose for treatment of chronic spasticity is 25 mg, twice daily. If needed, the dose can be raised to a maximum daily dose of 400 mg over a period of 3 to 4 weeks. If no response is demonstrated after a month, the drug should be discontinued.

The most frequent side effects of dantrolene are drowsiness, dizziness, muscle weakness, and occasional fatal or nonfatal hepatotoxicity. It is advisable to conduct liver function tests before initiating therapy and monitor liver function through the course of treatment.

Intravenous dantrolene is indicated in the treatment of malignant hyperthermia, a potentially life-threatening condition triggered by succinylcholine and inhalation anesthetics.

Oral or intravenous dantrolene is a useful adjunct to dopamine agonists in the treatment of neuroleptic malignant syndrome, brought about by dopamine-depleting agents, such as psychotropic drugs. The syndrome is characterized by encephalopathy, muscle rigidity, fever, autonomic disturbance, leukocytosis, and elevated creatine phosphokinase concentration. By its direct action on the muscle, dantrolene reduces muscle rigidity and limits muscle fiber breakdown and elevation of creatine phosphokinase levels.[16, 17]

Tizanidine (Zanaflex)

Mechanism of Action

Tizanidine is a newly introduced muscle relaxant. Structurally it is an imidazoline derivative. Pharmacologically it is a centrally acting α_2-adrenergic agonist. Because of pharmacologic and clinical evidence of its concomitant antinociceptive properties, it has gained acceptance in the treatment of both spasticity and rheumatologic conditions associated with painful muscle spasm.[18]

Animal experiments have revealed that tizanidine suppresses polysynaptic excitation of dorsal horn neurons in the spinal cord and depresses polysynaptic reflexes and spontaneous neuronal activity, probably by reducing the release of excitatory neurotransmitters from presynaptic sites.[19]

Tizanidine exhibits high affinity for α_2-adrenergic receptors. This property, along with the structural similarity of tizanidine to the α_2-agonist clonidine (which has a mild antispastic action of its own), raises the possibility that the muscle relaxant function is at least partly mediated by the adrenergic system. The action of tizanidine may include inhibition on locus ceruleus firing and subsequent inhibition of the cerulospinal pathways, which normally exert a facilitatory effect on synaptic activity in the spinal cord. Finally, evidence suggests possible postsynaptic action at excitatory amino acid receptors.[19] Because of its unique and various actions at different levels, tizanidine induces hypotonia without undue muscle weakness.

Animal studies have demonstrated antinociceptive activity of tizanidine, mediated by inhibition of A- and C-fiber activity, as well as selective inhibition of dorsal horn neurons to nociceptive stimulation.[20, 21]

Well-controlled studies have revealed the effectiveness of tizanidine as an antispastic agent in about a third to half of patients with multiple sclerosis, spinal cord injury, motor neuron disease, and stroke.[22, 23] It is most beneficial in reducing the frequency of muscle spasms and clonus, but is less consistent in improving the muscle tone. Assessments of neurologic functions and functional disability scores have failed to reveal consistent and significant treatment effects. Tizanidine provided little impact on scores of activities of daily living. When compared with baclofen, the results with tizanidine were about equal in most parameters assessed, except tizanidine caused less muscle weakness. Comparison with diazepam favors tizanidine in all parameters, including side effects (particularly sedation). Tizanidine was better tolerated than diazepam and baclofen.[24]

Tizanidine is supplied in 4-mg tablets. It is completely absorbed through the gastrointestinal tract, and has a half-life of approximately 2.5 hours. Peak plasma levels are reached in 1.5 hours after a single dose. It is 30% bound to plasma proteins, metabolized by the liver, and excreted in the urine and feces.

Reported side effects include asthenia, headache, digestive disturbance, somnolence, dry mouth, and hallucinations. About 80% of patients complain of at least one of the side effects, and 25% discontinue taking it. Although blood pressure and pulse rate are not adversely affected by tizanidine, it is recommended to administer the drug very carefully with other antihypertensive agents and not with other α_2-agonists. No consistent hematologic crises have been encountered in clinical trials, but mild elevations of liver enzymes have been observed.

The recommended starting dose is 4 mg, once daily. The dose may be raised in increments of 4 to 6 mg/week to a total daily regimen of 36 mg. Tizanidine can be used as a single agent or given in combination with diazepam or baclofen, although the efficacy of the combination doesn't differ significantly from that of the single agent. In some patients, combination therapy may offer long-term benefit if it allows reduction of each medication's daily dose and, therefore, its side effects.

Clonidine (Catapres)

Clonidine is another α_2-agonist that has antispastic action. Because of its effect on the cardiovascular system, it is not widely used to treat spasticity.

DRUGS USED IN SHORT-TERM RELIEF OF PAIN AND MUSCLE SPASM

Cyclobenzaprine Hydrochloride (Flexeril)

Cyclobenzaprine is a tricyclic amine salt. It relieves skeletal muscle spasm of local origin without interfering with muscle strength. It is indicated for relief of muscle spasm and pain associated with acute, painful musculoskeletal conditions. It is ineffective in spasticity due to CNS disease. Cyclobenzaprine does not act directly on

muscle or neuromuscular junction. Studies indicate that the primary action of cyclobenzaprine is on the brain stem. Pharmacologic studies in animals show a similarity between the effects of cyclobenzaprine and those of tricyclic antidepressants, such as norepinephrine potentiation, sedation, and peripheral and central anticholinergic effects. Cyclobenzaprine improves signs and symptoms of skeletal muscle spasm, reduces local pain and tenderness, and helps increase the range of motion. It is recommended for short-term therapy, as information is not available on its long-term effectiveness. Cyclobenzaprine is available in 10-mg tablets. The standard daily dose is 30 to 40 mg, taken for 2 to 3 weeks. The most common side effects are drowsiness, dizziness, and dry mouth. It may interact with monoamine oxidase (MAO) inhibitors.

Chlorzoxazone (Paraflex)

Chlorzoxazone is a centrally acting agent, although its exact mode of action has not been clearly identified. Experimental data suggest that the primary site of action is the spinal cord, where it inhibits polysynaptic reflex pathways that are involved in the production of increased muscle tone.

Chlorzoxazone is indicated for short-term treatment of muscle spasm associated with acute, painful musculoskeletal conditions. Spasticity due to CNS disease is not relieved by this agent.

Chlorzoxazone is available in 250-mg caplets. The usual effective dose is 1000 to 2000 mg/day. It is generally well tolerated; rare side effects include digestive disturbance, dizziness, drowsiness, and hepatotoxicity.

Carisoprodol (Soma)

Carisoprodol produces muscle relaxation, probably by inhibiting interneuronal activity in the descending reticular activating system and spinal cord. Some of its effect may be related to its sedative action. No direct action on skeletal muscle or neuromuscular junction has been identified.

Carisoprodol is recommended for use of relief of discomfort and pain in acute musculoskeletal conditions. It is not indicated to treat spasticity.

Carisoprodol is marketed in 350-mg tablets. A combination of 200 mg of carisoprodol and 325 mg of aspirin is also available. The usual recommended daily dose is 350 mg, three to four times daily. The most frequent side effects are drowsiness, ataxia, tremor, irritability, insomia, confusion, and disorientation. An occasional patient may experience tachycardia and postural hypotension.

Methocarbamol (Robaxin, Robaxisal)

The mechanism of action of methocarbamol is not clear. Although it is primarily used for relief of discomfort associated with acute painful musculoskeletal conditions, methocarbamol has no proven muscle-relaxant effect. It is believed that methocarbamol acts as a primary CNS depressant.

Methocarbamol is available in 500- and 750-mg tablets. The usual recommended daily dose is 3 to 4 g. Side effects include drowsiness, light-headedness, dizziness, and nausea.

REFERENCES

1. Ragan CI, McKernan RM, Wafford K, et al: Gamma-aminobutyric acid-A (GABA-A) receptor/ion channel complex. Biochem Soc Trans 21:622–626, 1993.
2. Twyman RE, Rogers CJ, Macdonald RL: Differential regulation of gamma-aminobutyric acid receptor channels by diazepam and phenobarbital. Ann Neurol 25:213–220, 1989.
3. Biggio G, Costa E (eds): Symposium: GABA and benzodiazepine receptor subtypes: Molecular biology, pharmacology and clinical aspects. Adv Biochem Psychopharmacol 46:1–239, 1990.
4. Pole P: Electrophysiology of benzodiazepine receptor ligands: Multiple mechanisms and sites of action. Prog Neurobiol 31:349–423, 1988.
5. Roth T, Roches TA: Issues in the use of benzodiazepine therapy. J Clin Psychiatry 53 (suppl 6):14–18, 1992.
6. Woods JH, Katz JL, Winger G: Benzodiazepines: Use, abuse and consequences. Pharmacol Rev 4:15–347, 1992.
7. Bowery NG, Hill DR, Hudson AL, et al: Baclofen decreases neurotransmitter release in the mammalian CNS by action at a novel GABA receptor. Nature 283:92–94, 1980.
8. Krain JS, Penn RD, Bissinger RL, et al: Reduced spinal reflexes following intrathecal baclofen in the rabbit. Exp Brain Res 54:191–194, 1984.
9. Mueller H, Zierski J, Drake D, et al: The effect of intrathecal baclofen in electrical muscle activity in spasticity. J Neurol 234:348–352, 1987.
10. Blaxter TJ, Carlen PL: Pre- and post-synaptic effects of baclofen in the rat hippocampal slices. Brain Res 341:195–199, 1985.
11. Hwang AS, Wilcox GL: Baclofen, gamma aminobutyric acid B receptors and substance P in the mouse spinal cord. J Pharmacol Exp Ther 248:1026–1033, 1989.
12. Penn RD: Intrathecal baclofen for spasticity of spinal origin: Seven years of experience. J Neurosurg 77:236–240, 1992.
13. Coffey RJ, Cahill D, Steers W, et al: Intrathecal baclofen for intractable spasticity of spinal origin: Results of a long-term multicenter study. J Neurosurg 78:226–232, 1993.
14. Van Winkle WB: Calcium release from skeletal muscle sarcoplasmic reticulum: Site of action of dantrolene sodium? Science 193:1130–1131, 1976.
15. Rosenberg H, Fletcher JE: Malignant hyperthermia. In Azar I (ed): Muscle Relaxants: Side Effects and Rational Approach to Selection (clinical pharmacology series), vol 7. New York, Marcel Dekker, 1987, pp 115–148.
16. Addonizio G, Susman VL, Roth SD: Neuroleptic malignant syndrome: Review of analysis of 115 cases. Biol Psychiatry 22:1004–1020, 1987.
17. Pearlman CA: Neuroleptic malignant syndrome: A review of the literature. J Clin Psychopharmacol 6:257–273, 1986.
18. Coward DM: Tizanidine: Neuropharmacology and mechanism of action: Neurology 44 (suppl 9):6–11, 1994.
19. Davies J: Selective depression of synaptic transmission of spinal neurons in the cat by a new, centrally acting muscle relaxant, 5-chloro- 4- (2 imidazolin-2-yl-amino) -2, 1, 3, -benzothiadiazole (DS 103-282). Br J Pharmacol 76:473–481, 1982.
20. Davies J, Johnston SE: Selective antinociceptive effects of tizanidine (DS 103-282), a centrally acting muscle relaxant on dorsal horn neurons in the feline spinal cord. Br J Pharmacol 82:409–421, 1984.
21. Villanueva L, Chitour D, LeBars D: Effects of tizanidine (DS 103-282) on dorsal horn convergent neurons in the rat. Pain 35:187–197, 1988.
22. Smith C, Birnbaum G, Carter JL, et al and U.S. Tizanidine Study Group: Tizanidine treatment of spasticity caused by multiple sclerosis: Results of a double-blind, placebo-controlled trial. Neurology 44 (suppl 9):34–43, 1994.
23. Nance PW, Baugaresti J, Shellenberger K, et al, and the North American Tizanidine Study Group: Efficacy and safety of tizanidine in the treatment of spasticity in patients with spinal cord injury. Neurology 44 (suppl 9):44–52, 1994.
24. Lataste X, Emre M, Davis C, et al: Comparative profile of tizanidine in the management of spasticity. Neurology 44 (suppl 9):53–59, 1994.

Therapeutic Interventions

Chapter 19

● Diagnostic Nerve Blocks

Robert E. Molloy, M.D.

It is important to make as exact a diagnosis as possible in patients with persistent pain. A complete history in a patient with chronic pain will include a detailed history of the pain problem and a review of all previous diagnostic testing and therapeutic interventions. After a careful pain-oriented physical examination and formulation of a differential diagnosis, any necessary specialty consultations and laboratory or radiologic studies should be obtained. Psychological testing by an expert in the field is necessary to make an accurate psychological assessment and diagnosis. At this point, a specific diagnosis can be made and an appropriate treatment plan instituted, without the use of diagnostic blocks in most circumstances.[1,2]

Classically, differential nerve blocks have been recommended as an objective diagnostic tool that can differentiate among the various mechanisms by which pain is mediated in a particular patient in whom diagnosis has proven to be difficult.[3,4] Differential neural blockade is reported to quickly and precisely differentiate among sympathetic, somatic, and central or psychogenic pain mechanisms in the vast majority of cases.[5] Two basic approaches to differential neural block have been outlined by Winnie: a pharmacologic approach and an anatomic approach. The pharmacologic approach is best represented by the differential spinal block.[6-8] This technique presumes that the concentration of local anesthetic required to block spinal nerve fibers is directly proportional to the fibers' diameters. Therefore, increasing concentrations of local anesthetic will block specific nerve fibers in this order: (1) preganglionic sympathetic; (2) somatic pain and temperature; and (3) motor, touch, and proprioception. In the classic technique, four solutions are injected: (1) saline, (2) 0.25% procaine, (3) 0.5% procaine, and (4) 1% procaine. Response to each of these solutions is interpreted as a response, respectively, to placebo, sympathetic, somatic sensory, and motor blocks (Table 19-1). This technique has been modified by Winnie to include only placebo and 5% procaine injections. The interpretation differs from that of the classic technique only when the second injection relieves pain: a somatic mechanism is diagnosed when

pain returns with return of sensation, and a sympathetic mechanism is identified when pain relief persists well after analgesia resolves. The pharmacologic approach may be used with spinal, epidural, or plexus blockade.

The anatomic approach uses three injections: a placebo, a sympathetic block, and a somatic sensory and motor block. The second injection is made at sites where the sympathetic fibers are anatomically separate from sensory and motor fibers and can thus be blocked independently. The various sympathetic and somatic block procedures vary depending on the painful area to be evaluated (Table 19-2). The responses to these blocks are interpreted in a similar fashion to those of differential spinal block. The anatomic approach has been preferred for better differentiation of sympathetic from somatic pain mechanisms and for pain located in the upper body. The pharmacologic (epidural) approach may be preferred for thoracic pain to avoid the risk of pneumothorax with diagnostic paravertebral blocks. Differential nerve blocks have been recommended for patients with intractable pain who exhibit no demonstrable cause of pain.

The current role of nerve blockade for diagnostic purposes is, in fact, fairly limited.[1] Nerve blocks do not allow for diagnosis of specific disease states, either physical or psychological. Nerve blocks may be used as

TABLE 19-1. CLASSIC DIFFERENTIAL SPINAL BLOCK INTERPRETATION

Solution	Blockade	Pain Relief	Interpretation
Saline	None	If yes	Placebo responder or psychogenic mechanism
0.25% Procaine	Sympathetic	If yes	Sympathetic mechanism
0.5% Procaine	Sensory	If yes	Somatic mechanism, organic pain
1% (5%) Procaine	Motor	If none	Central mechanism*

*Implies a CNS lesion, psychogenic pain, malingering, or central encephalization of peripheral mechanism
Data from Winnie and Collins,[3] Ramamurthy and Winnie,[4] and Winnie.[5]

TABLE 19–2. ANATOMIC APPROACH TO DIAGNOSTIC
NERVE BLOCKS

Painful Area	Order of Blocks: First After Placebo	Sympathetic Block	Somatic Block
Head	Sympathetic	Stellate ganglion	Greater occipital nerve, trigeminal nerve
Neck	Sympathetic	Stellate ganglion	Cervical plexus
Arm	Sympathetic	Stellate ganglion	Brachial plexus
Chest	Somatic	Thoracic sympathetic (or epidural sympathetic)	Intercostal nerve
Abdomen	Somatic	Celiac plexus	Intercostal nerve
Pelvis	Somatic	Hypogastric plexus	Paravertebral somatic or intercostal nerve
Leg	Sympathetic	Lumbar sympathetic	Lumbar plexus and nerves, sacral plexus and nerves

Data from Winnie AP: Differential neural blockade for the diagnosis of pain mechanisms. *In* Waldman SD, Winnie AP (eds): Interventional Pain Management. Philadelphia, WB Saunders, 1996, p 129.

tools to assist in the overall evaluation of patients with chronic pain. They may provide some information about the source and other aspects of pain, such as the pathway by which it is mediated by nociceptive input. To provide an accurate conclusion about various components of the patient's pain, the observations derived from blocks must be combined with all other information obtained about the patient.

ROLE OF DIAGNOSTIC BLOCKS

In an excellent review of the appropriate use of diagnostic neural blockade, Boas and Cousins[1] have listed seven aspects of a patient's pain that may be profitably investigated with nerve blocks (Table 19–3); these are addressed in the following discussion.

Anatomic Location of Pain Source

Injection of local anesthetic into tender superficial or deep tissues may clearly delineate the source of pain. Examples include nerve entrapment syndromes, post-traumatic neuroma formation, myofascial trigger points, and focal muscle spasm. Prompt, complete pain relief on at least two occasions may confirm the diagnosis.

TABLE 19–3. DIAGNOSTIC NERVE BLOCKS

Questions to Be Addressed by Nerve Blocks

1. Anatomic location and source of pain
2. Visceral vs. somatic origin of trunk pain
3. Sympathetic vs. somatic origin of peripheral pain
4. Identify referred pain syndromes
5. Segmental levels of nociceptive input
6. Painful muscle spasm vs. fixed contracture deformity
7. Diagnosis of central pain states

Data from Boas RA, Cousins MJ: Diagnostic neural blockade. *In* Cousins MJ, Bridenbaugh PA (eds): Neural Blockade in Clinical Anesthesia and Management of Pain, ed 2. Philadelphia, JB Lippincott, 1988, p 885.

Similarly, deeper injection into painful joints or adjacent tissues may allow localization of the source of pain. Low back pain may be evaluated in this fashion with deep muscle, nerve root, and facet joint injections.[9-11] The potential for future use of more extensive diagnostic spinal nerve blocks has been reviewed by Stolker.[12] The efficacy of these diagnostic blocks has not been validated. Headache may be evaluated with occipital nerve block and muscle injections to distinguish cervicogenic from myofascial etiologies.[13] Again, repeated relief after local anesthetic injection into a specific deeper body structure can provide valuable diagnostic information.

Visceral vs. Somatic Trunk Pain

The origin of pain in the chest, abdomen, or pelvis can be investigated. A somatic source may be confirmed by injections into costochondral tissue, truncal muscles, or intercostal nerves. Persistent postoperative truncal wound pain may also be evaluated by muscle and neuroma infiltration. Rectus abdominis muscle entrapment of cutaneous nerves may also be isolated.[14] Pain relief after local injection or intercostal nerve block can identify somatic pain arising from the abdominal or thoracic wall rather than from visceral structures, as is often initially suspected.[15] If somatic pain cannot be confirmed with these blocks, a visceral source of pain can be presumed if a specific visceral pathologic lesion has been identified. When no disease process can be identified, celiac or hypogastric plexus blocks may be used to confirm that visceral pain is present, but they do not provide specific diagnostic information about the etiology of chronic visceral pain.

Sympathetic vs. Somatic Peripheral Pain

When sympathetic efferent activity is suspected to play an important role in a patient with chronic pain, sympathetic blocks may help to confirm the diagnosis. Diagnostic sympathetic blocks should be performed at anatomic sites separate from somatic nerve fibers. These include the cervicothoracic and lumbar sympathetic chain. Confirmation of pain relief and complete sympathetic block on two occasions with different local anesthetics may establish the presence of a sympathetically maintained pain state. Failure to obtain pain relief is consistent with sympathetically independent pain (SIP). This distinction is descriptive of a pattern of response with potential therapeutic implications; however, it does not indicate a separate disease process. Somatic blocks may assist in diagnosis of specific pain syndromes, such as local stump pain, myofascial pain, and meralgia paresthetica, as described previously. Differentiation of sympathetic from somatic pain by a pharmacologic approach, using incrementally increasing or gradually decreasing concentrations of local anesthetics intraspinally or at major nerve plexuses, has been described.[3-5] This approach has been challenged and is no longer considered reliable.[1] There does not appear to be a concentration of local anesthetic that produces complete block of all sympathetic fibers in the absence of any somatic sensory block.

Referred Pain States

Somatic-somatic pain referral patterns may be identified if injection of the original pain site simultaneously relieves pain in the referral zone. This phenomenon can be seen when medial branch nerve blocks for facet disease relieve distal buttock and thigh pain, or when injection of active trigger points for myofascial pain syndrome provides relief of distant somatic referred pain.

Segmental Levels of Nociceptive Input

Determining the spinal segments associated with somatic or visceral pain, coupled with a knowledge of the segmental innervation of body tissues, may indirectly aid in locating the bodily structures involved. Either paravertebral somatic or intercostal nerves may be progressively blocked until all pain is relieved. Repeated blocks with fluoroscopic guidance are essential to making an accurate diagnosis.

Central Pain States

Central pain arises from the brain or spinal cord. It may occur after a central lesion or as a result of abnormal central modulation of nociceptive and non-nociceptive input. Examples include thalamic syndrome after cerebrovascular accident and traumatic spinal cord injury. The classic response seen with a central pain state is inadequate analgesia after multiple peripheral blocks. Inadequate pain relief is expected after epidural anesthesia to a segmental level that supplies the painful area, as well as poor analgesia with systemic or intraspinal opioids. However, temporary relief of central pain has followed diagnostic spinal anesthesia, such as relief of lower but not upper extremity pain in a patient with painful hemiplegia after a cerebral infarction.[16] Neuropathic pain associated with lesions of the peripheral nervous system may also be associated with altered central processing of nociception. They are often relieved with spinal or plexus anesthesia, and they may have a partial response to opioid analgesics.[17,18] Both peripheral and central neuropathic pain may be relieved by intravenous local anesthetic administration.[19,20]

Psychogenic pain has been given an important place in the interpretation of differential blocks. Failure to relieve pain with complete sensory and motor block of the segmental levels associated with the painful area suggests the presence of supraspinal mechanisms. It does not of itself allow the specific diagnosis of either central pain or a psychogenic pain syndrome. Temporary pain relief after a placebo block is a common phenomenon, which allows only for the diagnosis of placebo responder. Observations of unusual responses, such as prolonged dramatic analgesia after a placebo injection, or the presence of excessive pain behaviors

may correlate with the clinical impression formed during the initial history and physical examination.

Prognostic Blocks

Local anesthetic blocks may be used to evaluate patients with cancer pain as potential candidates for neurolytic blocks, such as celiac plexus block for the visceral pain of pancreatic cancer.[2] Opioid or local anesthetic injections may help predict the response to an implanted apparatus for intraspinal drug administration in similar patients with cancer pain. A single block or repeated local anesthetic blocks may be used before a contemplated neurodestructive procedure is undertaken. Failure to obtain adequate analgesia will prevent an unnecessary operation. Once initial postblock analgesia is achieved, the patient can experience the extent of pain relief and the presence of any unpleasant side effects, such as numbness and dysesthesias prior to accepting a neurodestructive procedure. However, positive prognostic blocks do not reliably predict long-lasting analgesia, without deafferentation pain, after neurodestructive procedures in patients with chronic nonmalignant pain.[21,22]

TECHNIQUES OF DIAGNOSTIC BLOCK

Local infiltration of painful surgical scars, neuromas, or muscle trigger points may provide reliable diagnostic information about the patient's pain. Infiltration of the piriformis or scalene muscles may relieve apparent radicular lower or upper extremity pain that is due to nerve compression by muscle rather than to spinal pathologic lesion. Repeat lumbar facet joint injections may indicate facet syndrome, but this conclusion is controversial.[9,10]

Somatic nerve blocks may include greater occipital, lateral femoral cutaneous, obturator, intercostal, paravertebral somatic, and medial branch nerve blocks.[23-25] Brachial plexus block may be useful to evaluate a painful extremity with restricted range of motion. This produces sensory, sympathetic, and motor block. Both analgesia and increased range of motion are evaluated after the block. Near normal passive range of motion in a previously deformed, restricted extremity suggests that lack of mobility is due primarily to pain and muscle spasm, not "fixed" soft tissue contractures and bone pathologic conditions. This information may be helpful to the physical therapist and important for the patient's management.

Sympathetic blocks of the upper extremity include stellate ganglion block and dilute brachial plexus block.[26] Lumbar sympathetic blocks provide lower extremity sympathetic block. Abdominal pain can be evaluated by celiac plexus and hypogastric plexus blocks of preaortic ganglia at the L1 and L5–S1 levels, respectively. It is essential to assess the extent of sympathetic block and to confirm the absence of incidental somatic block. Adequate temperature increase, loss of sympathogalvanic response, and absence of sweating are three tests used to document the presence of complete sympathetic block in an extremity. The presence of Horner's syndrome does not confirm that upper extremity sympathetic block has occurred after stellate ganglion block. The possibility of incomplete sympathetic block must always be entertained.

Intravenous regional sympathetic blocks are more useful as therapeutic than diagnostic blocks. Their interpretation is clouded by the concomitant analgesia that results from tourniquet compression of nerves during the block and systemic local anesthetic effects after tourniquet deflation.[20] Intravenous local anesthetic infusions may be used to evaluate suspected neuropathic pain syndromes.[19] Relief of paroxysmal lancinating pain particularly may suggest responsiveness to oral local anesthetic therapy and the presence of a neuropathic pain syndrome.[27]

Differential spinal blockade was intended to distinguish sympathetic, somatic, psychogenic, and central pain states.[3-8] It assumes the ability to produce selective, complete block of one category of nerve fibers with simultaneous absence of any block of other categories of nerve fiber. The three type of nerves that are important here are (1) B fibers (preganglionic sympathetic nerves); (2) Aβ and C nociceptive fibers; and (3) Aβ and Aα tactile and motor fibers. This assumption has been challenged, as discussed previously.[1] It is now clear that there is no reliable way to provide isolated block of each fiber type in a sequential fashion using successive intrathecal injections of saline and preselected concentrations of a local anesthetic. Similarly, after complete neural blockade produced by modified differential spinal or epidural block, recovery of sensory function does not occur without any regression of sympathetic block. In fact, sympathetic function often recovers while sensory block persists. A sympathetically maintained pain state may be suspected only if there is persistent pain relief, after sensory recovery, in the presence of persistent sympathetic block as evidenced by elevated skin temperature and absence of sweating and sympathogalvanic response.

Differential epidural block with various concentrations of local anesthetic has been used to allow functional assessment of the patient's pain with movement, which is facilitated by placement of an epidural catheter for repeated injections. This technique is fraught with most of the same problems as diagnostic spinal anesthesia. It may be used to slowly increase the level of block to assess the segmental levels needed to relieve pain. Neither spinal nor epidural block can reliably differentiate sympathetic from somatic pain. Persistence of pain within an area of complete blockade does suggest a supraspinal pain mechanism. Differential spinal and epidural blocks in patients with chronic low back pain have produced this result in 10%, 36%, 25%, and 30% of patients in four large series.[28-31]

Diagnostic epidural opioid blockade aims to eliminate unintended cues to patients that result from the obvious sensory and motor block that occurs.[32] It assumes that nociception at a site peripheral to the dorsal horn will be relieved, but that central pain will not be relieved. However, intraspinal opioids produce typical central side effects that patients will notice. They relieve deep, constant somatic or visceral pain most reliably, but they relieve episodic somatic and visceral pain variably; they may also provide relief to some patients with neuropathic pain associated with lesions of the peripheral nervous system.[33]

Prognostic epidural opioid block, used as a trial of opioid responsiveness prior to implanting a system for intraspinal opioid administration, seems much more reasonable. Similarly, diagnostic epidural electrode stimulation is recommended before implanting a permanent spinal cord stimulator. The pattern of response to both opioids and local anesthetics, given intraspinally and intravenously, may supplement the clinical evaluation of patients suspected of having neuropathic, central, or somatic pain; but they are of limited diagnostic value when considered in isolation. Prognostic spinal block has a limited role; it uses small doses of intrathecal local anesthetic to assess patients for intrathecal neurolytic block. Prognostic epidural local anesthetic block is similarly indicated before epidural neurolysis with alcohol or phenol.

PREREQUISITES FOR OPTIMAL DIAGNOSTIC BLOCK

The physician must make a complete evaluation of the patient prior to any procedure. A comprehensive history should include a pain diary, a history of the pain problem, and all previous workup and therapy information. A complete examination should include neurologic testing and functional evaluation. Results of diagnostic studies and psychological evaluations are reviewed. A physician who is knowledgeable about pain syndromes and diagnostic procedures must then determine if a diagnostic block is indicated and document the specific goal to be achieved with the selected procedure. Communication with the patient is necessary to obtain informed consent, ensuring that the true goals and limitations of the block are understood. The patient must be prepared and monitored as for any major regional anesthesia induction.

The following modifications to regional anesthesia procedures may improve the reliability of diagnostic block:

1. Limit the use of preblock sedatives and analgesics.

2. Use very small volumes of local anesthetic.

3. Locate target nerves precisely with the assistance of x-ray, fluoroscopy, contrast material, ultrasonography, computed tomography, or a peripheral nerve stimulator.

4. Repeat positive blocks with a local anesthetic of different duration, to correlate duration of pain relief to that of the block.[31]

5. Maintain thorough records of the block procedure.

6. Record the patient's pain scores at rest and with function, vital signs, sensory and motor examination findings, signs of sympathetic function, and presence of pain behaviors, before and after the diagnostic block procedure.

7. Ask the patient to keep records of neurologic

symptoms, degree of pain relief, pain scores, activity levels, and drug intake after discharge.

Interpretation of Block Results

It is important to understand the limits of diagnostic blocks. They are not intended to be therapeutic, and they have little diagnostic value unless considered within the framework of all other information obtained about the patient. Careful observation of the patient's response to blockade must be made and recorded. The extent of motor, sensory, and sympathetic block must be assessed by neurologic testing and correlated with the degree of pain relief and functional improvement over time. Conclusions about various aspects of the patient's pain may then be made, considering all of the information mentioned previously (Table 19–4).

Pitfalls in Evaluating Results

Pain relief due to an unintended action of a block can be classified as a false-positive response. False-positive responses may occur due to a placebo response, systemic effects of local anesthetic, spread of drug to other nerves, unreliable patient report of block effects, and temporary alterations in central processing due to lack of normal afferent input.[1] Placebo response occurs in about 30% of patients. A report of differential spinal block for chronic back pain has noted this response in just under 20% of patients.[28] Confirmatory facet blocks with different local anesthetics have documented a false-positive rate for uncontrolled blocks in 27% to 38% of patients.[9,10] The presence of a placebo response has no reliable diagnostic significance. Systemic effects of local anesthetics may be expected to influence neuropathic pain states, particularly after use of large doses of local anesthetic agents.[34] Distal block of afferent sensory input to the cord may temporarily relieve pain due to a proximal or central lesion.[16-18,35] This implies that normal sensory input is activating a sensitized central neuronal pathway, and it is temporarily interrupted by the diagnostic block.

False-negative responses may occur when a block fails to relieve pain. This may result from an incomplete block, the presence of alternate pain pathways, unappreciated referred pain syndromes, unreliable patient report of block effects, and diagnostic testing at inappropriate times.[1] Blocks may be incomplete due to deficiencies in technique, particularly when reduced volumes of local anesthetic are used to achieve selective block. Failure to select all the appropriate neural pathways may result in apparent failure, particularly for painful joints that have extensive innervation. Failure to document complete block of desired nerve fibers in the expected location will also lead to apparent failure. Referred somatic pain phenomena may lead to failure to block the correct source of somatic pain initially. For example, back and leg pain may be due to disc herniation, piriformis syndrome, facet joint disease, sacroiliac disease, ligament tear, or myofascial pain, requiring different diagnostic somatic blocks. Diagnostic blocks should not be performed unless the patient is experiencing significant pain; the extent of pain relief should be evaluated when maximum local anesthetic effect has been achieved.

Diagnostic nerve blocks can be useful tools to supplement and confirm clinical impressions based on an extensive patient evaluation, when the specific diagnosis remains in doubt. It is essential to document completeness and duration of blockade, absence of unwanted block, and degree and duration of pain relief and to confirm the response to local anesthetics of different durations.[2]

REFERENCES

1. Boas RA, Cousins MJ: Diagnostic neural blockade. *In* Cousins MJ, Bridenbaugh PO (eds): Neural Blockade in Clinical Anesthesia and Management of Pain, ed 2. Philadelphia, JB Lippincott, 1988, p 885.
2. Bonica JJ, Buckley FP: Regional anesthesia with local anesthetics. *In* Bonica JJ (ed): The Management of Pain, ed 2. Philadelphia, Lea & Febiger, 1990, p 1883.
3. Winnie AP, Collins VJ: Differential neural blockade in pain syndromes of questionable etiology. Med Clin North Am 52:123, 1968.
4. Ramamurthy S, Winnie AP: Diagnostic maneuvers in painful syndromes. Int Anesthesiol Clin 21:47, 1983.
5. Winnie AP: Differential neural blockade for the diagnosis of pain mechanisms. *In* Waldman SD, Winnie AP (eds): Interventional Pain Management. Philadelphia, WB Saunders, 1996, p 129.
6. Arrowood JG, Sarnoff SJ: Differential spinal block: V. Use in the investigation of pain following amputation. Anesthesiology 9:614, 1948.
7. McCollum DE, Stephen CR: The use of graduated spinal anesthesia in the differential diagnosis of pain of the back and lower extremities. South Med J 57:410, 1964.
8. Brothers MA, Finlayson DC: Evaluation of low back pain by differential spinal block. Can Anaesth Soc J 15:478, 1968.
9. Barnsley L, Lord S, Wallis B, et al: False-positive rate of cervical zygapophyseal joint blocks. Clin J Pain 9:124, 1993.
10. Schwarzer AC, April CN, Derby R, et al: The false-positive rate of

TABLE 19–4. INTERPRETATION OF DIAGNOSTIC BLOCK PROCEDURES

Classification	Results of Block
Placebo responder	Pain relief with sham block or saline injection
Sympathetic maintained pain	Relief with effective, complete sympathetic ganglion block; relief with confirmatory, comparative blocks
Visceral pain	No relief with trunk wall blocks; relief with celiac or hypogastric plexus block
Somatic pain	Repeated relief with local nerve, muscle, or joint injection; relief with confirmatory, comparative blocks*
Neuropathic pain	Relief with nerve block and IV local anesthetic; less relief with opioids
Central pain	Transient or no relief with peripheral or spinal block; better relief with local anesthetics than opioids
Psychogenic pain	Diagnosis by psychologist or psychiatrist after consultation and psychological testing

*An initial positive block is repeated with another local anesthetic that has a different duration. Pain relief should occur after both blocks, and the duration of relief should be significantly greater with the longer-acting local anesthetic.

uncontrolled diagnostic blocks of the lumbar zygapophyseal joints. Pain 58:195, 1994.

11. Traycoff RB, Crayton H, Dodson R: Sacrococcygeal pain syndromes: Diagnosis and treatment. Orthopedics 12:1373, 1989.
12. Stolker RJ, Vervest ACM, Groen GJ: The management of chronic spinal pain by blockades: A review. Pain 58:1, 1994.
13. Bovim G, Sand T: Cervicogenic headache, migraine without aura and tension-type headache: diagnostic blockade of greater occipital and supra-orbital nerves. Pain 51:43, 1992.
14. Applegate WV: Abdominal cutaneous nerve entrapment syndrome. Surgery 71:118, 1972.
15. Gallegos NC, Hobsley M: Recognition and treatment of abdominal wall pain. J R Soc Med 82:343, 1989.
16. Crisologo PA, Neal B, Brown R, et al: Lidocaine-induced spinal block can relieve central poststroke pain: Role of the block in chronic pain diagnosis. Anesthesiology 74:184, 1991.
17. Kibler RF, Nathan PW: Relief of pain and paresthesiae by nerve blocks distal to a lesion. J Neurol Neurosurg Psychiatry 23:91, 1960.
18. Loh L, Nathan PW, Schott G: Pain due to lesions of the central nervous system removed by sympathetic block. Br Med J 282:1026, 1981.
19. Boas RA, Covino BG, Shahnarian A: Analgesic response to iv lignocaine. Br J Anaesth 54:501, 1982.
20. Woolf C, Wiesenfeld-Hollin Z: The systemic administration of local anesthetics produces a selective depression of C-afferent fiber evoked activity in the spinal cord. Pain 23:361, 1985.
21. Loeser JD: Dorsal rhizotomy for the relief of chronic pain. J Neurosurg 36:745, 1972.
22. Tasker R: Deafferentation and causalgia. In Bonica JJ (ed): Advances in Pain Research and Treatment. New York, Raven Press, 1980, p 305.
23. Hong Y, O'Grady T, Lopresti D, et al: Diagnostic obturator nerve block for inguinal and back pain: A recovered opinion. Pain 67:507, 1996.
24. Dooley JF, McBroom RJ, Taguchi T, et al: Nerve root infiltration in the diagnosis of radicular pain. Spine 13:79, 1988.
25. Barnsley L, Lord S, Bogduk N: Comparative local anesthetic blocks in the diagnosis of cervical zygapophyseal joint pain. Pain 55:99, 1993.
26. Durrani Z: Role of brachial plexus block after negative response from stellate ganglion block for RSD. Anesthesiology 73:A837, 1990.
27. Tanelian DL, Brose WG: Neuropathic pain can be relieved by drugs that are use-dependent sodium channel blockers: Lidocaine, carbamazepine, and mexiletine. Anesthesiology 74:949, 1991.
28. Jacobson L, Chabal C, Mariano AJ, et al: Persistent low-back pain is real: However, diagnostic spinal injections are not helpful in its evaluation. Clin J Pain 8:237, 1992.
29. Ghia JN, Duncan G, Toomey TC, et al: The pharmacologic approach in differential diagnosis of chronic pain. Spine 4:447, 1979.
30. Sorensen J, Aaro S, Bengtsson M, et al: Can a pharmacologic pain analysis be used in the assessment of chronic low back pain? Eur Spine J 5:236, 1996.
31. Stanley D, Stockley I, Davies GK, et al: A prospective study of diagnostic epidural blockade in the assessment of chronic back and leg pain. J Spinal Disord 6:208, 1993.
32. Cherry DA, Gourlay GK, McLachlan M, et al: Diagnostic epidural opioid blockade and chronic pain. Pain 21:143, 1985.
33. Arner S, Arner B: Differential effects of epidural morphine in the treatment of cancer related pain. Acta Anaesthesiol Scand 29:32, 1985.
34. Ekblom A, Hansson P, Lindblom U, et al: Does a regional nerve block change cutaneous perception thresholds outside the anesthetic area? Implications for the interpretation of diagnostic blocks. Pain 50:163, 1992.
35. Xavier AV, McDanal J, Kissin I: Relief of sciatic radicular pain by sciatic nerve block. Anesth Analg 67:1177, 1988.

Chapter 20

Local Anesthetic Infusions for Pain Management

Honorio T. Benzon, M.D.

MECHANISM OF ANALGESIC EFFECT

Leriche theorized that tissue injury resulted in reflex vasoconstriction, capillary dysfunction, and increased permeability. These vascular changes, in turn, cause anoxia, accumulation of metabolites, and irritation of peripheral nerve endings.[1,2] Local anesthetics produce vasodilatation, anesthetize the irritated nerve endings, and interrupt the reflex arc.[1,2]

Bigelow and Harrison[3] demonstrated that the analgesic action of the local anesthetic was secondary to its systemic effect and not from its direct action. They noted that the injection of procaine into the arms of normal subjects increased the pain threshold in the forehead.

Boas and colleagues[4] believed that the analgesic action of intravenous (IV) lidocaine resulted from a decrease in the rate of neuronal depolarization and from selective decreases in high-frequency impulse transmission. A decrease in high-frequency impulse transmission had been demonstrated previously by Condouris,[5] who showed that sub-blocking concentrations of lidocaine modified the information-carrying capacity of axons.[5]

The relief of vascular headache with intravenous lidocaine probably results from the local inhibition of nociceptive trigeminal afferents that innervate cranial blood vessels.[6] Vascular headaches, such as the common migraine and cluster headache, are characterized by vasoconstriction and vasodilatation as well as alterations in blood flow. Sensory trigeminal neurons innervating the cranial blood vessels may be important mediators of vascular headaches. A discrete population of brain stem trigeminal cells respond to stimulation of dural blood vessels.[7] Many of these cells also receive nociceptive somatic input from the first division of the trigeminal nerve. These trigeminovascular afferents are activated by nociceptive mechanical and chemical stimuli, including the local intravascular infusion of bradykinin. The response of individual brain-stem trigeminal neurons to perfusion of bradykinin into the sagittal sinus is abolished by pretreatment with 2 mg/kg of lidocaine.[8]

Although it is well known that adequate metabolic control may reduce the symptoms of painful diabetic neuropathy, the relief of the pain of diabetic neuropathy is not totally dependent on improved metabolic regulation. Kastrup and associates[9] showed that the patients who experienced relief after lidocaine infusion had the same blood glucose concentrations and hemoglobin A_{1c} levels during the infusions with lidocaine as with saline. There was no association between the actual concentration of the blood glucose and hemoglobin A_{1c} and the effect of the lidocaine. Finally, at no time during the study did any change occur in the objective signs of the patients' diabetic neuropathy.[9]

RELIEF OF EXPERIMENTAL PAIN

In contrast to findings in clinical studies, Rowlingson and others[10] showed that intravenous lidocaine, up to blood levels of 3 μg/mL, showed no analgesic effect on experimental tourniquet-induced pain.[10] They commented, however, that experimental pain is different from the unremitting, psychologically significant pain seen in the clinical setting.

TECHNIQUE AND CLINICAL RESULTS

Procaine has been used in the past because of its potency and low toxicity. Its short duration of action led investigators to employ other drugs. The local anesthetic is administered either in bolus doses or in infusions. Monitoring is the same as that for regional anesthesia, with continuous monitoring for central nervous system (CNS) toxic effects, which include lightheadedness, tinnitus, perioral numbness, drowsiness, and slurred speech.[10] Full resuscitation equipment should be available.

Schnapp and co-workers[11] injected 3% chloroprocaine in 44 patients. Their technique consisted of injecting increments of 1 to 2 mL of chloroprocaine every 30 to 60 seconds until the pain subsided or until 900 mg was injected. If the patients had pain relief greater than

50%, they proceeded with several infusions. They gave between 4 to 45 injections, 1 to 14 days apart, to the patients who reported a favorable response. The patients had postlaminectomy syndrome, complex regional pain syndrome (CRPS), or stump or phantom limb pain. Of the 44 patients, 43% had greater than 50% relief of pain for a period greater than 30 days following the last injection. Eight were totally pain-free for at least 7 months. The researchers noted that patients who had allodynia or spontaneous pain responded better than those who did not have these symptoms.

Phero and associates[12] infused 1% chloroprocaine at a rate of 1 mg/kg/minute until a dose of 15 mg/kg was administered. The rate was reduced by half if a patient showed signs of CNS toxic effects and the infusion was discontinued if the symptoms persisted. A total of four infusions were given to the patients at 14-day intervals. Pain relief greater than 25% that lasted an average of 2 weeks was obtained in 67% of patients. Most of the patients had musculoskeletal problems.

Edwards and co-workers[13] infused between 1 mg/kg and 5 mg/kg of 1% lidocaine over 1 hour (usually 5 to 10 mg/minute). Their rate of infusion was adjusted to minimize CNS toxic effects (e.g., circumoral numbness, drowsiness, slurred speech). Patients who had complete or partial pain relief had repeat infusions so long as they responded. Patients were not preselected; all patients referred to the pain clinic were offered the treatment. Of 182 patients, 83 (46%) were responders. Response rates, in relation to the etiology of the pain, were as follows: (1) radiculopathy, 75%; (2) peripheral neuropathy, 59%; (3) CRPS, 36%; (4) mechanical problems, 29%; (4) central lesions, 29%; and (5) other diagnoses, 3%.

The use of IV lidocaine for painful diabetic neuropathy has been described by Kastrup and colleagues.[9] Lidocaine was infused at a rate of 5 mg/kg of body weight over 30 minutes. Significant reduction of pain was noted, and nearly significant beneficial effect was seen on spontaneous pain, dysesthesia, paresthesia, and nightly exacerbation. Relief of pain, as measured by the visual analogue scale, lasted 3 days, whereas relief of symptoms (subjective pain, dysesthesia, paresthesia, nightly exacerbation, and sleep disturbances) lasted 14 days.

Maciewicz and associates[6] injected 100 mg of lidocaine (25 mg/minute) in patients with headache. They noted that patients with vascular headache (cluster headache and common migraine) had a reduction in the intensity of the headache. Relief occurred within 4 minutes and lasted for 20 minutes. In contrast, the patients with nonvascular headache (myofascial pain, temporomandibular joint pain/dysfunction syndrome, or atypical facial pain) had no response to the IV lidocaine.

REFERENCES

1. Leriche R: Intra-arterial therapy of infections and other diseases. Mem Acad Chir 64:220, 1938.
2. Leriche R: Simple methods of easing pain in the extremities in arterial diseases and in certain vasomotor disorders. Presse Med 49:799, 1941.
3. Bigelow N, Harrison I: General analgesic effects of procaine. J Pharmacol Exp Ther 81:368, 1944.
4. Boas RA, Covino BG, Shahnarian A: Analgesic responses to IV lignocaine. Br J Anaesth 54:501, 1982.
5. Condouris GA: Local anaesthetics as modulators of neural information. In Bonica JJ, Albe-Fessard DG (eds): Advances in Pain Research and Therapy. New York, Raven Press, 1976, p 663.
6. Maciewicz R, Chung RY, Strassman A, et al: Relief of vascular headache with intravenous lidocaine: Clinical observations and a proposed mechanism. Clin J Pain 4:11, 1988.
7. Strassman A, Mason P, Moskowitz M, et al: Response of brainstem trigeminal neurons to electrical stimulation of the dura. Brain Res 379:242, 1986.
8. Strassman A, Pile-Spellman J, Oot R, et al: Responses of trigeminal nucleus caudalis neurons to mechanical and chemical stimulation of cranial blood vessels. Soc Neurosci Abstr 13:11, 1987.
9. Kastrup J, Petersen P, Dejgard A, et al: Intravenous lidocaine infusion: A new treatment of chronic painful diabetic neuropathy? Pain 28:69, 1987.
10. Rowlingson J, DiFazio CA, Foster J, et al: Lidocaine as an analgesic for experimental pain. Anesthesiology 52:20, 1980.
11. Schnapp M, Mays KS, North WC: Intravenous 2-chloroprocaine in the treatment of pain. Anesth Analg 60:844, 1981.
12. Phero JC, McDonald JS, Raj PP, et al: Controlled intravenous administration of chloroprocaine for intractable pain management. Reg Anesth 9:50, 1984.
13. Edwards WT, Habib F, Burney RG, et al: Intravenous lidocaine in the management of various chronic pain states. Reg Anesth 10:1, 1985.

Chapter 21

 # Botulinum Toxin for Myofascial Pain Syndrome

Raghavender Thunga, M.D.

HISTORY

Myofascial pain syndrome was first mentioned in the medical literature in 1843 when the German physician Froeriep described tender spots in muscles of his "rheumatic" patients and referred to them as *muskelschwiele* (muscle calluses). In 1931, an orthopedic surgeon named Max Lange described these taut bands of muscle that produce pain in characteristic reference zones. The term *trigger point* was later coined by Arthur Steindler to describe the muscle band. The term m*yofascial pain syndrome* was originated and essentially perpetuated by Janet Travell, an internist, to encompass a vague muscular pain disorder characterized by these trigger points. David Simons, a physiatrist, and Travell distilled their experience in *Myofascial Pain and Dysfunction: The Trigger Point Manual.*[1,2]

DEFINITION

For most clinical purposes, myofascial pain syndrome can be described as a pain disorder that is characterized by a tender trigger point in a taut band of muscle, which may produce a local twitch response to snapping or palpation of the band and produces pain in a characteristic reference zone. Simons developed a more specific method for diagnosis by listing five major criteria and three minor criteria, claiming that the diagnosis could be made if patients fulfilled all of the five major criteria and at least one minor criterion[3] (Table 21-1).

DIFFERENTIAL DIAGNOSIS

Other regional pain syndromes should be ruled out, such as bursitis, tendinitis, nerve root irritation, and fibromyalgia. The distinction between myofascial pain syndrome and fibromyalgia, however, often becomes confused. Whether these disease processes are distinct entities or two extremes of the same process is uncertain. Typically, fibromyalgia has been characterized by

tender areas of muscle without distinct trigger points; it involves several regions of the body and includes nonmusculoskeletal symptoms such as fatigue, sleep disturbances, and irritable bowel.

PREVALENCE

Although proper epidemiologic studies have not been conducted, it has been estimated that up to 11% of visits to a general internist may involve patients suffering from some degree of myofascial pain syndrome. There appears to be a female predominance of the syndrome, with a female-to-male ratio as high as 3:1.

CLINICAL PRESENTATION

The pain, which patients describe as steady, deep, aching, and, occasionally, burning, results in stiffness,

TABLE 21-1. SIMONS' CRITERIA FOR THE DIAGNOSIS OF MYOFASCIAL PAIN SYNDROME

Major Criteria	Minor Criteria
1. Localized spontaneous pain	1. Reproduction of spontaneously perceived pain and altered sensation by pressure on the trigger point
2. Spontaneous pain or altered sensation in expected referred pain area for the given trigger point	2. Elicitation of a local twitch response of muscular fibers by transverse "snapping" palpation or by needle insertion into the trigger point
3. Palpable taut band in muscle	3. Pain relief obtained by muscle stretching or injection of the trigger point
4. Exquisitely localized tenderness in a precise point along the taut band	
5. Some measurable degree of reduced range of motion	

Adapted from Simons D: Muscular pain syndromes. *In* Fricton JR (ed): Advances in Pain Research and Therapy, vol 17. New York, Raven Press, 1990, p 1.

92

weakness, and decreased mobility in the affected region. Commonly, but not always, there is associated anxiety, depression, and sleep disturbance. The trigger points can be aggravated by the following circumstances: strenuous use of the involved muscle, passive stretch of the muscle, pressure on the trigger point, cold and damp weather, viral infection, stress, or fatigue.

The taut band is an area of muscle with a hard consistency, usually running parallel to the direction of the fibers of the involved muscle and assuming a linear or nodular shape. The so-called trigger point is a distinct localized tenderness within the taut band. Palpation of the trigger point can (1) reproduce the patient's pain; (2) elicit a zone of pain radiation or altered sensation (i.e., hypoesthesia, hyperesthesia, paresthesia, or anesthesia) that is typical of the particular muscle; or (3) elicit a local twitch response (an immediate contraction of the taut band and adjacent normal muscle). The twitch response can also be evoked by using a plucking motion on or direct insertion of a needle into the trigger point.

Trigger points have been subdivided as active or latent and as primary, secondary, or satellite. Patients with *active trigger points* have pain at rest or on palpation, and the pain complaint can be reproduced with firm compression of the trigger points. The more common *latent trigger points* are incidental findings that produce the typical zone of radiation pain when palpated, but do not otherwise cause pain in the patient. Whether the latent trigger points are evolving into active trigger points, are devolving from active trigger points, or are of unrelated significance has not yet been determined. *Primary trigger points* are independent sites unrelated to other trigger points, whereas *secondary trigger points* can develop in muscles that are overloaded from synergistic substitution for, or anatomic antagonism to, muscles that contain a primary trigger point. Finally, *satellite trigger points* are located in a zone of reference of another trigger point.[1]

PATHOPHYSIOLOGY

Most diagnostic studies have given little insight into the pathophysiology of myofascial pain syndrome. Muscle biopsies have provided limited information: disruption of myofibrillar structure, elevated amounts of ground substance and mucopolysaccharides, multifocal loss of selected oxidized enzymes, occasional "ragged red fibers" suggestive of mitochondrial damage, and decreased levels of high-energy phosphates. Electromyographic (EMG) studies show electrical silence in these areas unless they are stimulated (e.g., by palpation or dry needling), which then produces motor unit action potentials of 0.25 seconds at 500 μV. Thermograms of skin overlying active trigger points have occasionally shown areas of increased temperature. Plain x-rays and computed tomographic scans have been normal, and serum laboratory test findings, including erythrocyte sedimentation rate and levels of electrolytes, hemoglobin/hematocrit, and muscle enzymes, have been consistently reported to be within the normal range. Current theories of the etiology of this disease process, therefore, have been speculative.

Travell and Simons have claimed that the initial changes occur secondary to local trauma, muscle fatigue from overuse, chronic postural imbalance, and psychological distress. Theoretically, as a result of the perpetuating events, there is release and accumulation of Ca^{2+}. The increased Ca^{2+} results in initiation and maintenance of a sustained contracture, with eventual depletion of adenosine triphosphate (ATP), release of vasoactive and neuroactive substances (e.g., histamine, serotonin, kinins, prostaglandins), and local vasoconstrictive response. This ultimately results in a region of increased metabolism, decreased circulation, and shortened muscle fiber.[4,5] Pain may occur as a result of (1) local release of these sensitizing substances, (2) possible ischemia with accumulation of metabolic byproducts, and/or (3) actual impingement on nerve fibers within the contracted muscle.

Following the use of trigger point injections with local anesthetic solution (see following discussion), pain relief appears to outlast the effect of the local anesthetic. This brings into consideration other more sophisticated mechanisms, such as central sensitization and the so-called wind-up phenomenon seen in other chronic pain states. Additional research may give further insights into these mechanisms.

TREATMENT

The most prudent initial treatment of this often debilitating illness is identification, correction, and prevention of predisposing, aggravating, and perpetuating factors in the home and work environment. These include trauma, abnormal body mechanics and posture, unusual or repetitive movements, deconditioned states, and emotional stressors. As this syndrome can, and often does, become a chronic pain state, a multidisciplinary approach is often required, which includes aggressive physical therapy and psychological intervention.

The goal of treatment is to apply inactivation and counterstimulation techniques followed by active and passive stretching to restore the muscles to their normal length, posture, and range of motion. Several inactivation and counterstimulation techniques are available, including massage, acupressure and acupuncture, ultrasound, moist heat and ice, transcutaneous electrical nerve stimulation (TENS), fluoromethane spray, diathermy, and trigger point injections. In the popular "spray-and-stretch" technique, a vapocoolant spray, such as fluoromethane (seldom used now because of its environmental effect), is applied to the affected area, followed immediately by passive stretching of the muscle unit containing the trigger point.

Trigger Point Injections

The trigger point injection has become the most commonly used, and sometimes abused, technique for the treatment of myofascial pain syndrome. In this procedure a small-gauge needle (25 gauge) is inserted into the trigger point, guided by the reproduction of the patient's pain (both local and referred).

Several proposed mechanisms of action leading to relief of pain from the trigger point injection have been suggested.[1] They include the following:

1. Mechanical disruption of the contractile elements
2. Local release of intracellular potassium secondary to damage of the muscle fibers, resulting in a "depolarizing" block of nerve fibers
3. Dilution and "wash-out" of the sensitizing substances
4. Local vasodilation by certain local anesthetics, leading to increased circulation and removal of metabolites
5. Interruption of neural feedback mechanisms that may perpetuate nociceptive inputs
6. Release of endogenous opioid (as evidenced by reversal of pain relief with the administration of naloxone)
7. Possible myotoxic effects of the injected solutions (local anesthetics)

Absolute contraindications to trigger point injections are local infection at the site of needle insertion and allergy to the injected drug. Some relative contraindications are systemic infections, coagulopathies, anticoagulation therapy, and recent muscle trauma (acute phase).

Technique

1. The skin is cleansed with a suitable antiseptic, such as an alcohol wipe
2. The most sensitive point along the taut band (the trigger point) is localized and secured between the fingers
3. A 25-gauge needle is advanced between the fingers into the trigger point until the referred pain, a twitch response, or the "jump" sign is elicited
4. The entire volume may be injected at this location or the solution can be "peppered" or fanned along the muscle length

Many different solutions and volumes have been used, including saline, local anesthetic, steroid, and, most recently, botulinum toxin. No current study has definitively shown one solution to be superior to the others. Dry needling alone has been shown to give some degree of relief as well. A comparison to classic acupuncture sites has shown close correlation with typical trigger point sites.[6] A recent compilation of studies to date addressing this issue has been made by Han and Harrison.[7]

Local anesthetics have the advantage of providing some analgesia to the surrounding tissue. Several agents have been used, including procaine, chloroprocaine, lidocaine, bupivacaine, and etidocaine. Because analgesic effects using local anesthetic trigger point injections often outlast the usual duration of local anesthetic effects, the concentration and type of local anesthetic probably does not matter. The usual recommended toxic dose has to be kept in mind for the particular solution used. In fact, because bupivacaine appears to be a more myotoxic agent, lidocaine (1%) may be the safer choice.[8]

The addition of steroid preparations such as triamcinolone or dexamethasone in the trigger point injection solution is often made despite little evidence of the existence of an inflammatory component in the affected muscle. No clear benefit has been demonstrated to the routine use of steroid. Complications of local steroid injection include skin depigmentation, local irritation, tendon atrophy, decreased plasma cortisol levels, and increased glucose levels.[7]

After these local treatments, the actual therapeutic intervention for *ultimate* relief of the pain is undertaken: an immediate and aggressive program of graded active and passive muscle stretching and strengthening. The local treatments are simply means by which temporary relief is achieved in order that the patients may tolerate physical therapy.

Botulinum Toxin

Botulinum has been shown to be effective for the treatment of various dystonic conditions such as blepharospasm, spasmodic torticollis, spasmodic dysphonia, and facial spasm. After irreversibly binding to presynaptic cholinergic nerve terminals, botulinum toxin prevents the release of acetylcholine, resulting in sustained muscle relaxation that lasts until regeneration (reinnervation) of the nerve terminals is accomplished.[9] Botulinum toxin has recently been proposed and employed as an alternative to the standard medications used for trigger point injections in the treatment of myofascial pain syndrome. Its proposed advantage over the more common treatment, using local anesthetic trigger point injections, is a more prolonged, and thus more effective, treatment for myofascial pain.

Botulinum toxin type A is a sterile, lyophilized form of purified botulinum toxin, produced from a culture of the Hall strain of *Clostridium botulinum*. It is packaged as 100 mouse units per vial, where one mouse unit is the median lethal dose for a 20 to 30 g Swiss Webster (genetically bred) mouse. The most common side effect has been transient flu-like symptoms. There have been no reported cases of systemic toxic effects from injection of botulinum toxin type A. However, cases of transient dysphagia have been reported when the drug was injected into anterior neck muscles with resultant leakage into esophageal musculature. There has been evidence of the development of antibodies to the formulation, resulting in decreased effectiveness after repeated injections. The current recommended maximum dose is 200 mouse units in a 30-day period. However, doses of up to 400 mouse units have been used in one sitting without untoward effects.[10]

Denervation by the toxin appears to occur via a three-step process: (1) binding to the presynaptic membrane receptor molecule, (2) translocation of the toxin into the nerve terminal by receptor-mediated endocytosis, and (3) irreversible inactivation of normal neurotransmitter (acetylcholine) *release* via an enzymatic lytic process.[11]

The onset of effect of botulinum toxin appears to vary from 3 to 7 days after the injection. Peak effect can extend up to 6 weeks. The duration, which can last up to 12 weeks, may depend on the location and size of the trigger point injected, accuracy of placement, and dose injected. For relatively small muscles, such as the cervical paraspinal and scalene muscles, doses of 25 to 40 mouse units should suffice, whereas the splenius capitis, levator scapulae, and trapezius muscles require doses of 50 to 75 mouse units. For larger muscles, such as those of the gluteal region and the psoas, higher doses are used (100 to 200 mouse units).

To date no large-scale, prospective, randomized, double-blinded study has compared the effectiveness of botulinum toxin with local anesthetic for trigger point injections. Studies have been undertaken in which small groups of patients have been given botulinum toxin trigger point injections with relatively positive and prolonged results.[12,13] Further study is needed before widespread use of botulinum toxin can be suggested as the initial treatment of myofascial pain syndrome.

Systemic medications have also been used in the treatment of myofascial syndrome. Although little actual evidence exists of an inflammatory state, nonsteroidal anti-inflammatory agents may at times give relief. After the acute injury, muscle relaxants and narcotics have been beneficial. Their use beyond the initial phase is discouraged by most practitioners. Finally, antidepressants have improved sleep and mood disturbances as well as provided some pain relief via their central effects.

PROGNOSIS

Limited epidemiologic studies make prognosis of myofascial pain syndrome difficult to quantitate. Although most patients do relatively well with limited treatment, a significant number of patients suffer for years despite proper treatment. With the potential for chronicity in this syndrome, a true multidisciplinary approach may be helpful in all refractory cases.

REFERENCES

1. Travell JG, Simons DG: Myofascial Pain and Dysfunction: The Trigger Point Manual, vol. 1. Baltimore, Williams & Wilkins, 1983.
2. Travell JG, Simons DG: Myofascial Pain and Dysfunction: The Trigger Point Manual, vol. 2. The Lower Extremities. Baltimore, Williams & Wilkins, 1992.
3. Simons D: Muscular pain syndromes. In Fricton JR (ed): Advances in Pain Research and Therapy, vol 17. New York, Raven Press, 1990, p 1.
4. Raj PP: Prognostic and therapeutic local anesthetic blockade. In Cousins MJ, Bridenbaugh PO (ed): Neural Blockade in Clinical Anesthesia and Management of Pain, ed 2. Philadelphia, J B Lippincott, 1988.
5. Hartrick C: Pain due to trauma including sports injuries. In Raj PP (ed): Practical Management of Pain, ed 2. St. Louis, Mosby-Year Book, 1992.
6. Melzack R, Stilwell DM, Fox EJ: Trigger points and acupuncture points for pain: Correlations and implications. Pain 3:3, 1977.
7. Han SC, Harrison P: Myofascial pain syndrome and trigger-point management. Reg Anesth 22:89, 1997.
8. Foster AH, Carlson BM: Myotoxicity of local anesthetics and regeneration of damaged muscle fiber. Anesth Analg 58:727, 1980.
9. Sellin LC: The action of botulinum toxin at the neuromuscular junction. Med Biol 59:11, 1981.
10. Jankovic J, Brin MF: Therapeutic uses of botulinum toxin. N Engl J Med 324:1186, 1991.
11. Simpson LL: Origin, structure, and pharmacological activity of botulinum toxin. Pharmacol Rev 33:155, 1981.
12. Acquadro MA, Borodic GE: Treatment of myofascial pain with botulinum A toxin [Letter]. Anesthesiology 80:705, 1994.
13. Cheshire WP, Abashian SW, Mann JD: Botulinum toxin in the treatment of myofascial pain syndrome. Pain 59: 65, 1994.

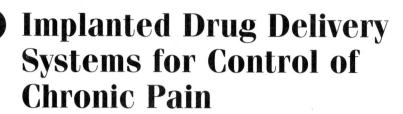

Chapter 22

Implanted Drug Delivery Systems for Control of Chronic Pain

Robert M. Levy, M.D., Ph.D.

RATIONALE

Although oral, parenteral, or transdermal narcotics can be extremely effective analgesic agents, systemic administration may have significant side effects (Table 22-1), and long-term use in sufficient doses may result in tolerance and increased potential for addiction. Thus, the control of chronic pain with systemic narcotics is often accompanied by a marked reduction in quality of life.

The discovery of opiate receptors in the substantia gelatinosa of the spinal cord first led to the recognition that opioids had a spinal, as well as supraspinal, analgesic action. Fields and Basbaum in the United States and Besson in France subsequently described and elucidated the descending pain inhibition system. This pathway begins with projections from the frontal cortex and hypothalamus to the periaqueductal gray matter (PAG) of the midbrain, projecting then to the dorsal pons and the rostroventral medulla and then through the dorsolateral funiculus to terminate in the substantia gelatinosa of the spinal cord dorsal horn. These efferents serve to inhibit the second-order ascending nociceptive neurons, thus blocking pain transmission. The understanding of the mechanism by which narcotics exerted their antinociceptive activity at the spinal level led to the first trials of direct intraspinal administration of these agents, with morphine administered epidurally[6] and intrathecally[28] for the treatment of cancer pain.[21]

Between the time of the discovery of opiate receptors in the substantia gelatinosa in 1976 and 1990, spinal opioids had been used in more than 120,000 patients.[27]

Intraspinal pharmacotherapy for pain largely restricts drug effects to regions associated with the source of noxious input. Systemic side effects are largely eliminated, and there is a much higher local analgesic concentration at the site of action, even at significantly lower doses. Morphine is particularly well suited for this application by virtue of its hydrophilicity and resulting slow absorption from the cerebrospinal fluid. Thus, analgesia from intrathecal injections of morphine not uncommonly last up to 24 hours.[6]

At the spinal level of *anti-nociceptive* processing, opiates presynaptically diminish primary afferent terminal excitability and inhibit substance P release. Postsynaptically, opiates act to suppress excitatory amino acid evoked excitatory postsynaptic potentials in dorsal horn neurons. There are at least five opioid receptor subclasses, three of which (μ, δ, and κ) are thought to mediate anti-nociception. Morphine, D-alanine-D-leucine enkephalin (DADLE), and dynorphin, respectively, are the prototypic agonists for these receptor subclasses.

The discovery of multiple receptor systems involved in nociceptive transmission and modulation has allowed for the testing and application of other receptor selective drugs (Table 22–2). Other than narcotics, α-adrenergic agonists have been the most widely used receptor agonists for intraspinal pain pharmacotherapy. α-Adrenergic receptors exist in the substantia gelatinosa of the spinal cord, situated on both presynaptic and postsynaptic terminals of small primary afferents. α-Adrenergic agonists appear to mediate nociception by indirectly decreasing the release of substance P. These agents have the particular advantage over opiates of having little or no effect on respiratory centers, thus largely eliminating the possibility of respiratory depression. A further potential advantage of adrenergic agents in this setting is their efficacy in the setting of neuropathic pain states. There is both experimental[18] and clinical[5] evidence that neuropathic pain states that respond poorly to morphine may be well treated by intrathecal α_2-adrenergic

TABLE 22–1. CNS AND PERIPHERAL EFFECTS OF OPIATES

CNS Effects	Peripheral Effects
Analgesia	*Decreased GI tract motility*
Mydriasis	*Constipation*
Euphoria or dysphoria	Urinary retention
Nausea and vomiting	Histamine release
Sedation	Pruritus
Confusion	Increased biliary duct pressure
Cough reflex depression	
Respiratory depression	

TABLE 22–2. SOME INTRASPINALLY ADMINISTERED DRUGS IN THE TREATMENT OF INTRACTABLE PAIN

Opiates
  Morphine
  Fentanyl
  Sufentanil
  Dilaudid
  Dynorphin
  β-Endorphin
  D-Ala-D-leu-enkephalin
α-Adrenoceptor agonists
  Clonidine
  Tizanidine
GABA-B Agonists
  Baclofen
Naturally occurring peptides and their analogues
  Somatostatin
  Octreotide
  Calcitonin
Local anesthetics

agents. Within this category, clonidine has been recently approved for instraspinal use, and tizanidine has been tested in clinical trials.

Although other agents, such as υ-aminobutyric acid-B (GABA-B) agonists, calcitonin, and somatostatin and its analogue octreotide have been investigated clinically, narcotics, local anesthetics, and adrenergic agonists are most often used clinically. At the present time, however, morphine and clonidine are the only agents approved by the U.S. Food and Drug Administration (FDA) for intraspinal analgesic use.

PATIENT SELECTION

To achieve optimal results, proper patient selection is crucial. Several factors must be taken into account that would indicate or contraindicate intraspinal analgesic treatment (Table 22–3).

Failure of Maximal Medical Therapy

If a noninvasive treatment program provides satisfactory pain relief without intolerable side effects, then intraspinal drug administration is not necessary. Thus, patients considered for intraspinal drug administration should have failed a multidisciplinary pain treatment program including analgesics and physical and psycho-

TABLE 22–3. INDICATIONS AND CONTRAINDICATIONS FOR CHRONIC INTRASPINAL ANALGESIC ADMINISTRATION

Indications
  Chronic pain with known pathophysiology
  Sensitivity of the pain to the agent to be infused
  Failure of maximal medical therapy
  Favorable psychosocial evaluation
  Favorable response to trial of intraspinal analgesic agents
Contraindications
  Intercurrent systemic infection
  Uncorrectable bleeding diathesis
  Allergy to agent to be infused
  Failure of a trial of intraspinal analgesic agents

logical therapies. In addition to anti-inflammatory agents, tricyclic antidepressants, and non-narcotic analgesics, chronic systemic narcotic therapy should be attempted prior to the consideration of implantation of a chronic infusion system. Should this or other therapies be effective and well tolerated, then intraspinal drug administration is not indicated. However, as is often the case with patients with pain of malignant origin, it is of great importance that failure of medical therapy be recognized early. Thus, patients on increasing oral, transdermal, or intravenous doses of morphine who have already been treated with anti-inflammatory and tricyclic analgesics should be referred for trial of intraspinal drug administration to limit their suffering and their exposure to extremely high doses of narcotics.

Favorable Psychosocial Evaluation

Although most investigators have highlighted the importance of a favorable psychosocial evaluation in the screening of potential implant candidates, the specific variables and their quantification and treatment are not widely agreed on. As part of this evaluation, most agree that both the patient and his or her support system need to be evaluated. Clearly, acute psychotic illnesses and severe untreated depression need to be diagnosed and effectively treated prior to the consideration of surgery. Other issues are less clearly accepted as reasons for delay or contraindication of surgery. A patient may have a behavioral abnormality that may affect his or her ability to adequately judge the degree of pain or pain relief. Deficiencies in social support systems may leave the patient without someone to provide aid in the event of a pain-related emergency or in the maintenance of the drug administration system (either drug administration or transfer of the patient for refilling of the drug-administration device).

Absence of Systemic Infection

The ramifications of infection of the drug administration system range from the need to remove the entire system, and thus to at least temporarily eliminate this option for pain control, to the potentially life-threatening complication of meningitis. Thus, any local infection at the placement site or the presence of systemic infection contraindicates the implantation of drug administration devices. Furthermore, the use of perioperative and postoperative prophylactic antibiotics is recommended.

Absence of Clotting Disorders

Coagulopathies, which are not uncommon in patients with malignancies, present a problem when one considers implanting a drug delivery system. Not only can the surgery be made difficult by bleeding that is difficult to control, but surgery can be then complicated by the development of subcutaneous, epidural, or intradural hematomas. All efforts should be made to reverse clotting disorders prior to surgery; significant uncorrectable coagulation disorders contraindicate the implantation of drug infusion systems.

Absence of Drug Allergy

Allergy to the analgesic agent to be infused obviously and absolutely contraindicates its use. With the advent of multiple potential intraspinal analgesic agents, however, this should much less frequently be a reason to abandon this mode of therapy. Nonallergic reactions to the infused agent, such as urinary retention or pruritus, are usually associated with acute exposure to the drug and may resolve with time or respond to specific treatment. These do not therefore represent absolute contraindications to chronic drug infusion.

Absence of Obstruction of Cerebrospinal Fluid Flow

Obstruction of cerebrospinal fluid (CSF) flow has been identified as a relative contraindication to intraspinal drug delivery, depending on the size, location, and cause of the obstruction. *In our experience, this has not been a significant problem, and patients have gotten excellent drug effects despite the presence of significant degrees of obstruction of CSF flow.* More important, the presence or absence of an obstruction of CSF flow is the response to an intraspinal drug trial at the level at which permanent catheter implantation is intended.

Life Expectancy Greater Than 3 Months

Although the expected length of life is not a contraindication to the intraspinal route of drug administration, *it does have a great bearing on the decision about which method of administration to employ.* Thus, percutaneous epidural catheters attached to external pumps, internalized passive reservoirs and catheters that require percutanous bolus administration of drug, patient-activated mechanical systems, constant-rate infusion pumps, and programmable infusion pumps are all options for intraspinal drug delivery. The choice of these approaches on the basis of ambulatory status and life expectancy is discussed later.

Favorable Response to an Intraspinal Narcotic Trial

Not all patients suffering from chronic pain syndromes will benefit from the intraspinal administration of narcotics. The response to acute intraspinal administration of analgesic agents is generally regarded as an excellent indicator of long-term efficacy.[22] The inability to achieve pain relief after such a trial is a contraindication to implantation.

Careful preoperative screening of candidates for indwelling drug administration systems for the relief of intractable pain can help to exclude patients who will not benefit from this technology and predict efficacy in others. Unfortunately, bias on the part of both the treating physician and the patient can inappropriately skew the results of subjective or improperly controlled trials

and lead to the implantation of drug administration systems in patients who will not benefit from chronic intrathecal narcotic administration.

Several approaches to the trial of intrathecal narcotics have been advocated, including single vs. multiple injections, administration via lumbar puncture vs. indwelling catheter, epidural vs. intrathecal routes, and bolus vs. continuous-infusion administration of the drug. Testing with a single intraspinal dose of an active agent raises the significant possibility that the strong desire of the physician and other health care personnel to help the patient and the patient's desperation to find some relief from intractable pain will lead to a significant placebo response to this injection, which may occur in at least 30% of cases. Attempts to control for patient bias by testing both morphine and saline and blinding the patient to which drug is being infused *still do not control for the bias of the health care team.* Furthermore, the conclusions arising from preimplantation drug trials are often based on completely subjective criteria. This subjectivity can negatively impact the validity and reliability of screening protocols. We have thus developed a quantitative, crossover, double-blind trial for the preimplantation screening of candidates for chronic drug infusion therapy for the control of intractable pain. Application of this protocol has resulted in the elimination of approximately 30% of potential implant candidates. *Of patients with a successful screening trial, about 70% have had good to excellent long-term pain relief.* This screening paradigm appears to be both reliable and easily applied.[19]

ROUTE OF ADMINISTRATION

Although no direct comparative study has been done to determine the relative efficacy of epidural vs. intrathecal administration, certain observations may be made by comparing the results of previous studies of both routes of administration (Table 22-4).

The equianalgesic epidural dose is roughly ten times that of an intrathecal dose. As 80% to 90% of an epidural injection is systemically absorbed, this larger dose re-

TABLE 22–4. INTRATHECAL AND EPIDURAL DRUG DELIVERY

Advantages	Disadvantages
Intrathecal Drug Delivery	
Lower dosage requirement (10 × epidural dose)	Increased risk of neural injury
Less systemic effect	Increased risk of spinal headaches
No dural fibrosis at tip of catheter	Increased risk of supraspinal distribution
Possible to sample spinal fluid for culture, diagnosis and drug levels	
Epidural Drug Delivery	
Reduced risk of respiratory depression	Greater dose requirement
Reduced risk of spinal headache	Higher systemic effect
Reduced risk of neural injury	Dural fibrosis possible
	Question of increased tolerance
	Limited reservoir volume

quirement may lead to greater systemic side effects, including constipation and urinary retention. These higher doses further increase the probability that narcotic tolerance will develop. In addition, in that there is a fixed maximum solubility of morphine in saline of approximately 55 mg/mL, and pump reservoirs are of limited size, the higher dose requirement necessitates refilling the reservoir on a more frequent basis. Epidural catheter placement has been associated with dural scarring, resulting in catheter failure due to occlusion, kinking, or displacement.

Although it avoids these complications, intrathecal drug administration carries the disadvantages of potential CSF leakage and associated postural spinal headaches, respiratory depression due to supraspinal redistribution of narcotic, and increased risk of meningeal infection or neural injury.

Thus, the major advantage of epidural administration is the theoretically lower risk of serious complications, although these complications with intrathecal drug administration are remarkably uncommon. Furthermore, epidural catheters can be placed at virtually any level, making it potentially more useful for the treatment of upper body pain. Anderson and others, however, have reported their excellent results with the treatment of pain of the trunk, the neck, and even the head, with lumbar intrathecal morphine administration.[1] The advantages of the intrathecal route (including the lower drug dosage requirements leading to increased intervals between pump refills and the lower risk of catheter failure) and the infrequency of potential complications suggest that this is the preferred route for intraspinal drug delivery.

DRUG DELIVERY SYSTEM

Despite the popularity of implantable drug pumps, there are a number of different methods by which intraspinal drug administration can be accomplished. These systems include percutaneous epidural catheters attached to external pumps, internalized passive reservoirs and catheters requiring percutanous drug administration, patient-activated mechanical systems, constant-rate infusion pumps, and programmable infusion pumps. In light of the significant expense of drug pumps and the surgery required for their implantation, the choice of drug administration system should be made with careful consideration of the benefits of bolus vs. continuous-drug infusion and the patient's general medical status, ambulatory status, and estimated life expectancy.

Several investigators have explored the question of continuous-flow vs. bolus infusion. Continuous spinal infusion results in lower peak CSF morphine concentrations and correspondingly lower plasma levels than bolus administration while providing stable steady-state levels at the spinal site of action of the agents. It has been further suggested that continuous infusion may result in a reduced rate of opioid receptor tachyphylaxis[8] and have a lesser risk of producing delayed respiratory depression.[7] Clinical studies, however, have not clearly confirmed the superiority of continuous over bolus intraspinal drug infusion.

In that there is no consistent evidence that continuous or bolus administration is more effective in the clinical setting, the type of drug delivery device should be chosen based on the patient's ambulatory status, general health, and estimated length of life. Thus, for patients with short life expectancy of days to weeks, especially those who are bedbound, an epidural tunneled percutaneous catheter attached to an external drug pump is a viable, inexpensive option. Although the risk of infection increases over time, these catheters can be maintained for several weeks to a few months without complication. Over time, the costs of renting the external drug pump and the required nursing and pharmacy services make this route quite costly. Taking care to tunnel the catheter and rigorous hygenic care of the catheter and its dressing help to ensure the viability of the drug infusion system.

For patients with limited life expectancy who are ambulatory, an implanted reservoir system attached to an intraspinal catheter is an attractive option. An intraspinal catheter is tunneled subcutaneously and attached to a reservoir placed over the anterior or anterolateral chest wall. Implanting the reservoir over the lower ribs allows for easy localization and stabilization of the reservoir during drug administration. Subcutaneous reservoirs are manufactured specifically for this application; they are rated to withstand hundreds of punctures, whereas other familiar reservoirs, such as the Ommaya reservoir, are rated only for several dozen punctures. These systems require daily percutaneous access of the reservoir, and as such are uncomfortable for the patient and engender an increased risk of infection. They do, however, allow for the patient to be unencumbered when moving about during the day and can be accessed for either bolus administration or for continuous infusion by attachment to an external pump.

Mechanical patient-controlled indwelling drug administration systems are a third option for intraspinal drug therapy. Unfortunately, these devices are presently in clinical trials and are only available for implantation in patients outside of the United States. One such device consists of an implanted drug reservoir and an intraspinal catheter, both of which are connected to a subcutaneously placed patient-activated control system. This panel consists of two Silastic chambers; depression of the first chamber allows for drug delivery when the second chamber is depressed. In that there is a fixed interval for refilling the drug delivery chamber, a maximum dose per unit time results. This is the functional equivalent to the patient lock-out times programmed into external patient-controlled analgesia pumps.

Two major types of implanted drug pumps are currently marketed. The device marketed by the Infusaid Company consists of a drug-filled bellows compressed by Freon gas under pressure; outflow is regulated by a high-resistance valve. The infused solution is then delivered at a fixed rate; dose changes are made by changing the concentration of the solution to be infused. Thus, there is some increased cost and patient discomfort when dose changes are indicated; furthermore, these devices are subject to small variations in drug-delivery rates with changes in temperature and atmospheric pressure.

Somewhat more expensive is the programmable, electronic drug pump. This pump can be programmed transcutaneously, and sophisticated drug dose regimens can be instituted. Dose changes can be made with noninvasive programming. Because these pumps are battery operated, they require surgical replacement when the batteries expire; under average conditions, this occurs about every 4 years. Both implanted pumps need to be refilled every 1 to 2 months, depending on the rate of drug delivery.

While careful controlled studies are lacking, several models have been explored to determine the relative costs of these drug administration systems over time. In general, *it appears that for patients whose life expectancy, and, thus, intraspinal drug use, will exceed 3 months,* it is cost-effective to use a fully implanted drug pump, whereas for patients with shorter life expectancy, a percutaneous catheter or implanted reservoir may be a more reasonable option.[9, 17] In light of current health care reform and the demands for greater cost containment in medicine, these issues must be considered in every patient who is deemed a candidate for intraspinal analgesic therapy.

RESULTS

Morphine

Several studies of the efficacy of intraspinally administered morphine for the treatment of intractable pain have appeared (Table 22-5). Although most studies suggest an efficacy of roughly 80% in the setting of cancer pain, the reported efficacy for nonmalignant pain states is much more variable. Although some investigators have reported poor results,[9, 17] several others have found significant success. Auld and co-workers have reported two studies of intraspinal narcotics for the treatment of nonmalignant pain; in the first,[4] 21 of 32 patients

TABLE 22–5. EFFICACY OF INTRASPINALLY ADMINISTERED MORPHINE FOR INTRACTABLE PAIN

No. of Patients*	Mode of Administration	Efficacy	Study (Year)
6	Epidural	3 had complete relief; 3 had better than 50% reduction in pain	Behar et al. (1979)
8	Intrathecal	2 had complete relief from separate saline and morphine injections; 6 had complete relief from morphine alone	Wang et al. (1979)
1	Intrathecal	1 had complete relief	Onofrio et al. (1981)
10 (5/5*)	Intrathecal	5 cancer patients had significant reduction in pain; 5 nonmalignant patients had poor reduction in pain	Coombs et al. (1983)
17 (16/1*)	Epidurally/intrathecally	16 cancer patients had 50%–70% reduction in pain; 1 nonmalignant patient had poor reduction in pain	Krames et al. (1985)
80	Epidural	25 patients had complete relief; 9 patients had partial pain relief	Yablonski-Peretz et al. (1985)
5	Intrathecal	3 had good relief; 2 had poor relief	Esposito et al. (1985)
43	Epidural	28 patients with nonmalignant pain had good to excellent relief	Auld et al. (1985)
6	Epidural	6 had sufficient pain relief	Andersen et al. (1986)
20	Epidural	15 patients with nonmalignant pain; 2 patients had excellent relief; 6 had good relief; 1 had fair relief; 2 had poor relief; 4 had no relief	Auld et al. (1987)
35	Intrathecal	35 patients had pain relief.	Madrid et al. (1987)
43 (35/8*)	Intrathecal	28 cancer patients had excellent to good relief; 8 noncancer patients had excellent to good relief	Penn et al. (1987)
26	Intrathecal	20 had excellent relief; 3 had good relief; 1 had poor relief; 1 had none; 1 was comatose	Brazenor (1987)
69	Intrathecal	41 patients had mean pain scores of 3.8, down from 8.6	Hassenbusch et al. (1990)
9	Intrathecal	9 patients had mean pain score of 7.6/10 at baseline; at 1 wk, 1.9/10; at 1 mo, 2.0/10; at 2 mo, 0.5/10 for surviving patients	Anderson et al. (1991)
28	Epidural	17 patients with deep somatic pain had mean 76% ± 15% improvement; 9 patients with visceral pain had 49% ± 43%; 4 patients with only radiating pain had poor relief (2% ± 37%); in combined pain types, significant pain relief was obtained if somatic pain was one of the types	Samuelsson & Hedner (1991)
37 (35/2)	Intrathecal	35 cancer patients had good relief; 2 nonmalignant patients had good pain relief	Follett et al. (1992)

*No. of patients with cancer-related pain/no. with non–cancer-related pain.

demonstrated adequate relief, while in the second,[5] 14 of 20 patients obtained satisfactory pain relief with intraspinal morphine.

At the present time, the data concerning intraspinal morphine for pain secondary to cancer appear to be compelling and consistent, with a success rate of approximately 80%. Data concerning use in the setting of nonmalignant pain are less clear and consistent. Although intraspinal morphine may provide pain relief in carefully selected patients with intractable benign pain, further work needs to be done before this should be considered a regular part of the neurosurgical armamentarium.

The most widely recognized side effects of intraspinal narcotics include urinary retention, pruritus, and, rarely, delayed respiratory depression. Respiratory depression is most often seen in the opioid-naive patient and results from supraspinal redistribution of the drug; this side effect is both dose dependent and naloxone reversible. Other potential side effects include a decrease in libido and decreased testosterone levels in men.[23]

Clinical experience has demonstrated that in a significant fraction of patients, increasing doses of narcotic are required over time to maintain a similar degree of pain control. Although this may reflect the development of tolerance at the receptor level, in many cases this apparent tolerance results rather from a change in the status of the patient's disease. In the setting of pain secondary to a malignancy, for example, tumor progression may occur, resulting in the involvement of new areas of pain, invasion of more pain-sensitive structures, or a change in the nature of the pain from predominantly nociceptive to neuropathic. Furthermore, changes in the patient's psychosocial status may result in a decreased ability to cope with the pain, resulting in a perceived increase in the degree of pain.

Several strategies have been advanced to deal with such apparent tolerance. First, simply increasing the drug dose may provide for excellent long-term pain control. When this fails, or when the drug dose is escalated to levels that are felt to be potentially problematic, some authors have suggested the temporary use of *systemic analgesics while the pump is turned off for a period of several days to a few weeks (a so-called drug holiday). If the decreased efficacy of intraspinal narcotics is due to receptor tolerance, the drug holiday often results in the downregulation of the opioid receptors and a return of efficacy when intraspinal narcotics are reinstituted.*

When confronted with apparent tolerance to intraspinal morphine, another strategy is the use of narcotics active at other opioid receptor subclasses. Like μ receptor agonists, δ receptor agonists appear to work through a G-protein system to hyperpolarize the neuronal membrane through an increase in potassium conductance and thus inhibit neuronal activity. κ-Receptor agonists appear to function differently than μ- or δ-receptor agonists. These agents appear to activate a different G-protein mechanism, which blocks calcium entry through a voltage-dependent calcium channel. Investigators have had some success with δ-receptor agonists or those with mixed receptor subclass activity.

A final strategy to deal with the development of apparent tolerance has been the concomitant administration of low-dose local anesthetics with the narcotic. The combination of morphine and a local anesthetic has been successfully tried and seems to provide equivalent relief to morphine while necessitating smaller amounts of the opiate. Hassenbusch and co-workers[15] had good results, which lasted more than 1 year, in four of seven patients whose pain was not of malignant origin, using an epidural infusion of morphine sulfate combined with bupivacaine. Although satisfactory results were achieved, it should be noted that a rather high concentration of epidural morphine was used. Eighty percent to 90% of this high dose is likely to have been systemically absorbed and would thus produce systemic levels of morphine similar to those seen with oral administration. Du Pen and co-workers[10] examined the efficacy of epidural morphine-bupivacaine in a series of 68 patients who found no relief from epidural opioids alone. Sixty-one patients (90%) were considered treatment successes, with chronic bupivacaine infusion concentrations ranging from 0.1% to 0.5% and infusion rates varying from 4 to 18 mL/hour. Sjoberg and colleagues[26] reported on the long-term results of intrathecal morphine-bupivacaine administration in 52 "refractory" cancer patients. They assessed the quality of analgesia as being adequate in 2, good in 12, very good in 31, and excellent in 7. Side effects of bupivacaine in this study included transient paraesthesias, motor blockade, and gait impairment.

Adrenergic Agonists

Eisenach and co-workers[11] treated 9 patients with intractable cancer pain tolerant to instraspinal opioids with epidural clonidine. Patients received between 100 and 1000 μg/day; clonidine produced analgesia lasting more than 6 hours but also decreased blood pressure by more than 30%. Hypotension was treatable with intravenous ephedrine. Clonidine also decreased heart rate by 10% to 30% and it produced a transient sedation in the patients receiving the larger doses. There were no opioid-like effects of respiratory depression, pruritus, or nausea. Several other studies have reported similar results. In part, as a result of a recent multicenter trial, intraspinal clonidine for the treatment of chronic pain has recently been approved by the FDA.

In contrast to clonidine, the α_2-adrenergic agonist tizanidine does not appear to induce hypotension. This agent has been demonstrated to be an effective analgesic agent when administered intrathecally in both experimental[18] paradigms. Tizanidine appears to be particularly useful in the treatment of narcotic-insensitive neuropathic pain syndromes.

COMPLICATIONS

Although implanted drug delivery systems offer a uniquely effective method for pain control in selected patients, they are not without significant potential complications. The risk of infection is common to all drug-delivery devices. Percutaneous catheters and implanted reservoirs appear to be particularly susceptible to infection in that there is either an ongoing communication to an external site or frequent injections through the skin. Infection may involve the surgical wound or the subcutaneous region surrounding the hardware, when it is effectively treated by removal of all implanted hardware and the administration of appropriate intravenous antibiotics. Cure is seldom accomplished without the externalization of the hardware. Reimplantation of the drug delivery system is usually delayed until 3 months after completion of antibiotic therapy.

Infusion of contaminated drug solution is of far greater concern, as it may lead to potentially life-threatening meningitis. The risk of this complication can be limited by the use of an in-line bacteriostatic filter; unfortunately, not all of these systems either allow for or provide such filters. Early recognition of this complication is critical; the hardware must be removed and appropriate antibiotic therapy administered.

Erosion of the hardware through the skin is a less common complication and may be more likely to occur in cachectic, poorly nourished patients. The risk of erosion can be limited by ensuring that the implant is placed deep enough, that the hardware does not lie directly underneath the surgical incision, and that a careful, multilayer closure has been performed.

The most frequently observed complications of implanted drug delivery systems involve failure of the system itself. Pump failures are uniquely uncommon, but they may occur, particularly with the complex electronics of programmable pumps. Problems with the catheter, however, are quite common, and have been observed in up to 25% of patients over time. These complications include kinking, obstruction, disconnection, or shearing of the catheter. Several techniques may be used to limit the risk of catheter failure. These include the use of fluoroscopy during catheter placement to ensure that the catheter is not looped, partially kinked, or placed with its tip lying in a dural nerve root sheath. Confirmation of CSF flow during each stage of the implant procedure helps to detect catheter obstruction during the surgery. The use of the paraspinous approach to catheter implantation limits the sharp angulation of the catheter as it exits and enters the interspinous ligament and guards against shearing at these sites. Securing the catheter with a purse-string suture as it exits the interspinous ligament, and again with a Silastic fixation device, helps to prevent CSF leak and migration of the catheter out of the subarachnoid space. The use of a loop of catheter distal to this point helps to relieve strain on the catheter and prevents catheter migration or dislocation. Finally, dissection of a small space above the fascia in which the catheter comfortably rests will help to prevent kinking when the wound is closed.

Despite great care during catheter implantation, these problems may still occur. *Drug delivery system failure is signaled by an increase in pain or the subcutaneous accumulation of infusate.* Initial evaluation includes the comparison of the expected and true residual volume in the pump reservoir; a significant disparity suggests further evaluation. Plain radiologic evaluation of the entire system detects catheter disconnection and may also demonstrate kinking or migration of the catheter from the subarachnoid space. Occasionally, the instillation and attempted intrathecal delivery of iodinated contrast material via the pump may be helpful in identifying a catheter or pump failure. Quantitative nuclear medicine studies may also be helpful; the pump may be filled with dilute solutions of radioactive material and the delivery of these materials can be followed over time. Even these diagnostic tests may be equivocal, requiring surgical exploration and revision of the pump and/or catheter. With such a rigorous approach, virtually all such mechanical problems can be corrected and pain relief restored.

Another problem common to all implanted drug delivery systems is the potential for overdose. With an externalized system, this may result from improper setting of the external drug pump or improper dilution of the infusate by the pharmacy. Great care must be taken to ensure that appropriate drug concentrations and delivery rates are maintained. *The incorrect reprogramming of indwelling drug pumps can be far more insidious, as these errors are potentially subtle and are not necessarily immediately recognized.* Drug overdoses resulting from programming errors or incorrect infusate concentrations have occurred.

A further risk is created by the presence in some pumps of a side port intended for either bolus drug injection or to test for catheter patency. There have been two reported deaths resulting from accidental access of the side port instead of the refill port; thus, the entire refill volume of the pump *was infused as a bolus* into the CSF. Modifications have recently been introduced to prevent access to the bolus port by needles intended for pump refilling; nonetheless, great care must be exercised to avoid this potentially life-threatening complication.

FUTURE DIRECTIONS

Although tremendous progress has been made in the past decade in the use of intraspinal analgesics for the treatment of intractable pain, several areas need to be addressed before the technique is more widely accepted and its clinical use is expanded. First, although its efficacy in the treatment of pain secondary to malignancy appears clear, the use of intraspinal drug administration for pain of nonmalignant origin remains to be elucidated. Properly controlled, large-scale trials are lacking; until such evidence is available, use in this setting should be considered investigational.

Second, patient selection criteria need to be better defined and validated. In particular, those aspects of the psychosocial evaluation that predict success or failure and the specific pain states that may respond to this intervention need to be better elucidated. In light of the cost and modest invasiveness of this approach, great attention must be paid to refining patient selection criteria to ensure a good chance of successful pain relief.

Finally, and perhaps most significantly, further development in analgesic pharmacology needs to be applied to intraspinal drug therapy. *Although dozens of analgesic agents for oral or parenteral use that capitalize on the complex neurochemistry of pain transmission and modulation pathways are currently available, only two such agents are available for intraspinal use.* With the development of newer and more specific agents designed particularly for intraspinal use, and with the utilization of agents active at a number of receptor systems involved in pain perception, intraspinal drug administration may help to limit the suffering of many more people with otherwise intractable pain.

REFERENCES

1. Anderson PE, Cohen JI, Everts EC, et al: Intrathecal narcotics for relief of pain from head and neck cancer. Arch Otolaryngol Head Neck Surg 117:1277-1280, 1991.
2. Andersen HB, Kjaergard J, Eriksen J: Subcutaneously implanted injection system for epidural administration. Acta Anaesthesiol Scand 30:473-476, 1986.
3. Arner S, Arner B: Differential effects of epidural morphine analgesia. Acta Anaesthesiol Scand 28:535-539, 1984.
4. Auld AW, Maki-Jokela A, Murdoch DM: Intraspinal narcotic analgesia in the treatment of chronic pain. Spine 10:778-781, 1985.
5. Auld AW, Murdoch DM, O'Laughlin KA: Intraspinal narcotic analgesia: Pain management in the failed laminectomy syndrome. Spine 12:953-954, 1987.
6. Behar M, Magora F, Olshwang D, et al: Epidural morphine in treatment of pain. Lancet 1:527, 1979.
7. Brazenor GA: Long term intrathecal administration of morphine: A comparison of bolus injection via reservoir with continuous infusion by implanted pump. Neurosurgery 21:484-491, 1987.
8. Coombs DW: Intraspinal analgesic infusion by implanted pump. Ann NY Acad Sci 531:108-122, 1988.
9. Coombs DW, Saunders RL, Gaylor MS: Relief of continuous chronic pain by intraspinal narcotics infusion via an implanted reservoir. JAMA 250:2336-2339, 1983.
10. Du Pen SL, Kharasch ED, Williams A, et al: Chronic epidural bupivacaine-opioid infusion in intractable cancer pain. Pain 49:293-300, 1992.
11. Eisenach JC, Rauck RL, Buzzaneli, et al: Epidural clonidine analgesia for intractable cancer pain: Phase I. Anesthesiology 71:647-652, 1989.
12. Esposito S, Bruni P, Delitala A, et al: Therapeutic approach to the pancoast pain syndrome. Appl Neurophysiol 48:262-266, 1985.
13. Follett KA, Hitchon PW, Piper J, et al: Response of intractable pain to continuous intrathecal morphine: a retrospective study. Pain 49:21-25, 1992.
14. Hassenbusch SJ, Pillay PK, Magdinec M, et al: Constant infusion of morphine for intractable cancer pain using an implanted pump. J Neurosurg 73:405-409, 1990.
15. Hassenbusch SJ, Stanton-Hicks MD, Soukap J, et al: Sufentanil citrate and morphine/bupivicaine as alternative agents in chronic epidural infusions for intractable non-cancer pain. Neurosurgery 29:76-82, 1991.
16. Kloke M: Somatostatin and neoplastic pain. *In* Recent Results in Cancer Research. Berlin, Springer-Verlag, 1993, p 129.
17. Krames ES, Gershow J, Glassberg A, et al: Continuous infusion of spinally administered narcotics for the relief of pain due to malignant disorders. Cancer 56:696-702, 1985.
18. Leiphart JW, Dills CW, Zikel OM, et al: A comparison of intrathecally administered narcotic and nonnarcotic analgesics in experimental chronic neuropathic pain. J Neurosurg 82:595-599, 1995.
19. Levy RM: Quantitative crossover double blind trial paradigm for patient screening for chronic intraspinal narcotic administration. Neurosurg Focus 2:2.1-2.4, 1997.
20. Madrid JL, Fatela LV, Lobato RD, et al: Intrathecal therapy: Rationale, technique, clinical results. Acta Anaesthesiol Scand 60-67, (suppl) 85: 1987.
21. Matsuki A: Nothing new under the sun—a Japanese pioneer in the clinical use of intrathecal morphine. Anesthesiology 58:289-290, 1983.
22. Onofrio BM, Yaksh TL, Arnold PG: Continuous low dose intrathecal morphine administration in the treatment of chronic pain of malignant origin. Mayo Clin Proc 56:516-520, 1981.
23. Paice JA, Penn RD, Ryan WG: Altered sexual function and decreased testosterone in patients receiving intraspinal opioids. J Pain Symptom Manage 9:126-131, 1994.
24. Penn RD: Use and abuse of drug pumps in cancer pain. Clin Neurosurg 35:409-421, 1987.
25. Samuelsson H, Hedner T: Pain characterization in cancer patients and the analgetic response to epidural morphine. Pain 46:3-8, 1991.
26. Sjoberg M, AppelorenL, Einarsson S, et al: Long term intrathecal morphine and bupivicaine in 'refractory' cancer pain: Results from the first series of 52 patients. Acta Anaesthesiol Scand 35:30-43, 1991.
27. Waldman SD, Yaksh TL: Historical overview and future horizons. J Pain Symptom Manage 5:1, 1990.
28. Wang JK, Nauss LE, Thomas JE: Pain relief by intrathecally applied morphine in man. Anesthesiology 50:149-151, 1979.
29. Yablonski-Peretz T, Klin B, Beilin Y, et al: Continuous epidural narcotic analgesia for intractable pain dure to malignancy. J Surg Oncol 29:8-10, 1985.

Chapter 23

Neuroablative Procedures for Treatment of Intractable Pain

Robert M. Levy, M.D., Ph.D.

Modern neurosurgical procedures for pain were first attempted in the latter part of the 19th century. Letievant first described sectioning of the cranial and peripheral nerves to alleviate pain in his book "Traite de Sections Nerveuses" in 1873. In 1891, Horsley performed a gasserian neurectomy for trigeminal neuralgia; Frazier perfected this technique in 1928. The first spinal dorsal rhizotomy was reported by Abbé in 1889 and the first successful cordotomy was performed by Spiller and Martin in 1912. Leriche, in his 1939 book "La Chirurgie de la Douleur," is credited with the development of sympathectomy. Moniz first performed frontal lobotomy for pain control in 1936. From these sentinel reports has grown a significant experience in the ablation of neural structures to control medically intractable pain. This chapter attempts to present a concise review of the current status of neuroablative procedures used in the management of chronic pain; neuromodulatory procedures are discussed elsewhere in this volume.

PERIPHERAL NERVE PROCEDURES

Spinal Dorsal Rhizotomy

Attempts at pain control through invasive procedures were initially directed at the peripheral nervous system. After Abbé performed the first spinal posterior rhizotomy in 1889, enthusiasm for the procedure spread quickly. At the height of its popularity, spinal dorsal rhizotomy was used for a wide variety of pain syndromes. Cervicothoracic dorsal rhizotomy was performed for angina pectoris, intractable headaches, and facial pain, and it became widely used for failed back surgery syndrome, postparaplegic pain, pelvic cancer pain, postherpetic neuralgia, and post-thoracotomy pain. More recently, percutaneous radiofrequency methods of spinal rhizotomy have been devised to minimize the risks of extensive laminectomies. Dorsal rhizotomy was thought to have great analgesic potential based on the early neuroanatomic principles that suggested that the dorsal roots carry only sensory fibers, whereas ventral roots carry only motor fibers. The more recent

demonstration of unmyelinated sensory fibers in the ventral root may explain the often unsatisfactory results of these procedures; sensory pain fibers entering via the ventral route escape interruption by dorsal rhizotomy. Histologic sprouting, both in the intact cutaneous nerves and the spinal cord dorsal horn adjacent to denervated regions, may also allow transmission of nociceptive information despite dorsal rhizotomy. The possibility that nociceptive afferents bypass the dorsal spinal roots and that dorsal horn neurons have modifiable receptive fields may further account for the poor success rate of dorsal rhizotomy for pain control.

Despite decades of experience, it is difficult to clearly define the indications for rhizotomy. Nonetheless, there is consistent failure of dorsal rhizotomy for post-thoracotomy pain, postherpetic neuralgia, failed back surgery syndrome, and postparaplegia pain. Current indications for open dorsal rhizotomy include neuropathic pain of the chest wall associated with allodynia, treated by thoracic rhizotomy; cancer pain of the pelvis, rectum, vulva, or cervix, treated by extradural sacral rhizotomy; and pain in a functionally useless limb, treated by multilevel rhizotomy.[1] Patients medically unfit for open laminectomy can benefit from percutaneous rhizotomy. Benign intractable monoradicular pain in the cervical, thoracic, or lumbar dermatomes as well as dermatomal thoracic pain of malignant origin may be effectively treated with percutaneous rhizolysis.

Prior to dorsal rhizotomy, a trial block of the selected roots with local anesthesia should be performed; nonetheless, transient pain relief with a local block does not guarantee long-term pain relief. If local blocks are successful, open dorsal rhizotomy is performed using a routine laminectomy technique. Due to overlapping dermatomal innervation, one or two roots above and below the targeted dermatome should be sectioned. The percutaneous approach for dorsal rhizotomy was introduced in 1974 by Uematsu and colleagues and the techniques in localization of intervertebral foramen are well described.[2-4] The technique combines the use of a thermistor-monitored electrode, a fluoroscopic image intensifier, a nerve stimulator, and a radiofrequency lesion generator. Uematsu and co-workers recommend graded increments of heating using the thermocoagulator at 50 to 90°C for 90 to 120 seconds. Potential but rare complications of rhizotomy include wound infection, meningitis, hemorrhage, spinal cord infarction, trauma to the spinal cord, and cerebral spinal fluid leak. Postrhizotomy dysesthesias and anesthesia dolorosa are also potential complications of this denervation procedure.

There is considerable variability in the reported effectiveness of open dorsal rhizotomy; few outcome studies of percutaneous dorsal rhizotomy are available. Ten studies published between 1969 and 1986 reported on a total of 1173 patients; the mean success rate was 59%, with a range from 28% to 100%. Four significant reports have been published on the results of percutaneous dorsal rhizotomy, but the number of subjects has been small and outcome definitions are not consistent. Nonetheless, these authors reported success rates ranging from 52% to 93%.

Dorsal Root Ganglionectomy

Scoville first reported an extradural approach to dorsal roots and dorsal root ganglions in 1966. Smith began performing dorsal root ganglionectomies using the rationale that simple dorsal rhizotomies failed because some of the pain impulses traveled via the dorsal root ganglia to the sympathetic chain and entered the spinal cord at a higher level.[5] With the exception of a small number of cell bodies of nociceptive fibers in the ventral root, dorsal root ganglionectomy should overcome the anatomic limitations of spinal rhizotomy by removing nearly all nociceptive cell bodies.

Possible indications for dorsal root ganglionectomy include perineal or chest wall pain secondary to cancer; peripheral pain of thoracic and abdominal origin; and thoracic postherpetic pain.[1] Although mixed results have been reported in the setting of failed back surgery syndrome,[6-9] North reported long-term follow-up of at least 5 years with only 15% success.

Preoperative screening with local anesthetic blockade of the spinal ganglia along with control placebo injection should be performed. Failure of the block should preclude ganglionectomy. However, complete pain relief from preoperative blockade does not guarantee surgical success. As with other segmental neuroablative procedures, ganglionectomy is performed at the involved level as well as at levels above and below, to cover the desired dermatomes. As with the dorsal rhizotomy, the risks of ganglionectomy may include disruption of the vascular supply, hemorrhage, infection, cerebrospinal fluid leak, wound dehiscence, and other possible complications of spinal surgery. Postganglionectomy dysesthesias and anesthesia dolorosa have been reported.[6-9] Eleven series have been reported from 1966 to 1991, representing 237 patients treated with dorsal root ganglionectomy. Reported success rates varied from 0% to 100%; the mean reported success rate was 61%.

Facet Denervation

Goldthwait first described pain from disorders of the facet joint in 1911. The innervation of the facet comes from radicular spinal nerves. The posterior primary ramus of the spinal nerve divides into a medial and lateral branch; the medial branch innervates the facet joint. With this anatomic understanding, Rees advanced the concept of percutaneous facet denervation and later communicated a 99.8% success rate without mortality or major morbidity in 1000 procedures.[10] Others have since reported lesser success with this procedure. Multiple modifications of the procedure, including the use of radiofrequency thermocoagulation, have since been described. Although no unanimity of opinion exists, patients with chronic mechanical back pain with no other treatable cause in whom conservative management has failed may be candidates for percutaneous facet denervation. Critical for patient selection is the response to a local, selective facet block with local anesthetic. Pain relief should be complete or nearly complete and should be achieved consistently with repeated trials. The technique for percutaneous facet denervation is well described.[11, 12] Repeating the procedure at least one level above and below the desired target is required for lasting pain relief. Complications from reported series are rare.[13-16] Beside the risks involved in all percutaneous operative procedures, superficial burns from failure of insulation and acute radiculitis have been reported. From 1971 until 1990, 10 reports were published of 1990 patients treated with facet denervation procedures. Success rates ranged from 21% to 99%; the mean success rate was 62%.

Peripheral Neurectomy

In 1828, Wood first used the term "neuroma" to describe the pathologic condition characterized by a bulbous terminal of injured nerves, and Mitchell coined the term "causalgia" in 1872 to describe the chronic pain after nerve injury experienced by veterans of the Civil War. Although resection of the involved peripheral nerve is, at first glance, an appealing approach, overwhelming clinical and physiologic evidence has accrued against the use of neurectomy for management of chronic pain.[4] Thus, most peripheral nerves consist of mixed motor and sensory fibers, and sectioning the nerve may result in both motor deficits and total anesthesia. With the resulting significant sensory loss, denervation hypersensitivity or anesthesia dolorosa may develop. Neuromas may form at the transsected nerve stump. Furthermore, pain relief following neurectomy is often short lived due to adjacent sprouting of sensory nerves.

Today, peripheral neurectomy has a limited role in the management of chronic pain. Cranial neurectomy has proved to be of little value in the treatment of trigeminal neuralgia, headaches, or atypical facial pain. Neurectomy has failed to consistently relieve phantom limb, chest wall, or abdominal pain. However, there are a few selected situations in which peripheral neurectomy may be of value, including pain due to a neuroma in a weight-bearing area, pain due to a neuroma in continuity from an entrapment or a traumatized nerve, and pain due to severe intractable meralgia paresthetica.[4] Proper patient selection is the most important predictor of successful neurectomy or neuroma excision. Thorough history and physical examination; sympathetic, thermal, and mechanical testing; electromyography/nerve conduction velocity studies; and diagnostic nerve blocks should be performed. At surgery, the neuroma can be best located with the help of the Tinel's sign. The neuroma is excised and the proximal nerve stump is implanted into muscle or bone marrow. External or internal neurolysis is reserved for treatment of neuroma-in-continuity, when preservation of function is desired. The addition of nerve transposition may be performed to avoid repeated trauma to the nerve stump or proximal nerve.

Postoperative dysesthesias following neurectomy are possible; anesthesia dolorosa is rare. For neuroma-in-continuity, the nerve function may be disrupted and a new neurologic deficit may occur. Between 1976 and 1995, seven large series have reported the results of peripheral neurectomy and/or neuroma resection in 443 patients. The mean reported success rate was 71%.

Sympathectomy

Leriche first performed a sympathectomy for lower extremity trophic ulcers and was the first to implicate the sympathetic nervous system in chronic pain states.[17] Pathogenetic studies of causalgia and sympathetic dystrophy soon postulated the formation of "artificial synapses" following nerve injury and suggested that tonic efferent sympathetic impulses jumped to the adjoining injured and poorly myelinated pain fibers. More recently, abnormal increases in the firing rate of regenerating transsected fibers, especially in response to norepinephrine, have been observed as has the successful use of regional guanethidine blocks in patients with causalgia and sympathetic dystrophy. The development of endoscopic approaches and both percutaneous radiofrequency and chemical techniques for the production of lesions have made sympathectomy a safer treatment option.

Sympathectomy for relief of chronic pain is currently indicated only in a handful of conditions involving the limbs and abdominal viscera. These include pain due to causalgia, reflex sympathetic dystrophy, peripheral vascular disease, and Raynaud's disease. Sympathectomy may also be considered for abdominal visceral pain due to chronic pancreatitis or pancreatic carcinoma. Failure of conservative therapy, a thorough preoperative assessment, and both therapeutic and diagnostic sympathetic blocks should be performed prior to surgical sympathectomy. The techniques for sympathectomy are well described and include upper thoracic ganglionectomy, lower thoracic sympathectomy or splanchnicectomy, and lumbar sympathectomy. Transthoracic endoscopic and stereotactic percutaneous approaches are also currently employed.[18, 19] Complications of upper thoracic ganglionectomy include wound infection, pneumonia, pneumothorax, cerebrospinal fluid leak, Horner's syndrome, spinal cord injury, and empyema. Pleural tears, wound infections, empyema, and paraplegia due to vascular disruption have been reported in splanchnicectomy. For lumbar sympathectomy, the major neurologic complication is sexual dysfunction in men who have undergone bilateral procedures. Postsympathectomy neuralgia consisting of severe, deep aching and burning pain in the proximal limb is not an infrequent complication of sympathectomy. Although it may occur in up to 20% of cases of sympathectomy, this phenomenon usually subsides spontaneously within 6 months. The reported success rate of sympathectomy varies from 59% to 89% for causalgia and sympathetic dystrophy and from 67% to 100% for pancreatic pain. For other chronic pain syndromes, the results of sympathectomy are less vigorous. Despite reports of 60% success for the treatment of pain from Raynaud's disease, other series report quite poor rates of success. Discouraging results have also been reported for postamputation pain. The effectiveness of lumbar sympathectomy for ischemic rest pain or claudication remains unclear.

Lesions of the Dorsal Root Entry Zone

With the knowledge that spontaneous discharges from neurons occurred within the spinal cord dorsal horn on deafferentation, Nashold and co-workers in 1976 attempted to produce a lesion in the substantia gelatinosa to alleviate phantom pain.[20] Sindou and colleagues[21] reported a similar operation using open microsurgical techniques. Current theory suggests that the pathologic responses associated with deafferentation, allodynia, hyperalgesia, and hyperesthesia result from the facilitation of incoming signals, which occurs in the dorsal horn. Thus, the goal of producing a lesion in the dorsal root entry zone (DREZ) is to destroy the site of pathologic processing at which such facilitation occurs.

DREZ is currently considered primarily for pain due to brachial or lumbosacral plexus avulsions. It may also be effective in treating the segmental pain secondary to spinal cord injury, postherpetic neuralgia, amputation or phantom limb pain, and pain due to malignancy and in certain facial pain syndromes.

A number of different methods have been devised to produce lesions in the DREZ, including the microsurgical ablation first described by Sindou and others,[21] laser destruction, and radiofrequency heating. Currently, radiofrequency lesioning is the most popular method; lesions are made by heating the electrode to 75°C for 15 seconds. Bernard and co-workers[22] have expanded the use of DREZ lesions to the nucleus caudalis for severe postherpetic neuralgia and severe intractable facial pain, in which the lesions are made from the upper rootlets of C2 to an area just rostral to the level of the obex.

Complications of DREZ lesioning include weakness of the ipsilateral leg, reduction of proprioception, and loss of pain and temperature sensation beyond the painful limb and impotence. In addition, the inherent risks of intradural spinal surgery such as cerebrospinal fluid leak, infection, hemorrhage, infarction, and wound dehiscence, may also be encountered.

DREZ lesions for pain control following brachial plexus avulsion injuries have been reported in 341 patients from 1984 until 1993. Success rates range from 29% to 100%; the mean reported success rate of these studies was 66%. Of the 130 reported cases of patients treated with DREZ lesions for spinal cord injury pain, 65 patients (50%) had good results. Pain relief was excellent for segmental pain and poor for distal pain. The results of DREZ lesions for postherpetic neuralgia are generally disappointing, ranging from 20% to 50%. Patients usually gain early relief only to experience recurrence of the pain. For phantom limb pain, the average success rate of DREZ lesioning is 37%. The experience of DREZ lesions in the nucleus caudalis for treatment of facial pain is very limited; good results may be obtained in patients with facial pain due to postherpetic neuralgia, brain-stem infarction, or multiple sclerosis, but not for anesthesia dolorosa or peripheral trigeminal neuralgia.

SPINAL CORD ABLATIVE PROCEDURES FOR CHRONIC PAIN

Commissural Myelotomy

Based on the anatomic concept that fibers carrying nociceptive information cross at the anterior commissure of the spinal cord, Armour in 1926 performed the first commissural myelotomy for pain. Commissural myelotomy involves interruption of decussating spinothalamic fibers in the anterior commissure with the expectation that this will produce bilaterally symmetrical analgesia at the level of myelotomy. Additional extensive areas of pain relief caudal to the lesion, without associated sensory changes, are often observed. The primary indication for commissural myelotomy is intractable bilateral pain in the lower half of the body, particularly due to malignancy. Myelotomy is especially valuable for patients with midline pelvic or perineal malignant pain that is unresponsive to spinal opioids.

Complications occur in 5% to 10% of patients and include dysesthesias, motor weakness, gait ataxia, and bladder dysfunction. The risks inherent to intradural spinal surgery must also be considered. Approximately 350 cases of open commissural myelotomy have been reported; the range of reported success rates varies from 20% to 100%, with a mean of approximately 65%. Although the total cases performed via percutaneous technique is smaller, the success rate is very similar.

The use of neuroaugmentative devices has reduced the use of the commissural myelotomy, and the indications for its use currently are quite limited. As has been suggested by the results just mentioned, this procedure has the potential to produce a favorable outcome in a selected group of patients who do have malignant disease and do not respond to other less invasive therapies.

Anterolateral Cordotomy

Spiller performed the first open thoracic cordotomy in 1912; since that time the procedure has been carefully described and refined.[23] Mullan and associates introduced the percutaneous method of performing an anterolateral cordotomy in 1963,[24] and Rosomoff and co-workers developed a percutaneous radiofrequency technique in 1965.[25] Anterolateral cordotomy leads to loss of contralateral pain and temperature sensation without loss of position or light touch sensation. In general, pain sensitivity is diminished within two to three levels below the level of cordotomy.

In the past, anterolateral cordotomy was used for a variety of painful conditions that were medically intractable. With greater knowledge of its long-term complications and newer neuroaugmentative techniques, anterolateral cordotomy is rarely used and is reserved for medically intractable pain due to cancer in patients whose life span is less than 3 years.

Numerous publications have described the techniques of open anterolateral cordotomy.[26] Following C2 hemilaminectomy or appropriate high thoracic bilateral laminectomy, the dura is opened and the dentate ligament identified. The lateral attachment of the dentate ligament is cut to allow for mobilization of the cord. A cordotomy knife is inserted just ventral to the dentate ligament, and this quadrant of the spinal cord is sectioned. In the percutaneous approach,[27] patients are placed in supine position and, under local anesthesia, an 18-gauge needle is introduced into the subarachnoid space under fluoroscopic guidance, aimed just anterior to the dentate ligament between C1 and C2. Following myelographic confirmation of the needle position, an electrode is introduced through the needle into the parenchyma of the cord, and the target location is confirmed with the use of electrical stimulation. When the appropriate target is identified, a radiofrequency lesion is made.

The mortality rate for open anterolateral cordotomy has been reported in different series to range from 3% to 20%. Cervical cordotomies and bilateral cordotomies have a higher mortality rate than that of thoracic and unilateral cordotomies. Respiratory complications occur in about 10% of the cases. Motor impairment is reported in 10% to 15% of patients for unilateral lesions and up to 39% when bilateral procedures are performed. Dysfunctions of micturition and defecation as a complication vary widely. Postcordotomy dysesthesias occur in up to 11% of patients. The complication rate for the percutaneous approach is much lower; motor deficit (3%), ataxia (3%), bladder or sexual dysfunction (3%), respiratory problems (1%), and postcordotomy dysesthesia (1%) are all uncommon following percutaneous cordotomy.

From 1966 to 1977, three large series reported the results of open cordotomy in 712 patients; the mean reported success rate was 75%. From 1966 to 1988, seven large series reported the results of percutaneous cordotomy in 6665 patients; the mean reported success rate was 73%. For bilateral procedures, the success rates were marginally lower. As with many other ablative procedures for pain, this rate of success decreases as the time of follow-up is lengthened. Thus, although 3-month pain control was reached in 84% of patients in one study, the long-term success rate at 5 to 10 years was 37%.[27]

INTRACRANIAL ABLATIVE PROCEDURES

The introduction of stereotactic techniques together with advances in neuroimaging and computer technology have revolutionized intracranial ablative procedures. Today, intracranial ablative procedures can be done accurately and safely under local anesthesia. Modern intracranial ablative techniques include producing lesions in the brain-stem pain pathways (trigeminal tractotomy, spinothalamic tractotomy, mesencephalotomy), the diencephalon (thalamotomy, pulvinarotomy, hypothalamotomy), the telencephalon (cingulotomy or cingulumotomy), and the pituitary gland (hypophysectomy).

Most patients considered for intracranial ablative procedures have medically intractable chronic severe pain secondary to cancer, although the procedures are rarely used for pain of nonmalignant origin. In these patients, in whom pain is unresponsive to medical therapy and less invasive surgical therapies have failed, intracranial ablative procedures are contemplated. Patients with diffuse, nociceptive pain and short life expectancy tend to have the best results; it is important that they have a sufficiently clear sensorium to provide meaningful informed consent.

Traditionally, ventriculography was the method of choice for localization of the target for the placement of the lesion. Today, computer tomography (CT) or magnetic resonance imaging (MRI) guided stereotactic methods are usually used. Modern stereotactic treatment planning software can allow for careful preoperative planning of target location and trajectory. Although radiofrequency thermal lesions are the standard for intracranial ablative procedures, noninvasive radiosurgical techniques are currently under active investigation.[28]

Trigeminal Tractotomy

Sjoqvist first developed the medullary trigeminal tractotomy in 1938, which was refined by both Grant in 1941 and Sweet in 1955. In the 1960s, Hitchcock and Crue developed percutaneous approaches to trigeminal tractotomy. The trigeminal nerve pain fibers traverse the medulla to the nucleus caudalis. These fibers are joined by pain fibers from cranial nerves VII, IX, and X. Medullary trigeminal tractotomy targets these fibers for pain control. This procedure has been particularly helpful in the relief of intractable pain caused by malignancy of the head and neck. For postherpetic neuralgia and anesthesia dolorosa, trigeminal tractotomy has been less effective.

Technically, this can be performed as an open or percutaneous procedure, with or without the aid of stereotaxy.[29, 30] The open procedure consists of a C1 and C2 laminectomy and durotomy followed by identification of obex and dorsolateral sulcus. After identification of the trigeminal tract by evoked potentials, a careful incision is made on the dorsolateral sulcus that is 3 mm in depth, extending from 2 mm below the obex to the accessory nerve filaments. Stereotactically, the procedure can be done under local anesthesia with radiofrequency lesioning.

Complications from trigeminal tractotomy include weakness and ataxia, usually of the ipsilateral upper extremity, analgesia in the contralateral leg, Horner's syndrome, dysarthria, and hiccups. Most of these are temporary. Including patients with advanced neoplastic disease, the overall mortality rate from this procedure may be as high as 5% to 10%. The overall success rate for a combined total of 669 cases for open medullary trigeminal tractotomy is 75%, whereas that for the 40 cases with the percutaneous approach is 82.5%; the overall complication rate is 22% to 25%.[31]

Pontine and Bulbar Spinothalamic Tractotomy

The first medullary spinothalamic tractotomy was described by Schwartz in 1941. Similar to the open anterolateral cordotomy, spinothalamic tractotomy at this level can relieve more rostral pain in the upper shoulder and neck. At the medullary level, the spinothalamic tract is located ventral to the descending trigeminal tract and dorsolateral to the inferior olivary nucleus. With the introduction of high percutaneous cervical cordotomy and DREZ lesions for the upper arm, this procedure is much less commonly used.

Current indications for medullary spinothalamic tractotomy include intractable unilateral cancer pain, especially in the upper arm shoulder and neck. Severe pulmonary compromise is a relative contraindication for this procedure. Technically, a suboccipital craniectomy is performed, the arch of C1 is removed, and the dura is opened on the side of the intended lesion. At a depth of 6 mm, a 4-mm incision is made transversely using the rootlets of the spinal accessory nerve as the dorsal limit. Risks may include ataxia, lateropulsion, weakness, loss of proprioception, bleeding, infection, and infarction. One hundred thirty-one cases have been reported in 14 series; the mean initial success rate was 87%, which dropped to 45% on long-term follow-up. Reported morbidity and mortality were 23% and 13%, respectively.

Mesencephalotomy

Walker, in 1942, was the first to perform an operation aimed at interrupting the spinothalamic pathway in the midbrain. With their introduction of newer stereotactic methods, Wycis and Spiegel performed the first stereotactic mesencephalotomy in 1947 and reported their long-term results in 1962.[32] The anatomic regions involved in a mesencephalotomy include the spinothalamic tract and the structures medial to it, the *quintothalamic tract*. As proposed by Wycis and Spiegel, the involvement of the reticulospinal fibers in the periaqueductal gray matter just medial to the quintothalamic tract in a mesencephalotomy improves the result of the procedure.

With similar indications as for medullary spinothalamic tractotomy, trigeminal tractotomy, or high cervical cordotomy, mesencephalotomy, by interrupting both the spinothalamic and quintothalamic tracts, affects both head and body or limb pain. In addition, there is no significant contraindication to its use in patients with pulmonary dysfunction. The patients most greatly benefiting from mesencephalotomy have unilateral head or neck pain secondary to cancer. Some authors advocate its use in central pain, facial dysesthesia, or anesthesia dolorosa after unsuccessful trigeminal surgery and in postherpetic facial pain.

Mesencephalotomy is performed using stereotactic methods. A twist drill or burr hole is performed and an electrode is passed into the midbrain. Once the target site is reached, stimulation should always be done for confirmation of location before the lesion is made.[30] Potential complications include gaze palsy, hemiparesis, and postoperative dysesthesia or anesthesia dolorosa. The overall complication rate is 22% and mortality rate is about 1.5%. In the 12 series reporting 501 cases, the mean success rate was 76%.[31]

Thalamotomy/Pulvinotomy

Wycis and Spiegel[32] first reported the use of dorsomedian thalamotomy for the treatment of pain in 1953. Several targets for thalamotomy have since been proposed including the area below the ventral posterior nuclei rostral to midbrain, the medial thalamus, the posteromedial thalamus and pulvinar, and the dorsomedial and anterior nuclei of the thalamus. Combination operations have been proposed in which lesions are placed at two different sites in the hope of controlling both the transmission of noxious stimuli and the affective component of pain.

Thalamotomy for intractable pain is controversial; some feel that this is best used for central noncancer pain, whereas others believe the only indication for thalamotomy is cancer pain. Thalamotomy is a stereotactic procedure and can be performed under local anesthesia with a low complication rate. Initial success rates for medial and basal thalamotomies have been reported to be as high as 80%, only to drop to 30% after 1 year.

Hypothalamotomy

Hypothalamotomy was first performed in 1962 by Sano for the treatment of violent aggressive behavior; in 1971 he performed posteromedial hypothalamotomy for intractable pain. The mechanism for pain relief following hypothalamotomy as well as the indications for hypothalamotomy remain unclear. In the past, this procedure has been used for cancer pain involving the face, especially when the pain is accompanied by affective features such as depression, anxiety, and suffering. The ventriculographic guided technique as described by Sano consists of placing the lesion 2 mm below the anterior commissure–posterior commissure midpoint and 2 mm lateral to the wall of the third ventricle. The reported success rate in a limited number of series is 65% to 80%. No operative mortality and a 10% transient complication rate were reported.

Hypophysectomy

In 1953, Luft and Olivecrona published their pioneering work on hypophysectomy for treatment of various conditions.[33] Based on their understanding of hormonal influence on cancer, they included a number of patients with advanced cancer of the breast and prostate. To their surprise, many of these cancer patients had relief of pain hours after the procedure. Since that time, numerous methods of pituitary destruction using the open transcranial or transsphenoidal approaches have been devised, including sectioning of pituitary stalk and the use of alcohol, radiofrequency, cryotherapy, and interstitial radiation. Currently, hypophysectomy is considered for patients with severe diffuse pain from cancer, especially of the prostate and breast.

Endocrinopathies, especially diabetes insipidus, are the most common side effects of hypophysectomy. Other potential complications include cerebrospinal fluid leak, ocular nerve palsy, visual field deficits, and, rarely, meningitis, carotid artery damage, headache, and hypothalamic dysfunction. Approximately 50% to 80% of hypophysectomy patients report excellent to good pain relief, regardless of technique;[34] this pain relief, however, appears to be relatively short lived. For treatment of severe cancer pain, the relatively safe and technically straightforward chemical hypophysectomy should be considered.

Cingulotomy

During follow-up of psychosurgical procedures performed in the 1940s, several investigators noted that some patients who complained bitterly about pain preoperatively no longer did so afterward. One consistent target for which pain relief was noted was the cingulate gyrus, which was chosen because this area represented the frontal lobe component in Papez's limbic lobe, and it was thought at the time that the best target for affective disorders and related intractable pain would be areas involved with emotional expression. In 1962, Foltz and White[35] and Ballantine and others[36] each developed stereotactic methods for cingulotomy. The patients for which cingulotomy may be of most benefit have diffuse nociceptive pain secondary to cancer. This is especially true when the patient has a significant affective component to the pain, with prominent features of emotional suffering and depression.

Cingulotomy may be performed under general or local anesthesia using image-guided stereotactic techniques. Two frontal burr holes are made, 1.3 cm from midline and 9.5 cm posterior to the nasion. The target site for the cingulum should be about 3 cm posterior from the tip of the lateral ventricles, 1.5 cm superior to the ventricles, and 1.5 cm from the midline. Radiofrequency lesions are then made at 75°C for 60 to 90 seconds or longer for larger lesions. Some authors recommend overlapping two lesions to produce a more discrete conical lesion consistent with the shape of the cingulate gyrus at this level.

Reported complications of cingulotomy include seizures, hemorrhage, transient mania, headaches, decreased memory, and hemiplegia. Extensive neuropsychiatric testing reveals very few and minor changes after cingulotomy.[37] Major morbidity is rare for this procedure, and mortality is extremely unusual (0.1%). The overall rate of successful pain relief from cancer pain for six modern series reporting a total of 87 patients was 31%, but a 92% success rate was demonstrated when the cingulotomy was combined with another central procedure that interrupted a pain pathway. For cingulotomies performed for chronic pain of nonmalignant origin, a long-term success rate of 38% was demonstrated.[38]

SUMMARY

Although the role of intracranial ablative procedures remains poorly defined, they are clearly of value for the treatment of some difficult intractable pain syndromes. In patients who have undergone multidisciplinary pain assessment and therapy, including pharmacotherapy, physical therapy, and psychological therapy, and in whom neuroaugmentative procedures for pain control have failed, neuroablative procedures offer what is often the last hope for the relief of pain and suffering. Taking advantage of advances in our understanding of neuroanatomy, surgical technique, neuroimaging, and computer technology, most of these procedures have a low complication rate, and many can be carried out under local anesthesia. In general, with appropriate patient selection, these procedures have success rates of 50% to 80%, which is similar to those reported for most neuroaugmentative procedures. Thus, with judicious use, neuroablative procedures remain an important part of the neurosurgical armamentarium in the treatment of intractable pain.

REFERENCES

1. Burchiel KJ: Neurosurgical procedures of the peripheral nerves. In North RB, Levy RM (eds): The Neurosurgical Management of Pain. New York, Springer-Verlag, 1997, p 133.
2. Uematsu S, Udvarhelyi G, Benson DW, et al: Percutaneous radiofrequency rhizotomy. Surg Neurol 2:319, 1974.
3. Sluijter ME, Mehta M: Treatment of chronic neck and back pain by percutaneous thermal lesions. In Lipton S, Miles J (eds): Persistent Pain: Modern Methods of Treatment. New York, Academic Press, 1981, pp 141-179.
4. Uematsu S: Percutaneous electrothermocoagulation of spinal nerve trunk, ganglion, and rootlets. In Schmidek HH, Sweet WH (eds): Operative Neurosurgical Techniques: Indications, Methods, and Results. New York, Grune & Stratton, 1988, pp 1207-1221.
5. Smith FP: Trans-spinal ganglionectomy for relief of intercostal pain. J Neurosurg 32:574-577, 1970.
6. Osgood CP, Dujovny M, Faille R, et al: Microsurgical lumbosacral ganglionectomy, anatomic rationale, and surgical results. Acta Neurochir 35:197-204, 1976.
7. Pawl RP: Microsurgical ganglionectomy for treatment of arachnoiditis related unilateral sciatica. Presented at the American Pain Society Meeting, Miami, 1982.
8. Taub A: Relief of chronic intractable sciatica by dorsal root ganglionectomy. Trans Am Neurol Assoc 105:340-343, 1980.
9. Taub A: Ganglionectomy lectures presented to the Massachusetts General Hospital (cited in Gybels JM, Sweet WH: Neurosurgical Treatment of Persistent Pain: Physiological and Pathological Mechanisms of Human Pain. Basel, S Karger, 1989, pp 122-123)
10. Rees WES: Multiple bilateral subcutaneous rhizolysis of segmental nerves in the treatment of intervertebral disc syndrome. Ann Gen Pract 26:126-127, 1971.
11. Bogduk N, Long DM: The anatomy of the so called "articular nerves" and their relationship to facet denervation in the treatment of low back pain. J Neurosurg 51:172-177, 1979.
12. Ingnelzi RJ: Radiofrequency lesions in the treatment of lumbar spinal pain. Contemp Neurosurg 12:1-6, 1980.
13. Lazorthes Y, Verdie JC, Lagarrugue J: Thermocoagulation percutanee des nerfs rachidiens a visee analgesique. Neurochirurgie 22:445, 1976.
14. Burton CV: Percutaneous radiofrequency facet denervation. Appl Neurophysiol 38:80-86, 1976.
15. Lora J, Long DM: So-called facet denervation in the management of intractable back pain. Spine 1:121-126, 1976.
16. Shealy CN: Percutaneous radiofrequency denervation of spinal facets: Treatment for chronic back pain and sciatica. J Neurosurg 43:448-451, 1975.
17. Leriche R: The Surgery of Pain. London, Bailliére Tindall, 1939.
18. Kux M: Thoracic endoscopic sympathectomy by transthoracic electrocoagulation. Br J Surg 67:71, 1980.
19. Wilkinson HA: Percutaneous radiofrequency upper thoracic sympathectomy: A new technique. Neurosurgery 15:811-814, 1984.
20. Nashold BS, Urban B, Zorub DS: Phantom pain relief by focal destruction of the substantia gelatinosa of Rolando. Adv Pain Res Ther 1:959-963, 1976.
21. Sindou M, Fischer G, Mansuy L: Posterior spinal rhizotomy and selective posterior rhizotomy. In Krayenbuhl H, Maspes PE, Sweet WH (eds): Progress in Neurological Surgery. Basel, S Karger, 1976, pp 201-250.
22. Bernard EJ, Nashold BS, Caputi F: Clinical review of nucleus caudalis dorsal root entry lesions for facial pain. Appl Neurophysiol 51:218, 1988.
23. Schwartz HG: High cervical cordotomy: Technique and results. Clin Neurosurg 8:282-293, 1960.
24. Mullan S, Harper PV, Hekmatpanah J, et al: Percutaneous interruption of spinal-pain tracts by means of a strontium needle. J Neurosurg 20:931-939, 1963.
25. Rosomoff HL, Carroll F, Brown J, et al: Percutaneous radiofrequency cervical cordotomy technique. J Neurosurg 23:639-644, 1965.
26. Poletti CE: Open cordotomy medullary tractectomy. In Schmidek HH, Sweet WH (eds): Operative Neurosurgical Techniques: Indications, Methods, and Results. New York, Grune & Stratton, 1988, pp 1155-1168.
27. Rosomoff HL: Percutaneous spinothalamic cordotomy. In Wilkins RH, Rengachary SS (eds): Neurosurgery. New York, McGraw-Hill, 1985, pp 2446-2451.
28. Young RF, Jacques D, Rand RW, et al: Medial thalamotomy for chronic pain: A comparison of gamma knife and radiofrequency stereotactic techniques (abstract). Neurosurgery 35:571, 1994.
29. King RB: Medullary tractotomy for pain relief. In Wilkins RH, Rengachary SS (eds): Neurosurgery. New York, McGraw-Hill, 1985, pp 2452-2454.
30. Nashold BS, Crue BL: Stereotaxic mesencephalotomy and trigeminal tractotomy. In Youmans JR (ed): Neurological Surgery, ed. 2. Philadelphia, WB Saunders, 1982, pp 3702-3716.
31. Loeser JD, Gildenberg PL: Medullary and mesencephalic tractotomy. In Bonica JJ (ed): The Management of Pain. Philadelphia, Lea & Febiger, 1990, pp 2086-2093.
32. Wycis HT, Spiegel EA: Long range results in the treatment of intractable pain by stereotaxic midbrain surgery. J Neurosurg 19:101-107, 1962.
33. Luft R, Olivecrona H: Experiences with hypophysectomy in man. J Neurosurg 10:301-316, 1953.
34. Ramirez LF, Levin AB: Pain relief after hypophysectomy. Neurosurgery 14:499-504, 1984.
35. Foltz EL, White LE: Pain relief by frontal cingulumotomy. Neurosurgery 19:89-100, 1962.
36. Ballantine HT, Bouckoms AJ, Thomas EK: Treatment of psychiatric illness by stereotactic cingulotomy. Biol Psychiatr 22:807-819, 1987.
37. Corkin S, Twitchell TE, Sullivan EV: Safety and efficacy of cingulotomy for pain and psychiatric disorder. In Hitchcock ER, Ballantine HT, Meyerson BA (eds): Modern Concepts in Psychiatric Surgery. Amsterdam, Elsevier, 1979, pp 253-272.
38. Ojemann G: Frontal lobe operations for pain. In Bonica JJ (ed): The Management of Pain. Philadelphia: Lea & Febiger, 1990, pp 2096-2100.

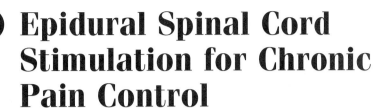

Chapter 24

Epidural Spinal Cord Stimulation for Chronic Pain Control

Sherwin E. Hua, M.D.,
and Robert M. Levy, M.D., Ph.D.

Only 2 years after Melzack and Wall[1] proposed the gate-control theory of pain, epidural spinal cord stimulation (SCS) was used by Shealy and co-workers[2] to treat patients with intractable pain. This was the first reversible, nondestructive procedure for the control of chronic pain, and, as an alternative to neuroablative procedures, it was met with great enthusiasm. Initially, the implantation of SCS electrodes involved laminectomy and was solely the domain of neurosurgeons. Through years of advancement in the design of implantable electrodes and refinement of percutaneous techniques, SCS has become a common procedure utilized by physicians in various specialties. Additionally, with the discovery that SCS is effective for the treatment of limb ischemia secondary to peripheral vascular disease and angina pectoris, SCS has recently become a focus of interest in cardiovascular medicine.

MECHANISM OF ACTION

Although the precise anatomic and physiologic substrates of SCS are still not well understood, the prevailing mechanistic theory involves selective stimulation of larger Aα and Aβ fibers. The overwhelming predominance of large-fiber activity then competitively inhibits the nociceptive input from smaller Aδ and C fibers, thereby closing the spinal "gate" and preventing nociceptive transmission.[1] The spinal gate model proposes that large dorsal root fibers activate spinal networks in the superficial layers of the dorsal horn that inhibit pain and sensory input to deeper layers. Stimulation of dorsal root fibers can directly modulate these inhibitory networks. Furthermore, stimulation of dorsal columns is thought to induce antidromic conduction to activate these inhibitory circuits through collateral processes of dorsal root and dorsal column fibers.

The inhibition to nociceptive transmission by SCS may also be mediated by neurochemical factors. In experimental pain models, SCS is associated with a significant increase in intrathecal γ-aminobutyric acid (GABA) levels over a 2- to 3-hour period.[3] The administration of adenosine has been demonstrated to potentiate the effects of SCS, which suggests a relationship between adenosine and SCS-induced pain relief.[4] The modulation by SCS of other factors, including glycine, substance P, serotonin, and neurokinin A, has been demonstrated. In contrast, naloxone administration does not decrease the effectiveness of SCS in humans, which suggests that endogenous opioids do not play a significant role in SCS-induced pain relief.[5]

In addition to the local effects on the spinal cord, SCS may elicit central inhibition through brain-stem centers. Activation of the anterior pretectal nucleus in the brain stem, causing descending inhibition through the dorsolateral funiculus, may induce longer-lasting inhibition of pain transmission in the spinal cord.

EFFICACY

Since its introduction in the 1960s, SCS has been found to be an effective procedure for the treatment of chronic, persistent pain. Dozens of studies have reported success with this procedure, although reported success rates range from 15% to 80%. Reasons for this great variance include differences in patient selection, pain syndromes treated, and definitions of success. One convention for the definition of a successful outcome is a reduction in pain by 50%. This criterion is often accompanied by asking the patient if he or she would go through the surgery again to achieve the same result. Changes in psychosocial factors that are associated with pain may be good indirect measures of the effectiveness of SCS-induced pain relief. Results on psychological test measures, such as the Minnesota Multiphasic Personality Inventory (MMPI) and the Beck Depression Inventory (BDI), have been used with some success to correlate with surgical outcome. Changes in functional aspects of daily living are also important indicators of success. Sleep habits, changes in amount and type of pain medications used, activities of daily living, and ability to return to work are all important factors that need to be considered when assessing the success of SCS.

Although many lack objective outcome measurements, the overwhelming majority of studies reporting the success rate of SCS are further plagued by problems in experimental design. Much needed are controlled, prospective, large-scale studies with long-term follow-up, for which pain ratings, psychosocial scale measurements, and other outcome measures are collected by a disinterested and "blinded" third party. Only a single prospective, randomized, crossover trial of SCS vs. another mode of therapy (spinal reoperation) has been performed.

Although a wide variation in results has been reported among investigators, most recent studies report a 50% to 60% long-term success rate for SCS. Two recent studies have provided particularly valuable information on the effectiveness of SCS in chronic pain therapy. North and co-workers[6] reported the results of SCS performed on 171 patients from 1972 until 1990. Of these patients, 52% reported at least 50% pain relief, with a mean follow-up period of 7 years. An increased percentage of patients younger than 65 years were actively working after SCS (54% vs. 41%), and 58% of patients reduced or eliminated their analgesic intake.

Burchiel and co-workers[7] performed a prospective, multicenter study of SCS and found that 56% of 66 patients treated with SCS experienced greater than 50% pain relief at 1-year follow-up. Patients also showed significant improvements in functional and psychosocial outcomes as measured by a number of objective outcome scales.

INDICATIONS

The most common indication for SCS is *failed back surgery syndrome* (FBSS), also known as *lumbar post-laminectomy syndrome*. The syndrome is defined as persistent back or leg pain after one or more reparative operations. Because of the broad definition, the syndrome encompasses a wide and heterogeneous population of patients with multiple potential etiologies for persistent pain. Thus, treatment of this population necessitates the use of diverse treatment strategies. Preliminary studies show that SCS is equal to or has better results than further reparative surgery in patients in the setting of FBSS.[8] Furthermore, studies have shown that 50% to 60% of patients have at least 50% pain reduction after 1 to 2 years of follow-up. Although a trial of percutaneous SCS is usually a prerequisite to the implantation of a permanent system, patients with FBSS tend to have a high rate (90%) of success with the trial electrode, as compared with patients with pain syndromes of peripheral origin.[6] These results are excellent when compared with the results of other methods of pain control used in these patients.

Reflex sympathetic dystrophy (RSD), also known as *complex regional pain syndrome, type 1* (CRPS-1) is a complex pain syndrome without universal consensus on definition, etiology, or treatment strategy. RSD can present with a wide spectrum of symptoms, including diffuse pain not confined to the distribution of a peripheral nerve, diminished function, joint stiffness, and skin or soft tissue changes that include swelling, changes in

temperature, hyperhidrosis, and atrophy. It is believed that most of these changes are related to dysfunctional sympathetic activity. Traditionally, pharmacologic therapy, physical therapy, and sympathetic blocks are tried first to manage the pain. If these conservative measures are not effective, neuroablative procedures (e.g., sympathectomy) and neuromodulatory procedures (e.g., SCS and intraspinal drug administration) may be considered.

SCS has been demonstrated to be effective for the long-term management of RSD. Fifty percent to 60% of patients with RSD experience pain control from SCS for 2 to 4 years of follow-up.[9] SCS may be preferable to sympathectomy for treatment of RSD because it is both reversible and efficacious, whereas the results of sympathectomy tend to fade over time. Other sympathetically maintained pain syndromes, including causalgia, appear similarly to benefit from treatment with SCS. Neuropathic pain secondary to peripheral nerve injury and phantom limb pain both appear to be effectively treated with SCS.

Experience with SCS for the treatment of pain related to spinal cord injury has been mixed. Most authors report good to excellent control of the well-circumscribed segmental pain of spinal cord injury with SCS, whereas the distal pain from spinal cord injury is poorly affected by SCS. The steady, burning pain following spinal cord injury appears to be more effectively treated than intermittent, lancinating, or touch-evoked pain.

SCS has become an important treatment modality especially in Europe for both the pain and ischemia related to peripheral vascular disease (PVD). SCS not only helps to control pain but may also improve blood flow and result in limb salvage. Both microcirculatory (transcutaneous partial pressure of oxygen at the dorsum of the foot) and macrocirculatory parameters (blood flow velocity at the femoral artery) have been found to be improved by SCS.[10] The improvement in circulation was seen within 6 weeks of stimulation, and this improvement regressed within 1 week after stimulation was stopped. European trials have found success rates of 50% to 60% for pain and circulation improvement.[11] Patients with PVD who qualify for SCS typically have PVD unresponsive to medical therapy, have been deemed unsuitable for revascularization, and do not have major psychosocial co-morbidities.

Recent studies have demonstrated that SCS is effective for the treatment of intractable pain due to angina pectoris. This stimulation effectively relieves angina pain without masking the pain of myocardial infarction. This effect is accompanied by improvement in exercise tolerance and myocardial metabolism and is thought to be mediated through sympathetic effects.

Thus, SCS is effective for a number of different chronic pain syndromes. Although SCS is more generally effective for limb rather than axial pain, several authors have reported success in treating axial pain using more complex stimulation configurations.

PATIENT SELECTION AND TRIAL ELECTRODE PLACEMENT

As with other interventional pain procedures, careful patient selection is the most crucial factor in achieving optimal results. Patients should have an objective diagnosis for their chronic pain complaints. A careful history and physical examination with relevant imaging studies needs to be performed. Multidisciplinary, conservative therapy, including physical therapy, psychological approaches, and pharmacologic therapy, including possibly nonsteroidal anti-inflammatory medications, tricyclic antidepressants, and anticonvulsants, should be initiated. A trial of chronic narcotic therapy may be considered. Should rehabilitation and medical therapy fail to adequately control the pain, invasive procedures should be considered. Psychosocial co-morbidities must be addressed before invasive therapies are initiated; psychological evaluation must be performed to rule out somatoform disorders, severe and inadequately treated depression, and other psychiatric disorders. Additionally, drug addiction and secondary gain issues should be addressed, as these psychosocial problems may reduce the efficacy of invasive therapies.

Prior to SCS implantation, a trial of percutaneous SCS should be performed. A percutaneous electrode is placed epidurally while the patient is under local anesthesia and monitored anesthesia care (MAC) with sedation. The patient is placed in a prone position and a 14 gauge Tuohy needle is inserted in the midline in the midlumbar region (for lower extremity pain) or in the upper thoracic region (for upper extremity pain). Using either the loss of resistance or hanging drop method, entrance into the epidural space is confirmed. Under fluoroscopic guidance, the lead is positioned in the epidural space so that the patient experiences paresthesia over the entire painful area with stimulation. The Tuohy needle is withdrawn and the electrode is anchored to the skin.

The stimulation trial usually lasts several days; a prolonged trial should be avoided due to the risks of infection or cerebrospinal fluid leak. Changes in the degree of pain relief, analgesic use, and activities of daily living are noted, as are any complications such as infection or altered neurologic function. A 50% decrement in pain is usually considered a successful trial, and as such warrants implantation of a permanent SCS system.

EQUIPMENT AND PERMANENT IMPLANTATION

Technical advances in the design of electrodes and pulse generators have improved the effectiveness and ease of use of SCS systems. Two main types of electrodes are used today: (1) the percutaneous electrode, which can fit through a Tuohy needle; and (2) the laminectomy or plate-type electrode. Percutaneous electrodes can be placed without an incision and are easier to internalize; they are, however, more likely to move in the epidural space. This movement may result in unpleasant positional alterations in perceived stimulation intensity or distribution. While the positional alteration of stimulation-induced paresthesia often diminishes after several weeks due to epidural scarring, some patients continue to have such problems and require replacement of the percutaneous electrode with a plate-

type electrode. These laminectomy electrodes are implanted under direct vision in the operating room at the time of a limited laminotomy. They are more resistant to migration and can be sutured to dura, thereby providing even more spatial stability. In patients with previous spine surgery at the level of desired electrode placement, laminectomy electrodes are often the only option, as percutaneous electrodes cannot be navigated through the scarred epidural space.

Both types of electrodes allow four to eight contacts distributed linearly along each electrode. Most electrodes used today employ a bipolar configuration with one or more anodes and cathodes. A four-contact electrode with the option of anode or cathode leads at each contact point allows 65 possible combinations of bipolar stimulation. An eight-contact electrode allows 6,000 combinations. Multiple contacts, combined with the placement of multiple electrodes, allow flexible stimulation parameters and modification of these parameters to optimize pain control. As the goal of electrode placement is to allow complete overlap between areas of stimulation paresthesia and the painful area, flexibility of the stimulation areas and parameters is of great importance. This flexibility may partially explain the vast improvement in long-term failure rates of multichannel electrodes compared with those of single-channel electrodes.[6] Most patients can be treated with a single quadripolar electrode and a simple bedside programming unit. Complex pain syndromes requiring multiple electrodes may require sophisticated computer systems for electrode selection and programming.

Power is supplied to the electrodes by way of external or implanted pulse generators. Two types of pulse generators are available: (1) a totally implantable lithium pulse generator and (2) a percutaneously powered radiofrequency-driven generator. The lithium battery-powered pulse generator is completely implanted and allows maximum convenience. The stimulator can be turned on and off and can be reprogrammed transcutaneously using a small telemetry device. The drawback of this unit is that at the end of the battery's life, the unit must be replaced at open surgery. Battery life is dependent on stimulation parameters and ranges from as little as 1 year to more than 7 years. Lithium-powered generators are also limited in terms of their maximum power output. External radiofrequency generators, however, require the patient to wear an external antenna and an alkaline battery-powered transmitter. This is cumbersome and may significantly limit freedom of motion. This inconvenience is balanced by the increased power and stimulation frequency allowed by the radiofrequency generator.

Several technical factors may contribute to the success of SCS. The complete overlap of the patient's pain area with stimulation-induced paresthesia is a critical requirement for successful SCS. For leg pain, the electrode is usually positioned between the T10 and L1 spinal levels. For angina pectoris, the pain involves the precordial area with frequent radiation to the left arm, so the electrode is usually positioned at the T1–2 level of the spinal cord. For arm pain, the electrode is usually positioned between the C4 and C7 spinal levels.

Stimulation parameters are also important for successful long-term SCS outcome. High-voltage stimulation can cause uncomfortable paresthesia and motor contractions; the voltage level at which stimulation becomes uncomfortable is labeled the *discomfort threshold*. In contrast, the voltage needs to be sufficiently high to be effective. The voltage at which the patient first perceives paresthesia is called the *perception threshold*. The range between the perception threshold and the discomfort threshold is the *usage range* and represents the usable range of voltage for stimulation. A wider usage range gives the patient more flexibility in identifying effective stimulation parameters. Other stimulation parameters, including frequency, pulse width, and pulse conformation, are also important and can be adjusted either at the time of implantation or, more commonly, at outpatient follow-up.

RISKS AND COMPLICATIONS

Overall, SCS implantation is quite safe and has a low rate of morbidity in experienced hands.[9] Isolated cases have been reported of direct penetration of the spinal cord during placement of the epidural needle. Epidural hematoma causing postoperative paraplegia has been reported. Both percutaneous and plate electrodes can also cause nerve root injury. The most minor complications include local pain overlying the hardware, electrode malfunction, lead migration, infection, cerebrospinal fluid leak, and muscle spasms. The incidence of all minor complications may be as high as 16%.[7] Most of these complications resolve spontaneously or can be addressed by altering stimulation parameters. Other complications, such as infection or lead repositioning, require surgical intervention. Infection rates have been reported to be as high as 5%[6]; these are best treated by removal of the hardware and institution of antibiotic therapy.

SUMMARY

SCS is an effective, nondestructive technique for the control of chronic pain. It is particularly effective for pain due to failed back surgery syndrome, RSD, peripheral nerve injury, peripheral vascular disease, and angina pectoris. SCS should be considered for carefully selected patients only when multidisciplinary, conservative therapy has failed to control pain.

REFERENCES

1. Melzack P, Wall PD: Pain Mechanisms: A New Theory. Science 150:971-978, 1965.
2. Shealy CN, Mortimer JT, Reswick JB: Electrical inhibition of pain by stimulation of the dorsal columns: Preliminary clinical report. Anesth Analg 46:489-491 1967.
3. Stiller CO, Cui JG, O'Connor WT, et al: Release of gamma-aminobutyric acid in the dorsal horn and suppression of tactile allodynia by spinal cord stimulation in mononeuropathic rats. Neurosurgery 39:367-375, 1996.
4. Cui JG, Sollevi A, Linderoth B, et al: Adenosine receptor activation suppresses tactile hypersensitivity and potentiates spinal cord stimulation in mononeuropathic rats. Neurosci Lett 223:173-176, 1997.
5. Freeman TB, Campbell JN, Long DM: Naloxone does not affect pain relief induced by electrical stimulation in man. Pain 17:189-195, 1983.
6. North RB, Kidd DH, Zahurak M, James, et al: Spinal cord stimulation for chronic, intractable pain: Experience over two decades. Neurosurgery 32:384-395, 1993.
7. Burchiel KJ, Anderson VC, Brown FD, et al: Prospective, multicenter study of spinal cord stimulation for relief of chronic back and extremity pain. Spine 21:2786-2794, 1996.
8. North RB, Kidd DH, Lee MS, et al: A prospective, randomized study of spinal cord stimulation versus reoperation for failed back surgery syndrome: Initial results. Stereotact Funct Neurosurg 62:267-272, 1996.
9. Barolat G: Spinal cord stimulation for persistent pain management. *In* Gildenbergand PL, Tasker RR (eds): Textbook of Stereotactic and Functional Neurosurgery. New York, McGraw-Hill, 1998, pp 1519-1537.
10. Kumar K, Toth C, Nath RK, et al: Improvement of limb circulation in peripheral vascular disease using epidural spinal cord stimulation: A prospective study. J Neurosurg 86:662-669, 1997.
11. Broseta J, Barbera J, de Vera JA, et al: Spinal cord stimulation in peripheral arterial disease: A cooperative study. J Neurosurg 64:71-80, 1986.

Chapter 25

Physical Medicine and Rehabilitation Approaches to Pain Management

Heidi Prather, D.O., Joel M. Press, M.D., and Jeffrey L. Young, M.D.

Physical medicine and rehabilitation practitioners use a comprehensive approach to pain management. The treatment they provide is guided by a specific diagnosis made in an acute, subacute, or chronic setting. Pain management programs may include using medications, flexibility and strengthening exercises, aerobic exercises, modalities, orthotics, injections, and adaptive equipment. A comprehensive rehabilitation program promotes improvement in function beyond simply resolving pain symptoms. Strong emphasis is placed on the patient being an active participant in the rehabilitation process. The purpose of this chapter, however, is to review briefly modalities and the application of therapeutic exercise.

OVERVIEW OF MODALITIES

Modalities are physical agents utilized to produce a therapeutic tissue response. Types of modalities include heat, cold, water, and ultrasound. Physical medicine and rehabilitation practitioners must have a good understanding of the physiologic effects of modalities to use them safely and appropriately. Modalities are most effective when applied in response to a specific diagnosis, with close monitoring of the patient's response. Most important, modalities are an adjunctive treatment included as part of a comprehensive rehabilitation program, not an isolated treatment option.

Heat

General Considerations. Tissue structures are warmed via three mechanisms: conduction, convection, and conversion. Conduction is the transfer of heat directly from one surface to another. Examples include hydrocollator packs and paraffin baths. Convection is the transfer of heat due to the movement of air or water across a body surface. Examples include hydrotherapy and fluidotherapy. Finally, conversion involves the transfer of heat via a change in energy. Examples are infrared lamps, ultrasound, and electromagnetic microwaves.

Heating a structure creates both local and distant effects. Vasodilation and increased metabolic demands promote increased blood flow with the delivery of leukocytes and oxygen and increased capillary permeability. The use of heat modalities is beneficial in assisting with pain control, muscle relaxation, and collagen extensibility. Table 25–1 summarizes the indications for heat modalities used for musculoskeletal pain management. The mechanism chosen is based on the specific diagnosis. Table 25–2 lists general contraindications and precautions for the use of therapeutic heat.

Superficial Heat. Direct heat penetration is greatest at an 0.5 to 2 cm depth from the skin surface and depends on the amount of adipose tissue. The more commonly used modes for musculoskeletal rehabilitation include hydrocollators, whirlpool, and contrast baths. Hydrocollator packs are made in three standard sizes and are heated in stainless steel containers in water with temperatures between 65 and 90°C. The highest temperatures found during use of the packs are at the skin's surface. Towels are applied with the packs to minimize skin trauma and to maintain heat insulation. Treatment sessions usually last 20 to 30 minutes.

Hydrotherapy is heating via submersion of small or large body surface areas. The risk of elevating core body temperature exists when large body surface areas are heated. Water temperature should not exceed 40°C when large body surfaces are heated in a Hubbard tank, whereas up to 43°C is acceptable when a patient submerges just a limb in a whirlpool. Hydrotherapy provides a gravity-eliminated environment that facilitates joint motion. Agitation created by the water flow provides sensory input.

Paraffin baths are a mixture of paraffin and mineral oil used as a treatment to deliver heat to small joints.

TABLE 25–1. INDICATIONS FOR THERAPEUTIC HEAT

Muscle spasm	Hyperemia
Pain	Increase collagen extensibility
Contracture	Accelerate metabolic processes
Hematoma resolution	

TABLE 25–2. CONTRAINDICATIONS FOR THERAPEUTIC HEAT

Acute inflammation	Edema
Hemorrhage or bleeding disorders	Ischemia
Decreased sensation	Atrophic skin or scarred skin
Poor thermal regulation	Inability to respond to pain
Malignancy	

Mineral oil creates a lower melting point for the paraffin, which provides increased thermal release when compared with the effects of water. The bath is kept at a temperature of 52 to 58°C for upper limb therapeutic sessions and between 45 and 52°C for lower limb sessions. Contraindications to paraffin baths include open wounds and severe peripheral vascular disease.

Fluidotherapy involves the placement of the extremity to be treated into a container through which hot air is blown within a medium of a dry powder of glass beads. Benefits include the heat plus mechanical stimulation that may further help in pain control.

Deep Heat. Conversion is used to heat deep tissue structures. Deep heating agents include ultrasound, phonophoresis, and shortwave and microwave diathermy. Ultrasound is most commonly used, however. Ultrasound is sound waves classified within the acoustic spectrum above 20,000 Hz. It is unique in that the production of heat is due to high-frequency alternating current (0.8 to 1.0 MHz), which is converted via a crystal transducer to acoustic vibration. Energy transfer occurs because of the piezoelectric effect, whereby the crystal undergoes changes in shape when voltage is applied. Selective heating is greatest when acoustic impedance is high, such as at the bone-muscle interface. Conversely, ultrasonic energy is readily conducted through homogeneous structures such as subcutaneous fat or metal implants with minimal thermal effects due to the rapid removal of heat energy. Ultrasound can be used safely near metal implants. However, in the presence of methyl methacrylate and high-density polyethylene, which is often used in total joint replacements, a higher amount of ultrasound energy is absorbed so there is potential for overheating. Ultrasound can heat to depths of 5 cm below the skin surface, thereby providing therapeutic benefit to bone, joint capsule, tendon, ligament, and scar tissue. Ultrasound also has some nonthermal effects. Gaseous cavitation involves gas bubbles created by high-frequency sound or turbulence. These bubbles may increase in size, causing pressure changes within the tissues. Cavitation may cause movement of material, mechanical distortion, and change in cellular function. Acoustic streaming causes movement of material secondary to pressure asymmetries produced by sound as it passes through a medium. Streaming has the potential to cause plasma membrane

TABLE 25–3. COMMON USES FOR THERAPEUTIC ULTRASOUND

Contractures	Degenerative arthritis
Tendinitis	Subacute trauma

TABLE 25–4. PRECAUTIONS FOR ULTRASOUND

Malignancy
Open epiphysis
Pacemaker
Laminectomy site
Radiculopathy
Near brain, eyes, or reproductive organs
Pregnant or menstruating uterus
Heat precautions in general
Caution around arthroplasties, methyl methacrylate, or high-density polyethylene

damage and acceleration of metabolic processes. Standing waves are produced by superimposition of sound waves and can cause heating at tissue interfaces at different densities.

Ultrasound dosage is measured in watts/cm_2. Intensities of 1.0 watts/cm^2 to 4.0 watts/cm^2 are most commonly used. Application is usually started at 0.5 watts/cm^2 and gradually increased while the practitioner monitors the patient's response. Duration of treatment is 5 to 10 minutes and is based on the size of the treatment area. Table 25-3 lists some common uses, and Table 25-4 lists precautions for ultrasound.

Cold

Cryotherapy. The physiologic effects of cold include vasoconstriction with reflexive vasodilation, decreased local metabolism, decreased enzymatic activity, and decreased oxygen demand. Cold decreases muscle spindle activity and slows nerve conduction velocity and therefore is often used to decrease muscle spasticity and guarding. Connective tissue stiffness and muscle viscosity are increased with cold. With these physiologic effects in mind, cryotherapy is often used during the first 48 hours after an acute musculoskeletal injury. However, care must be taken when applying cold over nerves owing to the potential development of neurapraxia. To minimize this, cold application should not exceed 30 minutes, and efforts should be made to protect peripheral nerves in the region being treated. Cryostretch and cryokinetics refer to the use of cryotherapy to facilitate joint motion. By decreasing pain and muscle guarding, improved flexibility and function can be achieved. Tables 25-5 and 25-6 summarize general indications and contraindications for cryotherapy.

Water

Contrast Baths. The alternating therapeutic use of heat and cold has been described as a form of vascular exercise because of the alternating vasodilation and vasoconstriction that occur. This alternation creates a hy-

TABLE 25–5. INDICATIONS FOR CRYOTHERAPY

Acute trauma	Pain
Edema	Muscle spasm
Hemorrhage	Spasticity
Analgesia	Reduction of metabolic activity

TABLE 25–6. PRECAUTIONS AND CONTRAINDICATIONS
FOR CRYOTHERAPY

Ischemia	Insensitivity to cold
Raynaud's disease or phenomenon	Inability to report pain
Cold intolerance	

peremic response, which improves circulation and fosters the healing response. Indications for contrast baths include improving range of motion, control of swelling, and assistance in pain control.

THERAPEUTIC EXERCISE

Therapeutic exercise is described in two broad categories: exercises that focus on muscle flexibility and strength and aerobic exercises. A rehabilitation program to manage musculoskeletal pain and dysfunction will include all of these in addition to patient education about proper biomechanics and ergonomics. The treatment program focuses on managing a particular diagnosis. Each program is customized to include specific work or sport activities.

When implementing an exercise program, the specific adaptation to imposed demand (SAID) principle should be applied. This principle states that the body responds to given demands with specific and predictable adaptations. Stronger muscles develop with strength training. Oxidative capacities of skeletal muscles increase with aerobic training. Pliability of connective tissue increases with flexibility exercises. With these outcomes in mind, exercise training parameters are implemented.

Flexibility Exercises. Maintaining or regaining muscle flexibility and range of motion is an important part of a rehabilitation program. Connective tissue stretches with a small amount of force and returns to its original length when the force is removed. When the muscle fibers are straightened, more force is required to apply a stretch. Furthermore, if connective tissues are stretched to a certain length and maintained, the tension within the tissue decreases. For best results, stretching should be maintained for 30 seconds, with the patient perceiving a pulling sensation rather than pain. Warming an area before stretching improves the elongation of the collagen fibers. Rapid or bouncing stretches promote tissue recoil, and a sustained stretch is not achieved. The risk of excessive loading and injury also occurs with bouncing. If too much force is applied with stretching, the patient will experience muscle soreness for more than 24 hours. Other potential problems with stretching include joint subluxation or overstretching during the healing phase of tissues such as tendons and ligaments. Improper timing of stretching in such instances may result in excessive laxity. With adherence to an appropriately applied stretching program, patient flexibility should improve within 1 to 2 months.

Types of Muscle Contractions. An isometric contraction is a muscle contraction without motion. Isometric contractions are used to stabilize a joint, such as when a weight is held at waist level without raising or lowering it. Dynamic contractions are muscle contractions with a fixed amount of weight. They are divided into concentric and eccentric contractions. A concentric contraction occurs when the muscle length is shortened during a contraction, for example, during a biceps curl. An eccentric contraction occurs when the muscle length is increased during the contraction, that is, the "negative" contraction. Eccentric contractions are used for decelerating or controlling motions. Isokinetic contractions are activated at a constant velocity and are created artificially by types of exercise equipment. Measurements of these contractions are often used in research settings, but little relevance has been demonstrated for real conditions. Plyometrics refers to a contraction sequence during which a rapid eccentric contraction precedes a concentric contraction, such as during a jump. An example is a jumper who lowers the body and eccentrically loads the gluteal muscles before the jump, which then requires concentric gluteal muscle contraction. Plyometric training can be especially useful in sport-specific rehabilitation. Strength is the maximal force generated during a single contraction, whereas power is the amount of force generated per unit of time. Power may be more important to emphasize for the athlete to return to maximal function. The amount of force generated by muscle contraction type from highest to lowest is: eccentric $\rightarrow$ isometric $\rightarrow$ concentric.

Strength Training. Muscle strengthening is a well-accepted part of any rehabilitation program. However, the practitioner must have a complete understanding of the functional anatomy so that the appropriate balance between agonist and antagonist muscle groups can be achieved. The amount of resistance to be applied is determined by the muscle's capability and should be assessed for each individual. Increases in cross-sectional area and hypertrophy of muscle are associated with increases in strength. Training is most effective when exercises focus on different muscle groups in rotating sessions. Improvements in strength observed during the first 2 weeks of training are related to neuromuscular re-education and more efficient recruitment of muscles. Initially, one to three sets of lifting weights 8 to 12 times per week is recommended. Resistance should not be increased by more than 10% per week. If progress is not made, the practitioner should evaluate whether the proper technique is being used, whether there is too little or too much training intensity, and whether there is neurogenic strength loss.

Aerobic Fitness. The patient must maintain cardiovascular fitness during rehabilitation. If the injury or dysfunction prohibits weight bearing, a non–weight-bearing aerobic activity needs to be implemented. To improve aerobic capacity, the oxidative metabolism of the muscle must be stressed. Oxygen consumption (Vo_2) increases in proportion to the intensity of the exercise. Vo_{2max}, the highest level of oxygen consumption achieved during exercise, is the best indicator of aerobic fitness. Intensity of exercise is the difficulty level of the exercise and is usually used in reference to maximal effort. This is typically at 40% to 85% of Vo_{2max}

for aerobic training and 25% to 95% of one repetition maximum for strength training. The duration of aerobic training is usually more than 15 minutes of continuous exercise. Frequency of aerobic training is usually three to six times per week, whereas frequency of strength training is typically three to five times per week. When prescribing an aerobic program, the practitioner must remember that if activity level is reduced beyond 1 week, aerobic conditioning decreases. Maximum oxygen consumption decreases by 25% when a patient takes 3 weeks of bed rest. Intensity, duration, and frequency parameters must be adjusted in the deconditioned patient. Benefits of aerobic conditioning measured by 10% to 20% increases in $V_{O_{2max}}$ can be noted within 8 to 12 weeks of training implementation. If improvements are not observed, their lack may be attributed to infrequent exercise sessions, too low an exercise intensity, or too short a duration of exercise sessions.

DEVELOPING A COMPREHENSIVE REHABILITATION PROGRAM

An individualized therapeutic program aims to correct soft tissue inflexibilities and to improve muscle strength deficits and imbalances, endurance, and power to the appropriate muscle groups. Consideration is given to the joint above and below the injured area, which are linked together and referred to as the kinetic chain. An individualized program should also include patient education about posture, body mechanics, and proprioception. A patient's return to activity should be monitored in a supervised setting so that any residual problems can be addressed.

A comprehensive rehabilitation program consists of an acute phase, a recovery phase, and a maintenance phase. During the acute phase, education about how to protect the injured tissue is important. A review of proper body mechanics and activities of daily living should be completed. Relative rest is important because excessive immobilization results in decreased muscle strength, endurance, and flexibility. Modalities can be used as described previously to help with pain management but should not be relied on as the only treatment application. Also, medications should be used to facilitate the rehabilitation program by decreasing pain and inflammation. Manual therapy techniques may help modify pain by assisting in early controlled motion of the injured tissue. Mechanoreceptor activation can assist in modifying muscle tone and pain. Although orthotics can help control range of motion, warm underlying tissue, and provide proprioceptive feedback, do not encourage the patient to rely on them. Therapeutic

exercise should begin during the acute phase. The direction of the initial movement pattern is based on the presumed pathologic condition, pain pattern, and functional anatomy.

Once acute inflammation and pain have been addressed, the program focuses on the subacute or recovery phase. Goals of this phase include achieving full range of motion that is pain-free to the affected tissue and surrounding tissues and regaining appropriate strength, balance, and proprioception. Manual techniques should focus on improving soft tissue extensibility that helps promote proper alignment of collagen fibers during healing and remodeling. These techniques may include massage, fascial stretching, traction, and joint mobilization. Myofascial release improves elasticity and motion by applying pressure in shear forces directed by fascial planes and assists with pain control. Mobilization is also used to facilitate motion at specific joints or joint segments. These techniques may facilitate a patient's progress but, again, should not be relied on solely because protracted passive treatment places the patient in a dependent role. Concern should also be given for the potential hypermobility that may result with extensively repeated treatment. A flexibility program is devised to achieve proper balance and allow the patient to achieve a neutral position, the least painful and best posture. While maintaining the posture, exercises progress from static to dynamic. Challenges to the neutral posture are afterward incorporated by gravity and then by a therapist or assistive device. Activity-specific retraining is initiated first by breaking the motion into components. Training for each component is completed before reassembling the entire motion. Cardiovascular training should be maintained, adapting the method to the specific injury. Aquatic training should be considered if a non–weight-bearing activity is necessary.

The final or maintenance phase is devised to promote continued cardiovascular fitness and to prevent reinjury as the patient returns to the work or sport-specific activity. Education about ergonomics and equipment or adaptive devices should be in place. The patient should be able to use a home exercise program independently and should know how to solve problems that may occur during this last stage of recovery.

BIBLIOGRAPHY

Basford JR: Physical agents. *In* DeLisa JA (ed): Rehabilitation Medicine: Principles and Practice, ed 2. Philadelphia, JB Lippincott, 1993, pp 404–423.

Young JL, Press JM, Cole AJ: Physical therapy options for lumbar spine pain. *In* Cole AJ, Herring SA (ed): The Low Back Pain Handbook. Philadelphia, Hanley and Belfus, 1997, pp 125–141.

Chapter 26

Psychological Interventions for Chronic Pain

Jennifer A. Haythornthwaite, Ph.D.,
and Leslie J. Heinberg, Ph.D.

Psychological factors, including cognitive and emotional variables, have long been recognized as influencing the experience of pain. A number of important historical events have contributed to the interest in these psychological factors. First, Beecher observed that the personal meaning of pain was an important determinant of the pain complaints he observed in soldiers wounded in combat.[1] Second, the work of Melzack and Wall[2] on the "gate-control" theory of pain stimulated much interest in the multidimensional and subjective aspects of the pain experience. Third, the pioneering work of Fordyce and colleagues[3] encouraged consideration of social and environmental factors both verbal and motor, that influence the expression of pain. Fourth, the taxonomy developed by the International Society for the Study of Pain introduced a definition of pain that included both sensory and emotional factors in the experience of pain.[4] And fifth, Turk and co-workers[5] published a comprehensive review of the literature demonstrating the influence of psychological factors on the experience of pain, which contained superb ideas for cognitive-behavioral interventions based on the existing empirical literature.

Psychological interventions for pain management have largely grown out of two important bodies of literature. First, early studies of laboratory pain demonstrated the importance of the influence of psychological factors on levels of reported pain and pain thresholds. Second, the psychotherapy literature has demonstrated the impact of psychological interventions on many areas of functioning and quality of life. This is particularly clear for anxiety and depression, which are two emotional states shown to influence the experience of pain. This chapter briefly reviews psychological interventions utilized for chronic pain, focusing primarily on the interventions that have been tested in clinical trials. General psychological interventions, such as psychotherapy, marital/family therapy, and group therapy, that have not been widely tested are not included in this overview. The overall *goals* for psychological treatment include reducing pain and pain-related disability; treating co-

morbid psychiatric illnesses, particularly depression; increasing perceptions of control and self-efficacy; and addressing pain-related psychosocial factors, such as the impact of pain on family and/or marital functioning.

BEHAVIORAL INTERVENTIONS

Learning theory provides the theoretical basis for behavioral interventions, incorporating the principles of operant conditioning (e.g., reinforcement and punishment). Many of the techniques are adapted from behavior therapy, which has been used extensively in managing anxiety and depression and behavioral aspects of other medical conditions.

Operant Interventions

In an operant model of pain, the primary focus of intervention is the behavior of the patient. These behaviors can include either verbal expressions of pain (e.g., complaints of pain or requests for medication) or gross motor movements that are indicators of pain (e.g., grimacing or limping). As overt behaviors, these responses are thought to be subject to the principles of operant conditioning, which focuses on the consequences of the behavior. Reinforcers increase the likelihood of a behavior occurring, and punishment decreases the likelihood of a behavior occurring. For example, when social attention from a loved one follows a grimace, grimacing may occur more frequently in the future. In this case, the social attention to the grimace serves to reinforce the behavior. Alternatively, pain as an aversive stimulus can serve as a punishment for an activity that increases the pain. If an individual experiences pain following sexual intercourse and decreases the frequency of sexual intercourse, then the pain serves to punish the sexual behavior.

The goal of operant interventions is to decrease learned pain behavior and to replace these maladaptive responses with adaptive behaviors inconsistent with the sick role. Operant interventions ideally occur in an environment in which the opportunity exists to control the social consequences of pain behavior and shape new "well" behavior. Most operant pain programs are based on inpatient units where this level of control is possible. "As-needed" prescriptions are changed to fixed time intervals to remove the contingent relationship between complaints of pain (i.e., the pain behavior) and pain relief (i.e., the reinforcer). Pain complaints are largely ignored, and well behaviors, including attending physical therapy and increasing activity level, are socially rewarded (i.e., reinforced).

Pacing and activity modulation are important components of operant behavioral pain programs. When an individual pushes the activity level to a point of pain exacerbation, he or she is more likely to decrease activity over time. That is, activity is punished by pain and therefore decreases over time. If an individual reports an exacerbation of low back pain after 30 minutes of sitting at a desk, an operant intervention would begin by having the individual get up after 20 minutes to stretch and move around for a period of time. After this duration of sitting with comfort is established, the duration of sitting is gradually increased, possibly by only 5-minute increments. Over a period of weeks, the individual may increase the comfortable duration of sitting to 60 minutes without shifting positions or standing up. This process of gradually increasing the nature, frequency, or duration of a behavior is called "shaping." The *goal* of such an intervention is to increase the behavior while managing the consequences, which includes removing any punishment (e.g., pain) and introducing reinforcement (e.g., social attention). The spouse or family is often involved in treatment and taught these principles of behavior—reinforcement/punishment and shaping. Inclusion of the family in treatment can facilitate generalization of treatment gains from the inpatient setting to the home environment.

Relaxation Interventions

An extensive number of publications in the literature documents the benefits of relaxation exercises, particularly in areas of anxiety and stress management. The goal for most relaxation techniques is nondirected relaxation, which is accomplished through two common components: (1) repetitive focus on a word, body sensation, or muscle activity; and (2) a passive attitude toward thoughts unrelated to the attentional focus.[6] Common methods used for teaching relaxation include systematically tensing and relaxing specific muscle groups (e.g., progressive muscle relaxation), focusing on breathing and emphasizing diaphragmatic breathing, and using guided imagery. A psychophysiologic model of pain, which has received some empirical support,[7] suggests that stress or pain leads to subtle increases in muscle tension, which can exacerbate pain at the site of an injury. A primary goal of relaxation training is to break such a pain–muscle tension–pain cycle.

A recent panel of experts, sponsored by the National Institutes on Health,[6] reviewed the empirical support for the use of relaxation techniques in the treatment of chronic pain. The panel concluded that the evidence supporting the use of these techniques for pain management was strong and recommended their broad integration with more traditional biomedical interventions for pain management.

Biofeedback

Biofeedback provides the individual with detailed information about a physiologic process of which he or she is not typically aware. Through this detailed feedback, the individual can learn to bring usually involuntary processes under control. The psychophysiological model briefly outlined above is an important underpinning for the use of biofeedback. Biofeedback for pain management usually entails providing feedback about muscle tension, typically using electromyographic (EMG) feedback from the site of the pain or from a standard location such as the frontalis muscles, or about skin temperature, typically using thermistors attached to the fingers.

Empirical support for the efficacy of biofeedback for pain management is limited to some specific painful conditions, including Raynaud's phenomenon, tension and migraine headaches, and low back pain. Although widely used within the pain field, particularly in conjunction with relaxation training, the empirical support for its specific efficacy beyond the general effects of relaxation strategies has been demonstrated only for migraine headaches. The NIH panel mentioned earlier[6] also reviewed the use of biofeedback for chronic pain management and concluded that moderate evidence supported its use, particularly within the area of headaches. Patients often respond favorably to the sophisticated technology required to implement this intervention, and the rationale often fits their own conceptualization of the pain problem, particularly because the intervention is focused on physiologic responses to pain and stress.

COGNITIVE-BEHAVIORAL INTERVENTIONS

The demonstration that cognitive and emotional factors influence the experience of pain has encouraged the application of cognitive-behavioral theory and treatment to the management of chronic pain. These interventions typically include components of the behavioral model, particularly relaxation training and some components of operant conditioning. However, an emphasis is also placed on cognitive factors, such as attitudes and beliefs that underlie maladaptive emotional and behavioral responses.[8] The recently convened NIH panel[6] concluded that the overall evidence was moderate for the use of cognitive-behavioral interventions for chronic pain management, providing the strongest support in treating patients with low back pain, rheumatoid arthritis, and osteoarthritis pain.

Coping Skills

Primary *goals* of these interventions include increasing perceptions of pain as a controllable experience and decreasing the use of maladaptive coping strategies, such as pain-contingent rest or use of medications. Specific pain coping skills often include some of the strategies outlined above, particularly relaxation and pacing. In this approach, the emphasis is on skill development and skill refinement. In the case of skill development, a new skill is introduced, and the patient is encouraged to develop and refine the skill during periods of lower pain, before applying the skill for actual pain management. Often the use of the skill is modified over time, so that the skill is gradually applied to increasingly challenging (i.e., painful) episodes. Therapy focuses on problem-solving discussions of skill application. A similar approach is taken to the application of many pain-coping skills, including cognitive or behavioral distraction, relaxation, pacing of activities, and the appropriate use of social support. Attention is paid to factors that increase or decrease pain, and these factors guide the application of pain coping skills.

Cognitive Restructuring

Cognitive restructuring focuses on the role of cognitive factors, such as attitudes, thoughts, and beliefs, in determining emotional and behavioral responses to pain. These interventions challenge negative self-talk, such as catastrophizing (e.g., "I can't stand the pain any more"), and replace these self-statements with more positive statements that reduce negative affect, emphasize control, and encourage adaptive coping (e.g., "this is a challenge that I have faced before, and I can handle it this time"). Catastrophizing is a particularly maladaptive response to pain that has been shown to correlate with depression and disability. In the context of treatment, patients are frequently asked to monitor their thoughts about the pain, or pain-related situations, identify negative thoughts, and generate accurate, adaptive thoughts to replace the negative thoughts. This monitoring process is supplemented with more in-depth discussions of the underlying attitudes and beliefs contributing to the negative thoughts.

HYPNOSIS

Hypnosis typically includes an attention-focusing component, similar to those identified earlier in the discussion of relaxation strategies, and a suggestion component, which outlines specific goals for outcome (e.g., analgesia). Hypnosis has been most widely applied and studied with pain due to cancer, and the recent NIH panel concluded that strong evidence supports the use of hypnosis in reducing chronic pain due to malignancies.[6] Other data support its efficacy in treating pain due to irritable bowel syndrome, temporomandibular joint disorders, and tension headaches.

MULTIDISCIPLINARY TREATMENT

Multidisciplinary programs typically include many or most of the procedures detailed above in conjunction with other nonpsychological interventions (e.g., physical therapy). A recent meta-analysis of the literature[9] to evaluate the efficacy of these programs demonstrated beneficial effects on pain, mood, and functioning. In addition to these important outcomes, return-to-work rates were higher (68% vs. 32%) and use of the health care system was lower in patients treated within these programs. Gains were found to extend well beyond treatment, lasting an average of almost 2 years. These patients were found to be functioning at a higher level than 75% of the patients treated within traditional unimodal treatment approaches.[9]

SUMMARY

A number of psychological interventions have been empirically demonstrated to reduce pain and suffering in patients with a wide variety of chronic pain syndromes. These treatments can be broadly identified as behavioral and cognitive and have become an integral part of multidisciplinary pain treatment programs. Although most patients with chronic pain may benefit from such interventions, certain subpopulations should be targeted for referral to these programs. For example, patients reporting depression or anxiety often require these interventions. In addition, patients reporting or demonstrating excessive disability should be referred for psychological treatment. Although this impairment may be due to negative affect, family/social factors, or "secondary gain," psychological interventions often minimize disability. Problematic medication use, including dose escalation, misuse, or underuse, can also be addressed. Certain pain disorders (e.g., headaches) may be highly responsive to psychological interventions such as biofeedback, and such treatments should be considered a standard part of medical management. Finally, specific patient groups may not be suitable candidates for some medical or pharmacologic treatment (e.g., chronic opioid therapy for a recovering substance abuser). For such individuals, psychological treatment, particularly multidisciplinary programs, may be considered an essential first-line treatment option.

REFERENCES

1. Beecher HK: Pain and some factors that modify it. Anesthesiology 12:633, 1951.
2. Melzack R, Wall PD: Pain mechanisms: A new theory. Science 150:971, 1965.
3. Fordyce WE, Fowler RS, Lehmann JF, et al: Operant conditioning in the treatment of chronic pain. Arch Phys Med Rehabil 54:399, 1973.
4. International Association for the Study of Pain: Pain terms: A list with definitions and notes on usage. Pain 6:249, 1979.
5. Turk DC, Meichenbaum D, Genest M: Pain and Behavioral Medicine: A Cognitive-Behavioral Perspective. New York, Guilford Press, 1983.

6. Pain and Insomnia—NIH Assessment Panel: Integration of behavioral and relaxation approaches into the treatment of chronic pain and insomnia. JAMA 276:313, 1996.

7. Ohrbach R, McCall WD: The stress-hyperactivity-pain theory of myogenic pain: Proposal for a revised theory. Pain Forum 5:51, 1996.

8. Turner JA, Romano JM: Psychological and psychosocial techniques: Cognitive behavioral therapy. *In* Bonica J (ed): The Management of Pain. Philadelphia, Lea & Febiger, 1990, p 1711.

9. Flor H, Fyndrich T, Turk DC: Efficacy of multidisciplinary pain treatment centers: A meta-analytic review. Pain 49:221, 1992.

Chapter 27

Acupuncture

Henry M. Liu, M.D.

Acupuncture involves the placement and manipulation of needles at various points in the body for the treatment of pain. Although the roots of acupuncture are deeply planted in China, acupuncture has increasingly been practiced in the Western Hemisphere. Acupuncture is an important option in today's multidisciplinary approach to the treatment of pain. However, due to the lack of scientific data, its use remains controversial.

HISTORY

Origin

Acupuncture originated in China more than 5000 years ago. Probably the first record of acupuncture therapy is in the *Huang-di-nei-jing (The Yellow Emperor's Classic in Internal Medicine)*, written by Chi Po around 200 B.C. Its popularity spread throughout ancient Egypt, the Middle East, the Roman Empire, and later into Western Europe. However, it remained essentially unknown in the United States until the 1970s, with the improvement of relations between the United States and China.

Acupuncture was born out of Taoist philosophy. Taoism, as described by Lao-tse in the *Tao-te-ching* around 500 B.C., assumes that nature is constantly changing. The *Tao*, or the way, is the source of all creation and is the force behind this ever-recurring change. It acts through two opposing but balancing forces, the *yin* and the *yang*. Because people exist in a dynamic interaction with nature, they exist within the tensions created by these opposing forces. According to the philosophy, sickness occurs when these opposing forces fall out of balance, and interventions are needed to restore the harmony.

Fundamental to the practice of classical acupuncture is the concept of *qi*, the energy flow that connects body structures and systems. The energy flows through a network below the skin, connecting the internal body with the external environment. This network is a set of pathways, or meridians, that run longitudinally in and around the body. Each meridian is categorized as being either *yin* or *yang* and is associated with one of the body's internal organs. There are 14 principal meridians, of which 12 are paired and 2 are unpaired. Thus, when the flow of *qi* is unobstructed, the body is in a healthy state of balance. Obstruction of *qi* results in a disequilibrium of *yin* and *yang*, which is manifested as disease or pain.

The meridians emerge at the surface of the body at certain places, known as *acupuncture points*. These points are areas where the *qi* may be affected and modulated by an external agent. There are a total of 361 classic acupuncture points, and they are located along the principal meridians. Acupuncture points are stimulated to balance the circulation of energy. Acupuncture involves choosing which points to stimulate as well as choosing how to stimulate these points, the needle being one method.

Schools of Acupuncture

Several different schools of acupuncture have developed. Although the meridians and points are universally accepted, each school differs in the choice of points as well as in the method of stimulation. These schools include classical acupuncture, formula acupuncture, acupuncture as a form of trigger-point therapy, and acupuncture as a procedure for electrical stimulation.

Classical acupuncture is the traditional practice according to the principles of Taoism. The goal is to reestablish the balanced energy state by restoring the flow of *qi*. Emphasis is on maintaining the wholeness of the patient. Treatment is individualized according to the patient's energy state at the time. Thus, points selected may differ from one patient to another, as well as from one treatment session to another. This individuality makes evaluations of efficacy difficult owing to the lack of comparable controls.

There are many variations of classical acupuncture. Among them is ear acupuncture, or auriculotherapy. The pinna of the ear contains a map of acupuncture points that represent the entire body. Although somatotropic mapping of musculoskeletal pain at the ear has been done,[1] controlled trials of auriculotherapy have failed to yield evidence supporting efficacy.[2]

Today, many practitioners in Asia and parts of Europe still practice classical acupuncture. However, most in the Western Hemisphere practice formula acupuncture. Formula acupuncture emphasizes standardized treatments. Routine sets of acupuncture points are used to treat specific pain problems. Practitioners have embraced this school partly because this approach is most often employed in acupuncture research.

Another application of acupuncture is essentially trigger-point therapy. Needles are inserted around symptomatic areas. Classical principles, meridians, and acupuncture points are not adhered to. The basis of this approach is that stress or injury causes local skeletal muscle contraction, which can result in neural changes. Needling provides relief by the release of these contractures. Trigger-point therapy and its mechanism were initially described by Bonica,[3] Travell and Simons,[4] Sola,[5] and others and is discussed elsewhere in this book

With the increasing use of acupuncture during prolonged operations in the early 1970s, Chinese practitioners began using electricity as a source of needle stimulation. At the same time, the growing popularity of the gate-control theory of pain by Melzack and Wall[6] led to electrical stimulation therapies for pain control, which in turn led to the development of the transcutaneous electrical nerve stimulation unit. Electrical stimulation is now commonly employed for needle stimulation.

Despite its initial popularity, acupuncture as a whole has remained in the realm of alternative medicine. Physiologic and clinical data to support diverse therapeutic claims have been scarce. The clinical database, although large, contains mostly anecdotal and biased information. After more than two decades of research, evidence to support the effectiveness of acupuncture in relieving pain is only beginning to surface.

MECHANISM

Research on the mechanism behind acupuncture has been problematic. During the 1970s, when interest in acupuncture began, enkephalins and endorphins were being discovered, and the roles played by the raphe-spinal structures were being elucidated. However, it has been difficult to prove an association between acupuncture and endorphin release. Animal studies of acupuncture analgesia cannot easily be extrapolated to human models. This is in part due to the difficulty in differentiating the effects of acupuncture analgesia with stress-induced analgesia.[7] Unlike in humans, acupuncture in animals is a stressful event, resulting in the release of hormones, including endorphins and cortisol. Furthermore, when animals are frightened they often fall into a state of insensibility and unconsciousness.[8, 9]

Human laboratory studies have been more helpful. In an extensive review, Pomeranz[10] concluded that acupuncture (1) appears to cause the release of various endorphins and monoamine neurotransmitters, and (2) involves both the peripheral and central nervous systems. According to Pomeranz, acupuncture activates sensory nerve fibers in muscles that, in turn, send signals to the spinal cord. This activates other centers in the midbrain and hypothalamic-pituitary axis, causing the release of neuropeptides. Enkephalin and dynorphin, released at the level of the spinal cord, block afferent pathways. Enkephalin, produced at the midbrain, stimulates the inhibitory raphe descending system, releasing the monoamines serotonin and norepinephrine. These neurotransmitters further block spinal cord pain transmission. Finally, β-endorphin, released from the hypothalamic-pituitary axis, produces analgesia through the systemic circulation and cerebrospinal fluid.

Peripheral nerve involvement in acupuncture had previously been established. Nathan,[11] and later Han and Terenius,[12] showed that infiltration of acupuncture points with local anesthetic abolished analgesia from subsequent needling. Furthermore, clinical observation showed that stimulation of denervated areas in patients with spinal cord injuries failed to produce analgesia in rostral regions. Both small and large fibers appear to be involved. It is interesting to note that acupuncture points are sites of low skin resistance and represent areas on the body where the peripheral nervous system is most accessible.[10, 13]

Proving critical to understanding acupuncture is understanding the role of the central nervous system. Acupuncture appears to increase the endorphin levels in various parts of the central nervous system.[14] During acupuncture analgesia, endorphin levels rise in the blood and cerebrospinal fluid. This correlates with an elevation of messenger RNA (mRNA) levels involved in the production of endorphins.[15] It also has been demonstrated that the opioid antagonist naloxone blocks acupuncture analgesia in animals and humans.[16] Also, antibodies to endorphins block acupuncture only if placed at known analgesic sites in the central nervous system.[15] Furthermore, lesions at the arcuate nucleus (a site of β-endorphin release) and at the periaqueductal gray matter (where high concentrations of opioid receptors reside) abolish acupuncture analgesia.[17]

It appears that different levels of stimulation produce different endorphins. Han and others[18] demonstrated that electrical stimulation at 4 Hz produces enkephalins, whereas stimulation at 100 Hz produces dynorphin A. Furthermore, acupuncture affects many other neuropeptides and neurotransmitters.[19, 20] These include dopamine, 5-hydroxytryptamine, acetylcholine, and norepinephrine. The importance of these neurotransmitters has yet to be defined. Moreover, the role of these neurotransmitters and neuropeptides in chronic pain still needs to be elucidated.

Needling tender areas as a form of trigger-point therapy is a poorly understood process. Trigger-point therapy has been reviewed by Travell and Simons[4] and Sola.[5] The goal of therapy is to release painful contractures. Studies have been performed comparing dry needling of a tender area to the injection of a local anesthetic, with or without steroids, and injection of placebo. Dry needling may be just as efficacious as injection of local anesthetics.[21] Interestingly, the relief of pain in a tender

TABLE 27–1. EFFECT OF ACUPUNCTURE ON DIFFERENT PAIN SYNDROMES*

Effective	Not Effective	Equivocal
Low back pain, nociceptive	Low back pain, neurogenic	Cervical neck pain
Fibromyalgia	Low back pain, psychogenic	Headache, migraine
Arthritic pain		Cancer pain
Muscle spasm		Reflex sympathetic dystrophy
Trigeminal neuralgia		Postherpetic neuralgia
Headache, tension		
Dysmenorrhea		
Abdominal pain		
Dental pain		

*Modified from Hsu DT: Acupuncture: A review. Reg Anesth 21:361, 1996.

area does not always relieve pain caused by a pathologic lesion at a remote site.[22] This suggests that the peripheral and central nervous systems are involved, and a tender area is just one manifestation.

INDICATIONS

The best documented effects of acupuncture are its beneficial effects on headache[23, 24] and backache.[25] However, acupuncture appears to provide some benefit in various other pain syndromes.[26] These include fibromyalgia, arthritic pain,[27, 28] pain from muscle spasms, trigeminal neuralgia,[29] chronic abdominal pain,[30] and dental pain.[31] Further evaluation is required for reflex sympathetic dystrophy,[32] cervical neck pain,[33] cancer pain,[34] herpetic neuralgia,[35] and migraine headache[24] (Table 27–1).

CONTRAINDICATIONS

Acupuncture has few absolute contraindications. However, reports of various adverse effects have generated a list of relative contraindications (Table 27–2). Pregnancy is a relative contraindication because acupuncture may induce premature labor.[36] Bleeding diathesis and anticoagulant therapy may result in prolonged bleeding and hematoma formation. Bacterial endocarditis has also been reported in patients with rheumatic heart disease.[37, 38] Steroids may attenuate the effects of acupuncture, and they should be discontinued prior to therapy if possible. Eating heavy meals or drinking alcohol before a treatment is inadvisable because of the risk

TABLE 27–2. RELATIVE CONTRAINDICATIONS TO ACUPUNCTURE

Pregnancy
Rheumatic heart disease/valvular heart disease
Bleeding diathesis/anticoagulant therapy
Severe lung disease
Cardiac pacemaker
Steroid use
Recent ingestion of food or alcohol

of vasovagal symptoms, including nausea, vomiting, and fainting. Caution should be exercised when performing acupuncture in the thoracic region in patients in whom a pneumothorax would be catastrophic, such as persons with severe lung disease. Care should be taken with electrical stimulation in patients with a cardiac pacemaker because of the risk of electromagnetic interference.[39] Finally, acupuncture can mask symptoms that are of medical importance. Therefore, treatment of certain pain syndromes, such as abdominal pain, should be performed only after a complete medical evaluation.

TECHNIQUE

No consensus exists about which of the many techniques of needle insertion is optimal. Some practitioners purport that different ways of placing the needle can produce different results. However, no evidence supports the efficacy of one technique over another.

Patients are positioned to allow adequate access for the therapist and optimal comfort for the patient. Positions include sitting as well as lying prone or supine. A lateral decubitus position may also be used. The skin is cleansed with an antiseptic, such as alcohol, and is stretched at the intended site. A sterile acupuncture needle is then inserted in a manner that minimizes discomfort. (This can be accomplished with or without rotating the needle.) Insertion can be rapid or slow. Some practitioners penetrate only the skin, whereas others penetrate to muscle and periosteum. Tubular guides are available for needle insertion.

The usual angle of insertion is perpendicular or oblique. Usually the deeper the penetration, the more perpendicular the needle ought to be angled. Horizontal insertion is often used in certain areas, such as the face and chest. Many classic acupuncturists slant the needle either in the same direction or in the opposite direction of the *qi* along the treated meridian.

There are a total of 361 classical acupuncture points. These are well described in the literature and various manuals. Most points are located linearly along the major meridians. Each point is identified by a Chinese name, its meridian, and a serial number. Two methods are used in locating a specific acupuncture site. One method uses anatomic landmarks, such as bony structures, muscles, and external features. The other method uses a defined unit of measurement to locate acupuncture points from identifiable landmarks. This unit of measurement is named *cun*, and is defined as the distance between the joint creases of the interphalangeal joints of the patient's flexed middle finger. This distance is also equivalent to the width of the patient's thumb.

The selection of acupuncture points follows certain basic rules. Tender spots, or pressure points, are used as local acupuncture points. These are also referred to as *trigger points*. Distal points are selected according to the involved meridian. Certain points are also selected according to specific symptoms present. Furthermore, certain points are chosen according to the acuteness or chronicity of the problem.

The insertion of the needle may be accompanied by

de qi, a painless sensation of heaviness and numbness at the site. Concomitantly, the therapist feels as if the muscle is grabbing and holding the needle. Classical therapists believe that *de qi* defines correct placement. Furthermore, the acupuncturist should not remove the needles until the *de qi* has dissipated. This is indicated by the ease with which the needle can be lifted from the underlying tissue. Others, however, report that patients who do not experience *de qi* often respond to acupuncture nevertheless.

After insertion, needles may be left in place or stimulated. According to traditional thinking, needle stimulation depends on the excess or deficiency of the *qi*. Stimulation can be continuous for a short course, such as 10 to 20 seconds, followed by the removal of the needle. The needle may also be stimulated intermittently for several seconds, with rest periods of a few minutes between each stimulation. A third method involves continuous stimulation of several minutes to hours or until the pain is resolved.

Stimulation of needles is most commonly accomplished manually or electrically. There are three basic techniques of manual stimulation: (1) rotation of the needle back and forth not more than 180 degrees, (2) thrusting the needle back and forth, and (3) twirling the needle with an up and down movement.

Manual techniques have largely been replaced by electrical stimulators. These consist of battery-operated units that deliver low to high frequencies of varying intensities. Following insertion of the needles, each needle is connected to an electrical lead. The electrical current is slowly increased. As with manual stimulation, the patient may feel numbness or heaviness at the acupuncture point. Optimal results occur at low frequencies with intense stimulation. *De qi* is usually elicited by a current that is just below the threshold of patient tolerance.

Needle removal is accomplished by applying pressure on the skin with one hand while withdrawing the needle with the other hand. Slowly twirling the needle during removal is often helpful.

Many types of needles are available. The most commonly used are stainless steel needles, but gold, silver, and copper needles are also available. The needle consists of a body or shaft with a handle. The needle shaft is used to base gauge and length measurements. Needles come in numerous sizes and lengths. Common sizes are 30 to 32 gauge, with lengths ranging from 20 to 125 mm. Shorter needles are useful with children or for shallow penetration, such as around the face. Longer needles are used for penetration of deeper structures, especially the limbs. Disposable stainless steel needles are now widely available.

Wide variation exists in the duration and course of therapy. Acute problems may involve one to three treatments a day. Chronic conditions may require several courses of treatment. A course may involve one treatment every 1 to 3 days for a total of 10 to 20 treatments. Each course of therapy is then separated by a rest period of 1 to 2 weeks.

Generalized body fatigue is a common side effect, and the patient may experience unusual sleepiness. Thus, patients should be advised to avoid strenuous activities after an acupuncture treatment. The fatigue may occur either immediately after a treatment or several hours later. The sleepiness has not been reported to interact with the somnolence that may be caused by some medications. Worsening of pain may occur 1 or 2 days after a treatment before relief is felt.

COMPLICATIONS

Although acupuncture has a long history of use and a paucity of complications has been documented, it is not free of risk (Table 27-3). In a review, Ernst and White[40] found a total of five documented fatalities related to acupuncture. Although these appear to be rare events, the actual incidence of adverse events is unknown. Probably the most common complications with needle placement result from a vasovagal response. Nausea, pallor, dizziness, and syncope may all occur. Conservative measures for the treatment of a vasovagal response are usually adequate, but occasionally oxygen, fluids, and medications are required.

Other concerns with needle insertion include tissue trauma, dermatitis, hematoma, and infection. Pneumothorax can occur when needles are placed in the thoracic region, including the upper trapezius muscle, and is the second most often reported serious complication.[40, 41] There have also been several reports of cardiac tamponade.[42] Injury to the spinal cord by an acupuncture needle has also been reported.[43] Contact and nickel dermatitis has been documented.[44, 45]

Another rare complication is the formation of a hematoma at the site of needle insertion. To prevent a hematoma, direct pressure can be applied over the acupuncture site on removal of the needle. Placing needles deeply or near vascular structures may increase the risk of hematoma formation; caution should be exercised with patients at risk for bleeding complications.

Infections can result from the improper sterilization of needles. Hepatitis B, hepatitis C, and human immunodeficiency virus (HIV) infections have all been reported. Rampes and James[41] reported 126 cases of hepatitis associated with acupuncture, making hepatitis transmission the most often reported serious complication of acupuncture. Transmission of HIV has also been linked to acupuncture, but is not well documented.[46, 47] Bacte-

TABLE 27-3. COMPLICATIONS OF ACUPUNCTURE

Trauma
    Pneumothorax
    Cardiac tamponade
    Spinal cord injury
Infection
    Hepatitis B, C
    HIV
    Bacterial infections
    Endocarditis
Miscellaneous
    Hematoma
    Dermatitis
    Cardiac pacemaker suppression

rial infections reported include *Propionibacterium acnes*,[37] *Pseudomonas aeruginosa*,[38] and *Staphylococcus aureus*.[48] These infections are especially significant in patients at risk for bacterial endocarditis. Infections may be minimized with the use of disposable needles.

CLINICAL DATA

Problems Associated With Acupuncture Research

Acupuncture has been difficult to evaluate as a form of therapy. This difficulty has several possible explanations.[26] First, studies determining the efficacy of acupuncture analgesia lack proper controls. In classic acupuncture, the therapist may select different points for patients with the same disease. Furthermore, the therapist may change points in the same patient with each visit, depending on the patient's prior responses. This approach is not amenable to rigorous analysis. Therefore, formula acupuncture, in which treatment consists of sets of points determined by the diagnosis, has gained widespread use in clinical trials. Even so, a comparable control in the form of sham acupuncture is less than ideal because of its possible therapeutic effects.

A second reason that evaluation is problematic is the difficulty in conducting a double-blind trial. A properly conducted double-blind study is optimal for the removal of bias. However, with acupuncture, "blinding" the therapist is not possible, because any qualified therapist can easily distinguish correct from sham points. Thus, a single-blind trial may be the best alternative.

Furthermore, no standards exist for correct acupuncture therapy. The frequency and number of treatments may affect patient response. Yet, there is no accepted minimum number of treatments that defines a treatment failure. Recent studies have used one to two acupuncture treatments a week for a duration of 2 to 4 months, each session lasting 20 to 30 minutes.[28, 49, 50] Follow-up evaluations should be long enough, preferably greater than 6 months, to establish long-term benefits.

Finally, chronic pain is complex, and often includes psychological components. Patients often have a history of failed therapies, such as surgery, and extensive medication use. Drug abuse and drug dependency are often present.

Results of Available Data

The evidence supporting the efficacy of acupuncture appears to be mixed. Mendelson[51] reviewed follow-up studies on acupuncture published before 1976. The studies were mostly uncontrolled and did not differentiate different pain syndromes. A recent review by Lewith and Machin[52] concluded that acupuncture benefited about 70% of chronic pain patients, whereas sham controls resulted in 50% positive response. Placebos gave a 30% positive response rate. In a later review, Lewith[53] concluded that acupuncture works to some extent in 60% of patients with chronic pain and that these effects were greater than those of random needling or placebo treatment. Furthermore, acupuncture was as effective as physiotherapy or pharmacologic therapy for musculoskeletal pain, but caused fewer adverse reactions.

In what is probably the most extensive review on acupuncture thus far, Richardson and Vincent[54] looked at acupuncture analgesic trials performed between 1973 and 1985. Headache and backache were the most commonly studied syndromes. Other studies included phantom limb pain, arthritic pain, and cervical neck pain. The extent of the therapeutic effect was mixed among the different studies. In the controlled studies, about 50% to 80% of the patients showed a therapeutic response, suggesting at least short-term effectiveness of acupuncture. Follow-up periods ranged from 2 weeks to 4 months. The few studies in which patients were followed up for more than 6 months were uncontrolled and showed a relapse rate of about 50%.

Carlsson and Sjolund[49] studied the long-term effects of acupuncture on several subtypes of pain. They demonstrated that patients with nociceptive low back pain improved the most, with nearly 50% of the patients experiencing long-term pain relief. Only 32% of patients with neurogenic pain and 15% of patients with psychogenic pain benefited from acupuncture.

SUMMARY

Acupuncture has been used as a treatment for pain for thousands of years. Although scientific data have not been able to support many of its diverse claims, there is evidence that acupuncture may be effective in relieving certain types of pain. Musculoskeletal problems, such as low back pain, and certain types of headaches seem to respond well to acupuncture. Furthermore, acupuncture appears to be effective with acute pain and spasm caused by injury. However, further clinical studies are needed to support this mode of treatment. Although the actual incidence of adverse effects is still unknown, acupuncture appears to have a low complication rate. Thus, acupuncture appears to be a safe alternative treatment for certain types of pain and has become an integral part of today's comprehensive pain therapy.

REFERENCES

1. Oleson TD, Kroenig RJ, Bresler DE: An experimental evaluation of auricular diagnosis: The somatotrophic mapping of musculoskeletal pain at acupuncture points. Pain 8:217, 1980.
2. Melzack R, Katz K: Auriculotherapy fails to relieve chronic pain: A controlled crossover study. JAMA 251:1041, 1984.
3. Bonica JJ: Management of myofascial pain syndromes in general practice. JAMA 165:732, 1957.
4. Travell J, Simons D (eds): Myofascial Pain and Dysfunction: The Trigger Point Manual. Baltimore, Williams & Wilkins, 1983.
5. Sola AE: Treatment of myofascial pain syndromes. *In* Benedetti C, Chapman CR, Moricca G (eds): Advances in Pain Research and Therapy, vol 7. New York, Raven Press, 1984, p 467.
6. Melzack R, Wall PD: Pain mechanisms: A new theory. Science 150:971, 1965.
7. Maier SF: The opioid/nonopioid nature of stress-induced analgesia and learned helplessness. J Exp Psychol 9:80, 1983.
8. Gellup GG: Animal hypnosis: Factual status of a fictional concept. Psychol Bull 81:836, 1974.

9. Carli G, Farabollini F, Fontani G: Effects of pain, morphine, and nalaxone on the duration of animal hypnosis. Behav Brain Res 2:373, 1981.
10. Pomeranz B: Scientific basis of acupuncture. *In* Stux G, Pomeranz B (eds): Acupuncture Textbook and Atlas. Berlin, Springer-Verlag, 1987, p 1.
11. Nathan PW: Acupuncture analgesia. Trends Neurosci 7:21, 1978.
12. Han JJ, Terenius L: Neurochemical basis of acupuncture analgesia. Annu Rev Pharmacol Toxicol 22:193, 1982.
13. Baldry PE: The deactivation of trigger points. *In* Baldry PE (ed): Acupuncture, Trigger Points, and Musculoskeletal Pain. London, Churchill Livingstone, 1993, p 91.
14. Han JJ: Central neurotransmitters and acupuncture analgesia. *In* Pomeranz B, Stux G (eds): Scientific Basis of Acupuncture. Berlin, Springer-Verlag, 1988, p 10.
15. Pomeranz B: Scientific basis of acupuncture. In Stux G, Pomeranz B (eds): Basics of Acupuncture, ed 2. Berlin, Springer-Verlag, 1991, p 4.
16. Mayer DJ, Price DD, Raffi A: Antagonism of acupuncture analgesia in man by the narcotic antagonist nalaxone. Brain Res 121:368, 1977.
17. Wang Q, Mao L, Han JJ: The arcuate nucleus of the hypothalamus mediates low but not high frequency electroacupuncture in rats. Brain Res 513:60, 1990.
18. Han JJ, Xie GX, Ding XZ, et al: High and low frequency electroacupuncture analgesia are mediated by different opioids. Pain 20 (suppl): S369, 1984.
19. Han JJ, Terenius L: Neurochemical basis of acupuncture analgesia. Annu Rev Pharmacol Toxicol 22:193, 1982.
20. Ungar G, Ungar A, Malin DH, et al: Brain peptides with opiate antagonistic action: Their possible role in tolerance and dependence. Psychoneuroendocrinology 2:1, 1977.
21. Frost FA, Jessen B, Siggaard-Andersen J: A control, double-blind comparison of mepivacaine injection versus saline injection for myofascial pain. Lancet 4:499, 1980.
22. Kellgren JH: Some painful joint conditions and their relation to osteoarthritis. Clin Sci 4:193, 1939.
23. Johansson V, Kosic S, Lindahl O: Effect of acupuncture in tension headache and brainstem reflexes. Adv Pain Res Ther 1:839, 1976.
24. Dowson DI, Lewith GI, Machin D: The effects of acupuncture versus placebo in the treatment of headache. Pain 21:35, 1985.
25. Thomas M, Lundberg T: Importance of modes of acupuncture in the treatment of chronic nociceptive low back pain. Acta Anaesthesiol Scand 38:63, 1994.
26. Hsu DT: Acupuncture: A review. Reg Anesth 21:361, 1996.
27. Man SC, Barager BD: Preliminary clinical study of acupuncture in rheumatoid arthritis. J Rheumatol 1:126, 1974.
28. Christensen BV, Iuhl IU, Vilbeck HC, et al: Acupuncture treatment of severe knee arthrosis: A long term study. Acta Anaesthesiol Scand 36:578, 1992.
29. Beppu S, Sato Y, Amemiya Y: Practical application of meridian acupuncture treatment for trigeminal neuralgia. Anesth Pain Control Dent 1:103, 1992.
30. Zhao J: Acupuncture at huatuojiaji points for treatment of acute epigastric pain. J Tradit Chin Med 11:258, 1991.
31. Sung YF, Kutner MH, Cerine FC, et al: Comparison of the effects of acupuncture and codeine on postoperative dental pain. Anesth Analg Curr Res 56:473, 1972.
32. Fialka V, Resch KL, Ritter-Dietrich D, et al: Acupuncture for reflex sympathetic dystrophy (letter). Arch Intern Med 153:661, 1993.
33. Petric JP, Langley GB. Acupuncture in the treatment of chronic cervical pain: A pilot study. Clin Exp Rheumatol 1:333, 1983.
34. Brule-Fermand S: Treatment of chronic cancer pain: Contribution of acupuncture, auriculotherapy and mesotherapy. Soins 568:39, 1993.
35. Lewith GT, Field J, Machin D: Acupuncture compared with placebo in post herpetic pain. Pain 17:361, 1983.
36. Dunn PA, Rogers D, Halford K: Transcutaneous electrical nerve stimulation at acupuncture points in the induction of uterine contractions. Obstet Gynecol 73:286, 1989.
37. Scheel O, Sundsfjord A, Lunde P, et al: Endocarditis after acupuncture and injection treatment by a natural healer. JAMA 267:56, 1992.
38. Jeffreys DB, Smith S, Brennand-Roper DA, et al: Acupuncture needles as a cause of bacterial endocarditis. Br Med J 287:326, 1983.
39. Fujiwara H, Taniguchi K, Ikezono E: The influence of low frequency acupuncture on a demand pacemaker. Chest 78:96, 1980.
40. Ernst E, White A: Life-threatening adverse reactions after acupuncture: A systematic review. Pain 71:123, 1997.
41. Rampes H, James R: Complications of acupuncture. Acupunct Med 1:26, 1995.
42. Hasegawa J, Noguchi N, Yamasaki J: Delayed cardiac tamponade and hemothorax induced by an acupuncture needle. Cardiology 78:58, 1991.
43. Ernst E: The risks of acupuncture. Int J Risk Saf Med 6:179, 1995.
44. Romaguera C, Grimalt F: Contact dermatitis from a permanent acupuncture needle. Contact Dermatitis 7:156, 1981.
45. Romaguera C, Grimalt F: Nickel dermatitis from acupuncture needles. Contact Dermatitis 5:195, 1979.
46. Vittiecoq D, Mettetal JF, Rouzioux C, et al: Acute HIV infection after acupuncture treatments. N Engl J Med 320:250, 1989.
47. Castro KG, Lifson AR, White CR: Investigation of AIDS patients with no previously identified risk factors. JAMA 259:1338, 1988.
48. Lee RJE, McIlwain JC: Subacute bacterial endocarditis following ear acupuncture. Int J Cardiol 7:62, 1985.
49. Carlsson CB, Sjolund BH: Acupuncture and subtypes of chronic pain: Assessment of long-term results. Clin J Pain 10:290, 1994.
50. Coan RH, Wang S, Ku SC, et al: The acupuncture treatment of low back pain: A randomized controlled study. Am J Clin Med 8:181, 1986.
51. Mendelson G: Acupuncture analgesia: I. Review of clinical studies. Aust NZ J Med 7:642, 1977.
52. Lewith GT, Machin D: On the evaluation of the clinical effects of acupuncture. Pain 16:111, 1983.
53. Lewith GT: How effective is acupuncture in the management of pain? JR Coll Gen Pract 34:275, 1984.
54. Richardson PH, Vincent C: Acupuncture for the treatment of pain: A review of evaluative research. Pain 24:15, 1986.

Chapter 28

Substance Use Disorders and Chronic Pain

Michael R. Clark, M.D., M.P.H., and Marc Fishman, M.D.

TERMINOLOGY

Substance use disorders are a significant problem. However, the various terms used to define these conditions are often confused. Terms such as *abuse*, *addiction*, *misuse*, and *dependence* have all been used inconsistently to describe drug-taking behavior. The American Society of Addiction Medicine has standardized the definitions of these terms (Table 28–1). Regardless of the setting, any use of alcohol, illicit drugs, or prescribed medications that results in distress or impairment in major life areas is a problem. This use should be of concern to physicians and other health care practitioners.

DEFINING THE PROBLEM

The use of opioids for the treatment of nonmalignant chronic pain remains a subject of considerable debate. A large number of opioids and several different medication delivery systems, such as implantable pumps and transdermal patches, with inherently less potential for abuse are now available. Fears of regulatory pressure, medication abuse, and the development of tolerance create a reluctance to prescribe these medications, and many studies have documented the underutilization of opioids. More recent studies of physicians specializing in pain, as well as of those who do not, have shown that prescription of long-term opioids is increasingly common in both groups. Clinical trials support the safety and effectiveness of opioids as well as reduced reports of pain and pain-related disability in patients with chronic nonmalignant pain.

The underreporting of medication use complicates accurate assessment of actual use patterns by patients with chronic pain. In patients with chronic pain who developed substance use disorders, the problem most commonly involved the medications prescribed by their physicians. The mechanisms are not well understood and probably involve multiple factors; however, a cycle of pain followed by relief after taking medications is

TABLE 28–1. DEFINITIONS APPROVED BY THE AMERICAN SOCIETY OF ADDICTION MEDICINE

Term	Definition
Abuse	Harmful use of a specific psychoactive substance
Addiction	Continued use of a specific psychoactive substance despite physical, psychological, or social harm
Misuse	Any use of a prescription drug that varies from accepted medical practice
Physical dependence	Physiological state of adaptation to a specific psychoactive substance characterized by the emergence of a withdrawal syndrome during abstinence, which may be relieved in total or in part by readministration of the substance
Psychological dependence	Subjective sense of need for a specific psychoactive substance, either for its positive effects or to avoid negative effects associated with its abstinence

a classic example of operant reinforcement of future medication use. Careful monitoring of patients is essential to prevent this complication of the treatment of chronic pain.

Research in patients with substance abuse has demonstrated abnormalities in pain perception and tolerance. Individuals with current opioid and cocaine abuse had significantly lower cold pressor pain tolerance than those with past abuse. Alcoholics have greater sensitivity to painful stimuli beyond the reported pain reduction induced by alcohol. These findings were present in nonalcoholic men with high familial genetic risk for alcoholism. Specifically, these men rated an aversive shock as more painful, but the differences from controls could be normalized with pharmacologically significant levels of ingested alcohol. An increased sensitivity to pain and the reinforcing effects of relieving pain with substance use suggest another mechanism for the development of substance abuse in patients with chronic pain.

THE RISKS OF TREATMENT
Opioids

Patients with chronic pain do have increased rates of substance use disorders. However, almost all occur in

129

individuals in whom substance abuse was a factor before the onset of chronic pain. Actual prevalence estimates vary owing to differences in the applied diagnostic criteria. Fishbain and colleagues reviewed 24 studies of drug and alcohol dependence or addiction in patients with chronic pain. Only seven studies met their standard of using acceptable criteria for these substance use disorders, and the prevalence ranged from 3% to 19%. In a study of patients with chronic low back pain, 34% had a substance use disorder, yet all cases were present before the onset of chronic pain. These individuals were found to be at increased risk for substance abuse during treatment for chronic pain as well as at increased risk of further physical injury. In another study of 414 chronic pain patients, 23% met criteria for active alcohol, analgesic, or sedative misuse or dependency; 9% met criteria for a remission diagnosis; and 13% were currently dependent on analgesics, which were the most commonly abused drugs.

Research investigating the risk of causing opioid abuse in patients with chronic pain has been reassuring. In one study of 12,000 medical patients treated with opioids, only 4 patients without a history of substance abuse developed dependence on the medication. Other studies of chronic opioid therapy found that patients who developed problems with their use of the medication all had a history of substance abuse. Even when the diagnosis of dependence was highly suspected in patients taking opioids for chronic pain, severe maladaptive behaviors, such as stealing or forging prescriptions, were rare.

Once the decision is made to prescribe opioids, several recommendations have been suggested to minimize risks of addiction and optimize the potential benefits of treatment. The Agency for Health Care Policy and Research has produced guidelines for the treatment of acute pain and cancer pain; however, no guidelines have yet been formulated for chronic nonmalignant pain. A consensus statement from the American Academy of Pain Medicine and the American Pain Society has been released for the use of opioids for the treatment of chronic pain. Education about addiction and medication interactions is important for monitoring the effects of treatment. The most important risk factor for developing a substance use disorder in relation to treatment for chronic pain is a previous history of a substance use disorder. Patients without this history have relatively low risk for the abuse of prescribed analgesics.

In patients with a higher risk of addiction, prevention begins with a treatment contract to clarify the conditions under which treatment with opioids will be provided. Elements of a contract emphasize a single physician being responsible for the prescription of the medication, and in advance, describing for the patient all of the conditions under which continued use of opioids will be inappropriate. The treating physician should always evaluate the patient's progress before refilling prescriptions. When there is concern that a patient will have difficulty taking medications as directed, a policy of prescribing small quantities of medications and not refilling lost supplies should be explicitly discussed and then followed. Random urine testing

may also be used to screen for nonprescribed medications and other drugs. Most experts agree that opioids with a slow onset of action and longer half-life are preferred to minimize the initial euphoria and interdose withdrawal symptoms. Oral and transdermal routes of administration also deemphasize these qualities. A constant, rather than intermittent ("as-needed") schedule should be followed to keep the time between dosages and the individual dose amounts equivalent.

In general, an active substance use disorder is a relative contraindication to chronic opioid therapy. However, opioid therapy can be accomplished successfully in individuals in whom clinical benefits are deemed to outweigh the risks. The treatment of this extraordinary subset of patients with chronic pain will always require considerably more effort, and probably frustration, on the part of the physician. In addition to all other monitoring for misuse of prescribed medications and abuse of illicit drugs, the patient should be actively participating in an addiction treatment program. This treatment needs to be closely coordinated with that provided for chronic pain. A strict treatment structure with therapeutic goals, landmarks to document progress, and contingencies for noncompliance should be made explicit and be agreed on by the patient and all practitioners of health care.

Benzodiazepines

Benzodiazepines are commonly prescribed for patients with chronic pain; however, clinical efficacy has not been established. In an extensive review by Dellemijn and Fields, only a limited number of chronic pain conditions, such as trigeminal neuralgia, tension headache, and temporomandibular joint disorders, were found to improve when treated with benzodiazepines. In addition, no studies have demonstrated any benefit for the associated insomnia and anxiety frequently reported by patients taking these drugs. Benzodiazepines have been used to gradually wean patients previously treated with sedative or hypnotic medications. Benzodiazepines are reported as superior to barbiturates for minimizing symptoms of withdrawal; however, no significant benefit in the prevention of increased anxiety has been documented.

Not only are the benefits of benzodiazepines difficult to document, but also the negative effects are well studied and extend beyond the usual concerns of abuse, dependence, withdrawal, and secondary effects on mood or affect. Benzodiazepines have been associated with exacerbation of pain and interference with opioid analgesia. They have also been found to cause cognitive impairment as demonstrated by abnormalities on neuropsychological tests and electroencephalograms. In general, unless patients have failed other established treatments for chronic pain, benzodiazepines should rarely be considered as a primary treatment; even then, they should be considered with caution. In all circumstances, benzodiazepines should be used only with very close monitoring.

THE DIAGNOSIS OF ADDICTION

The evaluation of a patient suspected of misusing medications should be thorough and include an assessment of the pain syndrome as well as other medical disorders, patterns of medication use, social and family factors, patient and family history of substance abuse, and a psychiatric history.

Reliance on medications that provide pain relief can result in a number of stereotyped patient behaviors that appear consistent with addiction. Persistent pain can lead to increased focus on opioid medications. Patients may take extraordinary measures to ensure an adequate medication supply, even in the absence of addiction. Patients understandably fear the reemergence of pain and withdrawal symptoms if they run out of medication. Drug-seeking behavior may be the result of an anxious patient's attempt to maintain a previous level of pain control. In this situation, the behavior results from therapeutic dependence and not addiction.

Many studies have also shown that tolerance leading to dosage escalation is generally not a problem in the management of patients taking long-term opioids. Recent evidence suggests tolerance is a complex phenomenon. The loss of analgesia over time can have many causes, and its cause should be carefully evaluated. It is most likely due to disease progression or other changes in the patient's condition, such as the development of delirium. True pharmacologic tolerance to the analgesic effects of opioids is an uncommon cause for the need to escalate the opioid dose. Tolerance to nonanalgesic effects occurs more reliably but may disappear when pain is eliminated by some unrelated mechanism.

Pseudoaddiction results in drug-seeking behavior when the patient with chronic pain cannot obtain tolerable relief from the prescribed dose of analgesic medication. This may be manifested as frequent requests for higher medication doses and larger quantities of medication or seeking medication from additional sources. This behavior resolves once adequate opioid therapy is prescribed. Opioid analgesia without side effects, not the avoidance of high doses of opioids, is the goal of treatment.

The *diagnosis* of addiction in the chronic pain patient must demonstrate certain drug-taking behavior that interferes with the successful fulfillment of life activities. In other words, the patient has lost control of the medication use, become preoccupied with the medication, and continues to insist on using the medication despite the presence of adverse consequences. Access to opioids may not be a specific problem because a physician has been prescribing them. If addiction is present, however, the patient may fear that opioid access will be limited and therefore try to conceal any problematic use of the medication. The presence of maladaptive behavior is emphasized to diagnose addiction, as physical dependence and tolerance are expected.

Types of behavior that raise serious concerns about addiction include selling or stealing medications, forging or losing prescriptions, using oral medications intravenously, concurrently abusing alcohol or illicit drugs, repeated noncompliance with the prescribed use of medications, and deterioration in the patient's ability to function in family, social, or occupational roles. Many other types of behavior are inconsistent with medication misuse and should prompt an evaluation for addiction, including requests for increasing amounts of medication, requests for specific medications, ongoing complaints of pain that are disproportionate to the identified pathologic condition, obtaining opioids from other sources, and combining opioids with other medications for the additive intoxicant effects or treatment of other symptoms.

Family and other professionals may note the patient repeatedly visiting the emergency room with complaints of pain exacerbation or repeatedly requesting hospitalization and treatment with intravenous opioids. Concerns by family or friends about the patient's pattern of medication use, an appearance suggesting intoxication, or the patient's having other difficulties with cognitive abilities should raise suspicion. Any unwillingness to discuss the possibility of addiction or changes in chronic pain management require in-depth discussion about the patient's worries and possible inappropriate behavior, including medication misuse.

THE TREATMENT OF SUBSTANCE USE DISORDERS IN CHRONIC PAIN

The first step in treatment is to stop the behavior of medication misuse. Then, sustaining factors must be assessed and addressed. These interventions include treating other medical diseases and psychiatric disorders, managing personality vulnerabilities, meeting situational challenges and life stressors, and providing support and understanding. Finally, the habit of taking the medication inappropriately must be extinguished by emphasizing the structure of taking medication as prescribed and examining the possible reasons for any inappropriate use that occurs. Relapse is common, and patients with addiction require ongoing monitoring even if the prescription of opioids has ceased.

The first step for the patient is to acknowledge the existence of a problem with medication use. Then, alternative pain treatment strategies can be utilized to assist the patient in decreasing the reliance on the problematic medications or their inappropriate use. Psychiatric risk factors for medication misuse, such as depression, anxiety, somatization, personality vulnerabilities, and demoralization, need to be addressed. The treating physician can adequately manage many problems, but psychiatric consultation will be required for the more complicated set of problems. Patients often experience a lack of interpersonal support, and family members should be actively involved in the treatment of addiction. Relapse prevention should rely on family members to assist the patient in getting prompt attention before further deterioration occurs. If relapse is detected, the precipitating incident should be examined and strategies to avoid another relapse should be implemented.

Although the misuse of medications is unacceptable,

complete abstinence is not always the most appropriate or optimal treatment of patients with chronic pain. Restoration of function should be the primary treatment goal, and this may improve with adequate, judicious, and appropriate use of medications. If detoxification is necessary, tapering the dosage of opioids often results in withdrawal symptoms, including exacerbation of the patient's primary pain symptoms. The concomitant administration of clonidine or other adjunctive medications can greatly reduce or eliminate many withdrawal symptoms. Traditional outpatient drug treatment or 12-step programs can provide support for recovery. However, treatment of addiction in patients with chronic pain must always include other appropriate treatments for chronic pain, including psychological treatment and physical therapy. Interdisciplinary programs for the treatment of chronic pain that include inpatient and partial hospitalization programs can provide the appropriate intensity of care required for some patients with addiction.

Careful ongoing documentation should be kept of the evaluation, diagnosis, treatment plan, and treatment response of all patients. This documentation is even more critical in patients with chronic pain, especially those given long-term opioid therapy. Pain severity and quality, the use of analgesics, involvement in nonpharmacologic strategies to decrease and cope with chronic pain, assessment of the level of functioning, evidence of medication misuse, and continuous reevaluation and updating of the treatment plan should be included.

SUMMARY

Patients with chronic pain are at increased risk of substance use disorders. However, it is crucial to appreciate that there are many causes for the nonprescribed use of medications. Medication misuse is a clinical problem that can be the result of dependence, but it is more likely to be the result of inadequate analgesia. This can be due to undertreatment with opioids and other analgesics, disease progression, or tolerance to medications. Eventually, instead of consulting the physician, the patient may simply take more medication, and without proper instruction, he or she will often take it inappropriately. The patient with an addiction is preoccupied with the medication, has lost control of its use, and continues to take it regardless of negative consequences. Such a patient requires specialized evaluation and treatment in addition to management of the chronic pain syndrome.

BIBLIOGRAPHY

Chabal C, Jacobson L, Chaney EF, et al: Narcotics for chronic pain: Yes or no? A useless dichotomy. Am Pain Soc J 1:276–281, 1992.

Dellemijn PL, Fields HL: Do benzodiazepines have a role in chronic pain management? Pain 57:137–152, 1994.

Fishbain DA, Rosomoff HL, Rosomoff RS: Drug abuse, dependence: Addiction in chronic pain patients. Clin J Pain 8:77–85, 1992.

Hoffmann NG, Olofsson O, Salen B, et al: Prevalence of abuse and dependency in chronic pain patients. Int J Addict 30:919–927, 1995.

Koenig TW, Clark MR: Advances in comprehensive pain management. Psychiatr Clin North Am 19:589–611, 1996.

Miotto K, Compton P, Ling W, et al: Diagnosing addictive disease in chronic pain patients. Psychosomatics 37:223–235, 1996.

Portenoy RK: Opioid therapy for chronic nonmalignant pain: Current status. In Fields HL, Liebeskind JC (eds): Progress in Pain Research and Management, vol 1. Seattle, IASP Press, 1994, pp 247–287.

Portenoy RK. Tolerance to opioid analgesics: Clinical aspects. Cancer Surv 21:49–65, 1994.

Porter J, Jick H: Addiction rate in patients treated with narcotics. N Engl J Med 302:123, 1980.

Sees KL, Clark HW: Opioid use in the treatment of chronic pain: Assessment of addiction. J Pain Symptom Manage 8:257–264, 1993.

Steindler EM: Addiction terminology. In Miller NS (ed): Principles of Addiction Medicine. Chevy Chase, Md, American Society of Addiction Medicine, 1994, chap 2, pp 1–3.

Turk DC, Brody MC, Okifuji EA: Physicians' attitudes and practices regarding the long-term prescribing of opioids for non-cancer pain. Pain 59:201–208, 1994.

C h a p t e r 2 9

Detoxification: Assessment and Methods

Marc Fishman, M.D., and
Michael R. Clark, M.D., M.P.H.

WHY IS DETOXIFICATION NECESSARY?

Needing detoxification does not mean that a patient has been given the diagnosis of addiction, abuse, or misuse of medications. Detoxification is simply the process of withdrawing a person from a specific psychoactive substance in a safe and effective manner. Although addiction may necessitate detoxification so that drug rehabilitation treatment can begin, patients undergo detoxification for many reasons. A carefully planned and monitored detoxification prevents a withdrawal syndrome in the patient who has become physiologically dependent on medications such as opioids or benzodiazepines.

The effects of any treatment should be assessed continuously. If the risks outweigh the benefits, the treatment should probably be discontinued. When pain is the problem being treated, the risks and benefits are particularly difficult to define and evaluate. Despite the substantial benefits of medications prescribed for most patients with pain, these medications can cause more harm than good. Patients with chronic nonmalignant pain syndromes are the most vulnerable to the risks of medications given to provide relief of suffering.

In the acute setting, the risk-benefit analysis is usually driven by the overwhelming potential for therapeutic gain. Most side effects are relatively tolerable because they will be temporary, as treatment will be short term. Intolerable side effects can be dealt with by reducing the dose, changing to another medication, or adding adjunctive medications. Tolerance, toxicity, and abuse rarely occur. Once the underlying condition has resolved, the medications are no longer required and are appropriately discontinued.

Although uncommon, the need for discontinuation of opioids and benzodiazepines can also arise in the treatment of cancer pain. Again, analgesia and symptomatic relief of insomnia or muscle spasms are almost always attainable therapeutic goals. Because treatment will probably be long term, the loss of analgesia or reemergence of symptoms becomes an ongoing concern. This phenomenon demands evaluation to determine the

cause. A change in the patient's condition such as disease progression or decreased gastrointestinal absorption is more likely than the development of actual tolerance to the medication. In some circumstances, the medication is no longer needed, or side effects have become intolerable. Because long-term treatment will have resulted in physiologic dependence, discontinuation or substantial dose reduction requires gradual tapering of the medication.

In the treatment of chronic nonmalignant pain, most patients can achieve functional gains and sustained analgesia from opioid therapy without developing aberrant drug-related behaviors. Nevertheless, the ongoing assessment of a therapeutic trial of long-term opioids may result in the conclusion that the risk-benefit ratio is no longer acceptable (Table 29–1). Of note, benzodiazepines and sedative-hypnotic agents are rarely indicated in the treatment of chronic pain syndromes. It is important, especially in this patient population, to distinguish between substance abuse and dependence.

The fourth edition of the *Diagnostic and Statistical Manual of Mental Disorders* of the American Psychiatric Association defines both substance abuse and dependence as maladaptive patterns of substance use leading to clinically significant impairment or distress. *Substance abuse* must be accompanied by any of the following: interpersonal problems, legal problems, failure to fulfill major role obligations, and recurrent substance use in hazardous situations.

Substance dependence is distinguished from abuse by

TABLE 29–1. INDICATIONS FOR DETOXIFICATION

Intolerable side effects
Inadequate response or benefit
Aberrant drug-related behaviors
   Noncompliance
   Loss of control of medication use
   Preoccupation with the medication
   Continued use despite adverse consequence
Refractory co-morbid psychiatric illness
Lack of functional improvement or impairment in role
   responsibilities

more than simply a continuum of severity. In contrast, substance dependence is manifested by tolerance, withdrawal, using the substance in larger amounts or over a longer period than was intended, persistent desire or unsuccessful efforts to decrease or control substance use, spending large amounts of time in activities necessary to obtain the substance, giving up or reducing time spent in important activities because of substance use, and continuing substance use despite knowledge of having physical or psychological problems caused or exacerbated by the substance. Making the distinct diagnosis of dependence is important because it reliably predicts more severe medical sequelae, poorer treatment outcomes, higher relapse rates, and worse overall prognosis.

OPIOID DETOXIFICATION

Although physiologic opioid dependence can be demonstrated experimentally within 7 days, most patients will not experience withdrawal symptoms unless they have been taking opioids continuously for at least several weeks. Patients with a history of physiologic opioid dependence, opioid withdrawal, or any other drug withdrawal are generally more likely to experience opioid withdrawal after shorter periods of treatment. Regardless of the total daily dose, once physiologic dependence is established, abrupt discontinuation of opioids precipitates acute withdrawal. Even a reduction in dose can precipitate withdrawal to a lesser degree.

Patients taking opioid analgesics on a variable schedule are at high risk for experiencing intermittent withdrawal. Even a long overnight dosing hiatus with short half-life agents can cause significant withdrawal symptoms. Relief of pain or relief from intermittent withdrawal symptoms by taking medications can reinforce medication use through operant conditioning. This is not an uncommon factor in the failure of detoxification. Patients require longer tapering schedules and more support to overcome this conditioned habit.

The essential element for successful opioid detoxification is the gradual tapering of the dose of medication. Opioid withdrawal is generally not dangerous except with patients at risk from increased sympathetic tone, such as those with increased intracranial pressure or unstable angina. However, opioid withdrawal is very uncomfortable and distressing to patients. Patients with pain are often particularly miserable during opioid withdrawal because of the phenomenon of rebound pain. Increases in pain can occur even if the analgesic effects of opioid therapy have not been appreciable. Although it is generally not possible to avoid discomfort completely, the goal of detoxification is to ameliorate withdrawal as much as is clinically practical.

Once the decision is made to proceed with detoxification, several clinical details must be determined. These include selecting a setting (inpatient vs. outpatient), choosing a pharmacologic agent, designing a taper and monitoring schedule, and making "next step" therapeutic goals. It is critical to give patients this treatment plan before the detoxification begins so that they know what to expect. Patients will tolerate discomfort better if it is expected, if it is in the service of an overreaching goal, and if it will be transient. In particular, patients should know to expect worsening of pain and should have a few concrete short-term goals to focus on, such as an improvement in withdrawal symptoms, an increase in functional abilities, or an alternate analgesic trial when withdrawal has resolved. The projected length of a taper is typically a balance between the expected severity of withdrawal symptoms (increased with faster tapers) and their expected duration (shorter with faster tapers).

Setting. Usually, opioid detoxification can be accomplished in the outpatient setting. Outpatient detoxification should be planned with a careful inventory of support and monitoring systems. Patients should plan not only for discomfort but also for temporary emotional lability and reduction in function. Compensatory planning might include warning family and work supervisors, planning for a decrease in workload on the job, and even taking vacation or sick leave days. Although opioid withdrawal might not be dangerous, it has been demonstrated clearly that extensive support with frequent monitoring substantially increases the likelihood of a successful taper. Higher success rates have been reported for patients with better therapeutic relationships or formal treatment programs that have usually been initiated by a period of stabilization on long half-life opioids and then proceed with a taper slowly over a period of months.

Office visits should be at least weekly, but sometimes daily contact with the patient proves a major advantage for ensuring success. Most contact with the patient does not have to involve the physician and often can be done over the telephone. A nursing visit to check vital signs and assess the severity of withdrawal can provide enormous help to the patient. The visit should include allowing the patient to express discomfort and frustration but then focusing on the treatment plan and the patient's progress. Formal checklists of signs and symptoms such as the Subjective Opioid Withdrawal Scale and the Objective Opioid Withdrawal Scale allow for the objective rating of withdrawal and documentation of the patient's condition over time (Table 29–2). Adjustment to the treatment plan is then based on several sources of information and not just the patient's complaints.

The inpatient setting offers more intensive monitoring, supervision, and other support that generally allows for a faster taper schedule. Indications for inpatient detoxification include the failure of outpatient detoxification attempts, medically unstable patients, co-morbid psychiatric illness, unreliable or noncompliant patients, and complicated pharmacologic regimens requiring taper of more than one medication or illicit drug. Increasingly, many facilities are utilizing less intensive or step-down settings such as intermediate care facilities, partial hospitalization programs, and intensive outpatient programs for opioid detoxification.

Agents. The primary principle for detoxification is that medication should not be prescribed by a "cookbook" approach but by careful patient evaluation and

TABLE 29–2. OPIOID WITHDRAWAL RATING SCALES

The objective opiate withdrawal scale (OOWS)
Score one point for each sign that is present during a 10-minute observation period.

_____Yawning (>1 yawn per observation period)
_____Rhinorrhea (>3 sniffs per observation period)
_____Piloerection (gooseflesh—observe patient's arm)
_____Perspiration
_____Lacrimation
_____Mydriasis
_____Tremors (hands)
_____Hot and cold flashes (shivering or huddling for warmth)
_____Restlessness (frequent shifts of position)
_____Vomiting
_____Muscle twitches
_____Abdominal cramps (holding stomach)
_____Anxiety (from mild fidgeting to severe trembling or panic)
Total Score _____
Maximum severity = 13

The subjective opiate withdrawal scale (SOWS)
Patients should rate each symptom statement on a scale of 0-4.
0 = not at all; 1 = a little; 2 = moderately; 3 = quite a bit; 4 = extremely

_____I feel anxious.
_____I feel like yawning.
_____I'm perspiring.
_____My eyes are tearing.
_____My nose is running.
_____I have goose flesh.
_____I am shaking.
_____I have hot flashes.
_____I have cold flashes.
_____My bone and muscles ache.
_____I feel restless.
_____I feel nauseous.
_____I feel like vomiting.
_____My muscles twitch.
_____I have cramps in my stomach.
_____I feel like taking [name of opioid] now.
Total Score _____
Maximum severity = 64

TABLE 29–3. SHORT HALF-LIFE OPIOID TAPER

Determine the total daily dosage being used by the patient.
Adopt a fixed interval schedule with equal doses every 4-6 hours for 48 hours.
Increase the prescribed dose until the patient has no opioid withdrawal symptoms for 48 hours.
Taper the amount of each dose without lengthening the interval between doses.
Taper the total daily dose approximately 10% every 3-7 days.
Slowing the taper may be accomplished by:
   Increasing the number of days at a given total dose.
   Decreasing a single dose amount while keeping the remaining doses the same.
   Increasing the time between doses only if the smallest individual dose has been reached.

tained-release morphine or transdermal fentanyl patches. Switching from short to long half-life opioids in anticipation of detoxification may serendipitously prove an effective analgesic strategy. Side effects, intermittent withdrawal, and rebound pain may all improve such that detoxification may not be needed. This strategy has the primary advantage of more constant opioid serum levels with less chance of intermittent withdrawal between doses. With a long half-life agent such as methadone, the onset of withdrawal symptoms should be expected at 12 to 24 hours, although 24 to 48 hours is the usually reported time course. The severity usually peaks at 36 to 96 hours but can occur up to 1 week later.

Substitution, which is often not exact, may require some initial titration to achieve dosing equivalence. An initial test dose of the agent can be given to determine the total dose needed. If the test dose does not sufficiently relieve or prevent withdrawal, it can be increased. If the test dose produces sedation, then the next dose should be held until the patient is fully alert and subsequent doses should be decreased.

A third detoxification strategy uses the opioid partial agonist-antagonists. The agent most commonly used in this category is buprenorphine (Table 29-5). The use of partial agonist-antagonists is designed to reduce the severity of withdrawal and cause fewer reinforcing drug effects. As a result, the taper should be easier and more successful. There is also less risk of respiratory depression, which is an infrequent consequence of overestimating the dosing equivalence with pure agonist

subsequent dosage titration. A number of variables are involved in the selection process of a specific opioid for detoxification. Pharmacologic strategies in opioid detoxification for chronic pain patients generally involve the gradual taper of an agent with pure opiate receptor agonist properties.

One strategy institutes a taper of the agent that the patient is currently using. This is usually a short half-life agent but may offer the advantages of using an agent already familiar to the patient, avoiding the imperfect calculation of dosage equivalence, and just simplifying an anxiety-filled process. Short half-life agents possess the disadvantage of pharmacokinetics that may not allow a smooth taper. Serum levels will fluctuate more with increasing dosing intervals. Patients usually experience mild withdrawal within 4 to 8 hours of a dosage reduction. The severity of withdrawal will usually peak with a short half-life agent at 8 to 36 hours; however, it can occur as late as 72 hours. When using these agents, certain procedures can minimize the risks of severe withdrawal symptoms (Table 29-3).

The preferable pharmacologic strategy is to choose a long half-life pure opioid agonist such as methadone (Table 29-4). Other long-acting agents include oral sus-

TABLE 29–4. LONG HALF-LIFE OPIOID TAPER

Determine the total daily dose of the prescribed agent being taken by the patient.
Estimate by conversion the equivalent total daily dose of the long half-life opioid.
Adopt a fixed interval schedule with equal doses every 6-8 hours for 48 hours.
Increase the prescribed dose of the long half-life opioid until the patient has no withdrawal symptoms for 3-5 days.
Taper the amount of each dose unless the patient can tolerate an interval schedule of dosing every 8-12 hours.
Taper the total daily dose approximately 10% every 3-7 days.
Increase the number of days at a given total daily dose to slow the taper.

TABLE 29–5. BUPRENORPHINE TAPER

Test for the precipitation of acute withdrawal symptoms by giving
  an initial dose of 0.1 mg SQ/IM or 1.0 mg SL.
Determine the total daily dose of the prescribed agent being taken
  by the patient.
Estimate the equivalent total daily dose of buprenorphine (0.2 mg
  SQ/IM = morphine 10 mg PO).
Adopt a fixed interval schedule with equal doses every 8–12 hours.
Titrate the dosage until the patient has no withdrawal symptoms for
  24–72 hours.
Taper the dose and interval to 0.1 mg SQ/IM or 1.0 mg PO qd.
Discontinue the medication when the patient experiences no or
  tolerable withdrawal symptoms.

SQ, subcutaneously; IM, intramuscularly; SL, sublingually; PO, orally; qd,
every day.

substitution. When using partial agonist-antagonists such as buprenorphine, it is important to give a small test dose under supervision because of the rare precipitation of withdrawal symptoms secondary to the partial antagonist effect. If patients tolerate the test dose, then the titration of dose-equivalence substitution can proceed.

Buprenorphine is currently available only as a parenteral preparation (intramuscular or subcutaneous) in the United States but is currently available as a sublingual tablet in Europe. It is likely to be available in the United States as a sublingual preparation. In its current parenteral form, buprenorphine may be appropriate for use in highly supervised settings such as inpatient units, specialty pain treatment centers, or intensive outpatient programs in which staff are available to administer injections. Once the sublingual preparation is available in the United States, it will probably be used more widely for detoxification in standard outpatient practice.

Adjunctive Agents. Several nonopioid pharmacologic agents are commonly used as adjunctive agents to provide patients with additional relief from withdrawal symptoms. Clonidine, an α_2-adrenergic agonist that decreases adrenergic activity, is the most commonly prescribed (Table 29–6). Clonidine can help relieve many of the autonomic symptoms of opioid withdrawal such as nausea, cramps, sweating, tachycardia, and hypertension, which result from the loss of opioid suppression of the locus ceruleus during the withdrawal syndrome. Other adjunctive agents include nonsteroidal anti-inflammatory drugs for muscle aches, bismuth subsalicylate (Pepto-Bismol) for diarrhea, dicyclomine hydrochlo-

TABLE 29–6. ADJUNCTIVE AGENTS FOR SYMPTOMS OF
OPIOID WITHDRAWAL

Diarrhea	Bismuth products	Pepto-Bismol
Rhinorrhea	Antihistamines	Diphenhydramine, loratadine
Muscle aches	Muscle relaxants	Methocarbamol
Abdominal cramps	Anticholinergics	Dicyclomine HCl
Insomnia	Antihistamines	Diphenhydramine
	Antidepressants	Trazodone, doxepin
Autonomic symptoms	α_2-adrenergic agonists	Clonidine

ride (Bentyl) for abdominal cramps, and antihistamines for insomnia and restlessness (see Table 29–6).

Schedule. Unless patients are involved with dangerous aberrant drug-taking behaviors, there is generally no urgency to decrease the duration of opioid detoxification. The longer a patient has been taking opioids, the more difficulty they are likely to have with withdrawal. The taper will then require more time to be completed. Other factors that tend to increase the difficulty and length of a taper are medical co-morbidity and complexity, older age, female gender, and detoxification from multiple agents simultaneously.

Detoxification is more difficult in the last stages of a taper, and it should be anticipated that decreases in the dose of opioids will be more gradual during this time. If a taper becomes more complicated, the schedule should be extended by decreasing the actual dosage reduction or increasing the intervals between reductions. Dosing titration at the end of the taper may be limited by the availability of smaller unit doses. At that point, only increases in time between doses can be implemented. As long as patients are demonstrating ongoing progress, there is generally no reason not to extend an opioid taper over several weeks. In some situations, months may be required. Progress can be demonstrated by simple compliance with taper instructions, not using other illicit substances, improvement in side effects of opioids, and maintenance of function in several different domains.

Accelerated withdrawal or rapid detoxification is based on the assumption that the dysphoria of opioid withdrawal contributes to continued opioid use and relapse. Methods to achieve rapid detoxification consist of treatment with opioid antagonists such as naltrexone. One approach involves gradually increasing doses over a period of several days. Usually adjunctive agents must be added to further reduce withdrawal symptoms. Another approach uses anesthetic levels of central nervous system depression and large doses of opioid antagonists to complete withdrawal within several hours. The evidence for longer-term advantages of these procedures is still lacking, although they are probably more cost efficient in the short-term phases of treatment.

Follow-up. The process of detoxification does not end with the completion of the opioid taper. Patients can have lingering subacute withdrawal symptoms for weeks. In rare circumstances, they can last for months. Insomnia and rebound pain are the most common symptoms. After the taper, patients who had difficulty with aberrant drug-taking behaviors continue to need increased levels of monitoring and supervision in their treatment because the risk of relapse is high. Patients without a history of addiction and aberrant drug-taking behaviors do not require addiction treatment. These patients should be reassured that they do not have an addiction or a diagnosis of substance abuse or dependence. However, anyone who undergoes detoxification that is precipitated by addiction or medication misuse should have further evaluation and treatment. Referral to an addiction specialist is usually a helpful first step. Furthermore, active ongoing participation in the treatment prescribed for addiction should be a condition of continued pain treatment. For these patients, the prevention of relapse requires a long-term outpatient program of rehabilitation.

BENZODIAZEPINE DETOXIFICATION

The principles of detoxification from benzodiazepines are much the same as those for opioids. There is very little evidence that benzodiazepines are beneficial in the treatment of chronic pain. They have a very unfavorable side effect profile with long-term use, including cognitive impairment, decreased psychomotor speed, and depression. The risk-benefit ratio usually favors their taper and discontinuation.

The general features of benzodiazepine withdrawal are similar to those of opioid withdrawal, with hyperarousal and hypersympathetic states. However, in its more specific features, the withdrawal syndrome is more like the one observed with alcohol (Table 29–7). Similarly, benzodiazepine withdrawal is much more dangerous than opioid withdrawal and includes the potential for seizures, hallucinations, hyperthermia, and delirium tremens. Like alcohol withdrawal when untreated, severe benzodiazepine withdrawal has a very high rate of morbidity and mortality.

The technique of a benzodiazepine taper also follows the same general principles of an opioid taper. If patients have been using benzodiazepines only intermittently, there is generally no need for a taper. However, anyone who has been using benzodiazepines continuously for more than 2 weeks should be tapered to avoid the unpleasant experience of mild withdrawal and the risk of unexpected major withdrawal symptoms. The higher the total daily dose and the longer the duration of use, the higher the risk of significant and potentially dangerous withdrawal with abrupt cessation.

The two main techniques for detoxification include a taper of the agent a patient has been taking and the substitution of an equivalent dose of a long half-life agent such as diazepam or clonazepam. It is important to note that infrequently the "second-generation" benzodiazepines (clonazepam, alprazolam, oxazepam, triazolam) are not fully cross-tolerant with one another or with the more traditional agents. A patient may require higher doses than expected to avoid significant withdrawal symptoms when taking these medications. Benzodiazepine tapers generally require more time than opioid tapers and use less frequent dose reductions. A taper of 6 weeks, especially with long half-life agents, is not unusual.

There is some evidence for the effectiveness of carbamazepine as an adjunctive agent to minimize benzodiazepine withdrawal symptoms, but conflicting research does not yet support its use as a standard treatment. Other anticonvulsants with GABAminergic actions, such as valproic acid and gabapentin, may offer similar benefits of minimizing withdrawal from benzodiazepines, but no consistent research has been performed to confirm this. The benzodiazepine receptor antagonist flumazenil has been used in the treatment of persistent withdrawal symptoms after discontinuation of long-term benzodiazepine treatment, but these results are still anecdotal.

Other strategies for benzodiazepine detoxification have included phenobarbital substitution, especially in cases of complex detoxification from multiple agents such as opioids, sedative-hypnotics, and alcohol. The phenobarbital dose should be determined by a series of test doses and subsequent observation to determine the level of tolerance. Another approach to complex detoxification involving both opioids and benzodiazepines focuses on the sedative-hypnotic drug and temporarily ignores the opioid component. The patient is stabilized with methadone, and then attention is directed to the more life-threatening sedative withdrawal. Opioid detoxification can then be initiated later.

SUMMARY

Clinical evaluation should precede the design of any treatment plan. If careful planning and common principles are applied, detoxification facilitates the transition from ineffective or problematic treatments to other potentially more effective treatments for pain. Treatment may include drug rehabilitation, but it should not be prescribed for every patient undergoing detoxification. By avoiding unpleasant or dangerous withdrawal syndromes and by providing the patient with the reinforcement that all treatments should result in benefits that outweigh their risks, the therapeutic relationship will be strengthened and the chances for successful treatment optimized.

TABLE 29–7. SIGNS AND SYMPTOMS OF SEDATIVE-HYPNOTIC WITHDRAWAL

Hyperarousal	Psychiatric
Agitation	Depersonalization
Anxiety	Depression
Hyperactivity	Hyperventilation
Insomnia	Malaise
Fever	Paranoid delusions
Neurologic	Visual hallucinations
Ataxia	**Gastrointestinal**
Fasciculation/myoclonic jerks	Abdominal pain
Formication	Constipation
Headache	Diarrhea
Myalgia	Nausea
Paresthesias/dysesthesias	Vomiting
Pruritus	Anorexia
Tinnitus	**Cardiovascular**
Tremor	Chest pain
Seizures	Flushing
Delirium	Palpitations
Genitourinary	Hypertension
Incontinence	Orthostatic hypotension
Loss of libido	Tachycardia
Urinary urgency, frequency	Diaphoresis

BIBLIOGRAPHY

Benzer DG: Management of sedative-hypnotic intoxication and withdrawal. *In* Miller NS (ed): Principles of Addiction Medicine. Chevy

Chase, Md, American Society of Addiction Medicine, 1994, Section XI, Chapter 4, pp 1-5.

Benzer DG, Smith DE, Miller NS: Detoxification from benzodiazepine use: Strategies and schedules for clinical practice. Psychiatr Ann 25:180-185, 1995.

Handelsman L, Cochrane KJ, Aronson MJ, et al: Two new rating scales for opiate withdrawal. Am J Drug Alcohol Abuse 13:293-308, 1987.

Jaffe JH: Pharmacological treatment of opioid dependence: Current techniques and new findings. Psychiatr Ann 25:369-375, 1995.

O'Brien C: Drug addiction and drug abuse. *In* Hardman JG, Gilman AG, Limbird LE (eds): Goodman and Gilman's The Pharmacologic Basis of Therapeutics, 9th ed. New York, McGraw-Hill, 1996, pp 557-578.

O'Conner PG, Koster TR: Management of opioid intoxication and withdrawal. *In* Miller NS (ed): Principles of Addiction Medicine. Chevy Chase, Md, American Society of Addiction Medicine, 1994, Section XI, Chapter 5, pp 1-6.

Postoperative Pain

Chapter 30

Preemptive Analgesia: Pathophysiology

Veronica D. Mitchell, M.D.,
and Srinivasa N. Raja, M.D.

During the past decade, many advances have been made toward understanding the pathophysiology of nociceptive pathways. Researchers have learned more about the presence and function of nociceptors and mediators that act in the periphery, as well as those that act at the level of the spinal cord. One such finding is the observation that noxious stimulus with resultant tissue injury leads to changes of prolonged excitability ("hypersensitivity") in the periphery and in the spinal cord. The characteristic changes leading to an increased excitability of neurons that signal pain are referred to as peripheral and central *sensitization*. These changes lead to a "hypersensitive state" within the nervous system that can persist for days and contribute to the postoperative pain state. Preemptive analgesia is the method of attenuating postoperative pain by preventing or inhibiting the occurrence of spinal sensitization.

POSTINJURY PAIN HYPERSENSITIVITY

Peripheral Sensitization

Postsurgical pain is an inflammatory pain state caused by peripheral tissue damage. The noxious stimulus of surgery and the resulting inflammatory response elicit changes in the periphery, leading to hypersensitivity of nociceptors. In addition, alterations in the spinal cord lead to central nervous excitability. In the periphery, activation of high-threshold nociceptors by tissue injury causes the release of several chemicals and mediators (Fig. 30-1). These substances, in combination with other mediators released by the inflammatory state and by activation of sympathetic terminals, form a "sensitizing soup." This soup modifies nociceptors so that they have an increase in sensitivity of their transduction mechanism. The threshold of nociceptors is lowered, and low-intensity stimuli can induce pain. As a result, clinically we observe allodynia—pain caused by a stimulus that is not normally noxious is also observed. Nonsteroidal anti-inflammatory drugs inhibit prostaglandin formation, which ameliorates this phenomenon of peripheral sensitization.

Peripheral Sensitization

Tissue Damage   Inflammation   Sympathetic Terminals

Sensitizing "Soup"

Hydrogen ions	Histamine	Purines	Leukotrienes
Norepinephrine	Potassium ions	Cytokines	Nerve Growth Factor
Bradykinin	Prostaglandins	5-HT	Neuropeptides

High-Threshold Nociceptor

Transduction Sensitivity

Low-Threshold 'Nociceptor'

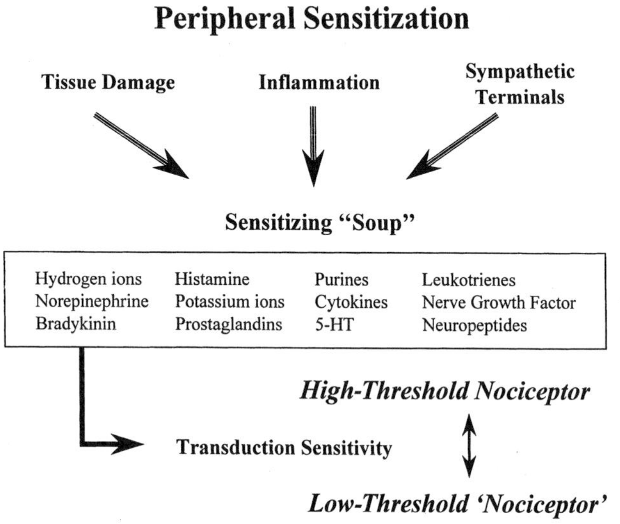

FIGURE 30–1. The transduction sensitivity of high-threshold nociceptors can be modified in the periphery by a combination of chemicals that act synergistically as a sensitizing "soup." These chemicals are produced by damaged tissue as part of the inflammatory reaction and by sympathetic terminals. 5-HT, 5-hydroxytryptamine.

Central Sensitization

Central nervous system hypersensitivity also occurs as a result of tissue injury and may outlast the duration of the initiating nociceptive stimulus. In rats, these spinal cord changes occur within minutes of exposure to a very brief noxious stimulus. Following a tissue injury, C-fiber nociceptors are activated and action potentials are transmitted toward the spinal cord. This C-fiber volley causes strengthening of synapses at spinal terminals. As a result, the response of dorsal horn neurons to a particular stimulus is increased in intensity as well as duration, and many dorsal horn neurons begin to respond to stimuli outside of their original border (known as receptive-field expansion). In addition, there is a reduction in the threshold necessary to elicit a response. Clinically, we may observe primary hyperalgesia (an area of pain and increased sensitivity to external

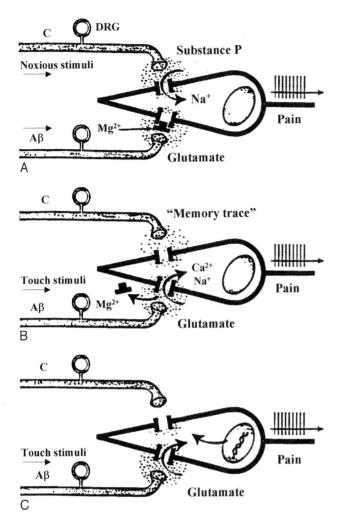

FIGURE 30–2. Proposed neural mechanisms of central sensitization. *A,* Noxious stimulus activates C-fibers and results in release of substance P and glutamate in the spinal cord. *B,* The substance P–induced depolarization of the neuron displaces the magnesium ion from the NMDA receptor and results in entry of Ca^{2+} into the cell. *C,* Ca^{2+} entry through NMDA receptors may alter gene expression in a way that makes central sensitization permanent and independent of ongoing nociceptor drive. The latter hypothesis needs further confirmation. Aβ, afferent Aβ fibers; C, afferent C fibers.

the periphery normally causes activation of dorsal horn neurons via the release of mediators such as substance P, a neuropeptide, and glutamate, an excitatory amino acid. Glutamate is also released after Aβ nociceptors are stimulated following a touch stimulus. However, the dorsal horn neurons are minimally activated by an Aβ source because the glutamate receptors (i.e., *N*-methyl-D-aspartate [NMDA] receptors) are blocked by Mg^{2+}. When C-fiber input occurs, a substance P–driven depolarization occurs, which in turn displaces Mg^{2+} and frees the NMDA receptor. This receptor can now respond to glutamate released from Aβ stimulation, activate dorsal horn neurons, and cause pain. With the release of the NMDA receptor, Ca^{2+} enters and elicits a phosphorylation process, which prolongs this touch-evoked pain state. It is also believed that C-fiber stimulation elicits genetic changes at the spinal cord level (e.g., *c-fos* gene) and may lead to excessive release of nitric oxide, causing cell death and further changes of dorsal horn neurons.

With the understanding of peripheral hypersensitivity, but more importantly of central sensitization, came the idea that the pain state may be lessened or inhibited if sensory input to the spinal cord were suppressed prior to the initiating stimulus. Most likely, central sensitization occurs, just as we believe peripheral sensitization occurs, as a warning mechanism to signal that tissue injury has occurred, therefore allowing us to protect that tissue until healing has taken place. However, in the postoperative period, the pain that occurs as a result of central sensitization is almost pathologic. Experimental studies have demonstrated a clear role of preemptive analgesia in diminishing postoperative pain. However, clinical studies have not been as definitive. Perhaps with this new knowledge of NMDA receptor–dependent mechanisms, gene expression, and nitric oxide–mediated processes occurring at the spinal cord level after an injury clinical studies will focus on new therapies directed toward antagonism of these processes. Preemptive analgesia may therefore have an important role in the management of acute postoperative pain.

BIBLIOGRAPHY

Abram SE: Importance of preincisional analgesia. Reg Anesth 21(6S):117–121, 1996.

Carpenter RL, Abram SE, Bromage PR, et al: Consensus statement on acute pain management. Reg Anesth 21(6S):152–156, 1996.

Cousins MJ: Prevention of postoperative pain. *In* Bond MR, Charlton JE, Woolf CJ (eds): Pain Research and Clinical Management. Vol. 4, Amsterdam, Elsevier, 1991, pp 41–52.

Kissin I, Raja SN: Preemptive analgesia: Concepts, controversies and caveats. Pain Digest 5:5–8, 1995.

McQuay HJ: Do preemptive treatments provide better pain control? Prog Pain Res Manage 2:709–723, 1994.

Niv D, Devor M: Preemptive analgesia in the relief of postoperative pain. Curr Rev Pain 1:79–92, 1996.

Treede RD, Meyer RA, Raja SN, et al: Peripheral and central mechanisms of cutaneous hyperalgesia. Prog Neurobiol 38:397–421, 1992.

Woolf CJ, Chong M: Preemptive analgesia—Treating postoperative pain by preventing the establishment of central sensitization. Anesth Analg 77:362–379, 1993.

stimuli where the noxious stimulus was applied) and an area of secondary hyperalgesia (increased sensitivity in the intact surrounding area). There is evidence that demonstrates C-fiber input from an injury also causes formation of anatomic connections at the spinal cord level between neurons that respond to Aβ fiber transmission and neurons that respond to Aδ and C-fiber transmission. A touch stimulus would then elicit pain (i.e., allodynia).

NEUROCHEMISTRY OF CENTRAL SENSITIZATION

Figure 30–2 illustrates a proposed mechanism for these central changes. Stimulation of C nociceptors in

Chapter 31

Preemptive Analgesia: Clinical Studies

Veronica D. Mitchell, M.D.,
and Srinivasa N. Raja, M.D.

The phenomena of peripheral and central sensitization (see Chapter 30) that occur following stimulation of nociceptors and the release of mediators as a result of tissue damage contribute to the postoperative pain state. Research has long compared the analgesic effects of certain techniques used in the postoperative period; however, the new understanding of central sensitization has evoked an interest in the postoperative analgesic effects of techniques applied preoperatively and intraoperatively.

Further widespread clinical interest in this subject occurred following publication of an editorial by Wall, in 1988,[1] based on clinical studies that suggested preoperative analgesic techniques may decrease postoperative pain. The hypothesis was that interrupting the pathway between the nociceptive stimulus and the spinal cord resulted in prevention of spinal cord changes, such as hyperexcitability. Thus was born the idea of "preemptive analgesia," that is, the prevention of central hypersensitivity and the subsequent prevention or reduction of postoperative pain by initiation of analgesic therapies prior to the noxious event (i.e., surgery).

The clinical importance of the phenomenon of preemptive analgesia, although based on a logical hypothesis and encouraging animal studies, has been very controversial. It is important to be familiar with the older studies that did not truly test the hypothesis of preemptive analgesia. They were not designed to compare the effects of an identical analgesic technique applied preoperatively or postoperatively to comparable patient groups. It is also important to be aware of the more recent clinical trials, which, although well-designed, have yielded inconsistent findings. Agents that have been used in these clinical studies include local anesthetics, opiates, nonsteroidal anti-inflammatory drugs (NSAIDs), and volatile anesthetic agents. Review of the clinical literature may help to design better studies to address the issue of preemptive analgesia, which not only has clinical implications in the treatment of postoperative pain but also perhaps in the prevention of the development of chronic neuropathic pain states.

CLINICAL EVIDENCE

A close review of the research in the area of preemptive analgesia reveals essentially three types of general approaches. The *first* category involves comparison between a specific preoperative therapy in one group of patients (experimental group) with an untreated second group (control group). The *second* type of study compares the efficacy of a specific therapy when given preoperatively vs. postoperatively. The *third* type of trial has involved observation of the effects of continuous analgesic therapy administered through the perioperative period. In addition, measurements for determining the efficacy of the therapy have varied. The most common components measured include patient reporting of pain based on visual analogue scale (VAS) ratings, total dose of postoperative analgesia requirements, and time to first request for analgesia following surgery.

Preemptive Analgesia vs. None

Several well-known studies have compared the effects of a particular treatment applied preoperatively with the results of no treatment. Although most of these studies support the hypothesis that preemptive analgesia decreases or abolishes postoperative pain, none of these have adequately addressed the question of whether the preoperatively administered therapy was more effective than the same therapy instituted after the surgery. However, this research has produced evidence suggestive of a potential clinical benefit, and thus has spurred further research in this area.

Presurgical vs. Postsurgical Intervention

Tables 31-1 to 31-3 summarize several studies that have compared administration of a local anesthetic, an opioid, or an NSAID prior to incision with the same analgesic technique applied after the surgical procedure.

TABLE 31–1. PRESURGERY VS. POSTSURGERY LOCAL ANESTHESIA

Study (Year)	Study Design	Treatment Tested	Surgical Procedure	No. of Patients	Preemptive Analgesia?
Ejlersen et al.[6] (1992)	DB/R	Lignocaine/wound infiltration	Inguinal herniorrhaphy	37	Yes
Dierking et al.[2] (1992)	DB/R	Lignocaine/wound infiltration	Inguinal herniorrhaphy	32	No
Ringrose and Cross[3] (1984)	NB	Bupivacaine/femoral nerve block	Knee joint surgery	20	Yes
Pryle et al.[24] (1993)	DB/R	Bupivacaine/epidural	Abdominal hysterectomy/myomectomy	36	No
Rice et al.[25] (1990)	DB/R	Bupivacaine/spinal	Herniotomy/orchidopexy/hydrocelectomy	40	No
Gunter et al.[26] (1990)	DB/R	Bupivacaine/caudal	Distal hypospadias repair	24	No
Katz et al.[4] (1994)	DB/R	Bupivacaine/epidural	Lower abdominal surgery	42	Yes
Nakamura et al.[5] (1994)	DB/R	Mepivacaine/epidural	Hysterectomy	90	Yes
Pasqualucci et al.[27] (1996)	DB/R	Bupivacaine/topical	Laparoscopic cholecystectomy	120	Yes

DB/R, double-blind randomized; NB, non-blinded.

Studies involving the use of local anesthetics can be categorized into trials of nerve blocks, epidural or intrathecal injections, and wound infiltrations (see Table 31-1). Dierking and co-workers[2] compared preoperative and postoperative inguinal field blocks in 32 herniorrhaphy patients. The study failed to support the efficacy of preemptive analgesia. Ringrose and Cross[3] reported a preemptive effect in patients who had a femoral nerve block prior to knee joint surgery under general anesthesia; however, the study was not performed in a blind fashion. Most of the studies looking at caudal, epidural, or spinal local anesthetics did not demonstrate any preemptive effects. However, two studies of adults undergoing lower abdominal surgical procedures under general anesthesia[4, 5] revealed a significant reduction in postoperative pain in those who received epidural local anesthesia prior to surgery. Several researchers have explored the effects of local anesthetic wound infiltration administered preoperatively and postoperatively. Most have not been able to demonstrate a preemptive effect; however, Ejlersen and others[6] showed a remarkable preemptive effect of preincisional local infiltration through a double-blind randomized trial of 37 herniorrhaphy patients.

Some studies involving presurgical vs. postsurgical administration of opioids have demonstrated a preemptive analgesic effect, whereas others have not (see Table 31-2). Richmond and colleagues[7] showed that intravenous morphine given prior to incision for 76 abdominal hysterectomy patients reduced the postoperative opiate requirement by 27% during the first 24 hours. Later, Collis and co-workers[8] performed a similar experiment using a higher dose of intravenous morphine and were able to demonstrate a better preemptive analgesic effect, however with the development of intolerable side effects. Mansfield and colleagues[9] and Wilson and others[10] studied the effect of preincision vs. postincision intravenously administered alfentanil in hysterectomy patients. Neither group was able to show a difference between control and experimental groups. The only trial that compared preincision vs. postincision epidural opioids without local anesthetics was performed by Katz and associates[11] in 30 thoracotomy patients. This study supported preemptive analgesia as demonstrated by the significantly reduced VAS pain scores in the preincision treatment group 6 hours postoperatively.

Most of the trials involving NSAIDs were performed in oral surgery patients (see Table 31-3). One well-

TABLE 31–2. PRESURGERY VS. POSTSURGERY OPIOID ADMINISTRATION

Study (Year)	Study Design	Treatment Tested (Route of Administration)	Surgical Procedure	No. of Patients	Preemptive Analgesia?
Richmond et al.[7] (1993)	DB/R	Morphine (intravenous)	Hysterectomy	60	Yes
Collis et al.[8] (1995)	DB/R	Morphine (intravenous)	Hysterectomy	60	Yes
Wilson et al.[10] (1994)	DB/R	Alfentanyl (intravenous)	Hysterectomy	40	No
Mansfield et al.[9] (1994)	SB/R	Alfentanyl (intravenous)	Hysterectomy	60	No
Katz et al.[11] (1992)	DB/R	Fentanyl (epidural)	Thoracotomy	30	Yes
Campbell and Kendrick[28] (1991)	DB/R	Pentazocine (intravenous)	Molar tooth extraction	80	No

DB/R, double-blind randomized; SB/R, single-blind randomized.

TABLE 31–3. PRESURGERY VS. POSTSURGERY NSAID ADMINISTRATION

Study (Year)	Study Design	Treatment Tested (Route of Administration)	Surgical Procedure	No. of Patients	Preemptive Analgesia?
Gustafsson et al.[15] (1983)	Crossover	Paracetamol (oral)	Third molar extraction	50	No
Flath et al.[12] (1987)	DB/R	Flurbiprofen (oral)	Pulpectomy	120	No
Sisk et al.[13] (1989)	WS	Diflunisal (oral)	Removal of impacted molar	20	No
Sisk and Grover[14] (1990)	WS	Naproxen (oral)	Removal of impacted molar	36	No
Fletcher et al.[16] (1995)	DB/R	Ketorolac (intravenous)	Hip replacement	60	Yes

DB/R, double-blind randomized; WS, within-subject design.

designed study by Flath and colleagues[12] that observed the effects of preoperative flurbiprofen in four groups of 30 patients undergoing pulpectomy revealed no preemptive effect. Within the four groups, preoperative and postoperative administration of flurbiprofen and placebo were varied. The preoperative and postoperative placebo group served as a control. Although this group demonstrated significantly higher pain scores than the remaining groups, no detectable difference was noted between the preoperative vs. postoperative NSAID groups. Three additional research groups were unable to demonstrate a preemptive effect of NSAIDs in patients undergoing oral surgery.[13-15] Fletcher and others,[16] however, showed that patients undergoing total hip replacement had less pain postoperatively if treated with intravenous ketorolac prior to incision.

Researchers have also looked at the effects of applying a continuous analgesic technique perioperatively for postoperative pain. Only one study compared the same technique initiated preoperatively vs. postoperatively. Dahl and associates[17] were not able to show a preemptive effect in the group that received an epidural bupivacaine and morphine infusion before colon surgery. In a study in patients undergoing radial retropubic prostatectomy, neuraxial blockade with epidural anesthesia resulted in decreased postoperative analgesic demands.[18] A more recent strategy has been the use of N-methyl-D-aspartate (NMDA) antagonists such as ketamine prior to the surgical incision.

Why then, despite convincing evidence for preemptive analgesia in experimental studies in animals, have we not been able to consistently demonstrate this phenomenon in humans? One such reason may lie in the fact that the clinical study design, in and of itself, may be somewhat faulty. The surgical incision is not a single, one-time noxious stimulus, but actually a constant source of C-fiber input to the spinal cord. Even if the analgesic technique applied prior to the incision initially blocked the C-fiber input from reaching the spinal cord, as the effects of the technique began to wear off, nociceptive information would reach the spinal cord, causing induction of hypersensitivity. It would be impossible in the postoperative period to determine if a beneficial effect has occurred. This is called the "Hydra problem" after the mythologic creature whose head would immediately regenerate when severed. Also, many of the studies performed involved the use of premedications or intraoperative analgesic adjuvants. These substances may have blunted the hypersensitive changes that would

have otherwise occurred in the spinal cord, thereby making it difficult to distinguish a significant difference between the control and experimental groups. In addition, studies have demonstrated that nitrous oxide has a preemptive analgesic effect.[20, 21] Therefore, clinical trials in which patients underwent general anesthesia with the use of nitrous oxide may not have shown a preemptive effect for this reason.

A second reason for the lack of strong evidence supporting preemptive analgesia in clinical studies may be that no objective standard exists to measure pain. Outcome measures usually involve such end points as 24-hour total opioid consumption using patient-controlled analgesia (PCA). However, a recent study by Jamison and co-workers[22] demonstrated that PCA consumption was not only a reflection of pain severity, but also a reflection of the patient's postoperative anxiety level, mood, expectations of recovery, and other psychosocial factors.

A third reason that preemptive analgesia is not an obvious phenomenon in clinical trials may be that it is extremely difficult to completely block noxious input from reaching the spinal cord. Researchers have used plasma cortisol levels as a determinant of the stress response to determine if complete neural blockade occurs during surgery. One researcher showed that only a block extending from T4 to S5 prevented a rise in cortisol levels following lower abdominal surgery.[23]

SUMMARY

Postoperative pain management has improved tremendously with the development of PCA and continuous epidural analgesia, yet it remains suboptimal for a subset of patients. The potential benefit of preemptive analgesia is great, but the optimal technique needs to be determined. Further studies need to be conducted after restructuring of study design and with novel analgesics, such as NMDA antagonists, and/or with multimodal therapies, given the recently acquired knowledge of acute pain mechanisms. Preemptive analgesia may not only prove to be a tool for managing acute postoperative pain, but it may also aid in the prevention of the development of chronic neuropathic pain states, which persist well beyond the postoperative period secondary to dysfunction of the nervous system.

REFERENCES

1. Wall PD: The prevention of postoperative pain. Pain 33:289-290, 1988.
2. Dierking GW, Dahl JB, Kanstrup J, et al: Effect of pre- vs. postoperative inguinal field block on postoperative pain after herniorrhaphy. Br J Anaesth 68:344-348, 1992.
3. Ringrose NH, Cross MJ: Femoral nerve block in knee joint surgery. Am J Sports Med 12:398-402, 1984.
4. Katz J, Clairoux M, Kavanagh BP, et al: Preemptive lumbar epidural anaesthesia reduces postoperative pain and patient-controlled morphine consumption after lower abdominal surgery. Pain 59:395-403, 1994.
5. Nakamura T, Yokoo H, Hamakawa T, et al: Preemptive analgesia produced with epidural analgesia administered prior to surgery. Masui 43:1024-1028, 1994.
6. Ejlersen E, Andersen HB, Eliasen K, et al: A comparison between preincisional and postincisional lidocaine infiltration and postoperative pain. Anesth Analg 74:495-498, 1992.
7. Richmond CE, Bromley LM, Woolf CJ: Preoperative morphine pre-empts postoperative pain. Lancet 342:73-75, 1993.
8. Collis R, Brandner B, Bromley LM, et al: Is there any clinical advantage of increasing the pre-emptive dose of morphine or combining pre-incisional with postoperative morphine administration? Br J Anaesth 74:396-399, 1995.
9. Mansfield M, Meikle R, Miller C: A trial of pre-emptive analgesia: Influence of timing of preoperative alfentanil on postoperative pain and analgesic requirements. Anaesthesia 49:1091-1093, 1994.
10. Wilson RJ, Leith S, Jackson IJ, et al: Pre-emptive analgesia from intravenous administration of opioids: No effect with alfentanil. Anaesthesia 49:591-593, 1994.
11. Katz J, Kavanagh BP, Sandler AN, et al: Preemptive analgesia: Clinical evidence of neuroplasticity contributing to postoperative pain. Anesthesiology 77:439-446, 1992.
12. Flath RK, Hicks ML, Dionne RA, et al: Pain suppression after pulpectomy with preoperative flurbiprofen. J Endodont 13:339-347, 1987.
13. Sisk AL, Mosley RO, Martin RP: Comparison of preoperative and postoperative diflunisal for suppression of postoperative pain. J Oral Maxillofac Surg 47:464-468, 1989.
14. Sisk AL, Grover BJ: A comparison of preoperative and postoperative naproxen sodium for suppression of postoperative pain. J Oral Maxillofac Surg 48:674-678, 1990.
15. Gustafsson I, Nystrom E, Quiding H: Effect of preoperative paracetamol on pain after oral surgery. Eur J Clin Pharmacol 24:63-65, 1983.
16. Fletcher D, Zetlaoui P, Monin S, et al: Influence of timing on the analgesic effect of intravenous ketorolac after orthopedic surgery. Pain 61:291-297, 1995.
17. Dahl JB, Hansen BL, Hjortso NC, et al: Influence of timing on the effect of continuous extradural analgesia with bupivacaine and morphine after major abdominal surgery. Br J Anaesth 69:4-8, 1992.
18. Shir Y, Raja SN, Frank SM: The effect of epidural versus general anesthesia on postoperative pain and analgesic requirements in patients undergoing radical prostatectomy. Anesthesiology 80:49-56, 1994.
19. Fu ES, Miguel R, Scharf JE: Preemptive ketamine decreases postoperative narcotic requirements in patients undergoing abdominal surgery. Anesth Analg 84:1086-1090, 1977.
20. Goto T, Marota JJ, Crosby G: Nitrous oxide induces preemptive analgesia in the rat that is antagonized by halothane. Anesthesiology 80:409-416, 1994.
21. Berkowitz BA, Finck AD, Ngai SH: Nitrous oxide analgesia: Reversal by naloxone and development of tolerance. J Pharmacol Exp Ther 203:539-547, 1977.
22. Jamison RN, Taft K, O'Hara JP, et al: Psychosocial and pharmacologic predictors of satisfaction with intravenous patient-controlled analgesia. Anesth Analg 77:121-125, 1993.
23. Kehlet H: Surgical stress: The role of pain and analgesia. Br J Anaesth 63:189-195, 1989.
24. Pryle BJ, Vanner RG, Enriquez N, et al: Can pre-emptive lumbar epidural blockade reduce postoperative pain following lower abdominal surgery? Anaesthesia 48:120-123, 1993.
25. Rice LJ, Pudimat MA, Hannallah RS: Timing of caudal block placement in relation to surgery does not affect duration of postoperative analgesia in pediatric ambulatory patients. Can J Anaesth 37:429-431, 1990.
26. Gunter JB, Forestner JE, Manley CB: Caudal epidural anesthesia reduces blood loss during hypospadias repair. J Urol 144:517-519, 1990.
27. Pasqualucci A, de Angelis V, Contardo R, et al: Preemptive analgesia: Intraperitoneal local anesthetic in laparoscopic cholecystectomy: A randomized, double-blind, placebo-controlled study. Anesthesiology 85:11-20, 1996.
28. Campbell WI, Kendrick RW: Postoperative dental pain—a comparative study of anti-inflammatory and analgesic agents. Ulster Med J 60:39-43, 1991.

FURTHER READING

Bridenbaugh PO: Preemptive analgesia: Is it clinically relevant? Anesth Analg 78:203-204, 1994.
Kehlet H, Dahl JB: The value of 'multimodal' or 'balanced analgesia' in postoperative pain treatment: A review. Anesth Analg 77:1048-1056, 1993.
Kissin I: Preemptive analgesia: Why its effect is not always obvious. Anesthesiology 84:1-5, 1996.
McQuay HJ: Do preemptive treatments provide better pain control? Prog Pain Res Manage 2:709-723, 1994.
McQuay HJ: Pre-emptive analgesia: A systematic review of clinical studies. Ann Med 27:249-256, 1995.
Woolf CJ, Chong M: Preemptive analgesia: Treating postoperative pain by preventing the establishment of central sensitization. Anesth Analg 77:362-379, 1993.

Chapter 32

 # Patient-Controlled Analgesia

Edward R. Sherwood, M.D., Ph.D.,
and Honorio T. Benzon, M.D.

Patient-controlled analgesia (PCA) is a method of administering narcotic analgesics for the purpose of pain control in a variety of settings. This technique is based on the use of a microprocessor-controlled infusion pump that delivers a preprogrammed dose of medication when the patient pushes a demand button. A timer within the pump is programmed to prevent administration of additional doses until a specified time period has elapsed. Modern PCA devices allow for the programming of demand dose, lockout interval, basal continuous infusions, and limitation of dose over a 1- to 4-hour period. These devices also provide information on patient usage, which includes number of demands and amount of medication delivered during the previous 1-hour and 24-hour periods. This information can be useful for optimizing the delivery of analgesics to individual patients. Most commonly, medication is delivered through an indwelling intravenous catheter, although techniques are available to deliver analgesics via the intramuscular, subcutaneous, and epidural routes using PCA technology.

PCA allows patients to titrate analgesics to their needs and bypasses the unavoidable delays that occur when analgesics are provided on request. These delays include the response time of a potentially busy nurse, screening of the appropriateness of the request, signout and preparation of the opioid, and, finally, administration of the medication. PCA, when used properly, allows patients to maintain a narrower range of plasma drug concentration compared with conventional intramuscular bolus dosing. Subtherapeutic troughs and excessive peak plasma concentrations, which can be associated with significant side effects including sedation and respiratory depression, are avoided. PCA also gives patients a sense of control over their analgesic needs; this is a major reason for the high degree of patient satisfaction with this modality of pain control. The ability to titrate analgesic dose to clinical effect is important. PCA allows patients to titrate their analgesic needs as their relative level of pain changes. Patients generally self-administer opioids appropriately, and several studies have shown that the total opioid requirements of patients using

PCA are less than those of patients using conventional intramuscular dosing.

A critical principle in the use of PCA is that the patient controls the amount of analgesic delivered. This is very important for the safe use of PCA technology. Sedation usually precedes respiratory depression as plasma opioid levels increase within a given patient. The sedated patient is unable to push the demand button and deliver additional opioid and therefore avoids opioid levels that could precipitate life-threatening complications. It is important for nursing personnel and family members to be aware of this principle so that the demand button is not pushed by anyone other than the patient. For optimal results, patients, family members, and nursing personnel should understand the basic principles of PCA use. Patients should be instructed on the use of PCA devices before therapy is initiated. The patient must be cooperative and able to understand the use of PCA and must have the ability to push the demand button. This requirement limits the use of PCA in children younger than 3 to 5 years of age and in persons with some mental or physical handicaps. It is the responsibility of physicians and nursing staff to monitor patients to ensure that adequate analgesia is obtained and that undesirable side effects are minimized. Because of pharmacokinetic and pharmacodynamic variability among patients, conventional PCA settings may need to be adjusted. In addition, PCA pumps are mechanical devices that can, on occasion, malfunction. Although the safety record of PCA pumps is excellent, several incidents of excessive medication delivery because of mechanical dysfunction or improper programming of PCA devices have been reported. However, there is no evidence to indicate an increased risk of adverse effects with PCA. In fact, experience has shown that sedation and respiratory depression are less common with PCA than with conventional intravenous or intramuscular dosing.

The use of a basal infusion with PCA is controversial. Studies have shown that addition of a basal infusion rate does not improve patients' ability to sleep or rest comfortably and does not alter scores for pain, fatigue, and anxiety.[1] The number of patient demands, number of supplemental bolus doses, and total opioid use were also the same. However, other studies have demonstrated improved patient comfort with a continuous basal infusion.[2] The disadvantage of a continuous infusion is that most programming errors that have resulted in adverse side effects occurred during the use of a continuous infusion. In addition, use of a continuous infusion bypasses the basic safety mechanism of patient control, which is important in the safe use of PCA technology. Specifically, in a sedated patient, delivery of opioid continues at a basal rate and may put the patient at higher risk for respiratory depression. The use of a continuous infusion in patients who have high opioid requirements may be safe and appropriate, but careful patient selection is essential.

Several opioids have been used effectively with PCA pumps. The ideal analgesic for use with PCA would have a rapid onset of action, high efficacy (no ceiling effect), and intermediate duration of action. Morphine, oxymorphone, and meperidine most closely satisfy these criteria and are the most widely used agents in PCA pumps. However, a variety of agonist opioids as well as agonist-antagonists have been used effectively in PCA pumps. The typical dosing, lockout, and infusion parameters for opiates that are used for PCA are indicated in Table 32-1.

APPLICATIONS OF PATIENT-CONTROLLED ANALGESIA

PCA is most commonly used for the management of postoperative pain. However, PCA also can be used for the management of labor pain, post-traumatic pain, cancer pain, and pain associated with myocardial infarction.

Labor Pain

Opioids are commonly administered for labor analgesia. However, many parturients wish to limit the use of medications and avoid excessive sedation before delivery. Compared with bolus intramuscular or intravenous dosing, PCA provides the ability to titrate analgesic needs as labor progresses and is better titrated against the large variability in analgesic requirements among parturients. Therefore, PCA provides a good alternative in laboring patients when epidural analgesia is not available or is contraindicated.

Compared with intramuscular or intravenous dosing, some advantages of PCA in the parturient include superior pain relief, less maternal sedation and respiratory depression, lower placental drug transfer, less need for antiemetics, and higher patient satisfaction. However, one major concern with the use of parenteral opioids during labor and delivery is the potential depression of fetal ventilation and neurologic activity during the postdelivery period. PCA has been shown to decrease cord opioid levels, compared with conventional bolus dosing, and most studies have not demonstrated significant fetal depression after its use for labor analgesia. In order to minimize fetal depression, many practitioners discontinue PCA once the mother's cervix is fully dilated. A disadvantage of PCA for labor pain is that parenteral narcotics are often ineffective in controlling the intermittently intense pain of uterine contractions.

Pain Control in Pediatric Patients

PCA is a safe and effective means of controlling pain in adolescents and young children. The most important factor in determining the success of PCA in pediatric patients is the ability of the patient to understand the basic principles of PCA use. Most children older than 7 years of age can use PCA independently. Children age 4 to 6 years usually can use PCA pumps with encouragement from parents and nursing staff. However, the failure rate in this age group is quite high. Children younger than 4 years of age are not good candidates for PCA use. Some investigators have advocated parental assistance for PCA use by young children. However, this practice bypasses the basic safety mechanisms of PCA and has been discouraged in the postoperative setting.

TABLE 32-1. GUIDELINES REGARDING BOLUS DOSES, LOCKOUT INTERVALS, AND CONTINUOUS INFUSIONS FOR VARIOUS PARENTERAL ANALGESICS WHEN USED WITH A PCA SYSTEM

Drug	Bolus (mg)	Lockout Interval (min)	Continuous Infusion (mg/hr)
Agonists			
Fentanyl	0.015-0.05	3-10	0.02-0.1
Hydromorphone	0.10-0.5	5-15	0.2-0.5
Meperidine	5-15	5-15	5-40
Methadone	0.5-3	10-20	—
Morphine	0.5-3	5-20	1-10
Oxymorphone	0.2-0.8	5-15	0.1-1
Sufentanil	0.003-0.015	3-10	0.004-0.03
Agonist-antagonists			
Buprenorphine	0.03-0.2	10-20	—
Nalbuphine	1-5	5-15	1-8
Pentazocine	5-30	5-15	6-40

The addition of a basal infusion is controversial (see text).
Adapted from Lubenow TR, Ivankovich AD, McCarthy RJ: Management of acute postoperative pain. *In* Barash PG, Cullen BF, Stoelting RK (eds): Clinical Anesthesia, ed 2. Philadelphia, JB Lippincott, 1992, p 1320.

TABLE 32–2. PCA DOSING IN CHILDREN

Drug	Bolus (μg/kg)	Lockout Interval (min)	4-hr Limit (μg/kg)	Infusion (μg/kg/hr)
Morphine	10–20	7–15	200–400	10–20
Demerol	100–200	7–15	2000–4000	100–200
Fentanyl	0.1–0.2	7–15	2–4	0.1–0.2

The addition of a basal infusion to PCA is controversial (see text).

Basal infusions also have been used in the pediatric population for control of postoperative pain. However, results from some studies show an increased incidence of hypoxemia in children receiving continuous opioid infusions in conjunction with PCA. Therefore, continuous infusions should be used with caution in the pediatric population and pulse oximetry, as a mechanism of assessing opioid-induced hypoxemia under these conditions, should be strongly considered (Table 32–2). Concurrent administration of drugs with respiratory depressant effects (e.g., antihistamines, antiemetics) should also be viewed with caution.

Cancer Pain

PCA is useful for cancer pain management in the inpatient setting in both children and adults. In contrast to postoperative pain management, the use of continuous opioid infusions for the management of cancer pain is very effective and is encouraged. In the pediatric cancer population, parental assistance with PCA use is also encouraged. The dosages of opioid used in the treatment of cancer pain often far exceed those used in the postoperative setting.

REFERENCES

1. Parker R, Holtmann B, White P: Effects of a continuous opioid infusion with PCA therapy on patient comfort and analgesic requirements after abdominal hysterectomy. Anesthesiology 76:362, 1992.
2. Smith G: Management of postoperative pain. Can J Anaesth 36:51, 1989.

SUGGESTED READINGS

Benzon H: Postsurgical pain. In Raj P (ed): Pain Medicine: A Comprehensive Review. St Louis, Mosby-Year Book, 1996, pp 359–365.
Houck C, Berde C, Anand K: Pediatric pain management. In Gregory G (ed): Pediatric Anesthesia. New York, Churchill Livingstone, 1994, pp 743–771.
Rawal N: Postoperative pain and its management. In Raj P (ed): Practical Management of Pain. St Louis, Mosby-Year Book, 1992, pp 367–390.
Wakefield M: Systemic analgesia: Opioids, ketamine and inhalational agents. In Chestnut D (ed): Obstetric Anesthesia: Principles and Practice. St Louis, Mosby-Year Book, 1994, pp 340–352.

Chapter 33

Intrathecal Opioid Injections for Postoperative Pain

Cynthia A. Wong, M.D.

Since the discovery of opioid receptors in the substantia gelatinosa of the spinal cord[1] and the first description of intrathecal opioid injection in humans to treat pain,[2] numerous studies of intrathecal opioid injection for the treatment of postoperative pain have been undertaken. Advantages of intrathecal administration of opioids, morphine in particular, include prolonged analgesia with a single injection, no adverse hemodynamic effects, no motor block, and no need to maintain an epidural catheter. Disadvantages include the lack of ability to reinject without repeating the procedure (although continuous intrathecal catheter techniques have been described) and serious or bothersome side effects, including respiratory depression, nausea and vomiting, pruritus, and urinary retention.

MECHANISM OF ACTION OF OPIOIDS

Opioid receptors are located in Rexed's laminae I, II, and V of the dorsal horn gray matter of the spinal cord.[3] Animal data suggest that μ- and κ-receptors mediate spinal cord analgesia.[4] Analgesia is reversed by naloxone. Agonist binding of spinal opioid receptors inhibits primary afferent transmission in the spinal cord. In an animal model, binding of μ- and κ-receptors mediates different types of pain.[5] Intrathecal opioids inhibit C-fiber nociceptive discharge more easily than Aδ-fiber discharge. Therefore, they block dull (C-fiber mediated) pain better than sharp (Aδ-fiber mediated) pain[6] and are excellent analgesics, but not anesthetics.

Drug injected into cerebrospinal fluid (CSF) diffuses across the pia into the spinal cord. Physical properties of the drug determine the onset of analgesia, dermatomal spread, duration of analgesia, and side effects. Speed of onset is directly related to the lipid solubility of the opioid. Dermatomal spread and duration of action are inversely related to lipid solubility. Duration of action is also directly related to dose. Because of its hydrophobic nature, morphine penetrates the spinal cord very slowly. Relatively high concentrations remain in the CSF, serve as a depot, and cause prolonged duration of action. For

example, in a cat study, time to maximum response for intrathecal morphine was 1.3 hours, compared to 0.4 hour for meperidine. In monkeys, equipotent doses of morphine and meperidine lasted 12 to 16 hours and 3 to 5 hours, respectively.[4] Morphine circulates in CSF to higher spinal cord levels and the brain stem, resulting in increased dermatomal spread and a different side effect profile (see following). In contrast, lipophilic opioids readily penetrate the spinal cord at the level of injection. Low concentrations remain in the CSF, little drug circulates to higher levels, and analgesia is more segmentally localized.[4]

ADVANTAGES OF INTRATHECAL OPIOIDS

Intrathecal administration of opioids, morphine in particular, has several advantages over systemic and epidural administration. A single intrathecal dose of morphine can provide hours of postoperative analgesia without the peaks and valleys associated with intermittent administration of systemic opioids. Cannulation of the intrathecal space is more reliable and is technically easier than cannulation of the epidural space, and there is no necessity to maintain an epidural catheter. Intrathecally injected opioids, compared to continuously infused epidural local anesthetics, do not block the sympathetic nervous system and are therefore not associated with adverse hemodynamic effects. Motor function is intact, which encourages early ambulation. The effective dose of intrathecal morphine is much lower than the systemic or epidural dose.[7] Intrathecal injections of morphine result in barely detectable systemic levels of the drug.[8] In contrast, after epidural injection or infusion, systemic analgesic levels of morphine (and other opioids) are achieved.[5] This can cause excessive sedation. Finally, intrathecal opioids administered prior to surgery improve intraoperative analgesia.[5, 9-11] A preemptive analgesic effect of intrathecal morphine has been demonstrated in a rat model.[12]

DISADVANTAGES AND SIDE EFFECTS

A disadvantage of intrathecal administration of opioids for postoperative analgesia is that is a single injection technique. Intrathecal catheters for reinjection or continuous infusion are not routinely used for postoperative analgesia. Other disadvantages include potentially serious or bothersome side effects, some of which are common to systemic and epidural administration of opioids.

Respiratory depression is a feared complication of intrathecal opioid injection. The risk is dose-dependent. Early studies reported high rates because high doses of morphine were utilized.[5] However, two studies in patients undergoing cesarean section[11, 13] found that low-dose intrathecal morphine was associated with less respiratory depression than that in control groups receiving systemic morphine.

The degree of lipophilicity dictates the timing of respiratory depression. Because morphine is hydrophilic, and the intrathecal dose is low, there is little vascular absorption after intrathecal injection. In contrast, the lipophilic opioids are readily absorbed, leading to significant systemic opioid levels shortly after injection. Therefore, early respiratory depression (within 30 minutes) does not occur after intrathecal morphine injection, but it may occur with injection of more lipophilic opioids.[5] In contrast, late respiratory depression (4 to 12 hours) is a risk with morphine that does not occur with lipophilic opioids. The late respiratory depression associated with intrathecal morphine is due to the rostral spread of morphine in the CSF to brain stem and cerebral respiratory centers.[4] The injection of morphine in a hyperbaric solution does not decrease the risk.[14]

Factors associated with increased risk of delayed respiratory depression include high doses of morphine (>0.5 mg),[5] advanced age, changes in intra-abdominal pressure (including positive-pressure ventilation), concomitant systemic administration of opioids or other central nervous system depressants,[4] obesity, hypermagnesemia,[5] and sleep apnea.[15] Tolerance to opioids is protective.[4]

Clinical signs and symptoms are not sensitive indicators of respiratory depression.[16] Respiratory rate, level of sedation, and pupil size did not predict respiratory depression as measured by pulse oximetry and ventilatory response to carbon dioxide.

The respiratory depression associated with intrathecal opioids is reversed by naloxone, but it may outlast a single dose. Continuous prophylactic infusions of naloxone have been described.[5] The continuous administration of supplemental oxygen prevents hypoxemia.[16]

Nausea and vomiting are also associated with intrathecal opioid administration. The incidence of nausea and vomiting in patients undergoing cesarean section who were treated with intrathecal morphine, 0.2 mg, ranged from 5%[17] to 40%.[18] The incidence may be dose-dependent[13, 18] and may depend on whether symptoms are actively elicited by the investigators. However, the incidence of nausea and vomiting may be as high as 30% in postoperative patients receiving systemic narcotics.[4]

Nausea and vomiting can be reversed by small doses of naloxone, without reversing analgesia.[4]

Pruritus complicates neuraxial administration of opioids more often than systemic administration. The incidence ranges from 40% to 100% and occurs more often with morphine than the lipid-soluble opioids.[5] The mechanism is unclear, but it is not secondary to histamine release. The incidence may be dose-related.[14, 18] The time course after intrathecal morphine parallels that of rostral spread of the drug.[14] Mild symptoms may respond to diphenhydramine (perhaps because of its sedative effects). More severe symptoms respond to doses of naloxone that do not reverse analgesia. A continuous infusion of naloxone may be necessary.[5]

Urinary retention is a side effect of intrathecal opioids that is not dose-dependent.[4] It may be caused by sacral parasympathetic inhibition, resulting in detrusor muscle relaxation and inability to relax the sphincter. Antagonism of epidural morphine-induced urinary retention requires large doses of naloxone, which may reverse analgesia.[5] Bladder catheterization may be necessary for treatment.

Epidural morphine increases the incidence of reactivation of herpes simplex virus labialis (HSV-1). It is not known whether other opioids are also associated with reactivated HSV-1 infections. In one study in a heterogeneous population, neither intrathecal nor epidural opioid administration was associated with an increased risk of HSV-1 recrudescence. No other studies of intrathecal opioids address this issue.[5]

Several authors have investigated means of decreasing the side effects associated with intrathecal opioids. In a small study, naloxone infusions shortened the duration of analgesia without decreasing the incidence of side effects.[19] Similarly, prophylactic oral naltrexone shortened the duration of analgesia, although naltrexone did decrease the incidence of pruritus and vomiting.[20] The serotonin antagonist tropisetron did not decrease the incidence of nausea and vomiting after intrathecal morphine administration.[21]

ADJUVANTS TO INTRATHECAL OPIOIDS

Several adjuvants to intrathecal opioids have been investigated. Epinephrine added to intrathecal lidocaine and fentanyl prolonged surgical anesthesia and duration of postoperative analgesia and decreased the incidence of pruritus in patients undergoing postpartum tubal ligation.[22] Similarly, epinephrine added to intrathecal bupivacaine and morphine prolonged motor block and duration of postoperative analgesia.[23]

Co-administration of intrathecal clonidine and morphine with bupivacaine for patients undergoing total hip replacement did not improve postoperative analgesia or the side effect profile.[24]

In patients undergoing major genitourinary procedures who received intrathecal morphine and fentanyl, the scheduled administration of intravenous ketorolac reduced supplemental analgesia requirements without affecting the incidence of side effects.[25]

CLINICAL USES OF INTRATHECAL OPIOIDS FOR POSTOPERATIVE ANALGESIA

Numerous studies have demonstrated that intrathecal opioids, primarily morphine, provide excellent analgesia after a variety of surgical procedures, including cesarean section and gynecologic, orthopedic, genitourinary, abdominal, thoracic, cardiac, peripheral vascular, head and neck, and pediatric procedures. Randomized and blinded studies are discussed below. However, adequate dose-response studies are lacking for most surgical procedures.

Intrathecal morphine analgesia has been studied most commonly in patients undergoing cesarean section with hyperbaric bupivacaine anesthesia.[5] Dose-response studies have identified an intrathecal morphine dose of 0.1 to 0.2 mg as the ideal dose (prolonged analgesia with the fewest side effects).[18, 26] Other opioids described for post-cesarean section analgesia include fentanyl, sufentanil, meperidine, and methadone.[5] Duration of analgesia is significantly shorter with these opioids (2 to 6 hours). Meperidine, which, unlike other opioids, has local anesthetic properties, has been used as a total spinal anesthetic and postoperative analgesic in patients undergoing postpartum tubal ligation.[5]

Two dose-response studies in patients undergoing abdominal hysterectomy vary markedly in dose recommendations. Yamaguchi and co-workers found morphine, 0.04 mg, to be the optimal intrathecal dose when combined with hyperbaric tetracaine spinal anesthesia.[27] In contrast, Sarma and Boström injected intrathecal morphine, diluted with saline, prior to emergence from general anesthesia.[28] They recommend intrathecal morphine, 0.3 mg, as the most effective dose, with an acceptable incidence of side effects.

Optimal dose-response studies of intrathecal morphine for postoperative analgesia in patients undergoing total joint replacement procedures have not been published. The current studies mix together patients undergoing total knee and total hip replacement. Postoperative pain may be markedly different for these two procedures. However, in this mixed patient population, the optimal intrathecal morphine dose is 0.3 to 0.4 mg.[29, 30] Intrathecal morphine, 2.5 mg, was associated with an unacceptably high incidence of respiratory depression.[30] In patients undergoing lumbar spine surgery, the optimal intrathecal morphine dose was 0.25 to 0.50 mg.[31]

In patients undergoing transurethral resection of the prostate with hyperbaric lidocaine anesthesia, the addition of intrathecal morphine, 0.1 mg, reduced postoperative pain while minimizing side effects.[32]

In coronary artery bypass surgery, intrathecal morphine, 0.5 mg, decreased the need for postoperative intravenous morphine and sodium nitroprusside.[33] Similarly, large-dose intrathecal morphine (4.0 mg) decreased postoperative intravenous morphine requirements.[34] However, stress response, as measured by norepinephrine and epinephrine levels, was not reduced. Intrathecal morphine, 10 μg/kg, when combined with a moderate-dose fentanyl/midazolam anesthetic, resulted in a significantly longer time to extubation compared to that in a control group of patients undergoing coronary artery bypass (10.9 vs. 7.6 hours).[35] Rigorous dose-response studies have not been done in cardiac surgery patients.

In a dose-response study of patients undergoing lower extremity revascularization procedures, postoperative administration of intrathecal fentanyl, 40 μg, resulted in 5 hours of analgesia.[36]

The intrathecal administration of morphine for post-thoracotomy pain, postcholecystectomy pain, and post–head/neck surgery pain has been described. Randomized and/or dose-response studies have not been done.

Intrathecal morphine has been used in pediatric surgery. Doses of 10 to 30 μg/kg have been described. A single randomized, double-blind dose-response study in children undergoing selective dorsal rhizotomy for cerebral palsy–associated spasticity found 10 μg/kg provided analgesia comparable to higher doses.[37] Lower doses were not studied.

MONITORING AND NURSING CARE AFTER INTRATHECAL OPIOIDS

Most patients who have received intrathecal opioids can be safely cared for on standard nursing units, provided the nursing staff has received adequate training and education. Standard orders to treat side effects should be available, as well as nursing policies and procedures and a physician to manage complications. Routine respiratory monitoring (e.g., apnea monitors, pulse oximetry) are associated with frequent false alarms and may be impractical. Frequent nursing checks may be the best monitor.[5] Patients at increased risk for respiratory depression should receive supplemental oxygen and may need monitoring in an intensive care setting.

SUMMARY

Intrathecal injection of opioids is a simple, practical, and effective means of providing postoperative analgesia. For most procedures and patients, morphine is the opioid of choice, as it provides the longest duration of analgesia. Delayed respiratory depression is the most serious side effect and is dose related. Dose-response studies for most surgical procedures are lacking.

REFERENCES

1. Yaksh T, Rudy TA: Analgesia mediated by a direct spinal cord action of narcotics. Science 192:1357, 1976.
2. Wang JK, Nauss LA, Thomas JE: Pain relief by intrathecally applied morphine in man. Anesthesiology 50:149, 1979.
3. Kitahata LM, Kosaka Y, Taub A, et al: Lamina-specific suppression of dorsal horn activity by morphine sulfate. Anesthesiology 41:39, 1974.
4. Cousins MJ, Mather LE: Intrathecal and epidural administration of opioids. Anesthesiology 61:276, 1984.

5. Sinatra RS: Postoperative analgesia: Epidural and spinal techniques. *In* Chestnut D (ed): Obstetric Anesthesia: Principles and Practice. St Louis, Mosby–Year Book, 1994, p 513.

6. Rawal N, Sjostrand UH: Clinical application of epidural and intrathecal opioids for pain management. Int Anesth Clin 24:43, 1986.

7. Stoelting RK: Intrathecal morphine—an underused combination for postoperative pain management. Anesth Analg 68:707, 1989.

8. Sjöstrom S, Tamsen A, Persson MP, et al: Pharmacokinetics of intrathecal morphine and meperidine in humans. Anesthesiology 67: 889, 1987.

9. Cohen E, Neustein SM: Intrathecal morphine during thoracotomy: I. Effect on intraoperative enflurane requirements. J Cardiothorac Vasc Anesth 7:154, 1993.

10. Swenson JD, Hullander M, Wingler K, et al: Early extubation after cardiac surgery using combined intrathecal sufentanil and morphine. J Cardiothorac Vasc Anesth 8:509, 1994.

11. Abouleish E, Rawal N, Fallon K, et al: Combined intrathecal morphine and bupivacaine for cesarean section. Anesth Analg 67: 370, 1988.

12. Abram SE, Yaksh TL: Morphine, but not inhalation anesthesia, blocks post-injury facilitation: The role of preemptive suppression of afferent transmission. Anesthesiology 78:713, 1993.

13. Abboud TK, Dror A, Mosaad P, et al: Mini-dose intrathecal morphine for the relief of post-cesarean section pain: Safety, efficacy, and ventilatory responses to carbon dioxide. Anesth Analg 67:137, 1988.

14. Nordberg G: Pharmacokinetic aspects of spinal morphine analgesia. Acta Anesthesiol Scand 79 (suppl):1, 1984.

15. Martin R, Lamarche Y, Tetrault JP: Epidural and intrathecal narcotics. Can Anaesth Soc J 30: 662, 1983.

16. Bailey PL, Rhondeau S, Schafer PG, et al: Dose-response pharmacology of intrathecal morphine in human volunteers. Anesthesiology 79:49, 1993.

17. Abouliesh E, Rawal N, Rashad MN: The addition of 0.2 mg of subarachnoid morphine to hyperbaric bupivacaine for cesarean delivery: A prospective study of 856 cases. Reg Anesth 16:137, 1991.

18. Uchiyama A, Ueyama H, Nishimura M, et al: Low dose intrathecal morphine and pain relief following cesarean section. Int J Obstet Anesth 3: 87, 1994.

19. Wright PM, O'Toole DP, Barron DW: The influence of naloxone infusion on the action of intrathecal diamorphine: Low-dose naloxone and neuroendocrine responses. Acta Anaesthesiol Scand 36:230, 1992.

20. Abboud TK, Lee K, Zhu J, et al: Prophylactic oral naltrexone with intrathecal morphine for cesarean section: Effects on adverse reactions and analgesia. Anesth Analg 71:367, 1990.

21. Pitkanen MT, Niemi L, Tuominen MK, et al: Effect of tropisetron, a 5-HT3 receptor antagonist, on analgesia and nausea after intrathecal morphine. Br J Anaesth 71:681, 1993.

22. Malinow AM, Mokriski BL, Nomura MK, et al: Effect of epinephrine on intrathecal fentanyl analgesia in patients undergoing postpartum tubal ligation. Anesthesiology 73:381, 1990.

23. Goyagi T, Nishikawa T: The addition of epinephrine enhances postoperative analgesia by intrathecal morphine. Anesth Analg 81:508, 1995.

24. Grace D, Bunting H, Milligan KR, et al: Postoperative analgesia after co-administration of clonidine and morphine by the intrathecal route in patients undergoing hip replacement. Anesth Analg 80:86, 1995.

25. Gwirtz KH, Kim HC, Nagy DJ, et al: Intravenous ketorolac and subarachnoid opioid analgesia in the management of acute postoperative pain. Reg Anesth 20:395, 1995.

26. Jiang CJ, Liu CC, Wu TJ, et al: Mini-dose intrathecal morphine for post-cesarean section analgesia. Acta Anaesthesiol Sin 29:683, 1991.

27. Yamaguchi H, Watanabe S, Fukuda T, et al: Minimal effective dose of intrathecal morphine for pain relief following transabdominal hysterectomy. Anesth Analg 68:537, 1989.

28. Sarma VJ, Boström UV: Intrathecal morphine for the relief of post-hysterectomy pain—a double-blind, dose-response study. Acta Anaesthesiol Scand 37:223, 1993.

29. Kalso E: Effects of intrathecal morphine, injected with bupivacaine, on pain after orthopaedic surgery. Br J Anaesth 55:415, 1983.

30. Jacobson L, Chabal C, Brody MC: A dose-response study of intrathecal morphine: Efficacy, duration, optimal dose, and side effects. Anesth Analg 67:1082, 1988.

31. Ross DA, Drasner K, Weinstein PR, et al: Use of intrathecally administered morphine in the treatment of postoperative pain after lumbar spinal surgery: A prospective, double-blind, placebo-controlled study. Neurosurgery 28:700, 1991.

32. Kirson LE, Goldman JM, Slover RB: Low-dose intrathecal morphine for postoperative pain control in patients undergoing transurethral resection of the prostate. Anesthesiology 71:192, 1989.

33. Vanstrum GS, Bjornson KM, Ilko R: Postoperative effects of intrathecal morphine in coronary artery bypass surgery. Anesth Analg 67:261, 1988.

34. Chaney MA, Smith KR, Barclay JC, et al: Large-dose intrathecal morphine for coronary artery bypass grafting. Anesth Analg 83: 215, 1996.

35. Chaney MA, Furry PA, Fluder EM, et al: Intrathecal morphine for coronary artery bypass grafting and early extubation. Anesth Analg 84:241, 1997.

36. Reuben SS, Dunn SM, Duprat KM, et al: An intrathecal fentanyl dose-response study in lower extremity revascularization procedures. Anesthesiology 81:1371, 1994.

37. Dews TE, Schubert A, Fried A, et al: Intrathecal morphine for analgesia in children undergoing selective dorsal rhizotomy. J Pain Symptom Manage 11:188, 1996.

Chapter 34

Epidural Morphine for Postoperative Pain

Sam Page, M.D.

Spinal opioids (epidural and subarachnoid) have been used clinically for management of postoperative pain since 1979, as single or multiple injections or as continuous infusions. They have been especially helpful in the management of postoperative pain associated with thoracic and abdominal surgery. Spinal opioids provide antinociceptive benefits without blocking the sympathetic nervous system, as local anesthetics do. Therefore, hemodynamic alterations in the postoperative period that are caused by loss of sympathetic tone or reflexes are minimized. In addition, absence of motor blockade allows early ambulation. This selective block of nociception without effect on other systems is called *selective spinal analgesia.* Opioids tend to be most effective for C-fiber–mediated pain (dull pain), rather than Aδ-fiber–mediated pain (sharp pain) associated with surgical incision. Morphine, a hydrophilic opioid, was the first agent used and is the standard of comparison for other opioids.

The single property of opioids that best predicts behavior is lipid solubility (Fig. 34–1). There are several routes of clearance for epidurally administered opioids. They can

- Bind to epidural fat.
- Enter posterior spinal radicular arteries to be delivered to the dorsal horn.
- Enter epidural venous system and systemic circulation.
- Penetrate the dura through arachnoid granulations, enter the cerebrospinal fluid (CSF), and diffuse into the spinal cord tissue.

Highly lipid-soluble opioids are presented to the opioid receptors in the dorsal horn via both rapid diffusion through the arachnoid granulations and delivery by spinal arteries. Diffusion into epidural veins leads to systemic distribution and analgesia from supraspinal mechanisms. Epidural fat may act as a "buffer" to store lipophilic opioids, providing a reservoir and leaving less opioid to diffuse into the other systems.

Hydrophilic opioids, such as morphine, are more predictable owing to less absorption into epidural fat and the epidural venous and arterial systems. Once present in the CSF, hydrophilic opioids may accumulate, leading to long duration of analgesia with potential for rostral flow.

The transfer of epidural morphine across the arachnoid granulations into the dura takes about 90 minutes. Morphine is a highly ionized and hydrophilic drug, so only a low concentration of the lipid-soluble, un-ionized drug is present for transfer across the arachnoid granulations. Blood concentrations peak about 10 minutes after epidural administration. High concentrations of un-ionized drug in the spinal fluid can move cephalad with CSF flow, leading to delayed respiratory depression. The presence of a low concentration of un-ionized, lipid-soluble drug in the CSF provides a low concentration for diffusion into the spinal cord dorsal horn tissue (Fig. 34–2).

Several factors may contribute to venous distention and increased epidural morphine uptake by epidural veins. Venous drainage of the epidural space is by way of the azygos vein and collateral veins to the inferior vena cava. Obstruction of the vena cava, increased intra-

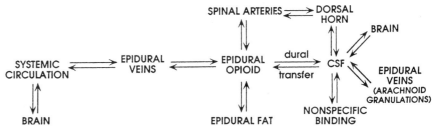

FIGURE 34–1. Routes of opioid absorption after epidural administration. (From Vade-Boncoeur TR, Ferrante FM: Epidural and subarachnoid opioids. *In* Ferrante FM, Vade-Boncoeur TR (eds): Postoperative Pain Management. New York, Churchill-Livingstone, 1993, p 280.)

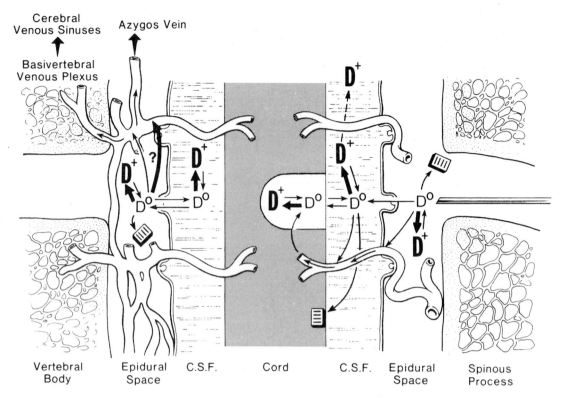

FIGURE 34–2. Pharmacokinetic model for the epidural injection of a hydrophilic drug such as morphine. D°, un-ionized lipophilic drug; D⁺, ionized hydrophilic drug. *Shaded squares* indicate nonspecific lipid binding sites. An epidural needle is shown delivering the drug to the epidural space. (From Cousins MJ, Cherry DA, Gourley GK: Acute and chronic pain: Use of spinal opioids. *In* Cousins MJ, Bridenbaugh PO (eds): Neural Blockade in Clinical Anesthesia and Management of Pain, ed 2. Philadelphia, JB Lippincott, 1988, p 987.)

abdominal pressure, or increased intrathoracic pressure may lead to epidural venous distention and redirection of venous flow to the azygos system. This may lead to an increased rate of systemic absorption of epidural morphine. A significant increase in intrathoracic pressure may redirect epidural blood flow from the azygos system to the basivertebral veins and to the brain.

Rostral progression of morphine in the CSF coincides with the ascending, dermatomal progression of analgesia, but not anesthesia, to pin-prick. The onset of nausea, vomiting, and respiratory depression due to epidural morphine coincides with trigeminal analgesia. The time delay for migration is similar to that of intrathecal morphine. As a rule, respiration should be monitored closely when parenteral opioids are given within 24 hours of epidural morphine, because of the concomitant effect on respiratory depression.

The epidural catheter usually is placed at the interspace corresponding to the middle dermatome of the surgical incision. Lipophilic opioids depend on the catheter location for optimal spread, whereas hydrophilic agents easily migrate into the CSF and are not dependent on the site of injection to reach the affected dermatomes. Hydrophilic opioids delivered to the lumbar epidural space provide good analgesia for thoracotomy pain. Lipophilic opioids (e.g., fentanyl) may be equianalgesic, but they depend on systemic absorption and suphraspinal effect for a large part of their analgesic efficacy.

Absolute contraindications to opioid analgesia in-

clude contraindication to epidural catheter placement and history of opioid intolerance. *Relative contraindications* are (1) history of significant opioid use preoperatively, (2) presence of dural puncture, and (3) central sleep apnea.

NONANALGESIC EFFECTS OF OPIOIDS

In patients receiving long-term opioids for chronic pain, the amount of opioids presented to the brain after epidural administration may not be enough to prevent *withdrawal*. In addition, the amount of opioid needed to effect analgesia after spinal opioid administration may be difficult to predict.

Spinal opioids have no major effect on motor function at doses used for spinal analgesia. Spinal opioids do *inhibit polysynaptic flexion reflexes* and therefore have been found to be helpful in the treatment of spasticity. Intense motor rigidity seen in experimental models from high-dose morphine may involve inhibition of the inhibitory neurotransmitter glycine.

Dysphoria and other central nervous system side effects are familiar complications of all parenteral opioids. *Sedation* is more common with hydrophilic opioids, although lipophilic opioids can cause a brief episode of sedation immediately after epidural administration. Sedation is less in patients who have recently been exposed to oral or parenteral opioids.

Regarding *cardiovascular effects*, spinal morphine

has no appreciable effect on heart rate or blood pressure.

Regarding *gastrointestinal function*, gastric emptying and gastrointestinal motility are delayed.

Hyperesthesia has been reported with high doses of spinal morphine for cancer pain but not with doses used for postoperative pain.

Regarding *bladder function*, the volume-evoked micturition reflex is inhibited by spinal morphine. This is not dose-dependent. Detrusor muscle tone is decreased, and urethral sphincter tone is slightly increased.

Generalized pruritus develops with epidural opioid administration owing to alteration in sensory modulation of upper cervical cord and trigeminal systems. The pruritus coincides with hypalgesia in these areas. It is most profound in the distribution of the trigeminal nerve. It is not caused by histamine release, since it occurs with fentanyl, which does not release histamine. Onset of pruritus is delayed up to 3 hours after epidural morphine administration. If asked, 50% of patients receiving epidural morphine for postoperative pain will complain of pruritus, but only 1% will find it significant.

Nausea and vomiting is seen in about 50% of patients receiving epidural morphine for postoperative pain. Onset usually occurs about 6 hours after injection, coinciding with the rostral spread of morphine in the CSF to the chemotactic trigger zone in the medulla.

Respiratory depression by hydrophilic opioids (e.g., morphine), is caused by cephalad migration in CSF or systemic absorption and delivery to the brain. Respiratory depression by lipophilic opioids (e.g., fentanyl), if present, is brief and develops early. This probably results from rapid venous absorption and systemic delivery of opioid to the brain. Late respiratory depression is most common with epidural morphine, especially when other parenteral opioids are given additionally (Table 34-1). Nausea, vomiting, generalized pruritus, and respiratory depression are the most common side effects of epidural opioids. They all are mediated by opioid receptors and are easily antagonized by intravenous naloxone, 5 µg/kg per hour, without affecting analgesia.

DOSING EPIDURAL OPIOIDS

There are no significant differences in the efficacy of spinal opioids given in equivalent doses. Morphine and other hydrophilic opioids given at the lumbar epidural space for thoracic incisional pain effect analgesia at

TABLE 34–1. PREDISPOSING FACTORS TO DEVELOPMENT OF DELAYED RESPIRATORY DEPRESSION AFTER SPINAL ADMINISTRATION OF OPIOIDS

Advanced age
Opioid-naive patient
Inferior vena cava obstruction
Large doses of opioids
Intrathecal opioids, or inadvertent dural puncture
Thoracic placement
High-risk patient
Use of water-soluble opioids

TABLE 34–2. DOSE, LATENCY, AND DURATION OF EPIDURAL OPIOIDS

Drug	Dose (mg)	Onset (min)	Duration (hr)
Meperidine	30–100	5–10	6 (4–20)
Methadone	1–10	10	6–10
Morphine	5	30–60	18
Hydromorphone	1	13	11
Fentanyl	0.1	4–10	2.6–4.0
Sufentanil	.01–.06	5	2–4

Data from VadeBoncoeur TR, Ferrante FM: Epidural and subarachnoid opioids. In Ferrante FM, VadeBoncoeur TR (eds): Postoperative Pain Management. New York, Churchill Livingstone, 1993, p 280, and Cousins M, Bridebaugh PO (eds): Neural Blockade in Clinical Anesthesia and Management of Pain, ed 2. Philadelphia, JB Lippincott, 1988, p 987.

lower equivalent doses than do lipophilic opioids, which rely at least in part on systemic absorption and supraspinal analgesia (Table 34–2).

Although morphine has been used extensively for epidural analgesia, there is significant experience with other opioids. Epidural opioids also are commonly combined with local anesthetics for optimal postoperative analgesia. This is more commonly done for total joint procedures, possibly because of the increased physical activity in the immediate postoperative period and the limited effect of opioid analgesia for sharp, Aδ-fiber–mediated pain. Intermittent injections of opioids for postoperative pain are more suitable to hydrophilic opioids, due to their long duration of action. Lipophilic opioids, which have a shorter duration of action, should be given by constant infusion and placed near the dermatomal level of surgery.

EFFICACY OF EPIDURAL OPIOIDS

There are extensive data to indicate that epidural morphine analgesia is superior to parenteral morphine for postoperative pain after extensive abdominal and thoracic procedures, although patients may prefer intravenous patient-controlled analgesia because of the control it gives them over dosing frequency. Patient-controlled epidural analgesia remains an alternative. When compared with local anesthetic infusions, similar analgesia is provided by infusion of epidural morphine, but without the risk of hypotension, lower extremity numbness, or lack of bowel and bladder control. Epidural morphine, when given early enough to allow for its onset, is an effective way to control postoperative pain.

BIBLIOGRAPHY

VadeBoncoeur TR, Ferrante FM: Epidural and subarachnoid opioids. *In* Ferrante FM, VadeBoncoeur TR (eds): Postoperative Pain Management, ed 1. New York, Churchill Livingstone, 1993, p 280.

Cousins MJ, Cherry, DA, Gourlay GK: Acute and chronic pain: Use of spinal opioids. *In* Cousins MJ, Bridenbaugh PO (eds): Neural Blockade in Clinical Anesthesia and Management of Pain, ed 2. Philadelphia, JB Lippincott, 1988, p 987.

SUGGESTED READINGS

Badner NH, Sandler AN, Colmenares ME: Lumbar epidural fentanyl infusions for postthoracotomy patients. Anesthesiology 71:A667, 1989.

Behar M, Magora F, Olshwang D, et al.: Epidural morphine in treatment of pain. Lancet 1:527-528, 1979.

Chaplan SR, Duncan SR, Brodsky JB, et al.: Morphine and hydromorphone epidural analgesia. Anesthesiology 77:1090-1094, 1992.

Cousins MJ, Mather LE, Glynn CJ, et al.: Selective spinal analgesia. Lancet 1:1141-1142, 1979.

Grant GJ, Zakowski M, Ramanathan S, et al.: Thoracic versus lumbar administration of epidural morphine for post operative analgesia after thoracotomy. Reg Anesth 18:351-355, 1993.

Marlowe S, Engstrom R, White PF: Epidural patient-controlled analgesia (PCA): An alternative to continuous epidural infusions. Pain 37:97-101, 1989.

Raj PP: Spinal opioids. In Raj PP: Practical Management of Pain, ed 2. St. Louis, Mosby-Year Book, 1992, pp 829-850.

Chapter 35

Epidural Opioid Infusion

*Hak Yui Wong, M.B.B.S.,
and Honorio T. Benzon, M.D.*

Epidural administration of opioids for analgesia follows the discovery of spinal opioid receptors and is an extension of intrathecal (subarachnoid) administration.[1]

Compared with intrathecal administration, the epidural route offers several advantages. Dural puncture and possible post–dural puncture headache are avoided. In contrast to the limited number of sites of subarachnoid injection, epidural administration (via needle or catheter) can be made as close as possible to the spinal cord segment in which pain transmission from the periphery originates, allowing higher drug concentration as well as combination with local anesthetics to achieve better analgesia. In postoperative analgesia, epidural injection is also a logical extension of use of the epidural catheter inserted for surgical anesthesia. A continuous mode of administration via catherer allows a wider choice of opioids, including the shorter-acting opioids.

However, the epidural infusion route is encumbered by potential technical problems associated with the epidural catheter, and the pharmacokinetic aspect is complicated by meningeal penetration, fat deposition, and systemic absorption. Because the meninges act as a diffusion barrier to the opioids, much larger doses (compared with intrathecal doses) are needed to achieve the same level in cerebrospinal fluid (CSF) and neural tissues. These large doses produce blood opioid concentrations that are similar to those from intramuscular injection of an equivalent dose and raise uncertainty and confusion about the site of analgesia of epidurally administered opioids. The large doses also expose the patient to possible toxic effects, should the epidural catheter unintentionally migrate into a blood vessel.

DISPOSITION OF OPIOIDS FROM EPIDURAL SPACE

The disposition of opioids deposited in the epidural space is influenced largely by their lipophilicity, which is characterized by the octanol-buffer partition coefficient and the ionized fractions. The routes of disposition include the following:

1. *Sequestration into the epidural fat tissues.*

2. *Uptake by epidural veins and radicular blood vessels—mechanism for systemic absorption and rise in blood opioid concentration.* Following epidural administration, blood fentanyl concentrations peak at about 5 to 10 minutes, whereas sufentanil blood concentrations peak even faster. In contrast, blood concentrations of morphine following epidural administration peak at about 10 to 15 minutes.

3. *Crossing the meninges into cerebrospinal fluid and neural tissues.*[2, 3] Although lipophilicity facilitates dural penetration, the arachnoid mater presents a hydrophilic barrier, and the speed of crossing, characterized by the meningeal permeability coefficient, is limited by very high lipophilicity. As a result, for example, the rank in ascending order according to octanol-buffer partition coefficient is morphine, alfentanil, fentanyl, and sufentanil, whereas the rank in ascending order according to meningeal permeability coefficient is sufentanil, morphine, fentanyl, and alfentanil.

4. *Distribution via rostral CSF flow.* The degree and speed whereby this process occurs depend on the dose of opioid and the balance between speed of meningeal crossing and vascular and/or neural tissue uptake of the particular opioid.[4] For example, fentanyl and sufentanil injected in the lumbar epidural space give rise to early and transient cervical CSF peak levels, whereas morphine has a delayed cranial CSF peak. Rostral spread of opioid in CSF is the main mechanism of adverse effects, such as pruritus, delayed somnolence, and delayed respiratory depression.

MECHANISMS OF ANALGESIA OF EPIDURAL OPIOIDS

Several factors have been identified as influencing mechanism of clinical analgesia from the pharmacokinetic aspect: lipophilicity and receptor affinity, dose and volume of drug dilution, and mode of delivery (bolus vs. continuous infusion). Continuous epidural infusions tend to be more efficacious, even with long-acting hydrophilic opioids such as morphine. There are likely fewer fluctuations in CSF drug level, and the risk of delayed respiratory depression may be reduced.

Spinal Level

With morphine and hydromorphone, and with lower doses of lipophilic opioids, selective spinal analgesia can be demonstrated. The analgesic effect is a result of at least two components: (1) presynaptic reduction of neurotransmitter release from dorsal root ganglia, and (2) hyperpolarization of dorsal horn neuron membrane and reduction of signal transmission (postsynaptic).[5]

Supraspinal Level

When higher doses of the more lipophilic opioids are administered, the resultant systemic blood opioid levels often approach therapeutic blood levels obtained with intravenous administration. The contribution of brain-opioid interaction to overall analgesia cannot, therefore, be discounted.

OPIOIDS AVAILABLE FOR EPIDURAL INFUSION

At equivalent doses, the different opioids are equally efficacious, although with the more lipophilic opioids, the clinical effects may vary depending on the anatomic proximity of the site of deposition to the origin of pain.[6–9]

Morphine

Morphine is the least lipophilic opioid, and after a single epidural injection, the clinical effect is slow in onset (20 to 30 minutes), long in duration (18 hours), dose-dependent, and anatomically widespread (lumbar epidural injection effective for post-thoracotomy pain).[10] It is therefore a popular choice for single or intermittent bolus injections. It can also be used in a continuous epidural infusion at 0.1 to 0.2 mg/hour with good analgesia and lower total dose.[11, 12] The resultant high and persistent morphine level leads to high incidence of side effects, which are attributed to presence of opioid in CSF: pruritus, urinary retention, nausea and vomiting, and delayed respiratory depression.

Hydromorphone

The analgesic effect of epidural hydromorphone (potency ratio to morphine, about 3:1) has faster onset (10 to 15 minutes) and shorter duration (11 hours) than that of morphine. Continuous infusion of hydromorphone is associated with a lower incidence of side effects than with morphine.[13]

Fentanyl

Fentanyl is 800 times as lipophilic as morphine and undergoes rapid vascular absorption from the epidural space. The analgesic effect has rapid onset (4 to 10 minutes) but limited duration (3 to 5 hours). The rapid vascular uptake results in low and short-lived CSF fentanyl levels and reduced potential for cephalad migration and, hence, a lower incidence of pruritus, nausea, and delayed respiratory depression. Rapid vascular and tissue uptake also limit the anatomic spread of analgesia; fentanyl must be injected close to the spinal levels at which pain originates, or a larger dose is needed.

Due to the short duration of action of single injections, fentanyl is preferably used as continuous epidural infusion. The concentration of 10 μg/mL appears to be optimal. When the epidural catheter is placed close to the spinal levels at which pain originates, 0.5 to 1.0 μg/kg/hour provides good analgesia without significant systemic blood fentanyl levels. When the epidural catheter is placed further away, a higher infusion rate (1.0 to 1.5 μg/kg/hour) is needed. At the higher infusion rates, the systemic blood fentanyl level can approach that obtained by intravenous infusion.[14]

Sufentanil

Sufentanil is twice as lipophilic as fentanyl. After single epidural injection, the analgesia has short onset (10 to 15 minutes) and a duration of 4 to 6 hours. Rapid-onset sedation and early respiratory depression can be seen. Due to the short duration of analgesia, sufentanil is also preferably used as a continuous epidural infusion. Used as a 1.0 μg/mL solution, the rate of infusion is 0.15 to 0.3 μg/kg/hour. Proximity of epidural catheter to spinal level of pain origin allows the use of a lower dose and reduces the systemic blood sufentanil level.[15]

Although the potency ratio of sufentanil to fentanyl is 10:1 when administered intravenously, it appears to be in the range of 3:1 to 5:1 when administered epidurally. This is probably related to the high lipophilicity of sufentanil, which hinders its penetration of arachnoid mater and facilitates sequestration in other adipose tissue.

Alfentanil[16]

Alfentanil is less lipophilic than fentanyl and has a higher unbounded un-ionized fraction. Analgesic effect after a single epidural injection has a short onset (5 to 10 minutes) and duration (2 to 3 hours). Therefore, alfentanil is preferably used as a continuous epidural infusion. Using a 250 μg/mL solution, the usual infusion rate is 10 to 18 μg/kg/hour. The analgesic and side effects profiles are similar to those of fentanyl.

Meperidine[12]

Meperidine is an opioid of intermediate lipophilicity (octanol-water partition coefficient of 39 compared to 1.4 for morphine). It is unique among the opioids as it also has antimuscarinic, local anesthetic, histamine-releasing, N-methyl-D-aspartate–receptor blockade actions. The time course of analgesic effect after epidural administration is similar to that of fentanyl (onset, 15 to 30 minutes; duration, 4 to 6 hours), although direct comparison with another opioid may be difficult due to its local anesthetic action (Table 35-1).

EFFECTIVE CONCENTRATION OF OPIOIDS FOR INFUSION

The effect of opioid concentration in epidural infusion has been studied for fentanyl. Epidural fentanyl is most effective (in terms of rapidity of onset and spread of analgesia) when given in concentration of at least 0.001% dilution.[17] Further dilution to 0.0005% and increasing the infusion rate may increase the spread of analgesia.[18]

COMBINATION WITH LOCAL ANESTHETICS

In laboratory experiments, a synergistic effect has been shown to exist between local anesthetics and opioids administered intrathecally. This effect was demonstrable whether the opioid was given at the same time,[19] or before the local anesthetic.[20] This synergism, however, has not been uniformly noted in clinical studies.

Clinical studies that compared the epidural opioid–local anesthetic combination with epidural local anesthetic showed a definite advantage in combining the drugs. The advantages included significantly better pain relief, comparable analgesia with lower concentration of the local anesthetic, shorter onset of analgesia, and increased duration of analgesia.[21-26] The studies dealt with patients who were in labor,[22, 23, 25] or who underwent cesarean section[26] or abdominal surgery.[22, 24]

Clinical studies that compared the epidural opioid–local anesthetic combination with the opioid alone showed different results. Several studies revealed no advantage of the combination when used in patients who had cesarean section,[27, 28] total knee replacement,[29] or abdominal or thoracic surgery.[30, 31] In contrast, other studies showed some advantage.[32-35]

It appears from the above mentioned studies that the addition of a local anesthetic to the epidural opioid is not always necessary. It is therefore advisable to start an epidural opioid infusion without a local anesthetic. The advantage of obviating the risks of epidural local anesthetic infusion (e.g., hypotension, lower extremity numbness, consequences of an intravascular injection) is obvious. If the patient's analgesia is inadequate or if high infusion rates are required, then a local anesthetic can be added.

ADVERSE EFFECTS OF EPIDURAL OPIOID ADMINISTRATION[36]

Many of the adverse effects of epidural opioid administration are believed to be related to the appearance of the opioid in CSF and the cephalic migration of CSF, resulting in interaction with opioid receptors in specific centers in the brain and brain stem. Hence, many of these effects have delayed onset and are readily reversible by intravenous administration of naloxone or another opioid antagonist.

Respiratory Depression

The incidence of clinically important respiratory depression requiring intervention after conventional doses of intrathecal and epidural opioids is approximately 1%, which is the same as that following conventional dosing of intramuscularly and intravenously delivered opioids. Respiratory depression has been associated with epidural morphine, intrathecal fentanyl, epidural fentanyl, intrathecal sufentanil, and epidural sufentanil. Respiratory depression may occur within minutes of injection of opioid or may be delayed for hours.

Early respiratory depression (within 2 hours of epidural injection) results from significant blood concentration of opioids secondary to systemic absorption by way of epidural veins and, possibly, rapid redirection to the brain by way of basilovertebral system; or it may result from rapid appearance of lipophilic opioids in cervicocranial CSF. Early respiratory depression is most commonly seen with fentanyl and sufentanil. Following epidural administration of sufentanil, cisternal cerebrospinal fluid concentrations of opioid are measurable within 1 minute.

Delayed respiratory depression (more than 2 hours, characteristically 6 to 12 hours after epidural injection) results from cephalad migration of opioid in CSF, which interacts with the ventral medulla. It is seen primarily with a single injection of morphine, but it can also be seen with continuous infusions or repeated doses of a more lipophilic opioid. It is usually not preceded by bradypnea (rendering the routine counting of respiratory rate useless). However, it is most often preceded by depressed sensorium.

TABLE 35–1. DOSE RANGE OF VARIOUS INFUSIONS

Drug	Solution	Bolus Dose	Infusion Rate	Breakthrough Bolus	Increment
Morphine	0.01%	4–6 mg	0.1–0.8 mg/hr	0.2–0.3 mg q 15 min	0.1 mg
Meperidine	0.25%	20–100 mg	5–20 mg/hr		
Hydromorphone	0.005%	0.8–1.5 mg	0.15–0.3 mg/hr	0.15–0.3 mg q 15 min	0.05 mg
Fentanyl	0.001%	0.5–1.5 μg/kg	0.5–1 μg/kg/hr	10–15 μg q 15 min	10 μg
Sufentanil	0.0001%	0.3–0.7 μg/kg	0.15–0.3 μg/kg/hr	5–7 μg q 15 min	5 μg
Alfentanil	0.25%	10–15 μg/kg	10–18 μg/kg/hr	250 μg q 10 min	250 μg

Sedation and Other Neurologic Effects

Sedation after epidural opioid administration results from cephalad migration of opioid in CSF, but it may also be related to blood level attained with the more lipophilic opioids, such as sufentanil. It appears to be dose-related, and although it is possible with all opioids, it is seen particularly with sufentanil. Sedation often heralds the onset of delayed respiratory depression.

Other mental changes are rare and may include paranoid psychosis, catatonia, euphoria, anxiety, and hallucinations. Rarely, tonic muscle rigidity, myoclonic activity, and hypertonic reflexes may follow epidural administration of opioids.

Miosis, late-onset nystagmus, vertigo, and a Ménière-like syndrome have also been reported following epidural administration of morphine. These are all naloxone-reversible and are related to cephalad migration of opioid in CSF.

Pruritus

Pruritus is the most common side effect of epidural opioid administration. It is usually localized to the face, neck, or upper thorax, and its onset corresponds with the appearance of opioid in the cervical CSF and the vicinity of the trigeminal nucleus. Because the trigeminal nucleus descends into the cervical region of the spinal cord and becomes continuous with the substantia gelatinosa of the dorsal horn, opioid interaction in the substantia gelatinosa may initiate an "itch reflex" through indirect action on the trigeminal nucleus.

Nausea and Vomiting

Nausea and vomiting following epidural infusion of opioids is likely due to appearance of opioid in CSF and interaction with the vomiting center (area postrema). They are therefore somewhat delayed, usually occurring within 4 hours of injection. Sensitization of the vestibular system to motion and decreased gastric emptying produced by opioids may also play a role. Nausea and vomiting are more frequent in women than in men and in those experiencing pain, and the overall incidence (30%) is similar to that after intravenous administration.

Urinary Retention

Urinary retention is much more common following epidural administration than after intravenous or intramuscular administration of equivalent doses of opioids. It is much more common in males. It is most likely related to local (spinal cord level) inhibition of sacral parasympathetic outflow and relaxation of detrusor muscle. It is readily reversible with naloxone.[37]

Gastrointestinal Dysfunction

Epidural opioids may delay gastric emptying and prolong intestinal transit time by interacting with opioid receptors in the spinal cord. The resultant ileus may in turn contribute to the symptoms of nausea and vomiting.[38]

Other Effects

Decreased shivering has led to hypothermia after epidural sufentanil administration.

Stimulation of the posterior pituitary and release of vasopressin, with resultant water retention and peripheral edema, have been reported following administration of intrathecal and epidural morphine.

Use of epidural morphine in obstetric patients has been linked to reactivation of HSV-1 2 to 5 days later, characteristically in the same sensory innervation area as the primary infection (usually facial areas innervated by the trigeminal nerve).

REFERENCES

1. Cousins MJ, Mather LE: Intrathecal and epidural administration of opioids. Anesthesiology 61:276, 1984.
2. Bernards CM, Hill HF: Physical and chemical properties of drug molecules governing their diffusion through the spinal meninges. Anesthesiology 77:750, 1992.
3. McEllistrem RF, Bennington RG, Roth SH: In vitro determination of human dura mater permeability to opioids and local anesthetics. Can J Anaesth 40:165, 1995.
4. Gourlay GK, Cherry DA, Plummer JL, et al: The influence of drug polarity on the absorption of opioid drugs into CSF and subsequent cephalad migration following lumbar epidural administration: Application to morphine and pethidine. Pain 31:297, 1987.
5. Dickenson AH: Mechanisms of analgesic actions of opiates and opioids. Br Med Bull 47:690, 1991.
6. Guinard JP, Mavrocordatos P, Chiolero R, et al: A randomized comparison of intravenous versus lumbar and thoracic epidural fentanyl for analgesia after thoracotomy. Anesthesiology 77:1108, 1992.
7. Chrubasik J, Wust H, Schulte-Monting J, et al: Relative analgesic potency of epidural fentanyl, alfentanil, and morphine in treatment of postoperative pain. Anesthesiology 68:929, 1988.
8. Coda B, Cleveland-Brown M, Schaffer R, et al: Pharmacology of epidural fentanyl, alfentanil and sufentanil in volunteers. Anesthesiology 81:1149, 1994.
9. deLeon-Casasola OA, Lema MJ: Postoperative epidural opioid analgesia: What are the choices? Anesth Analg 83:864, 1996.
10. Ionescu TI, Taverne RHT, Drost RH, et al: Epidural morphine anesthesia for abdominal aortic surgery—pharmacokinetics. Reg Anesth 14:107, 1989.
11. Logas WG, El-Baz N, El-Ganzouri A, et al: Continuous thoracic epidural analgesia for postoperative pain relief following thoracotomy: A randomized prospective study. Anesthesiology 67:787, 1987.
12. Sjöström S, Hartvig P, Persson MP, et al: Pharmacokinetics of epidural morphine and meperidine in humans. Anesthesiology 67:877, 1987.
13. Chaplan SR, Duncan SR, Brodsky JB, et al: Morphine and hydromorphone epidural analgesia. Anesthesiology 77:1090, 1992.
14. Badner NH, Sandler AN, Koren G, et al: Lumbar epidural fentanyl infusions for postthoracotomy patients: Analgesic, respiratory, and pharmacokinetic effects. J Cardiothorac Vasc Anesth 4:543, 1990.
15. Hansdottir V, Woestenborghs R, Nordberg G: The cerebrospinal fluid and plasma pharmacokinetics of sufentanil after thoracic or lumbar epidural administration. Anesth Analg 80:724, 1995.
16. Burm A, van der Lely FH, van Kleef JW, et al: Pharmacokinetics of alfentanil after epidural administration: Investigation of systemic absorption. Anesthesiology 81:308, 1994.
17. Birnbach D, Johnson M, Arcario T, et al. Effect of diluent volume on analgesia produced by epidural fentanyl. Anesth Analg 68:808, 1989.

18. Thomson CA, Becker DR, Messick JM, et al: Analgesia after thoracotomy: Effects of epidural fentanyl concentration/infusion rate. Anesth Analg 81:973, 1995.
19. Akerman B, Arwestrom E, Post C: Local anesthetics potentiate spinal morphine antinociception. Anesth Analg 67:943, 1988.
20. Wang C, Chakrabarti MK, Whitman JG: Specific enhancement by fentanyl of the effects of intrathecal bupivacaine on nociceptive afferent but not on sympathetic efferent pathways in dogs. Anesthesiology 79:766, 1993.
21. Hjortso NC, Lund C, Mogensen T, et al: Epidural morphine improves pain relief and maintains sensory analgesia during continuous epidural bupivacaine after abdominal surgery. Anesth Analg 65:1033, 1986.
22. Niv D, Rudick V, Golan A, et al: Augmentation of bupivacaine analgesia in labor by epidural morphine. Obstet Gynecol 67:206, 1986.
23. Chestnut DH, Owen CL, Bates JN, et al: Continuous infusion epidural analgesia during labor: A randomized, double-blind comparison of 0.0625% bupivacaine/0.0002% fentanyl versus 0.125% bupivacaine. Anesthesiology 68:754, 1988.
24. Scott NB, Mogensen T, Bigler D, et al: Continuous thoracic extradural 0.5% bupivacaine with or without morphine: Effect on quality of blockade, lung function and the surgical stress response. Br J Anaesth 62:253, 1989.
25. Hunt CO, Naulty JS, Malinow AM, et al: Epidural butorphanol-bupivacaine for analgesia during labor and delivery. Anesth Analg 68:323, 1989.
26. King MJ, Bowden MI, Cooper GM: Epidural fentanyl and 0.5% bupivacaine for elective cesarean section. Anaesthesia 45:285, 1990.
27. Douglas MJ, McMorland GH, Janzen JA: Influence of bupivacaine as an adjuvant to epidural morphine for analgesia after cesarean section. Anesth Analg 67:1138, 1988.
28. Parker RK, Sawaki Y, White PF: Epidural patient-controlled analgesia: Influence of bupivacaine and hydromorphone basal infusion on pain control after cesarean delivery. Anesth Analg 75:740, 1992.
29. Badner NH, Reimer EJ, Komar WE: Low-dose bupivacaine does not improve postoperative epidural fentanyl analgesia in orthopedic cases. Anesth Analg 72:337, 1991.
30. Badner NH, Komar WE: Bupivacaine 0.1% does not improve postoperative epidural fentanyl analgesia after abdominal or thoracic surgery. Can J Anaesth 39:330, 1992.
31. Benzon HT, Wong CA, Wong HY, et al: The effect of low-dose bupivacaine on postoperative epidural fentanyl analgesia and thrombelastography. Anesth Analg 79:911, 1994.
32. George KA, Wright PMC, Chisakuta A: Continuous thoracic epidural fentanyl for postthoracotomy pain relief: With or without bupivacaine? Anaesthesia 46:732, 1991.
33. Hanson AL, Hanson B, Matousek M: Epidural anesthesia for cesarean section: The effect of morphine-bupivacaine administered epidurally for intra and postoperative pain relief. Acta Obstet Gynecol Scand 63:135, 1984.
34. Dahl JB, Rosenberg J, Hansen BL, et al: Differential analgesic effects of low-dose epidural morphine and morphine-bupivacaine at rest and during mobilization after major abdominal surgery. Anesth Analg 74:362, 1992.
35. Badner NH, Bhandari R, Komar WE: 0.125% Bupivacaine is the optimum concentration for continuous postoperative epidural fentanyl analgesia. Reg Anesth 18(2S):27, 1993.
36. Chaney MA: Side effects of intrathecal and epidural opioids. Can J Anaesth 42:891, 1995.
37. Peterson TK, Husted SE, Rybro L, et al: Urinary retention during intramuscular and extradural morphine analgesia. Br J Anaesth 54:1175, 1982.
38. Wattwil M: Postoperative pain relief and gastrointestinal motility. Acta Chir Scand 550:140, 1988.

Chapter 36

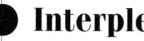

Interpleural Analgesia

Kathleen A. O'Leary, M.D.

Interpleural analgesia (IPA) is a relatively new technique that was first described in 1986 by Reiestad and Stromskag.[1] Since then it has enjoyed some favor but generally has not gained tremendous popularity because of its limitations.

ANATOMY OF PLEURAL SPACE

The pleura is divided into visceral and parietal pleura: the visceral pleura covers the lungs, and the parietal pleura lines the inside of the chest wall and the diaphragm. The pleural space extends at its most superior border to approximately 4 cm above the midclavicular line. Its most inferior border extends to just below the 12th thoracic vertebra posteriorly. It moves up to the 10th rib at the midaxillary line and to the 8th rib at the midclavicular line.

MECHANISM OF ACTION

There are several theories as to the mechanism of action of IPA. The most likely of these[1] involves analgesia from multiple intercostal nerve blocks. This is thought to occur by diffusion of local anesthetic from the pleural space to the subpleural space, then through the innermost muscles to reach a large number of intercostal nerves.

Another proposed mechanism is blockade of the thoracic sympathetic chain and splanchnic nerves.[2] This is theorized to occur by diffusion of local anesthetic, ultimately into the paraspinal space. There, it reaches the sympathetic chain and the splanchnic nerves (arising from the roots of T5 to T12).

The third mechanism of action, thought to be a minor one, is analgesia mediated by brachial plexus blockade.[3]

INDICATIONS

IPA has been used with varying degrees of success for the management of acute postoperative pain after unilateral surgery of the chest or upper abdomen that does not cross the midline.[4-7] It has also been quite successful for management of pain after multiple rib fractures.[8] Its best effects have been seen in patients with chronic pain syndromes, especially cancer pain,[9-11] postherpetic neuralgia,[12] chronic pancreatitis,[13] and reflex sympathetic dystrophy of the upper extremity.[3]

CONTRAINDICATIONS

Absolute contraindications to IPA are coagulopathies, local anesthetic allergy, and infection at the site of catheter insertion (Table 36–1). Those conditions in which the distribution and/or diffusion of local anesthetic in the pleural space may be altered are relative contraindications. They include pleuritis, pleural fibrosis or adhesions, pleural effusions, hemothorax, and recent pulmonary infections.

Other relative contraindications are those situations that increase the risk of pneumothorax at the time of catheter insertion. Pulmonary fibrosis and/or adhesions that make identification of the interpleural space difficult, bullous emphysema, and the use of mechanical ventilation with positive end-expiratory pressure all increase this risk.

TABLE 36–1. CONTRAINDICATIONS TO PLACEMENT OF AN INTERPLEURAL CATHETER

Coagulopathy
Local anesthetic allergy
Infection at site of catheter insertion
Conditions affecting distribution and/or diffusion
    of local anesthetic in the pleural space
  Pleuritis
  Pleural fibrosis
  Pleural adhesions
  Hemothorax
  Recent pulmonary infections

TECHNIQUE OF INSERTION OF AN INTERPLEURAL CATHETER

The patient is positioned in the lateral decubitus position with the affected side up. The area of insertion is identified, usually posteriorly in the eighth intercostal space, approximately 10 cm from midline. Placement of the needle should be over the superior border of the rib, so as to avoid trauma to the neurovascular bundle that runs along the inferior border of each rib.

Using an aseptic technique, the area should be sterilely prepared and draped. Interpleural kits or epidural kits with soft-tipped catheters and blunter needles should be used to reduce the risk of pneumothorax. Local anesthesia should be introduced, making sure to anesthetize the periosteum of the rib. The needle is introduced in a slightly medial direction, with the bevel facing cephalad, walking off the superior border of the ninth rib. After removal of the stylet, a well-lubricated glass syringe with 3 to 4 mL of air is attached.

The needle and syringe are advanced slowly, and a loss of resistance technique is used, without applying positive pressure on the syringe plunger. The interpleural space usually is reached at a distance of 2 to 4 cm from the skin. Once the interpleural space is reached, the plunger will move inward as the air is entrained due to the negative intrathoracic pressure. The use of positive pressure on the plunger has been associated with an increased incidence of pneumothorax. As the parietal pleura is penetrated a "clicking" sensation may be felt. However, the inward movement of the plunger is a more reliable sign.

The catheter is then threaded approximately 5 cm through the hub, taking care to cover the hub with a finger after the syringe is removed to minimize air entrainment. Slight resistance to the catheter may be noted and is normal. After negative aspiration of blood and air, a test dose of lidocaine with epinephrine is given, and if the result is negative the catheter is secured in place for use.

DOSING

Numerous methods of dosing have been used (i.e., continuous infusion vs. bolus dosing), as have varied concentrations of local anesthetic with or without epinephrine. Additionally, various volumes have been described.[1, 4-6, 15-19]

In general, bupivacaine appears to be the agent of choice, because of its longer duration of effect. Concerns regarding the toxicity of this agent are well known. Yet reports of systemic toxicity due to intravascular absorption are rare, even when plasma bupivacaine levels are found to be in the toxic range.[14]

Continuous infusions seem to be associated with better pain control and less toxicity than bolus dosing, although this conclusion remains controversial. Continuous techniques definitely require less manpower and are attractive for that reason, especially in a busy postoperative setting.

If a bolus dosing regimen is to be used, it is probably best to start with 20 or 30 mL of 0.25% bupivacaine with epinephrine every 4 to 6 hours. If this is not effective, then increasing the concentration to 0.5% may be worthwhile, keeping in mind that the risk of systemic toxicity will be increased.

With continuous infusion, a bolus dose should be given first to achieve adequate analgesia. An initial dose of 20 mL of 0.25% bupivacaine with epinephrine, followed by an infusion of the same concentration at 5 mL/hour, is a good starting point. The rate may be titrated as needed up to 10 mL/hour, and the concentration may be increased to 0.5% bupivacaine as needed. Again, increasing the concentration or rate, or both, increases the risk of systemic toxicity.

Dosing regimens in patients with chronic pain are varied, and their requirements are frequently much less than those of patients with acute pain. Generally, the initial bolus dose should be titrated until pain relief is achieved. Then, based on the patient's response and duration of effect of the analgesia, a decision is made about the use of continuous infusion vs. bolus dosing. Duranni et al.[9] reported complete relief of intractable abdominal pain due to pancreatic cancer with an 8-mL dose of 0.5% bupivacaine which was repeated once in 24 hours. Ultimately, the patient had adequate analgesia for 3 months.

PATIENT POSITION FOR DOSING

A patient's position during bolus dosing of an interpleural catheter ultimately determines the area of effect of the local anesthetic. If the goal is to provide postoperative analgesia, as with a subcostal or flank incision, or analgesia after rib fracture, then the patient should be positioned with the affected side up at an angle of about 20 degrees. After the 5 to 6 minutes required for the injection, the patient should be repositioned supine. This procedure results in both sympathetic and intercostal nerve block of the affected side.

If the goal is to provide surgical anesthesia of the chest wall, as for breast surgery, then the patient should be placed in the full lateral decubitus position with the affected side down. The table also should be tilted about 20 degrees in the head-down position.[20] Twenty to 30 minutes after injection of the local anesthetic, the patient may be positioned for surgery. This procedure results in a complete unilateral block of the intercostal nerves from T1 to T9.

If the goal is to achieve sympathetic blockade, then the patient should be positioned in the lateral decubitus position with the affected side up. If blockade of cervical and superior thoracic segments is desired, as with treatment of reflex sympathetic dystrophy of the upper extremity, then the bed should be tilted head-down. If blockade of the splanchnic nerves is desired, then the bed should be placed in the head-up position. The patient should remain in the appropriate position for about 20 to 30 minutes after dosing. The patient should be placed in the same position for repeat bolus injections.

TABLE 36–2. COMPLICATIONS OF INTERPLEURAL ANALGESIA

Pneumothorax	Horner's syndrome
Systemic toxicity from large local anesthetic dose	Catheter breakage
	Catheter migration into tissue
Intravascular injection	Bleeding
Phrenic nerve block	Infection

COMPLICATIONS

The most bothersome complication of interpleural catheter placement is pneumothorax. A minor pneumothorax should be expected, because a small amount of air is entrained through the needle before threading. This typically is of no clinical significance. However, a larger pneumothorax must be observed closely and possibly treated. If the patient is stable, aspiration of air via the interpleural catheter should be attempted. If this is unsuccessful, the pneumothorax is increasing in size, or the patient becomes unstable, then a chest tube should be placed.

Systemic toxicity from local anesthetic use is another complication of IPA. However, as discussed previously, there is an overall lack of signs of toxicity in patients with high plasma bupivacaine levels. It has been theorized that the toxic plasma concentration is more dependent on the rate of change in concentration than on any specific concentration.[21] In any event, all patients should be monitored closely for signs of toxicity.

Other complications are bleeding, infection, intravascular injection, phrenic nerve block, Horner's syndrome, catheter breakage, and migration of the catheter into lung parenchyma with possible formation of a bronchopleural fistula (Table 36–2).

INTERPLEURAL NEUROLYSIS

In cases of severe, intractable pain (usually malignancy-related), neurolysis can be used to improve quality of life. Alcohol and phenol are the most commonly used neurolytic agents. A case report of the use of 6% to 10% phenol via an interpleural catheter documented successful treatment of severe pain from metastatic esophageal carcinoma.[22] A postmortem examination at the time of the patient's death 4 weeks later revealed no gross or histologic evidence of tissue or nerve damage from a total of 3 to 4 g of injected phenol.

CONCLUSION

IPA in the acute setting can be used for management of pain associated with rib fractures or with unilateral chest, abdominal, or flank incisions. Pain from an incision that crosses the midline will not be relieved by this method, which is its main drawback. However, the use of IPA in management of chronic pain syndromes affect-

ing these areas has been quite successful. As a result, it has gained popularity in the field of pain management.

REFERENCES

1. Reiestad F, Stromskag KE: Interpleural catheter in the management of postoperative pain: A preliminary report. Reg Anesth 11:89, 1986.
2. Thompson GE, Moore DC: Celiac plexus, intercostal and minor peripheral blockade. *In* Cousins MJ, Bridenbaugh PO (eds): Neural Blockade in Clinical Anesthesia and Management of Pain, ed 2. Philadelphia, JB Lippincott, 1988.
3. Reiestad F, McIlvaine WB, Kvalheim L, et al.: Interpleural analgesia in treatment of upper extremity reflex sympathetic dystrophy. Anesth Analg 69:671, 1989.
4. Scheinin B, Lindgren L, Rosenberg PH: Treatment of post-thoracotomy pain with intermittent installations of intrapleural bupivacaine. Acta Anaesthesiol Scand 33:156, 1989.
5. Kambam JR, Handke RE, Flanagan J, et al.: Intrapleural anesthesia for post-thoracotomy pain relief. Anesth Analg 66:S90, 1987.
6. Rosenberg PH, Scheinin BM, Lepentalo MJ, et al.: Continuous interpleural infusion of bupivacaine for analgesia after thoracotomy. Anesthesiology 67:811, 1987.
7. Symreng T, Gomez MN, Rossi N: Intrapleural bupivacaine vs. saline after thoracotomy—Effects on pain and lung function—A double blind study. J Cardiothorac Anesth 3:144, 1989.
8. Rocco A, Reiestad F, Gudman J, et al.: Intrapleural administration of local anesthetics for pain relief in patients with multiple rib fractures. Reg Anesth 12:10, 1987.
9. Duranni Z, Winnie AP, Ikuta P: Interpleural catheter analgesia for pancreatic pain. Anesth Analg 67:479, 1988.
10. Myers DP, Lema MJ, deLeon-Casasola OA, et al.: Interpleural analgesia for the treatment of severe cancer pain in terminally ill patients. J Pain Symptom Manage 8:505, 1993.
11. Fineman SP: Long-term post-thoracotomy cancer pain management with interpleural bupivacaine. Anesth Analg 68:694, 1989.
12. Reistad F, Kvalheim L, McIlvaine WB, et al.: Interpleural analgesia in the treatment of severe thoracic postherpetic neuralgia. Reg Anesth 15:113, 1990.
13. Ahlburg P, Noreng M, Molgaard J, et al.: Treatment of pancreatic pain with interpleural bupivacaine: An open trial. Acta Anaesthesiol Scand 34:156, 1990.
14. McIlvaine WB, Knox RF, Fennessy PV, et al.: Continuous infusion of bupivacaine via intrapleural catheter for analgesia after thoracotomy in children. Anesthesiology 69:261, 1988.
15. Stromskag KE, Minor BG, Lindeberg A: Comparison of 40 milliliters of 0.25% intrapleural bupivacaine with epinephrine with 20 milliliters of 0.5% intrapleural bupivacaine with epinephrine after cholecystectomy. Anesth Analg 73:397, 1991.
16. VanKleef JW, Logeman A, Burm AGL, et al.: Continuous interpleural infusion of bupivacaine for postoperative analgesia after surgery with flank incisions: A double-blind comparison of 0.25% and 0.5% solutions. Anesth Analg 75:268, 1992.
17. Brismar B, Pettersson N, Tokics L, et al.: Postoperative analgesia with intrapleural administration of bupivacaine-adrenaline. Acta Anaesthesiol Scand 31:515, 1987.
18. Laurito CE, Kirz LI, VadeBoncoeur TR, et al.: Continuous infusion of interpleural bupivacaine maintains effective analgesia after cholecystectomy. Anesth Analg 72:516, 1991.
19. Stromskag KE, Reiestad F, Holmquist EL, et al.: Intrapleural administration of 0.25%, 0.375%, and 0.5% bupivacaine with epinephrine after cholecystectomy. Anesth Analg 67:430, 1988.
20. Schlesinger TM, Laurito CE, Baughman VL, et al.: Interpleural bupivacaine for mammography during needle localization and breast biopsy. Anesth Analg 68:394, 1989.
21. Scott DB: Evaluation of clinical tolerance of local anesthetic agents. Br J Anaesth 47:328, 1975.
22. Lema MJ, Myers DP, deLeon-Casasola OA: Neurolytic interpleural block in the treatment of advanced cancer pain from metastatic esophageal carcinoma. Reg Anesth 17:166, 1992.

Chapter 37

Outcome Studies in Postoperative Pain Control

Hak Yui Wong, M.B.B.S.,
and Honorio T. Benzon, M.D.

OUTCOME STUDIES

Abolition of pain during surgical procedures is central to the practice of anesthesiology. Relief or minimization of pain postoperatively is another imperative of modern anesthesia practice. There are now a multitude of drugs, as well as different (some innovative) ways of administering them. Some of these are extensions of techniques of surgical anesthesia (regional local anesthetic blocks and local anesthetic nerve blocks). In addition, nonpharmacologic physical treatment modalities exist. Most of these available methods of treatment have some proven efficacy; i.e., they reliably reduce pain under well-controlled, essentially ideal circumstances. Much less is known about their effectiveness, i.e., how well they work under ordinary circumstances with average practitioners and typical patients. Effectiveness of a particular treatment modality is a more complex quality to ascertain because it encompasses the technical complexity and risk of the modality, availability and skill of the personnel, side effects, and acceptance by the average patient (for example, many patients have an automatic aversion to "spinal" procedures).

Conceptually, the study of effectiveness of different postoperative analgesic modalities involves the application of medical technology assessment to the various alternative analgesic technologies (e.g., intravenous versus epidural infusion of opioids), comparing differences in efficacy, cost, ease of use, risks, and impact on the well-being of patients.[1] From the standpoint of an institution providing a menu of options for pain control, the markedly different apparent costs of the various interventions demand careful cost-benefit analysis, because the difference may diminish or may be outweighed by cost-saving in other areas of patient care. The various services would also need to be evaluated for their quality, a procedure that encompasses study of the structure, process, and outcome of the service(s).

It is for all of these reasons—namely, effectiveness study, technology assessment, cost-benefit analysis, and quality assurance—that outcome studies are of particular interest. Performing an *outcome study* has been defined as "linking the type of care received by a variety of patients with a particular condition to positive and negative outcomes in order to identify what works best for which patient."[2]

Problems in Studying the Impact of Postoperative Analgesia on Outcome

There are good reasons to suspect that inadequate pain relief will lead to adverse outcomes, considering the many undesirable physical effects of acute postoperative pain, including activation of the neuroendocrine (stress) response, stressful changes in the cardiovascular system and coagulation, impairment of pulmonary and gastrointestinal functions, sleep disturbance, impaired ambulation, and risks of immobility. However, there is now growing realization that relief of pain per se plays only a limited role in attenuation of these postoperative responses and morbidity. Currently, few conclusive studies or convincing data support the positive influence of postoperative pain relief on outcome, let alone the cost-effectiveness of the more complex modalities, such as epidural anesthesia and opioid administration. The uncertainties arise largely because of difficulties in defining meaningful or useful outcome, as well as in defining the analgesic intervention.

Choice of Meaningful Outcome Measure

For an outcome study to be relevant, the outcome variables studied must be of some real import and there must be a valid link between the process and the outcome variable.[3] Classically, outcome measures have been described as involving "the five Ds": death, disease, disability, discomfort, and dissatisfaction. With the emergence of emphasis on outcome in the past two decades, the definition of medical outcome has been broadening and is now clothed in more positive terms.[4] Medical outcome can be defined as "change in a patient's current and future health status"[5] and encompasses many areas: survival, functional status, general well-being, quality of life, length of stay, and patients' satisfaction with care. These definitions and requirements pose significant difficulties for outcome study of postoperative pain relief, primarily because postoperative pain (and its relief), relative to the entire sickness period, is a time-limited event and does not occur without the many other extraneous factors that make up the total experience of recovery from surgery and hospital stay.

In the study of acute pain relief, there is an inverse relationship between the "meaningfulness" of the outcome variable and the ease of establishing the linkage to the process of pain relief. The more dramatic outcomes that have undisputed meaning—death and major morbidity (such as pneumonia, thromboembolism, congestive heart failure, and long stay in the intensive care unit [ICU])—are uncommon events for all patients undergoing elective surgery, and proof of linkage to any particular therapeutic process will require studying a very large sample of patients. Death and major morbidity also tend to occur in a delayed fashion, days or even weeks after surgery and pain relief. In general, the longer the period of observation, the weaker the link between outcome and the process of care, because many extraneous factors besides postoperative pain (or lack of relief thereof) would have affected the patient and the health care environment during this period.

In lieu of profound outcome variables, intermediate outcomes[6] or physiologic outcome variables such as hypoxemia, pulmonary function tests, myocardial ischemia, return of bowel function, and so forth are often used. These possess several advantages in that they occur more frequently, can be clearly defined and timed, and can be more directly attributable to the process of pain relief. However, the use of intermediate outcome variables is not without problems, the most troubling of which is that the relationship between intermediate outcomes and true outcomes (e.g., major morbidity and death) is neither direct nor invariable.

At present, instruments designed to measure other outcome variables such as general well-being, quality of life, and disability are geared toward a longer time frame than the inhospital period. Again, the long time period of observation makes linkage to the acute event of inhospital pain relief at best conjectural. Patient satisfaction is increasingly being viewed as a valid outcome measure of the process of care. For postoperative pain relief, patient satisfaction likely reflects, besides efficacy, respect for patient's choice of treatment modality and well-being. However, patient satisfaction is also likely to be clouded by other parts of the patient's entire perioperative experience.

Analgesia Induction as an Intervention

Despite all the accompanying physical manifestations, pain and (postoperative pain in particular) is very much a subjective experience. Likewise, the definition of adequate/acceptable relief of postoperative pain is highly subjective and dependent on a patient's expectation and motivation. This subjectiveness is likely to complicate efforts at quantifying pain and analgesic end point. For example, attempts at correlating physiologic parameters

to the degree of analgesia may yield inconsistent results. Likewise, the amount of supplemental opioid consumed via patient-controlled analgesia (PCA) has been proposed as a comparative instrument for different analgesic modalities. However, it is now known that patients often have widely different pain scores, and they often use PCA independent of their pain scores.[7, 8]

The interventions used to induce analgesia (e.g., local anesthetic epidural infusion) may well have other physiologic effects unrelated to pain relief that may affect patient outcome. For example, sympatholysis and vasodilation caused by epidural local anesthetic infusion may be responsible for the decreased incidence of thromboembolism independent of pain relief.

Finally, it is often difficult to separate the effects of intraoperative intervention from that of postoperative analgesic intervention. For example, the suppression of endocrine stress response and hypercoagulability by intraoperative epidural anesthesia may completely overshadow the role (or lack thereof) of any postoperative analgesic modality.

CURRENT STATE OF THE LITERATURE

The main bulk of current literature on postoperative analgesia and outcome has focused on the beneficial effects of regional anesthesia and analgesia techniques. The subject was recently exhaustively reviewed by Liu and colleagues.[9]

Because of the low incidence of death and severe morbidities in the general population, most published studies of analgesic techniques do not have sufficient power (i.e., sample size) to detect clinically significant differences in terms of these events. Studies of sufficient size to achieve the requisite power will likely require multi-institutional cooperative efforts.

Studies of intermediate outcomes, although more likely to have sufficient sample size and power, are not problem-free. Many have not prospectively identified the (meaningful) outcome variables or adequately controlled the type and duration of the analgesic interventions. The effect of intraoperative anesthetic care cannot be controlled or ruled out in many of the studies. Most of them by necessity suffer from the inherent difficulties of defining and quantifying analgesia.

Many studies are not randomized controlled studies (RCTs), and there is a bias against non-RCTs in the literature. However, with increasing interest in outcome studies, it is now recognized that whereas the RCT design is excellent in demonstrating efficacy of a treatment, it may be too restrictive for studying the effectiveness of a treatment intended for use in a less controlled setting and a less-selected population of patients. For example, although epidural analgesia has been shown to reduce the incidence of major morbidities in a selected group of high-risk patients, the same advantage could not be reproduced in less-selected, all-inclusive groups of patients. There is thus a need to design studies to delineate subsets of patients who may be matched to and derive the most benefits from the various analgesic interventions.

Some Questions Regarding Outcomes, and Studies That Address the Questions

Does Intensive Analgesia (As Opposed to No or Minimal Analgesia) Make a Difference in Outcome?

Studies performed in two unique situations addressed this question, but they cannot be extrapolated to the majority of surgical patients.

Mangano and coworkers[10] found lower incidence and severity of myocardial ischemia after coronary artery bypass surgery in patients who received prolonged intensive analgesia via intravenous sufentanil infusion. (However, the incidence of overt adverse cardiac events was unchanged.)

Anand and Hickey[11] showed fewer major complications and lower mortality in neonates who received high-dose sufentanil during and after cardiac surgery.

Do Improved Methods of Systemic Analgesic Administration Make a Difference?

Patient-controlled analgesia bypasses interpatient variability in pharmacokinetics and pharmacodynamics and problems of administrative delays and judgment. The most prominent impact of PCA is in improved quality of analgesia and satisfaction and acceptance by patients and caregivers.[12, 13] Some data show a shorter hospital stay[14] and improved patient mobility with PCA. Beneficial effect on the respiratory system has not been consistently demonstrated.[15]

Do the More Specialized (i.e., Invasive and Costly) Forms of Analgesia Make a Difference?

Regarding this topic, interest has centered around central neuraxial (epidural or intrathecal) analgesia using opioids with or without local anesthetics.

There are reasons for hypothesizing that neuraxial analgesia may affect outcome: efficacy in pain relief, effective deafferentation, decreased stress response, and sympathetic activation in response to surgery.[16–18]

There are also many problems in proving the impact of neuraxial analgesia on outcome: It is often used in conjunction with intraoperative neuraxial anesthesia; effects of opioids and local anesthetics are different to separate; varying degrees of sympatholysis are achieved; and study sample size is often small and lacks statistical power.

Mortality and Major Morbidity Outcomes

Yeager and colleagues[19] showed a lower incidence of major cardiorespiratory complications, shorter ICU stays and reduced hospital cost in high-risk patients undergoing major surgeries who received epidural anesthesia combined with general anesthesia and epidural opioid plus local anesthetics postoperatively. In a small study of thoracotomy patients,[20] more rapid improvement in pulmonary function, shorter hospital stay, and duration of ileus were seen with epidural fentanyl use. Tuman

and associates[21] saw a lower incidence of adverse cardiac events in vascular surgical patients who received epidural anesthesia and analgesia. However, these salutary effects have not been consistently reproduced by others for patients undergoing abdominal aortic,[22] abdominal,[23] or peripheral vascular[24] surgery, and repair of femoral neck fracture.[25]

Length of Stay in the Hospital and Intensive Care Unit

The length of ICU stay was shorter for patients who had general or epidural anesthesia followed by postoperative epidural fentanyl analgesia (mean, 1.5 days) for major vascular surgery, compared with general anesthesia and postoperative intramuscular opioid analgesia (mean, 3.3 days).[21]

The length of hospital stay after gastroplasty was reduced from 9 to 7 days with epidural morphine injections, compared with intramuscular morphine.[26] Likewise, the length of hospital stay after thoracotomy was shorter after thoracic epidural fentanyl infusion (11 days) compared with lumbar epidural fentanyl infusion (14 days) or intravenous fentanyl infusion (15.6 days).[20] Another study, however, showed the same length of hospital stay for patients who underwent abdominal surgery, whether they received epidural morphine and bupivacaine or subcutaneous morphine for postoperative pain.[27]

Intermediate Outcomes and Process Variables

Deep vein thrombosis and thromboembolism after hip fracture repair and replacement surgery are reduced with epidural anesthesia and analgesia.[16]

Vascular graft failure and immediate reoperation are reduced in patients who received epidural anesthesia with or without general anesthesia plus postoperative epidural analgesia.[16, 24] This may be related to the ability of epidural anesthesia to reduce hypercoagulation and facilitate fibrinolysis.[28]

Pulmonary mechanics after thoracic and abdominal surgery are compromised. The effort-dependent components (FVC, FEV_1, PEF) are more liable to be improved with effective analgesia, and pulmonary complications are less frequent. Existing data do not support a definitive position.

In the majority of published studies, failure rates of the analgesic technique and requirement for rescue, patient satisfaction and other measures of physical and psychological well-being, and general feasibility have not been addressed.

CONCLUSIONS

Many techniques of analgesia are available and are generally efficacious in relieving acute postoperative pain. Data on the effect of analgesia on outcome are limited and debatable. In the overall technology assessment of a technique or service, risks to the patient and provider (especially of the more invasive methods), material and personnel cost in instituting and maintaining these interventions, and appropriate indications for the technique all will have to be taken into consideration and elucidated.

REFERENCES

1. Bunker JP: Is efficacy the gold standard for quality assessment? Inquiry 25:51, 1988.
2. Guadagnoli E, McNeil BJ: Outcomes research: Hope for the future or the latest rage. Inquiry 31:14, 1994, p 14.
3. Lohr KN: Outcome measurement: Concepts and questions. Inquiry 25:37, 1988.
4. Epstein AM: The outcomes movement—Will it get us where we want to go? N Engl J Med 323:266, 1990.
5. Donabedian A: The definition of quality and approaches to its assessment. *In* Explorations in Quality Assessment and Monitoring, vol 1. Ann Arbor, Mich, Health Administration, 1980, p 79.
6. Orkin FK, Cohen MM, Duncan PG: The quest for meaningful outcomes [editorial]. Anesthesiology 78:417, 1993.
7. Johnson LR, Magnani B, Chan V, Ferrante FM: Modifiers of patient-controlled analgesia efficacy. I. Locus of control. Pain 39:17, 1989.
8. Jamison RN, Taft K, O'Hara JP, Ferrante FM: Psychosocial and pharmacologic predictors of satisfaction with intravenous patient-controlled analgesia. Anesth Analg 77:121, 1993.
9. Liu S, Carpenter RL, Neal JM: Epidural anesthesia and analgesia: Their role in postoperative outcome. Anesthesiology 82:1474, 1995.
10. Mangano DT, Siliciano D, Hollenberg M, et al.: Postoperative myocardial ischemia. Therapeutic trials using intensive analgesia following surgery. Anesthesiology 76:342, 1992.
11. Anand KJS, Hickey PR: Halothane-morphine compared with high-dose sufentanil for anesthesia and postoperative analgesia in neonatal cardiac surgery. N Engl J Med 326:1, 1992.
12. Eisenach JC, Grice SC, Dewan DM: Patient-controlled analgesia following cesarean section: A comparison with epidural and intramuscular narcotics. Anesthesiology 68:444, 1988.
13. Harrison DM, Sinatra R, Morgese L, et al.: Epidural narcotic and patient-controlled analgesia for post-cesarean section pain relief. Anesthesiology 68:454, 1988.
14. Finley RJ, Keeri-Szanto M, Boyd D: New analgesic agents and techniques shorten postoperative hospital stay. Pain 2:S397, 1984.
15. Rosenberg PH, Heino A, Scheinin B: Comparison of intramuscular analgesia, intercostal block, epidural morphine and on-demand IV fentanyl in the control of pain after upper abdominal surgery. Acta Anaesthesiol Scand 28:603, 1984.
16. Kehlet H: Epidural analgesia and the endocrine-metabolic response to surgery: Update and perspectives. Acta Anaesthesiol Scand 28:125, 1984.
17. Weissman C: The metabolic response to stress: An overview and update. Anesthesiology 73:308, 1990.
18. Salomaki TE, Leppaluoto J, Laitinen JO: Epidural versus intravenous fentanyl for reducing hormonal, metabolic, and physiologic responses after thoracotomy. Anesthesiology 79:672, 1993.
19. Yeager MP, Glass DD, Neff RK, Brinck-Johnson T: Epidural anesthesia and analgesia in high-risk surgical patients. Anesthesiology 66:729, 1987.
20. Guinard J, Mavrocordatos P, Chiolero R, Carpenter RL: A randomized comparison of intravenous versus lumbar and thoracic epidural fentanyl for analgesia after thoracotomy. Anesthesiology 77:1108, 1992.
21. Tuman KJ, McCarthy RJ, March RJ, et al.: Effect of epidural anesthesia and analgesia on coagulation and outcome after major vascular surgery. Anesth Analg 73:696, 1991.
22. Baron JF, Bertrand M, Barre E, et al.: Combined epidural and general anesthesia versus general anesthesia for abdominal aortic surgery. Anesthesiology 75:611, 1991.
23. Hjortso NC, Neumann P, Frosig F, et al.: A controlled study on the effect of epidural analgesia with local anesthetics and morphine on morbidity after abdominal surgery. Acta Anaesth Scand 29:790, 1985.
24. Christopherson R, Beattie C, Frank SM: Perioperative morbidity in patients randomized to epidural or general anesthesia for lower extremity vascular surgery. Anesthesiology 79:422, 1993.
25. Sorenson RM, Pace NL: Anesthetic techniques during surgical repair of femoral neck fractures. A meta-analysis. Anesthesiology 77:1095, 1992.
26. Rawal N, Sjostrand U, Christofferson E, et al.: Comparison of intramuscular and epidural morphine for postoperative analgesia in the grossly obese: Influence on postoperative ambulation and pulmonary function. Anesth Analg 63:583, 1984.
27. Jayr C, Thomas H, Rey A, et al.: Postoperative pulmonary complications. Epidural analgesia using bupivacaine and opioids versus parenteral opioids. Anesthesiology 78:666, 1993.
28. Rosenfeld BA, Beattie C, Christopherson R, et al.: The effects of different anesthetic regimens on fibrinolysis and the development of postoperative arterial thrombosis. Anesthesiology 79:435, 1993.

Chapter 38

Pediatric Postoperative Pain

Patrick K. Birmingham, M.D.

Although pediatric pain has historically been under-recognized and undertreated, its management has improved dramatically over the last 10 to 15 years. Advances in pain assessment, pharmacokinetic studies of opioid and nonopioid analgesics in children, and development of physician-directed hospital-based acute pain services have been important factors in this improvement.

PEDIATRIC ANATOMY AND PHYSIOLOGY

The rational use of analgesics in pediatric patients, particularly neonates and infants, requires a recognition of maturational changes that take place after birth in both body composition and core organ function.

Total body water represents about 80% of body weight in full-term newborns. This drops to 60% of body weight by 2 years of age, with a large proportional decrease in extracellular fluid volume. The larger extracellular and total body water stores in infancy lead to a greater volume of distribution for water-soluble drugs. Newborns have smaller skeletal muscle mass and fat stores, decreasing the amount of drug bound to inactive sites in muscle and fat. These stores increase during infancy.

Cardiac output is relatively higher in infants and children than in adults and is preferentially distributed to vessel-rich tissues such as the brain, allowing for rapid equilibration of drug concentrations. Immaturity of the blood-brain barrier in early infancy allows increased passage of more water-soluble medications such as morphine. This combination of increased blood flow to the brain and increased drug passage through the blood-brain barrier can lead to higher central nervous system drug concentrations and more side effects at a lower plasma concentration.

Renal and hepatic blood flow also are increased in infants relative to adults. As glomerular filtration, renal tubular function, and hepatic enzyme systems mature, generally reaching adult values within the first year of life, increased blood flow to these organs leads to increased drug metabolism and excretion.

Both the quantity and the binding ability of serum albumin and α_1-acid glycoprotein (AAG) are decreased in newborns relative to adults. This may result in higher levels of unbound drug, with greater drug effect and toxicity at lower overall serum levels. This consideration has led to lower local anesthetic dosing recommendations in neonates and young infants, although neonates have shown the ability to acutely increase AAG levels while receiving continuous local anesthetic infusions. The difference in serum protein quantity and binding ability disappears by approximately 6 months of age.

Neurotransmitters and peripheral and central pathways necessary for pain transmission are intact and functional by late gestation, although opiate receptors may function differently in the newborn than in adults. Cardiorespiratory, hormonal, and metabolic responses to pain in adults have also been well documented to occur in neonates.

The spinal cord and dura mater in the newborn infant extend to approximately the third lumbar (L3) and third sacral (S3) vertebrae, respectively, and reach the adult levels of approximately L1 and S1–2 by about 1 year of age. The lower-lying spinal cord in young infants is theoretically more vulnerable to injury during needle insertion at middle to upper lumbar levels. The intercristal line connecting the posterior superior iliac crests, used as a surface landmark during needle insertion, crosses the spinal column at the S1 level in neonates but at the L4 or L5 level in adults. There is less fat in the epidural space in infants than in adults, and it is more loosely connected, explaining in part the relative ease with which epidural catheters inserted at the base of the sacrum can be threaded to lumbar or thoracic levels in infants and small children.

PAIN ASSESSMENT

Depending on developmental age and other factors, the pediatric patient may be unable or unwilling to

TABLE 38–1. AGE AND MEASURES OF PAIN INTENSITY

Age	Self-report Measures	Behavior Measures	Physiologic Measures
Birth to 3 yr	Not available	Of primary importance	Of secondary importance
3 to 6 yr	Specialized developmentally appropriate scales available	Primary if self-report not available	Of secondary importance
>6 yr	Of primary importance	Of secondary importance	

From McGrath PJ, Beyer J, Cleeland C, et al.: Report of the subcommittee on assessment and methodologic issues in the management of pain in childhood cancer. Pediatrics 86:816, 1990.

verbalize or quantify pain as an adult would. Nonetheless, a number of developmentally appropriate pain assessment scales have been designed for use with both infants and children (Table 38-1). Specialized self-reporting scales are available for children and can be used in patients as young as 3 years of age (Fig. 38-1). Behavioral or physiologic measures are available for younger ages (Table 38-2).

NONOPIOID ANALGESICS

Acetaminophen

Acetaminophen (paracetamol) is very commonly used in pediatric patients, alone or in combination with other analgesics. It is often administered rectally in the perioperative period in infants or children for whom oral intake is not an option. Higher dosing, at least initially, is needed if the drug is given rectally (Table 38-3). Suppository insertion before surgical incision does not appear to significantly alter acetaminophen kinetics and may result in more timely analgesia in the early postoperative period. Higher-dose rectal acetaminophen has been shown to be equianalgesic to intravenous ketorolac after tonsillectomy. An intravenous prodrug form of acetaminophen is also available in some parts of the world.

Acetaminophen dosing in premature and full-term neonates is less well defined. Despite age-related differences in elimination pathways, overall elimination in small studies was similar in neonates, children, and adults. Dose-dependent hepatotoxicity is the most serious acute side effect of acetaminophen administration. Acute hepatotoxicity appears to be less common and less likely to be fatal in children than in adults.

Nonsteroidal Anti-inflammatory Drugs

Nonsteroidal anti-inflammatory drugs (NSAIDs) also are widely administered to children. Studies of intravenous, intramuscular, and rectal NSAID administration in pediatric surgical patients demonstrate reduced postoperative pain scores and decreased supplemental analgesic requirements. Intravenous ketorolac is used widely in children and has a generally good safety record. The clinical significance of NSAID effects on bleeding remains controversial, leading some to avoid it in procedures such as tonsillectomy. Bleeding, renal damage, and gastritis are more likely to occur with prolonged administration and in the presence of coexisting disease. The clinical significance of NSAID inhibitory effects on osteogenesis after bone surgery, as documented in animal studies, remains unclear. Acetaminophen and NSAIDs are often given in combination; they work by different mechanisms, and their toxicity does not appear to be additive.

Aspirin (Acetylsalicylic Acid)

Aspirin is not used for postoperative pain management in infants and children because of a highly signifi-

Faces Pain Rating Scale

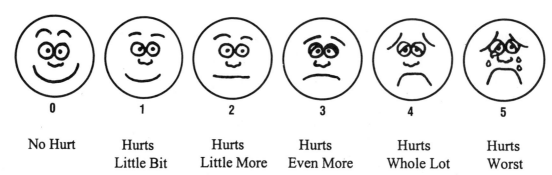

0	1	2	3	4	5
No Hurt	Hurts Little Bit	Hurts Little More	Hurts Even More	Hurts Whole Lot	Hurts Worst

FIGURE 38–1. The Wong-Baker Faces Pain Rating Scale is recommended for children age 3 years and older. Explain to the child that the faces show a person who feels happy because he or she has no pain (hurt) or sad because he or she has some or a lot of pain. Ask the child to choose the face that best describes how he or she is feeling. (From Wong D: Whaley and Wong's Essentials of Pediatric Nursing, ed 5. St Louis, Mosby–Year Book, 1997, p 1215.)

TABLE 38–2. OBJECTIVE PAIN-DISCOMFORT SCALE

Observation	Criteria	Points
Blood pressure	± 10% of preoperative value	0
	10%–20% > preoperative value	1
	20%–30% > preoperative value	2
Crying	Not crying	0
	Crying but responds to tender loving care (TLC)	1
	Crying and does not respond to TLC	2
Movement	None	0
	Restless	1
	Thrashing	2
Agitation	Patient asleep or calm	0
	Mild	1
	Hysterical	2
Verbal evaluation or body language	Patient asleep or states no pain	0
	Mild pain (cannot localize)	1
	Moderate pain (can localize) verbally or by pointing	2

From Broadman LM, Rice LJ, Hannallah RS: Testing the validity of an objective pain scale for infants and children. Anesthesiology 69:A770, 1988. Reproduced with permission from Lippincott-Raven.

cant association with Reye's syndrome. Reye's syndrome is an acute, fulminant, and potentially fatal hepatoencephalopathy that occurs in children with influenza-like illness or varicella who ingest aspirin-containing medications.

OPIOID ANALGESIA

Oral, parenteral, and epidural opioids are widely employed in infants and children to optimize postoperative comfort. Codeine is given orally in a dose of 1 mg/kg and often in combination with acetaminophen for mild to moderate pain. Parenteral opioids are still given on an as-needed basis to some patients, but alternative means of opioid delivery have been employed increasingly over the last 10 years.

Patient-Controlled Analgesia

Patient-controlled analgesia (PCA) is used in children as young as 5 or 6 years of age, with morphine the most commonly used and studied opioid and meperidine and

TABLE 38–3. DOSING OF ACETAMINOPHEN (PARACETAMOL) AND NONSTEROIDAL ANTI-INFLAMMATORY DRUGS

Oral acetaminophen	10–15 mg/kg q 4–6 hr
Rectal acetaminophen	35–45 mg/kg loading dose,* then 20 mg/kg every 6–8 hr thereafter†
Intravenous acetaminophen	15–30 mg/kg q 4–6 hr‡
Oral ibuprofen	4–10 mg/kg q 6–8 hr
Intravenous/intramuscular ketorolac	0.5 mg/kg (maximum 15 mg if <50 kg or 30 mg if >60 kg) q 6 hr for <5 days

*Dosing in neonates and young infants is not well defined and may be less.
†No evidence of accumulation at 24 hr.
‡Lower range of this dose is recommended in infants younger than 10 days old.

fentanyl among the more commonly used alternatives. Dose guidelines for morphine are listed in Table 38–4. Compared with as-needed intramuscular injection of opioids, PCA has been shown to be safe in children and to provide more effective analgesia with greater patient satisfaction. A low-dose continuous or "background" infusion is sometimes added for patients who have undergone major surgery to optimize analgesia.

Parent- or Nurse-Assisted Analgesia

The concept of PCA has been expanded to allow parent- or nurse-assisted analgesia in selected cases in which the patient is unwilling or unable—because of age, developmental delay, or physical disability—to operate the PCA button. This technique is used with caution because it does away with one of the safety features of PCA, the low likelihood of self-overdose with patient-controlled administration. Although parent- or nurse-assisted analgesia is most commonly used in infants and children with pain related to cancer treatment (e.g., oral mucositis with bone marrow transplantation), it has been used safely for postoperative analgesia as well.

Continuous Intravenous Infusions

Continuous intravenous opioid infusions are used, alone or in combination with PCA, to provide pain relief after pediatric surgery. Compared with adults given morphine, neonates and premature infants have a longer elimination half-life, lower plasma clearance, and marked interindividual variability in plasma morphine concentration. For a given dose, such young children achieve a higher plasma concentration for a longer duration. By approximately 6 to 12 months of age, the kinetics of morphine and fentanyl approach adult values, and children soon thereafter demonstrate increased plasma clearance and a shorter elimination half-life. Continuous morphine infusion rates and patient age ranges are summarized in Table 38–5.

TABLE 38–4. PARAMETERS FOR PATIENT-CONTROLLED ANALGESIA

Opioid	Morphine	Meperidine	Fentanyl
Loading dose over 1-10 min (mg/kg)	0.05-0.20	0.5-2.0	.0005-.002
Demand dose (mg/kg)	0.01-0.02	0.1-0.2	.0002-.0004
Lockout time (min)	5-15	5-15	5-15
Four-hour limit* (mg/kg)	0.30-0.40	3.0-4.0	.006-.008
Continuous infusion* (mg/kg/hr)	0.01-0.20	0.1-0.2	.0002-.0004

Dose ranges are approximate; selection of opioid & actual parameters depends on assessment of individual patient.
*Optional.
Adapted from Birmingham PK: Recent advances in acute pain management. Curr Prob Pediatr 25:99–112, 1995. Reproduced with permission.

REGIONAL ANALGESIA

Single-Shot Caudal Administration

One of the most widely used techniques for pediatric postoperative regional analgesia is the so-called single-shot caudal administration. Its popularity stems in part from the readily palpable landmarks and relative ease of caudal block insertion in infants and children compared with adults. This technique is used in infants and children up to 8 or 10 years of age who have undergone surgery from lumbosacral to midthoracic dermatome levels with anticipated moderate postoperative pain. Bupivacaine in concentrations of 0.125% to 0.25% is the most commonly used and studied local anesthetic for single-shot caudal administration. Injection volumes of 0.5 to 1.5 mL/kg provide analgesia for lower lumbar to midthoracic levels, respectively. An upper volume limit of 20 mL is generally used. The maximum recommended dose is 2.5 to 3.0 mg/kg, with an upper limit of 1.25 mg/kg recommended in infants younger than 4 months of age. A test dose of 0.1 mL/kg (maximum 3 mL) of local anesthetic with 1:200,000 epinephrine (5 μg/kg) is used to ensure correct needle or catheter position. It is unclear whether block placement at the beginning instead of the end of the procedure prolongs postoperative analgesia.

Although it usually is used alone, bupivacaine can be combined with 1 to 2 μg/kg epidural fentanyl or 20 to 50 μg/kg epidural morphine. Delayed respiratory depression up to 22 hours can occur with epidural morphine. Greater risk is seen in children younger than 1 year of age and when parenteral opioids have also been given. Preliminary studies of α_2-adrenergic agonists such as clonidine hold some promise for more widespread epidural use in children.

Continuous Epidural Infusions

Epidural local anesthetic infusions with or without opioids have been used in children, infants, and even newborns for postoperative analgesia. Bolus and infusion rate recommendations for bupivacaine, fentanyl, and morphine are listed in Table 38-6. In general, lower infusion rates are recommended in neonates and infants younger than 4 to 6 months old. This is because of lower protein binding and consequently higher free fractions of drug, and because of pharmacokinetic differences that potentially could result in higher plasma levels and prolonged drug half-life. Substitution of other opioids, such as those with mixed agonist-antagonist effects, may minimize clinical side effects. As a rule, optimal analgesia is obtained with the catheter tip posi-

TABLE 38–5. CONTINUOUS INTRAVENOUS MORPHINE INFUSION FOR POSTOPERATIVE ANALGESIA IN INFANTS AND CHILDREN

Age Range of Subjects (EGA)	Infusion (μg/kg/hr)	Comments	No. of Subjects
1-18 days (32-40 wk)	15	Some patients mechanically ventilated	20
1-49 days (35-41 wk)	6-40	Some patients mechanically ventilated; seizures at 32 and 40 μg/kg/hr; recommend rate of 15 μg/kg/hr	12
3 mo-12 yr	14-21	Less total morphine than with time-contingent IM morphine	20
<1-14 yr	10-40	Spontaneously ventilating	121
14 mo-17 yr	10-30	Postoperative cardiac; able to wean from mechanical ventilation	44
1-15 yr	20	Superior to IM morphine	20
1-16 yr	10-40	Superior to IM morphine	46
3-22 yr	20-40	Cerebral palsy patients	55

EGA, estimated gestational age at birth; IM, intramuscular.
Adapted from Birmingham PK, Hall SC: Drug infusions in pediatric anesthesia. In Fragen RF (ed): Drug Infusions in Anesthesiology, ed 2. Philadelphia, Lippincott-Raven, 1996, pp 193–224. Reproduced with permission.

TABLE 38–6. SUGGESTED PEDIATRIC EPIDURAL DOSING GUIDELINES

Medication	Age Group	Bolus	Infusion
Bupivacaine	Infants <4 mo	≤1.25 mg/kg initial bolus	≤0.2 mg/kg/hr
	Older infants and children	≤2.5–3.0 mg/kg initial bolus	≤0.4–0.5 mg/kg/hr
Fentanyl	Infants and children	1–2 μg/kg initial bolus	0.2–2.0 μg/kg/hr
Morphine	Infants <6 mo	10–25 μg/kg q 6–24 hr	≤2.5 μg/kg/hr
	Older infants and children	20–50 μg/kg q 6–24 hr	≤5.0 μg/kg/hr

These are approximate dose ranges. Actual dose selected depends on individual patient assessment.

tioned at or near the dermatomes to be blocked. It is possible in infants and smaller children to thread caudally inserted catheters to lumbar or thoracic levels. This can also be done in older children with the use of styletted catheters.

Peripheral nerve blocks also play an important role in relief of pediatric postoperative pain. Ilioinguinal-iliohypogastric, penile, femoral, digital, and other nerve blocks are often done to provide analgesia in suitable candidates.

BIBLIOGRAPHY

Dalens B: Regional Anesthesia in Infants, Children, and Adolescents, ed 1. Baltimore, Williams & Wilkins, 1995.

Schechter NL, Berde CB, Yaster M: Pain in Infants, Children and Adolescents, ed 1. Baltimore, Williams & Wilkins, 1993.

Chronic Pain Syndromes

Chapter 39

Classification of Headache Disorders

Jan Slezak, M.D., and Milan Stojanovic, M.D.

The classification system of chronic headaches created over the years by the Ad Hoc Committee of the National Institute of Neurologic Diseases and Blindness was a standard from 1962 until 1988, when the International Headache Society (IHS) proposed a new set of guidelines for categorizing headaches. The new classification was elaborated by the Headache Classification Committee of the IHS and published in the journal *Cephalalgia*. This system helps to standardize diagnostic headache criteria throughout the world.

The IHS classification is hierarchically constructed. It contains 13 diagnostic groups which are subdivided to allow for coding up to a four-digit level. Because it is very detailed, it may seem somewhat awkward for clinical use. A simplified version of the IHS classification is presented here. The chapter then focuses on the diagnostic criteria of the primary headaches.

The vast majority of patients with recurrent head pain suffer from a primary headache disorder (i.e., no structural, infectious, or systemic abnormalities are identified). Secondary headaches (i.e., those in which an organic cause is present) are a symptom of an underlying condition; they should be diagnosed promptly and treated accordingly.

Considering the severity of headaches, the classification distinguishes between a mild, a moderate, and a severe pain intensity. A mild pain is one that does not inhibit daily activities; a moderate pain restricts but does not prevent daily activities, and severe pain suspends daily activities.

I. PRIMARY HEADACHE DISORDERS
   A. *Migraine*
      1. Migraine without aura (common migraine)
      2. Migraine with aura (classic migraine)
         a. Migraine with typical aura
         b. Migraine with prolonged aura
         c. Familial hemiplegic migraine
         d. Basilar migraine
         e. Migraine aura without headache
         f. Migraine with acute-onset aura
      3. Ophthalmoplegic migraine

4. Retinal migraine
      5. Childhood periodic syndromes that may be precursors to or associated with migraine
         a. Benign paroxysmal vertigo of childhood
         b. Alternating hemiplegia of childhood
      6. Complications of migraine
         a. Status migrainosus
         b. Migrainous infarction
      7. Migrainous disorder not fulfilling the above criteria
   B. *Tension-type* headache
      1. Episodic tension-type headache (acute scalp muscle contraction headache)
      2. Chronic tension-type headache (chronic scalp muscle contraction headache)
      3. Headache of the tension type not fulfilling the above criteria
   C. *Cluster* headache and chronic paroxysmal hemicrania
      1. Cluster headache
         a. Episodic
         b. Chronic
      2. Chronic paroxysmal hemicrania
      3. Cluster headache–like disorder not fulfilling the above criteria
II. SECONDARY HEADACHE DISORDERS
   A. Headache associated with *head injury*
   B. *Miscellaneous* headaches not associated with structural lesion (idiopathic stabbing headache, exertional headache, coital headache)
   C. Headache associated with *vascular* disorders (hemorrhage, stroke, arteritis)
   D. Headache associated with *nonvascular intracranial* disorders (neoplasms)
   E. Headache associated with *substances* or their withdrawal
   F. Headache associated with *noncephalic infection* (diffuse viral infection)
   G. Headache associated with *metabolic* disorders (hypoxia and hypoglycemia)
   H. Headache associated with facial pain and disorders of cranium, neck, ears, nose, sinuses, teeth,

mouth, and other *facial* or *cranial* structures (temporomandibular joint dysfunction, sinusitis, glaucoma)
I. *Cranial neuralgia* (trigeminal neuralgia)
J. Headache *not classifiable*

PRIMARY HEADACHE DISORDERS

Migraine

Migraine Without Aura (Common Migraine)

The headache must fulfill at least two of the four characteristics listed in group A and at least one of the two characteristics in group B. The patient also must have experienced at least five similar episodes with pain lasting 4 to 72 hours.

Group A:

Unilateral location
Pulsating quality
Moderate or severe intensity (inhibits or prohibits daily activities)
Aggravation by stair walking or similar routine physical activity

Group B:

Nausea and/or vomiting
Photophobia and phonophobia

Migraine With Aura (Classic Migraine)

In addition to the group A and group B criteria listed for common migraine, the patient must have experienced at least two previous attacks with three out of the following four characteristics:

1. One or more reversible aura symptoms
2. Aura symptoms that develop over more than 4 minutes
3. Aura that lasts not more than 60 minutes
4. Headache that follows within 60 minutes of aura termination

Aura symptoms can manifest as visual disturbances, hemisensory changes, hemiparesis, dysarthria, and so on.

Ophthalmoplegic migraine is characterized by paralysis of the third, fourth, or sixth cranial nerve. Retinal migraine manifests as a reversible monocular visual change of less than 60 minutes' duration.

Miscellaneous Benign Headaches

The following headache subtypes are seen more often in migraine patients.

Exertional headache can be induced by any form of exercise.
Idiopathic stabbing headache manifests as a series of sharp, jabbing pains ("like an ice pick") lasting seconds to minutes; patients may experience up to 30 episodes per day.

Hemicrania continua is a constant unilateral headache that resembles chronic tension-type headache.

Other syndromes include cold-induced headache, orgasm-induced headache, and benign cough headache.

TENSION-TYPE HEADACHE

Episodic Tension-Type Headache

Diagnostic criteria include more than 10 previous episodes and fewer than 15 headache days per month. Duration of headache ranges from 30 minutes to 7 days. At least two of the following characteristics must be fulfilled:

1. Pain is pressing or tightening, not pulsating.
2. Mild to moderate intensity may decrease but does not abolish activities.
3. Pain is bilateral.
4. Pain is not aggravated by stair walking or routine physical activity.

In addition, both of the following criteria must be fulfilled:

1. Nausea and vomiting are absent.
2. Photophobia and phonophobia are absent, or one but not the other is present.

Chronic Tension-Type Headache

The pain must be present for more than 15 days per month and for more than 6 months. The rest of the diagnostic criteria are identical to those for episodic tension-type headache, except that nausea may be present.

Chronic Daily Headache

This category is often used by headache specialists although it is not officially included in the IHS classification. It is characterized by daily, mild to moderately severe headache with superimposed migrainous episodes.

Benign Recurring Headache

This category also is not included in IHS classification.

Some reports suggest that migraine and tension-type headaches have certain similarities in (1) clinical symptoms, (2) pathophysiology, and (3) response to both pharmacologic and nonpharmacologic therapies. The IHS authors propose use of the term "benign recurring headache" instead of arbitrary separation of "migraine" and "tension-type" headaches. They suggest redefining these categories as a single entity of varying intensity.

CLUSTER HEADACHE

Cluster headache is also known as *Horton's headache* or *histamine cephalalgia*. The following diagnostic criteria must be fulfilled:

1. At least five attacks of severe unilateral, orbital, supraorbital, or temporal pain lasting 15 to 180 minutes without treatment have occurred.
2. At least one of the following signs is ipsilaterally associated with the headache.

   Conjunctival injection
   Lacrimation
   Nasal congestion
   Rhinorrhea
   Forehead and facial sweating
   Miosis
   Ptosis
   Palpebral edema

3. Attacks occur with a frequency of up to eight per day.

Most patients have the episodic form, with 4- to 12-week cluster periods followed by symptom-free intervals lasting 1 or more years. In contrast to the patient with migraine, these patients cannot stay still. Cluster headache is seen five times more often in men than in women.

Chronic paroxysmal hemicrania consists of a brief unilateral attack of pain around the eye associated with ipsilateral autonomic signs.

BIBLIOGRAPHY

Cutrer M: Headache. *In* Borsook D, LeBel A, McPeek B (eds): The Massachusetts General Hospital Handbook of Pain Management. Boston, Little, Brown, 1996.

Marcus DA: Migraine and tension-type headaches: The questionable validity of current classification system. Clin J Pain 8(1):28–36, 1992.

Olesen J (ed): IHS classification and diagnostic criteria for headache disorders, cranial neuralgias and facial pain. Cephalalgia 8(suppl 7):1–96, 1988.

Olesen J, Rasmussen BK: Classification of primary headaches. Biomed Pharmacother 49:446–451, 1995.

Rapoport AM, Sheftell FD: Headache Disorders: A Management Guide for Practitioners. Philadelphia, WB Saunders, 1996.

Chapter 40

Differential Diagnosis of Headache

Onassis A. Caneris, M.D.

Headache is a common and ubiquitous symptom. There exist more than 300 conditions that can produce headache. Headaches can be classified as either *primary headache disorders* or *secondary headache disorders*. The primary headache disorders are those in which headache represents the primary pathologic entity, and in general there is a genetic predisposition to acquiring these disorders. Included are cluster and migraine headache; this group is discussed elsewhere in this book (Chapters 41 and 43).

The secondary headache disorders include those in which headache is a symptom of another condition. From the many entities that can produce headache, a differential diagnosis of headache can be derived. This classification can be organized from a number of different viewpoints. One method is to organize headache with respect to its temporal evolution. Three such arbitrary categories include *headaches of sudden onset; headaches of subacute onset, recurrent in nature;* and *headaches of subacute onset, progressive in nature.*

HEADACHES OF SUDDEN ONSET

Sudden onset of the "worst headache of my life" or "first headache"—the so-called *first or worst headache*—is a neurologic emergency and should be assumed to be the result of a neurologic event, even though its cause is frequently a primary headache disorder. A concomitant neurologic deficit or change in level of consciousness suggests an intracranial process as the cause of headache. Clinical features that suggest a worrisome process include an *abrupt, unexpected* headache with symptoms rapidly progressing over seconds to minutes and *associated symptoms* including stiff neck, fever, diminished level of consciousness, papilledema, and nausea and vomiting. This type of headache usually is the most serious and requires the clinician to be thoroughly familiar with the differential diagnosis of this category.

Subarachnoid Hemorrhage

The most common cause of subarachnoid hemorrhage (SAH) is rupture of a saccular arterial intracranial cerebral aneurysm. Autopsy studies indicate an overall frequency of 0.2% and 9.9%, with the incidence of symptomatic SAH being approximately 10 to 15 per 100,000 population in North America. Patients most often are between 40 and 60 years of age. The typical presentation is that of an acute, severe, bilateral headache of sudden onset, often associated with nausea and vomiting, photophobia, nuchal rigidity, and transient or persistent loss of consciousness. The headache probably relates to an abrupt increase in intracranial pressure with distortion of pain-sensitive structures as well as meningeal irritation. Physical examination reveals signs of meningismus (nuchal rigidity, Kernig's sign, Brudzinski's sign) and often focal neurologic deficits. Occasionally patients may experience warning leaks before a major hemorrhage, with a sudden but milder headache termed a *sentinel hemorrhage* or *sentinel headache*. A noncontrast computed tomographic scan of the brain is the neuroimaging procedure of choice for a suspected acute SAH, with high-density material seen in the subarachnoid space confirming the diagnosis. However, a normal scan does not completely exclude the diagnosis of SAH: computed tomography is 95% sensitive if performed within the first 2 days and about 50% sensitive if performed after 5 days. If there remains a high index of suspicion, a lumbar puncture should be performed, with either frank blood or xanthochromia being diagnostic. Conventional cerebral angiography is important in defining the location of the aneurysm. Definitive treatment includes surgical clipping of accessible aneurysms and the prevention of cerebral vasospasm.

Acute Parenchymal Intracranial Hemorrhage

The occurrence of headache with an acute cerebral or cerebellar hemorrhage is variable. Acute parenchymal intracranial hemorrhage is very likely to be associated with an acute neurologic deficit and alteration in level of consciousness. This type of hemorrhage is often associated with hypertension or amyloid angiopathy. The character of the headache is nonspecific and usually is related to increased intracranial pressure.

Cerebral Ischemia

Transient cerebral ischemia or cerebral infarction may result in episodic or persistent headache that precedes, accompanies, or follows the acute neurologic event. The neurologic accompaniment usually is apparent within 48 hours of the headache. Approximately 35% of patients with cerebral infarction and 25% of those with transient ischemic attacks present with headache. The headache is nonspecific.

Meningeal Infection

Both acute bacterial and viral infections of the meninges produce headache by causing an inflammatory reaction in the arachnoid and pia, in the cerebrospinal fluid (CSF), and in the ventricles. Clinical features usually include severe global headache with signs of meningeal irritation, photophobia, fever, alteration in level of consciousness, and occasionally convulsions. CSF examination reveals a pleocytosis. Additional agents that can cause headache related to central nervous system infection include toxoplasmosis fungi, the human immunodeficiency virus, and the agent that causes Lyme disease.

Acute Systemic Hypertension

Acute severe systemic hypertension or hypertensive encephalopathy can produce a severe, sudden-onset headache. A rise in diastolic pressure of more than 25% or a combined pressure greater than 200/130 mm Hg usually is required; more moderate elevations do not cause headache. Pressor responses to medications (including monoamine oxidase inhibitors) and systemic illness (including pheochromocytoma) can produce this phenomenon.

Arterial Dissection

Dissection of the *internal carotid artery* is an uncommon but important cause of both headache and neurologic deficit. The headache is frequently unilateral, orbital, periorbital, or frontal. An associated Horner's syndrome is not infrequently present. *Cervical vertebral artery* dissection causes headache, usually high in the neck or occiput, often accompanied by signs of lateral medullary syndrome. Dissection can be spontaneous or associated with trauma; it usually occurs in patients younger than 50 years of age.

Acute Angle-Closure Glaucoma

Acute glaucoma can manifest with sudden-onset eye and orbital pain associated with frontal headache. Associated symptoms include conjunctival injection, pupillary changes, and clouding of the lens. The diagnosis is confirmed by demonstration of increased intraocular pressure. This may be precipitated by the use of anticholinergic agents.

Coital Headache

The term *coital headache* refers to the sporadic occurrence of a sudden, high-intensity, excruciating, throbbing occipital headache, usually just before or at orgasm. Duration of symptoms is a few minutes to a few hours. Men are affected more commonly than women. This headache can be difficult to distinguish from the headache that occurs with SAH. Coital headache should lack nuchal rigidity, alteration in level of consciousness, and focal neurologic deficit; if any of these is present, other causes should be investigated.

Benign Cough Headache

Benign cough headache causes severe, short-lived pain after coughing, lifting, bending, stooping, or sneezing. The headache arises after the stimulus reaches peak intensity and subsides over several seconds to minutes. Structural pathology in the posterior fossa should be excluded. This disorder primarily affects middle aged men and usually has a self-limited course lasting several years.

RECURRENT HEADACHES OF SUBACUTE ONSET

Arteriovenous Malformations

Arteriovenous malformations may manifest with SAH and acute-onset headache, but more commonly patients present with episodic, migraine-like headaches that are associated with neurologic symptoms. Diagnosis is confirmed by neuroimaging studies.

Cerebral Sinus or Venous Thrombosis

Thrombotic occlusion of the dural sinuses or cerebral veins can produce either paroxysmal or persistent headache. The headache is usually global, results from increased intracranial pressure, and is frequently associated with papilledema, focal neurologic deficit, partial seizures, and alteration in level of consciousness. Risk factors include hypercoagulable states, dehydration, and pregnancy.

Cavernous sinus thrombosis causes retro-orbital pain, periorbital pain, or pain around the forehead. Associated symptoms include proptosis, conjunctival injection, ptosis, ophthalmoparesis, and papilledema. Cavernous sinus thrombosis frequently originates from suppurative processes of the orbit or nasal sinuses but can also occur in the context of hypercoagulable states. Diagnosis is confirmed by neuroimaging studies.

Obstructive Hydrocephalus

Obstructive hydrocephalus can produce paroxysmal or, more frequently, continuous headaches that are often worsened by supine posture, exertion, or cervical posture. Associated symptoms include disturbance of gait, cognitive impairment, and urinary incontinence. Neuroimaging studies reveal hydrocephalus and the obstructing lesion. The headache resolves with normalization of the elevated intracranial pressure.

SUBACUTE PERSISTENT PROGRESSIVE HEADACHES

Benign Intracranial Hypertension (Pseudotumor Cerebri)

The term *idiopathic benign intracranial hypertension* describes a heterogeneous group of disorders characterized by increased intracranial pressure for which other organic causes, including intracranial mass lesions and obstructive hydrocephalus, have been excluded. The headache is often continuous, worse on awakening, and aggravated by coughing and straining. Associated symptoms are visual obscurations and papilledema. The condition is most common in obese women. A variety of associations, including Addison's disease, adrenal steroid withdrawal, hypoparathyroidism, vitamin A, lithium carbonate, and connective tissue disorders, have been noted. Diagnosis is established with demonstration of elevated CSF pressure by lumbar puncture with careful manometry. Headaches typically improve after lumbar puncture.

Chronic Subdural Hematoma

Chronic subdural hematoma can cause the insidious onset of a mild or severe, unilateral or bilateral headache. This is often associated with focal neurologic signs or alterations in consciousness or personality. In 50% of cases there is a reported history of head trauma. There may be percussion tenderness over the site of the hematoma.

Cerebral Neoplasm

Headache occurs as the presenting symptom in 40% of patients with a brain tumor. It usually is mild to moderate in severity and global in character. In 50% of cases it is accompanied by nausea and vomiting. Position, exertion, and coughing often aggravate the headache. Morning headache is common, and increased intracranial pressure is frequently found.

Intracranial Abscess

The headache of intracranial abscess is similar to that of an intracranial neoplasm, but the temporal progression usually is more rapid. Fever and focal neurologic deficit are frequently associated.

Giant Cell Arteritis (Temporal Arteritis)

Giant cell arteritis is the painful granulomatous inflammation of extracranial and intracranial arteries. The headache may localize to anywhere on the scalp but is most frequently located temporally. Associated symptoms include arthralgia, myalgia, malaise, anorexia, jaw claudication, and a palpable, tender temporal artery. Most patients are older than 50 years of age. The onset usually is insidious. Visual loss and cerebral infarction are the most serious complications. An elevated erythrocyte sedimentation rate supports the diagnosis, but this value is normal or only mildly elevated in 25% of the patients. Granulomatous inflammation found on temporal artery biopsy confirms the diagnosis. Corticosteroids are the treatment of choice. Temporal arteritis should be suspected in any elderly patient who presents with new-onset headache.

Chronic Meningitides

Chronic fungal, infectious, or inflammatory granulomatous or carcinomatous meningitis gives rise to a persistent headache, not infrequently associated with mild nuchal rigidity and multiple cranial neuropathies. Diagnosis is confirmed by CSF examination with appropriate analysis.

Sinusitis

The role of sinusitis as a contributing cause or aggravating factor of headache is controversial. Most agree that acute sinusitis can cause or contribute to headache syndromes. The contributing role of chronic sinusitis is more controversial.

BIBLIOGRAPHY

Raskin NH: Headache. New York, Churchill Livingstone, 1988.
Spence J: Migraine and other causes of headache. Ann Emerg Med 27:448–450, 1996.
Wall PD: Textbook of Pain. New York, Churchill Livingstone, 1994, pp 495–520.
Wolff HG: Wolff's Headache and Other Head Pain. New York, Oxford University Press, 1987.

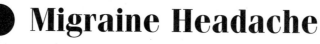

Chapter 41

Migraine Headache

Jack M. Rozental, M.D., Ph.D.

EPIDEMIOLOGY

Migraine headache represents an extremely common, benign headache syndrome sometimes referred to as a *vascular headache*. Approximately two thirds of migraines occur in women. The prevalence of migraine in North America, ascertained through epidemiologic studies, is 12% to 17.6% in females and 4% to 6% in males. Before puberty, migraine prevalence in boys is similar to or higher than in girls; during and after adolescence, prevalence increases more rapidly in girls. Prevalence increases until age 40, after which it declines altogether, a decline that is steeper in women as they approach menopause. Among those with severe migraine, about 25% have four or more migraines per month, 35% have one to three migraines per month, and the rest experience one or fewer migraines per month. More than 80% of patients with severe migraine experience headache-related disability which ranges from decreased productivity to time off work during an attack. The cost in productivity may be as high as $18 billion per year in the United States. The risk of migraine is about 50% higher among those who have relatives with migraines; however, genetic factors seem to account for fewer than one half of all migraine cases. Very often there is a family history for migraine. The cause of migraine is unknown.

PATHOPHYSIOLOGY OF MIGRAINE

The pain-generating structures of the head include the venous sinuses, meningeal and large cerebral arteries, basal meninges, muscles, skin, and cranial nerves V, IX, and X. A plexus of largely unmyelinated fibers arises from the trigeminal ganglion and innervates the cerebral and pial arteries, the venous sinuses, and the dura mater; this plexus is referred to as the *trigeminovascular system*. A similar plexus arises from the dorsal roots of the upper cervical nerves to innervate comparable structures in the posterior fossa. The neurons of the trigeminovascular system contain substance P, one of

the major nociceptive neurotransmitters of primary sensory neurons; calcitonin gene-related peptide (CGRP); and neurokinin A. When the trigeminal ganglion is stimulated these peptide transmitters are released, resulting in neurogenic extravasation of plasma or so-called *sterile neurogenic inflammation*, the end result of which is the perception of pain. Elevated venous levels of CGRP during migraine and cluster headache have been described. Neurogenic inflammation is blocked by ergot alkaloids (ergotamine, dihydroergotamine), sumatriptan, aspirin, valproate, indomethacin, and substance P antagonists. Stimulation of pain-generating structures in the head activates neurons in the trigeminal nucleus caudalis and in the dorsal horn of upper cervical levels.

The trigeminovascular system, through release of neurotransmitters such as substance P and CGRP, provokes vasodilatation. Thus, stimulation of the trigeminal ganglion causes an increase in cerebral and extracerebral blood flow. Stimulation of the dorsal raphe nucleus in the midbrain, a serotoninergic nucleus, also increases cerebral blood flow. In contrast, stimulation of the nucleus caeruleus, the major source of central noradrenergic input, causes a decrease in cerebral blood flow. The major drugs used to abort migraine attacks are agonists at a specific subset of serotonin (5-HT) receptors—5-HT_{1D} and 5-$HT_{1\beta}$. Drugs that act as agonists at these sites are thought to reduce neurogenic inflammation; they also produce vasoconstriction.

Pain interneurons in the spinal cord and brain stem use enkephalins, and perhaps γ-amino butyric acid (GABA), as neurotransmitters. An ascending serotoninergic pathway in the midbrain raphe region relays painful stimuli to the ventroposteromedial thalamus via the quintothalamic tract. A descending endogenous pain-modulating system originates in the periaqueductal gray region of the midbrain, one of its major relay structures being the nucleus raphe magnus in the medulla. After this relay, the descending pain-modulating system connects with the spinal tract of the trigeminal nerve and the dorsal horns of the first through third cervical nerves. Stimulation of the periaqueductal gray region causes headache. The major neurotransmitters of this modulating system are norepinephrine, serotonin, and enkephalins.

The aura phase of migraine is associated with an electrical *spreading depression* in the cortex. This spreading depression is concurrent with a phenomenon of spreading oligemia, which moves across the cortex at a rate of 2 to 3 mm/minute. Neither spreading depression nor spreading oligemia respects vascular territories. Spreading oligemia has been documented with positron emission tomography during the headache phase of a migraine in a patient who did not have a classic aura. The exact relation between spreading depression, spreading oligemia, aura, and the headache phase of migraine is not clear. The trigeminovascular system might be activated by the aura or by the same mechanism that causes the aura. Phosphorus magnetic resonance spectroscopy of patients with migraine headache has revealed a reduced phosphocreatine level, increased concentration of adenosine diphosphate (ADP), and a high rate of synthesis of adenosine triphosphate (ATP). These results suggest a relative failure of ATP production by mitochondria, similar to that found in patients with cluster headache; however, the exact mechanism by which this happens is not understood.

A growing body of evidence points to the importance of dopamine in the pathophysiology of migraine. Dopamine receptor hypersensitivity may be responsible for the nausea, vomiting, hypotension, and dizziness that frequently accompany and sometimes characterize attacks of migraine. These symptoms can be elicited by low doses of dopamine and dopamine agonists in migraineurs and are common toxic effects of dopaminergic drugs. In addition, antiemetics, most of which are dopamine receptor antagonists (especially at the D2 receptor), are efficacious in treating migraine attacks.

DIAGNOSIS

The diagnosis of migraine is made by a suggestive clinical history and a normal neurologic examination. Migraines can be divided into those with aura (*classic migraine*) and those without aura (*common migraine*). The usual migrainous aura consists of visual symptoms such as bright spots (sometimes like champagne bubbles) or dark spots, tunnel vision, or zigzag lines (so-called fortification spectra). Other common auras include numbness or paresthesias in one arm or one side of the body in a stereotypic pattern. Some patients present with complicated auras or with neurologic dysfunction during the headache (*complicated migraine*). These headaches are preceded or accompanied by transient neurologic signs such as oculomotor or limb palsy, which may resemble signs of a transient ischemic attack or a major neurologic catastrophe. The aura is followed by an intense, crescendo head pain, frequently unilateral and retro-ocular, which may be pounding, throbbing, pressure-like, vise-like, stabbing, or jabbing; patients may describe pain so intense that it feels like their head is about to explode. The migrainous aura may also occur independently of pain (*migraine equivalent*). The headache phase lasts from about 30 minutes to a day; occa-

sionally, a headache becomes intractable and lasts 1 week or longer. A migraine usually is accompanied by other symptoms, such as photophobia or phonophobia (or both) and nausea and vomiting, but it should resolve without lasting complications. Although there may be a very slightly increased risk of stroke in some migraineurs, that relation is not yet clear.

Given reasonable clinical judgment, most migraine headaches can be recognized and treated as such, but occasionally a patient or clinical circumstance requires that the physician be more circumspect. Although in any given individual the headaches may occur predominantly on the same side of the head, if a headache has not at least once involved the opposite side it is reasonable to search for vascular pathology (e.g., aneurysm, malformation). Some patients develop vascular or migrainous headaches of an exploding nature related to exertion (*exertional migraine*), for example while doing heavy work or lifting weights or during sexual climax. Occasionally a new-onset headache, or a change in the usual pattern of a patient's headache, is the presenting symptom of a brain tumor. In such cases—strictly unilateral headache, exertional migraine, recent change in clinical condition, and others dictated by the judgment of the treating physician—a magnetic resonance imaging study of the brain, angiography, electroencephalography, or some combination may be indicated.

TREATMENT

Migraines can be treated prophylactically (i.e., with preventive intent) or with abortive intent after they begin. Dosages listed are meant to serve only as general guidelines.

I. Drugs that are useful for treatment of acute migraine headaches (abortive drugs)
   A. Ergotamine tartrate (Wigraine): two tablets at the onset of the headache or aura, followed by one tablet every 30 minutes until the headache is gone or until a maximum of 5 tablets per headache or 10 tablets per week have been consumed. If consumed in excess, ergotamine-containing preparations can cause complications related to vasospasm and also are emetogenic. (The similar preparation Cafergot has been removed from the market.)
   B. Isometheptene (Midrin): two capsules at the onset of the headache or aura, followed by one capsule every 60 minutes until the headache is gone or until a maximum of 5 capsules per headache or 10 capsules per week have been consumed. If consumed in excess, isometheptene can cause complications related to vasospasm.
   C. Preparations containing butalbital (a barbiturate), caffeine, and acetaminophen (Fioricet, Esgic) or aspirin (Fiorinal): one to two tablets every 4 hours as needed. These barbiturate preparations cause drowsiness and may be habit-forming if used excessively.

D. Narcotic-containing preparations such as codeine plus acetaminophen (Tylenol No. 3), butorphanol nasal spray (Stadol), or meperidine (Demerol). Narcotics, in the emergency room or any other setting, should be used only as drugs of last resort. These drugs bind at opiate receptors and temporarily mask the pain but do not bind serotonin receptors; therefore, narcotics do not directly deal with the putative pathophysiologic basis of the migraine pain (described previously). Narcotic-containing preparations can cause drowsiness or euphoria, may be habit-forming, and cause hypotension and respiratory depression if used excessively. Accumulation of meperidine's metabolite from repeated administration can cause or aggravate seizures.

E. Sumatriptan (Imitrex), 6 mg injectable subcutaneously or in 25-mg or 50-mg tablet form or 20 mg of nasal spray. Sumatriptan is administered either as one 6-mg subcutaneous injection or as an initial oral dose of 25 to 100 mg; either dose may be repeated in 1 to 2 hours if symptoms persist and then not again for 24 hours. Sumatriptan should not be administered within 24 hours of a vasoconstricting or an ergot drug (ergotamine, dihydroergotamine, methysergide) or isometheptene; it should not be administered within 2 weeks after discontinuation of a monoamine oxidase inhibitor or to patients with cardiac disease. Because of its cardiotoxic potential, the first dose should be administered under medical supervision.

F. Antinauseants such as prochlorperazine (Compazine), chlorpromazine (Thorazine), or metoclopramide (Reglan). These drugs, by virtue of their effect on serotonin receptors, are effective against the migraine pain. Their action as antagonists at the D2 dopamine receptors helps control the nausea and vomiting that frequently accompanies migraines and makes them excellent adjuvant drugs.

G. Dihydroergotamine (DHE), 0.5 to 1 mg, previously was available only by injection; it is now available as a 4 mg/mL nasal spray.

H. Other nonsteroidal anti-inflammatory drugs (NSAIDs) work for some patients with milder migraine. Ketorolac (Toradol), 30 or 60 mg administered intramuscularly, may be particularly effective. It should not be administered for longer than 5 days.

I. Corticosteroids may be used for a very limited time period and only under strict medical supervision. Corticosteroids are useful mainly as adjuvants to other specific drugs to break an intractable migraine (status migrainosus). Both short- and long-term use of corticosteroids entails significant potential for morbidity.

II. Drugs that are useful for prophylactic treatment

A. β-blockers, such as propranolol (Inderal), may be used as first- or second-line drugs for migraine prophylaxis. In most healthy people, 60 to 80 mg once per day of the long-acting propranolol preparation may be started; lesser doses tend to be ineffective. Side effects include dizziness from bradycardia and/or hypotension, depression, worsening shortness of breath in patients with asthma or chronic obstructive pulmonary disease, gastrointestinal distress, blunting of hypoglycemic symptoms in diabetics, and vivid dreams. Dosages of propranolol up to 400 mg/day, in divided doses, may be necessary. Sometimes, if the initial β-blocker used proves ineffective, another may be tried; efficacy has been reported for metoprolol, atenolol, and nadolol.

B. Tricyclic antidepressants, particularly amitriptyline (Elavil) at a starting dose of 10 to 25 mg at bedtime (10 mg for elderly, frail, or sensitive persons and for those with a history of sensitivity to medications), are very active. Other useful tricyclics include imipramine (Tofranil), nortriptyline, desipramine, and protriptyline. Most patients who respond to amitriptyline, imipramine, nortriptyline, or desipramine do so at doses of 75 to 200 mg at bedtime; occasionally, patients require up to 300 mg/day. The major side effects from these drugs relate to their anticholinergic effects and include dry mouth, dizziness, difficulty waking up in the morning, urinary retention, glaucoma in patients with narrow angles, and cardiac arrhythmias. Tricyclics induce sleep, which may constitute one of the mechanisms by which they help migraineurs. If excessive morning sleepiness is a side effect, protriptyline may be tried.

C. The specific serotonin reuptake inhibitors (SSRIs) such as paroxetine (20 to 40 mg/day) and fluoxetine (20 to 40 mg/day) are worth a try in patients who do not respond to tricyclics or have intolerable toxic effects from them. These SSRIs may be used alone or in combination with a tricyclic. The major side effects of the SSRI drugs include jitteriness, tremors, gastrointestinal distress, and occasionally headaches.

D. Calcium channel blockers—verapamil (Calan) and others. These drugs may occasionally be useful in migraineurs, but they tend to be more specifically indicated for patients with cluster headache, for which, if one considers the natural history of the disease, they may or may not be particularly efficacious. Calcium channel blockers are worth a try when other first-line agents prove ineffective.

E. Anticonvulsants—valproic acid (Depakote), phenytoin (Dilantin), carbamazepine (Tegretol). Valproic acid, in doses up to 1000 mg/day, alone or in combination with other prophylactic agents, is particularly useful. Valproic acid has been reported to reduce headache frequency or severity by about 50% in half of the patients who try it.

F. Methysergide (Sansert), an antiserotoninergic agent, should not be used longer than 3 months without an interruption of several weeks, because it can cause irreversible retroperitoneal, lung, and heart valve fibrosis. Its major acute toxicity is gastrointestinal distress.

G. Cyproheptadine (Periactin) is an antihistamine with serotoninergic activity; it can be used in doses up to 6 mg twice per day. Cyproheptadine is frequently used as a drug for pediatric migraine prophylaxis, but is quite useful in adults as well.

H. Lithium carbonate may be useful for patients with intractable migraine, but its major indication is in the prophylaxis of cluster headache.

I. Sometimes one or two regular-strength aspirin tablets or 25 to 50 mg of indomethacin taken at bedtime is an effective adjuvant to other prophylactic medications.

J. Among the antiemetics, metoclopramide in oral doses of 10 to 20 mg three times per day may be used.

III. Women who have migraines around the time of their menses (catamenial or menstrual migraine) may benefit from prophylactic treatment timed for the days of the month during which they are at risk. During that time, they may benefit from a temporary increase of their prophylactic medication, ergotamine or isometheptene taken once or twice per day, or addition of an NSAID once or twice per day. Since the onset of a menstrual migraine relates to the precipitous drop in estrogen levels, addition of an estrogen patch beginning a few days before the predicted onset of headache sometimes is effective.

IV. Self-help strategies aimed at minimizing the incidence of migraines

A. Regularize the intake of caffeine-containing beverages (coffee, tea, soda, cocoa), including weekends, holidays, and vacations.

B. Avoid foods high in tyramine, a substance metabolized to serotonin that is thought to play a role in triggering migraines. Some foods high in tyramine are chocolate, aged cheeses, yogurt, sour cream, soy sauce, chicken liver, bananas, avocados, nuts, and yeast extracts (including beer).

C. Avoid foods high in nitrates, including processed meats (e.g., hot dogs, salami, sausage) and other canned, smoked, or aged meats.

D. Some patients are sensitive to certain food additives. Two examples are monosodium glutamate, a flavor enhancer frequently added to oriental food that is the cause of "Chinese restaurant syndrome," and the artificial sweetener aspartame (Nutrasweet). These substances contain glutamate, an excitatory neurotransmitter.

E. Many migraineurs are sensitive to alcoholic beverages because alcohol tends to dilate blood vessels. Among alcohol-sensitive people, darker beverages (e.g., red wine, champagne, beer) are the worst.

F. New migraines or exacerbations of an existing migrainous condition may occur as a reaction to medication; implicated drugs include SSRIs such as fluoxetine (Prozac), aminophylline, or birth control pills.

G. The overuse of any pain killer, including all NSAIDs, acetaminophen, narcotics, barbiturates, and drugs indicated specifically for the abortive treatment of migraine (e.g., sumatriptan, ergots, isometheptene) causes rebound or withdrawal headaches (discussed later).

H. Miscellaneous but not unusual causes of migraine include a poststress situation, lack of adequate rest or changes in sleep habit, allergies, hypoglycemia, and noncompliance with medications intended for prophylaxis against headaches.

I. During the headache, patients should lie down in a darkened, quiet room. It is important not to become dehydrated.

J. If bright light is an irritant, patients should wear optical-quality sunglasses that block at least 85% of incident light (as well as 100% of ultraviolet light) while driving or engaging in outdoor activities.

REBOUND HEADACHE AND TRANSFORMED MIGRAINE

Overuse of pain killer should be considered in patients who consistently use any pain-killing drug three or more times per week for headache. Typically, patients awaken with a headache or develop one in the morning or at any time of the day, prompting consumption of pain killers on an almost regular schedule several times per day. This phenomenon is called rebound headache. Frequently, the characteristics or the description of the rebound headache is different from that of the syndrome that prompted the overuse; this is called transformed migraine. More often than not, rebound headache and transformed migraine coexist and are refractory to standard treatment.

The treatment for both rebound headache and transformed migraine is discontinuation of all pain killers. Pain killer withdrawal generally results in a temporary, dramatic exacerbation of the pain which usually lasts several days. The physiologic washout period, during which the patient may continue to experience symptoms resulting from drug overuse, lasts at least 2 to 3 weeks and may extend for up to 3 months. Patients should be counseled to refrain from reverting to the uncontrolled use of pain medicines out of frustration.

TREATMENT OF INTRACTABLE MIGRAINE (STATUS MIGRAINOSUS)

An intense, incapacitating migraine lasting longer than 72 hours, unresponsive to standard interventions, and during which nausea and/or emesis precludes maintenance of adequate hydration, requires inpatient treatment with intravenous (IV) dihydroergotamine. Dihydroergotamine also is indicated for treatment of menstrual migraine or cluster headache and during the acute detoxification phase of ergot-induced rebound headache.

1. Start with a test dose of dihydroergotamine, 0.25 to 0.5 mg IV given over a period of 2 minutes.

2. If the test dose is tolerated and the headache persists, proceed with 0.5 to 1 mg of IV dihydroergotamine given 1 hour after the test dose; then schedule 0.5 to 1 mg IV dihydroergotamine every 8 hours for up to 5 days if needed and as tolerated.

3. If nausea and/or emesis limit tolerance or constitute prominent elements of the presentation, an antiemetic must be administered parenterally. For example, prochlorperazine, 10 mg IV in saline or as a slow push, is effective as an antiemetic and frequently treats the headache as well; it may be scheduled before the dihydroergotamine as needed. Prochlorperazine's pharmacologic action at dopamine receptors may cause an acute dystonia which is treatable with IV diphenhydramine (Benadryl). Similarly, metoclopramide, 10 mg IV, may be administered before the dihydroergotamine although it is not by itself as effective in treating the headache.

4. In the inpatient setting, a corticosteroid often is administered as an adjuvant. Dexamethasone (4 mg IV every 6 hours, tapered over 2 to 3 days) or hydrocortisone (100 mg IV every 6 hours, tapered in the same way) is most commonly used.

5. Dihydroergotamine should be tapered gradually over 1 or 2 days once the patient is headache free. For example, the drug can be decreased to 0.5 mg every 8 hours for several doses and then to 0.25 mg every 8 hours, with or without metoclopramide, for several doses before discontinuation.

6. Dihydroergotamine mainly produces venous constriction but may cause significant arterial constriction. Chest pain, a significantly elevated blood pressure, and leg cramps represent important indicators of arterial vasospasm and call for discontinuation of the drug.

7. Parenteral hydration and an adequately quiet, dark environment should not be neglected.

8. Ketorolac (Toradol), 30 to 60 mg intramuscularly, can be used up to three times per day for up to 5 days, with or without an antiemetic, instead of dihydroergotamine.

9. Narcotics are particularly ineffective drugs for the management of this condition.

BIBLIOGRAPHY

Denier HC, Limmroth V: The management of migraine. Rev Contemp Pharmacother 5:271–284, 1994.

Hering R, Kuritzky AA: Sodium valproate in the prophylactic treatment of migraine: A double blind study versus placebo. Cephalalgia 12:81–84, 1992.

Holroyd KA, Penzien DB: Propranolol in the management of recurrent migraine: A meta-analytic review. Headache 31:33–44, 1991.

International Headache Society: Classification and diagnostic criteria for headache disorders, cranial neuralgias, and facial pain. Cephalalgia 8(suppl 7):1–96, 1988.

Lauritzen M: Pathophysiology of the migraine aura: The spreading depression theory. Brain 177:199, 1994.

Lipton RB, Silberstein SD, Stewart WF: An update on the epidemiology of migraine. Headache 34:319–328, 1994.

Lipton RB, Stewart WF: Migraine in the United States: Epidemiology and healthcare use. Neurology 43(suppl 3):6–10, 1993.

Mathew NT, Reuveni U, Perez F: Transformed or evolutive migraine. Headache 27:102–106, 1987.

Montagna P, Lodi R, Cortelli P, et al.: Phosphorus magnetic resonance spectroscopy in cluster headache. Neurology 48:113–118, 1997.

Moskowitz MA: Neurogenic inflammation in the pathophysiology and treatment of migraine. Neurology 43(suppl 3):16–20, 1993.

Moskowitz MA: Neurovascular and molecular mechanisms in migraine headache. Cerebrovasc Brain Metab Rev 5:150–177, 1993.

Peroutka SJ: Dopamine and migraine. Neurology 49:650–656, 1997.

Silberstein SD, Silberstein JR: Chronic daily headache: Long-term prognosis following inpatient treatment with repetitive IV DHE. Headache 32:439–445, 1992.

Stewart WF, Lipton RB: Work related disability: Results from the American Migraine Study. Cephalalgia 16:231–238, 1996.

Stewart WF, Lipton RB, Ottman R: Familial risk of migraine: A population-based study. Neurology 41:166–172, 1997.

Warner JS: Analgesic rebound as a cause of hemicrania continua. Neurology 48:1540–1541, 1997.

Chapter 4 2

Tension Headache

Jack M. Rozental, M.D., Ph.D.

EPIDEMIOLOGY

Tension headache is not only the most common headache type, but also perhaps the most difficult of the head pain syndromes to classify. Adding to the classification chaos are the multiple terms that have been or are applied to what probably represent variants of the same syndrome. If one considers that headaches in general affect more than 90% of the population and that only about 15% of those fit the description of migraine, then up to 70% of the population suffer tension or tension-like headache. Moreover, almost all patients with migraine, cluster headache, trigeminal nerve neuralgias, and other forms of recurring cephalgic syndromes have interposed tension headaches.

DIAGNOSIS

The pain of tension headache tends to be duller and less intense than that of a migraine or a cluster attack; it also is more diffuse, even circumferential or bandlike. The pain usually lasts for several hours or even for a day but may continue for days or weeks. During a severe tension headache, patients may experience photophobia, phonophobia, nausea, and emesis. Pain referred to the neck is common, but the neurologic examination results should be normal. A common variety of tension-like headache occurs in patients with headaches of any sort in whom these temporarily exacerbate and become more frequent. Patients begin taking analgesics (e.g., nonsteroidal anti-inflammatory drugs [NSAIDs], acetaminophen, narcotics, ergot derivatives, sumatriptan) on a regular basis and eventually develop rebound or transformed headaches, or both.

The major variants of tension headache are those with disorder of the pericranial muscles, those without disorder of the pericranial muscles, and chronic tension-type headache (with and without disorder of the pericranial muscles). Those with disorder of the pericranial muscles are characterized by tenderness on palpation of those muscles, increased activity on an electromyo-

gram, or both. Tension-type headaches without disorder of the pericranial muscles lack those characteristics. Chronic tension-type headache is also called chronic daily headache and is diagnosed in a patient with a headache frequency of 15 days per month or 180 days per year averaged over a 6-month period.

A particularly severe, persistent, or unusual headache should always prompt consideration of alternative explanations, and, when appropriate, these should be investigated thoroughly. For example, temporal arteritis should be considered in an elderly patient with a chronic headache of recent onset whether or not other typical elements are present in the history and physical examination; an erythrocyte sedimentation rate should be ordered immediately, and consideration should be given to a temporal artery biopsy. Likewise, one would not wish to miss an infectious meningitis or idiopathic intracranial hypertension (pseudotumor cerebri), with or without papilledema, when the diagnosis can be made with a lumbar puncture. We must be vigilant for the sentinel bleed of an aneurysm, an undiagnosed intracranial vascular malformation, a subdural hematoma, a hydrocephalus, or an arterial dissection. Therefore, when dictated by the judgment of the treating physician, magnetic resonance imaging or computed tomography of the brain, angiography, electroencephalography, or several of these tests may be indicated.

PATHOPHYSIOLOGY OF TENSION HEADACHE

The physiologic mechanism by which tension headaches occur is unknown. Some investigators believe that, clinically, tension headache lies at one end of a continuum of head pains and that severe migraine is located at the other. Thus, at least to some degree, the underlying pathophysiologic mechanism of most chronic recurring headache syndromes would be shared.

The precise relationship between cervicogenic disorders and headache is unclear, although most painful cervical pathologic conditions are associated with some sort of headache. Cervical pain can be referred to the head from intervertebral disks, interspinous ligaments, zygapophyseal joints, the periosteum, paracervical muscles, major arteries of the posterior circulation, and irritation of the C1, C2, and C3 nerve roots (which supply sensory innervation to the neck and to the scalp caudal to the innervation of the trigeminal nerve and to the meninges and arteries of the posterior fossa). In addition, headache can arise from foramen magnum pathology. Some examples of the latter include Chiari I malformation, Dandy-Walker syndrome, atlantoaxial dislocation (as may occur in rheumatoid arthritis), Paget's disease of the bone, and basilar invagination.

The muscle contraction theory of headaches relates the pain of tension-type headaches to prolonged contraction or spasm of cervical or pericranial muscles. No objective data support the theory, and the observation of more cervical and/or pericranial muscle contraction during migraine than during tension-type headache has been used as a basis to dispute it. Another ill-defined condition that warrants some consideration is fibromyalgia or myofascial pain syndrome.

TREATMENT

As in other headache types, both abortive and prophylactic strategies are available for treatment. For the occasional tension-type headache, over-the-counter analgesics are all that is required. The patient usually has a good idea of which analgesic is effective and what dose is required. The number of over-the-counter drugs has increased significantly in the past several years, and although they are generally safe, the lay population has little basis on which to decide how to choose among them or how to use them properly. If aspirin or acetaminophen becomes ineffective in controlling the headaches, the choice of an alternative analgesic should proceed in an orderly fashion by testing in turn members of different NSAID chemical categories at adequate doses. Indomethacin may be more effective than alternative NSAIDs for pain of cephalic origin. Occasionally, biofeedback is helpful, but it is impossible to predict accurately whom it will help. The major chemical categories of NSAIDs include the following:

1. Carboxylic acids—This group includes aspirin, which is an acetylated acid, as well as salsalate and choline magnesium trisalicylate, which are nonacetylated.
2. Propionic acids—ibuprofen, naproxen, ketoprofen, and fenoprofen.
3. Aryl and heterocyclic acids—indomethacin, diclofenac, sulindac, and tolmetin.
4. Fenamic acids—mefenamic acid and meclofenamate.
5. Enolic acids—piroxicam and phenylbutazone.
6. Pyrrolo-pyrrole—ketorolac.

Fortunately, most chronic or daily tension-type headaches respond to the first-line drugs used in migraine prophylaxis. It is possible that this reflects on the presumed common pathophysiologic mechanism that is felt to underlie both disorders. The most common drugs used for prophylaxis include the following:

1. Tricyclic antidepressants, particularly amitriptyline (Elavil), at a starting dose of 10 to 25 mg at bedtime (10 mg at bedtime for elderly or frail individuals or those highly sensitive to medication effects), are very active. Other useful tricyclics include imipramine (Tofranil), nortriptyline, desipramine, and protriptyline. Most patients who respond to amitriptyline, imipramine, nortriptyline, or desipramine do so at doses of 75 to 150 mg at bedtime; occasionally, patients require doses up to 300 mg/day. The major adverse effects from these drugs are related to their anticholinergic effects and include dry mouth, dizziness, difficulty waking up in the morning, urinary retention, glaucoma (in patients with narrow angles), and cardiac arrhythmias (at toxic doses). Tricyclics induce sleep, which may contribute to their beneficial effect. If excessive morning sleepiness is bothersome, protriptyline may be tried.
2. The specific serotonin reuptake inhibitors (SSRIs) such as paroxetine (20 to 40 mg/day) and fluoxetine (20 to 40 mg/day) are worth a try in patients who do not respond to tricyclics or have intolerable side effects from them (e.g., excessive morning sleepiness). However, there is no good evidence that SSRIs are effective against tension-type headaches. These drugs may be used alone or in combination with a tricyclic. The major adverse effects of the SSRI drugs include jitteriness, tremors, gastrointestinal distress, and, occasionally, headaches.
3. β-Blockers, such as propranolol (Inderal), may be used as either first- or second-line drugs for headache prophylaxis. In most healthy people, 60 to 80 mg once a day of the long-acting propranolol preparation may be started; lesser doses are usually not as effective. Adverse effects include dizziness from bradycardia, hypotension, or both; depression; worsening shortness of breath in patients with asthma or chronic obstructive pulmonary disease; gastrointestinal distress; blunting of hypoglycemic symptoms in diabetics; and vivid dreams. Dosages up to 400 mg/day, in divided doses, may occasionally be necessary. Sometimes, if the initial β-blocker proves ineffective, another may be tried; efficacy has been reported for metoprolol, atenolol, and nadolol.

BIBLIOGRAPHY

International Headache Society: Classification and diagnostic criteria for headache disorders, cranial neuralgias, and facial pain. Cephalalgia 8(suppl 7):1–96, 1988.

Mathew NT: Transformed migraine, analgesic rebound, and other chronic daily headaches. Neurol Clinics 15:167–186, 1997.

Pini L, Bigarelli M, Vitale G, et al: Headaches associated with chronic use of analgesics: A therapeutic approach. Headache 36:433–439, 1996.

Sheftell FD: Role and impact of over the counter medications in the management of headache. Neurol Clinics 15:199–208, 1997.

Silberstein SD, Lipton RB, Solomon S, et al: Classification of daily and near daily headaches: Proposed revisions to the IHS criteria. Headache 34:1–7, 1994.

Chapter 43

Cluster Headache

Jack M. Rozental, M.D., Ph.D.

EPIDEMIOLOGY

Cluster headache, unlike migraine, affects predominantly males in a ratio of 3 or 4:1 (males-to-females). The prevalence is 0.1% to 0.3% of the population. A family history of cluster is not as frequent as a family history of migraine; however, most patients with cluster have a history of smoking and alcohol consumption. In the majority of cases, attacks begin between the ages of 20 and 40.

PATHOPHYSIOLOGY OF CLUSTER HEADACHE

The physiologic mechanism by which cluster headaches occur is unknown. Some investigators believe that, clinically, cluster lies within a continuum of head pains that include severe migraine at one extreme and tension headache at the other. Thus, at least to some degree, the underlying pathophysiologic mechanism between most chronic recurring headache syndromes would be shared. Some of the clinical features of cluster, which seem to reflect local vasoactive phenomena, support an involvement of neurogenic inflammation in its pathophysiology. Phosphorus magnetic resonance spectroscopy of patients with cluster headache (although not studied during an actual headache) revealed a reduced phosphocreatine level, an increased concentration of adenosine diphosphate, and a high rate of adenosine triphosphate synthesis. These results suggest a relative failure of adenosine triphosphate production by mitochondria similar to that found in migraineurs; however, the exact mechanism by which this happens is not understood.

DIAGNOSIS

The diagnosis of cluster headache is made by its clinical features. Typically, a severe pain, which lasts between 10 and 90 minutes, wakes the patient from sleep. The pain is unilateral, periorbital, or over the temple, forehead, or cheek. The syndrome is usually accompanied by lacrimation, conjunctival injection, nasal stuffiness, ptosis, and miosis ipsilateral to the pain. During a cluster phase, the headaches, which may be single or multiple, occur with circadian predictability and have a similar duration. Unlike patients with migraine, who seek a dark, quiet environment, patients with cluster tend to pace, scream, and appear agitated; nausea and emesis are uncommon with cluster. A bout of cluster may last from several days to several months. Characteristically, an attack will be provoked by alcohol. The neurologic examination results, except for abnormalities during the headache as noted earlier, should be normal.

Chronic paroxysmal hemicrania is considered by some to be a variant of cluster. Its clinical description is similar to that of cluster, including the presence of autonomic signs. The major differences between these syndromes is that chronic paroxysmal hemicrania occurs primarily in women and the duration of pain is shorter, lasting less than half of what the average cluster headache does.

TREATMENT

Cluster headache should be treated prophylactically, that is, with preventive intent, because most attacks are over or nearly so by the time an abortive agent has exerted its effect. However, the same drugs that are effective at aborting migraine are effective for cluster. Dosages listed are meant to serve only as general guidelines.

1. Ergotamine tartrate (Wigraine [Cafergot was recently removed from the market]): 2 tablets at the onset of the headache followed by 1 tablet every 30 minutes until the headache is gone or until a maximum of 5 tablets per headache or 10 per week have been consumed.

2. Isometheptene (Midrin): 2 capsules at the onset

of the headache followed by 1 capsule every 60 minutes until the headache is gone or until a maximum of 5 capsules per headache or 10 per week have been consumed.

3. Preparations containing butalbital (a barbiturate), caffeine, and acetaminophen (Fioricet, Esgic) or aspirin (Fiorinal): 1 to 2 tablets may be taken, but the onset of action might occur after the current episode of head pain has run its course. These barbiturate preparations may be habit forming if used excessively.

4. Narcotic-containing preparations such as codeine plus acetaminophen (Tylenol No. 3) or butorphanol nasal spray (Stadol): These can be habit forming if used excessively.

5. Sumatriptan (Imitrex): 6 mg injectable, given subcutaneously; the onset of action of the oral formulation might occur after the current episode of head pain has run its course. The dose may be repeated in 1 to 2 hours if symptoms persist and then not again for 24 hours. Sumatriptan should not be administered within 24 hours of a vasoconstricting or an ergot drug (ergotamine, dihydroergotamine, methysergide) or isometheptene; it should not be administered within 2 weeks after discontinuation of a monoamine oxidase inhibitor. Because of its cardiotoxic potential, the first dose should be administered under medical supervision.

6. Oxygen inhalation: 100% oxygen should be administered at 8 L/minute through a nonrebreather mask for 10 to 15 minutes as soon after the onset of the attack as possible. If relief was incomplete, the treatment may be repeated after a 10 to 15 minute interval.

7. Dihydroergotamine (DHE): 0.5 to 1 mg, previously only available by injection; now available as a 4 mg/mL nasal spray.

8. Other nonsteroidal anti-inflammatory drugs: These may work for some patients with milder clusters. The onset of action of oral formulations might happen after the current episode of head pain has run its course. However, ketorolac (Toradol), 30 or 60 mg administered intramuscularly, may be effective.

9. Corticosteroids (for a very time-limited period and only under strict medical supervision): Corticosteroids are mainly useful as adjuvants to break a cluster and should be started simultaneously with a prophylactic agent.

10. Narcotics, such as meperidine (Demerol): In the emergency department or any other setting, these should be used only as drugs of last resort.

Drugs that are useful for prophylactic treatment:

1. Calcium-channel blockers (verapamil [Calan] and others): These drugs are frequently employed but usually require administration at relatively high doses, 240 to 480 mg/day, to be effective.

2. Anticonvulsants (valproic acid [Depakote], phenytoin [Dilantin], carbamazepine [Tegretol]): Valproic acid, in doses up to 1000 mg/day, alone or in combination with other prophylactic agents, may be useful.

3. Lithium carbonate: The initial dose is 300 mg at bed time. It may be increased to 300 mg two or three times daily. The drug has a small therapeutic window.

4. Methysergide (Sansert): This drug should not be used longer than 3 months without an interruption of several weeks because it can cause irreversible retroperitoneal, lung, and heart valve fibrosis. Its major acute side effect is gastrointestinal distress.

5. Beta blockers, such as propranolol (Inderal): These may be used as either first- or second-line drugs for cluster headache prophylaxis. In most healthy people, 60 to 80 mg once a day of the long-acting propranolol preparation may be started; lesser doses are usually ineffective. Side effects include dizziness from bradycardia, hypotension, or both; depression; worsening shortness of breath in patients with asthma or chronic obstructive pulmonary disease (COPD); gastrointestinal distress; blunting of hypoglycemic symptoms in diabetics; and vivid dreams. Dosages up to 400 mg/day, in divided doses, may be necessary.

6. Tricyclic antidepressants: These drugs, particularly amitriptyline (Elavil) at a starting dose of 10 to 25 mg at bedtime (10 mg at bedtime for elderly or frail persons or individuals who are highly sensitive to medications), are very active. Other useful tricyclics include imipramine (Tofranil), nortriptyline, desipramine, and protriptyline. Most patients who respond to amitriptyline, imipramine, nortriptyline, or desipramine do so at doses of 75 to 150 mg at bedtime; occasionally, patients require doses up to 300 mg/day. The major side effects from these drugs are due to their anticholinergic effects and include dry mouth, dizziness, difficulty waking up in the morning, urinary retention, glaucoma in patients with narrow angles, and cardiac arrhythmias. Tricyclics induce sleep, and this may be one of the mechanisms by which they help patients with cluster. If excessive morning sleepiness is a side effect, protriptyline may be tried.

7. The specific serotonin reuptake inhibitors such as paroxetine (20 to 40 mg/day) and fluoxetine (20 to 40 mg/day): These are worth a try in patients who do not respond to tricyclics or who have intolerable side effects from them. However, there is no compelling evidence that they are effective against cluster. They may be used alone or in combination with a tricyclic. The major side effects of the specific serotonin reuptake inhibitors include jitteriness, tremors, gastrointestinal distress, and occasionally headaches.

8. Ergotamine or isometheptene: Given the regularity and circadian predictability of headache onset during the cluster, a preparation containing ergotamine or isometheptene may be administered up to several hours before the anticipated attack, for example, at bedtime. This strategy, in addition to being part of a prophylactic regimen, is quite effective for a limited time until the prophylaxis becomes active.

9. Indomethacin: Among the nonsteroidal anti-inflammatory drugs, indomethacin appears to be more active than others, especially in patients with chronic paroxysmal hemicrania. Indomethacin can be administered in doses up to 150 mg/day.

BIBLIOGRAPHY

Fogan L: Treatment of cluster headache: A double blind comparison of oxygen vs. air inhalation. Arch Neurol 42:362–363, 1985.

Gabe IJ, Spiering CLH: Prophylactic treatment of cluster headache with verapamil. Headache 29:167-168, 1989.

International Headache Society: Classification and diagnostic criteria for headache disorders, cranial neuralgias, and facial pain. Cephalalgia 8(suppl 7):1-96, 1988.

Kudrow L: Response of cluster headache attack to oxygen inhalation. Headache 21:1-4, 1981.

Montagna P, Lodi R, Cortelli P, et al: Phosphorus magnetic resonance spectroscopy in cluster headache. Neurology 48:113-118, 1997.

The Sumatriptan Cluster Headache Study Group: Treatment of acute cluster headache with sumatriptan. N Engl J Med 325:322-326, 1991.

Wilkinson F, Pffafenrath V, Schenen J, et al: Migraine and cluster headache: Their management with sumatriptan: A critical review of the current clinical experience. Cephalalgia 15:337-357, 1995.

Chapter 44

Trigeminal Neuralgia

Carmen L. Dominguez, M.D.,
and Milan Stojanovic, M.D.

DEFINITION

Trigeminal neuralgia or tic douloureux is a chronic disorder manifested as severe, paroxysmal, recurrent, lancinating pain in the trigeminal nerve (cranial nerve V), the distribution of which is not associated with any sensory or motor dysfunction. The term *tic douloureux* (painful tic) was first used by Nicolas André in the 17th century to describe the grimacing and facial muscle spasms that accompanied episodes of severe pain of trigeminal neuralgia.

INCIDENCE

The average incidence of trigeminal neuralgia in the United States is 5 per 100,000 persons.[1] Although an infrequent occurrence, trigeminal neuralgia is 400 times more common among patients with multiple sclerosis than among the general population.[1] Most patients with trigeminal neuralgia are between 50 and 70 years of age.[2] However, younger patients have been found to suffer from this disorder. In the past, the diagnosis of tic douloureux in a young person implied the presence of undiagnosed multiple sclerosis. New information reveals that this is not the case.

SIGNS AND SYMPTOMS

1. The sudden onset, stabbing, sharp, "electric shock"–like pain in one or more divisions of the trigeminal nerve is a hallmark of trigeminal neuralgia. The mandibular and maxillary divisions are more commonly affected (V3, V2, and V1, in descending order). In a minority of patients, the distribution of pain can include the intermedius branch of the facial nerve (pain localized to the ear or posterior pharynx) or the glossopharyngeal nerve (pain localized to the posterior tongue, tonsillar fossa, or larynx).[2]
2. The pain is unilateral in 97% of patients.[3]
3. Intermittent episodes of pain usually last seconds to minutes. The frequency of episodes is variable, but it can be increased by emotional and physical stress.
4. Nonpainful stimulus to certain areas (trigger zones) of the face, head, lips, tongue, and upper neck can precipitate an attack. Environmental (cold) and tactile stimuli and simple daily functions such as chewing, talking, swallowing, and smiling can act as triggering factors. Severe prolonged attacks can lead to depression, dehydration, anxiety, sleep deprivation, and suicide.
5. Minimal or no sensory deficits are present in the painful areas.

DIAGNOSIS

The diagnosis of trigeminal neuralgia is based on the clinical history and physical examination findings. A complete history of the symptoms can help the physician to differentiate this condition from other types of facial pain originating from diseases of the jaw, teeth, sinuses, muscles of mastication, pharynx, and blood vessels. Important syndromes to consider in the differential diagnosis of trigeminal neuralgia include atypical facial pain, postherpetic neuralgia, cluster headaches, and temporomandibular joint disease. Although these syndromes can present as unilateral facial pain, classic trigeminal neuralgia is characterized by the lancinating and intermittent nature of pain (Table 44–1).[2]

Magnetic resonance imaging (MRI) of the head that focuses in the area of the pons can help identify any pathologic condition of the trigeminal nerve root. This test is not very specific for trigeminal neuralgia, because a third of the patients that have an MRI for an unrelated condition have abnormalities in the area of the trigeminal nerve root. A computed tomographic (CT) scan can also be helpful when an MRI is not available to detect tumor, angiomas, or bony abnormalities of the base of the skull.

ETIOLOGY

The cause and pathophysiology of tic douloureux is not entirely clear. In 85% of patients the trigeminal

TABLE 44–1. FACIAL PAIN SYNDROMES

	Trigeminal Neuralgia	**Atypical Facial Pain**	**TMJ Disease**
Duration	Seconds to minutes, weeks to years	Weeks to years	Constant, weeks to years
Quality	Lancinating, electric, shock–like, stabbing, intense	Diffuse burning, aching, dull	Deep
Location	Unilateral, trigeminal nerve distribution	Can be bilateral in the trigeminal nerve and upper neck area; usually does not follow a nerve distribution	Unilateral in the area of the temporomandibular joint
Triggering factors	Noxious stimulation of rare facial trigger zone areas	Stress, fatigue	None
Associated symptoms	Minimal or no facial tenderness; usually no sensory deficits	No tenderness; facial dysesthesias, paresthesias	No sensory dysfunction
Classic treatment	Carbamazepine	Tricyclic antidepressants	Nonsteroidal anti-inflammatory drugs

Data from Melzack R, Wall P: Textbook of Pain., ed 3. New York, Churchill Livingstone, 1994, pp 699–710.

nerve root is compressed at the level of the pons by aberrant or tortuous blood vessels, tumor (including acoustic neuroma, cholesteatoma, and meningioma), or bony abnormalities.[2]

In patients with multiple sclerosis (2% to 3%), trigeminal neuralgia is thought to be due to demyelinating plaques in the trigeminal posterior root.[2] However, these plaques can occur anywhere on the trigeminal tract or nucleus.

Some researchers have proposed that tic douloureux is due to hyperactivity in the trigeminal nucleus. It is thought that the structural lesion that compresses the trigeminal nerve can lead to demyelination of the trigeminal root, leading to ectopic unregulated electrical activity at the level of the nuclei and the peripheral nerve, which translates into painful sensations.[3]

PHARMACOLOGIC TREATMENT

Carbamazepine

Carbamazepine (Tegretol) is considered the first-line drug for treatment of trigeminal neuralgia. It acts by suppressing synaptic transmission at the trigeminal nucleus. It is thought to be effective in 50% of patients.[2] The recommended starting dose is 100 to 200 mg at nighttime to three times daily. The maximum dose is 1200 mg/day. Common side effects include nausea, drowsiness, dizziness, rash, diplopia, hepatic dysfunction, and aplastic anemia. Close monitoring of the liver function and hematologic parameters throughout treatment is essential.

Phenytoin

Phenytoin (Dilantin) can be used as a second-line drug if carbamazepine is not effective. The initial dose is 100 mg/day and should be gradually increased to a maximum of 300 to 400 mg/day (100 mg three times a day).

Baclofen

Baclofen (Lioresal), an antispasmodic agent and muscle relaxant, can be useful in patients who do not respond to anticonvulsants. It is usually used in combination with anticonvulsants due to its synergistic effect. The initial dose is 5 to 10 mg, three times daily, to a maximum of 40 to 80 mg/day. Side effects include drowsiness, confusion, weakness, and hepatic dysfunction. Many patients are intolerant of these side effects. Some studies suggest that the use of a specific stereoisomer, L-baclofen, can be more effective and produce fewer side effects than the usual racemic mixture.

Mexiletine

Mexiletine, an antiarrhythmic agent, can be useful if the patient responds to an intravenous lidocaine test. The initial dose is 150 mg, three times daily, to a maximum of 1200 mg/day.

Other neuropathic pain medications, such as gabapentin or dextromethorphan, can be used if the aforementioned oral medication regimens are ineffective or only partially effective. However, the efficacy of these medications has not been adequately studied.

Opioids

Opioids can be helpful during episodes of severe pain; however, their long-term efficacy is low for the treatment of trigeminal neuralgia as well as for other kinds of deafferentation pain. If there is a clear benefit to the patient, the fear of prescribing opioids for nonmalignant pain is unsubstantiated. If opioids are found to be helpful for a particular patient, long-acting preparations are preferable.

INVASIVE TREATMENT

Trigeminal Nerve Blocks

Trigeminal nerve blocks with local anesthetics and/or steroids can provide temporary pain relief while oral medication doses are gradually maximized. A minority of patients might experience prolonged pain relief after one or more nerve blocks.

Gasserian Ganglion Alcohol Injections

Gasserian ganglion alcohol injections usually provide longer-lasting pain relief than blocks with local anesthetic. Patients can be pain-free for up to 1 year.[5] Repeated injections can lead to loss of sensation in the trigeminal nerve distribution. The main disadvantage of this technique is a high recurrence rate.

Gangliolysis

Radiofrequency gasserian ganglion ablation (gangliolysis) is performed under fluoroscopy in patients with intractable trigeminal neuralgia. The purpose of this procedure is to destroy the pain fibers by coagulation of the nerve via a percutaneous electrode. About 80% of the patients have 1 year of pain relief and 50% have up to 5 years of pain relief. The complication rate is less than 0.5% and the recurrence rate is 15% to 20%.[2] Among the most common complications are painful paresthesias, painful loss of facial sensation (anesthesia dolorosa), and keratitis secondary to corneal denervation. In general, there is an inverse relationship between the degree of facial numbness that a patient experiences after this procedure and the likelihood of recurrence. The probability of dysesthesias in the hypoalgesic area increases with profound facial numbness.

Jannetta's Procedure

Microvascular decompression of the trigeminal nerve root (Jannetta's procedure) consists of a retroauricular craniotomy or craniectomy in which the trigeminal nerve root at the level of the pons and the compressing blood vessel (usually the superior cerebellar artery) are identified. A small piece of Dacron sponge or a small piece of muscle tissue is interposed between the two structures to avoid recompression. The mortality rate is 0.5% and the morbidity rate is 5% to 15%. The success rate at 5 years is 70% to 80%.[2] The most common complications include unilateral facial paresis, deafness, and ataxia.

REFERENCES

1. Reder AT, Arnason B: Trigeminal neuralgia in multiple sclerosis relieved by a prostaglandin E analogue. Neurology 45(6):1097-1100, 1995.
2. Melzack R, Wall P: Textbook of Pain, ed 3. New York, Churchill Livingstone, 1994, pp 699-710.
3. Raj PP: Pain Medicine: A Comprehensive Review. St Louis, Mosby-Year Book, 1996, pp 394-395.
4. Rovit R: Trigeminal neuralgia. Compr Ther 18:17-21, 1992.
5. Slettebo H, Hirschberg H, Lindegaard KF: Long term results after percutaneous retrogasserian glycerol rhizotomy in patients with trigeminal neuralgia. Acta Neurochir 122:231-235, 1993.

SUGGESTED READINGS

Cheng TM, Cascino TL: Comprehensive study of diagnosis and treatment of trigeminal neuralgia secondary to tumors. Neurology 43:2298-2302, 1993.
Dyck PP: Peripheral Neuropathy, ed 3. Philadelphia, WB Saunders, 1993, pp 810-814.
Fromm G, Terrence CF: Comparison of L-baclofen and racemic baclofen in trigeminal neuralgia. Neurology 37:1725-1728, 1987.
Fromm G: Trigeminal neuralgia and related disorders. Neurol Clin 7:305-319, 1989.
Rappaport ZH: Trigeminal neuralgia: The role of self-sustaining discharge in the trigeminal ganglion. Pain 56:127-138, 1994.
Rowland L: Merritt's Textbook of Neurology. Philadelphia, Lea & Febiger, 1989, pp 419-421.

Chapter 45

Pharmacologic Treatment of Headache

Gary M. Reisfield, M.D.,
and David Borsook, M.D., Ph.D.

Despite our incomplete knowledge of the pathogenesis of most headache types, identification and modification of risk factors and important advances in pharmacologic therapies have greatly decreased suffering. We discuss several headache types notable because of their frequency or dramatic response to specific treatments.

MIGRAINE

Migraine is a common cause of primary headaches, affecting perhaps 20% of the population. The disorder is three times as prevalent in females and there is a positive family history in about 70% of cases. A prodrome, consisting of lethargy, hyperactivity, or other symptoms, often occurs 1 or 2 days before the headache onset. Migraine without aura (common migraine) is typically a moderate to severe, throbbing, unilateral headache lasting from 4 hours to 3 days. It is associated with nausea, vomiting, photophobia, and phonophobia. Migraine with aura (classic migraine), which affects a distinct minority of migraineurs, includes phenomena such as visual scotoma, unilateral numbness or weakness, and visual disturbances, usually within 1 hour of headache onset.

Acute Treatment

Nonsteroidal Anti-inflammatory Drugs

A variety of nonsteroidal anti-inflammatory drugs (NSAIDs), especially in combination with an antiemetic, can be effective treatment, especially if introduced early in the attack. Naproxen, 500 to 1000 mg, and ibuprofen, 400 to 800 mg, as well as diclofenac, mefenamic acid, ketoprofen, and tolfenamic acid have been shown to be beneficial in double-blind trials, although the benefits have often been marginal.[1] Side effects are referable primarily to the gastrointestinal system. Contraindications include peptic ulcer disease, renal disease, and oral anticoagulant therapy.

Sumatriptan

Sumatriptan is a selective agonist at 5-HT$_{1D}$ receptor sites. Eight randomized, controlled clinical trials have demonstrated the efficacy of this drug administered by either oral or subcutaneous routes.[2] The oral dose is 25 to 100 mg, with a maximum daily dose of 300 mg. The subcutaneous dose is 6 mg, with a maximum recommended daily dose of 12 mg. Side effects include tingling or warm sensations, flushing, chest pain or pressure, and throat tightness. Coronary vasospasm has been reported after both oral and subcutaneous administration, making coronary artery disease a contraindication to sumatriptan administration.[2]

Dihydroergotamine

Dihydroergotamine, an ergot alkaloid, has been shown to be effective in randomized, controlled trials. It is thought to carry a lower risk than ergotamine of causing rebound headaches during chronic use.[3] The dose is 0.5 mg, given intravenously, or 1 to 2 mg, given subcutaneously, intramuscularly, or transnasally, and may be repeated once. Side effects include nausea and vomiting and sinus tachycardia or bradycardia. Contraindications include coronary artery disease, significant peripheral vascular disease, and uncontrolled hypertension.

Prophylactic Treatment

Prophylactic treatment is indicated for attacks that occur with a frequency of at least twice monthly, are not responsive to abortive treatments, and are severe enough to cause physical or psychological impairment of normal activities.

β-Blockers

The clinical effectiveness of β-blockers, specifically atenolol, metoprolol, nadolol, propranolol, and timolol, in reducing the frequency and severity of migraines has been demonstrated repeatedly. Several well-controlled studies have demonstrated the efficacy of propranolol

197

in oral doses starting at 80 mg/day and increasing incrementally to a maximum of 320 mg/day.[4] The relatively low potential for side effects is important because of the likely long-term administration of the drug. Contraindications include asthma, diabetes, congestive heart failure, and certain atrioventricular conduction defects.

Calcium-Channel Blockers

Double-blind, placebo-controlled studies have shown calcium-channel blockers to be of benefit in migraine prophylaxis. Nimodipine, nifedipine, and verapamil have all shown benefit in terms of reduction of frequency and severity of headaches. The studies were remarkable for a high dropout rate, perhaps due to the side effects of constipation and orthostasis. Tolerance has also been a problem with these agents.[4]

Valproic Acid

Valproic acid has been demonstrated as effective prophylaxis in placebo-controlled, randomized clinical trials.[2] The dose is titrated to achieve plasma levels of 70 to 120 mg/L. Side effects, which tend to be mild, include nausea and vomiting, asthenia, and somnolence. The rare occurrence of hepatotoxicity mandates periodic checks of liver function. The drug is contraindicated during pregnancy.

TENSION-TYPE HEADACHE

Tension-type headache is the most common headache type, with a lifetime prevalence of 69% in men and 88% in women.[5] It exists in both episodic and chronic types. The pathogenesis is incompletely understood. International Headache Society diagnostic criteria for tension-type headache require more than ten headaches that meet the following criteria:

1. Duration of 30 minutes to 7 days
2. At least two of the following:
   a. Pressing or tightening (nonpulsatile) quality
   b. Mild-to-moderate intensity, not interfering with normal functioning
   c. Bilateral location
   d. Not exacerbated by normal physical activity
3. No associated nausea or vomiting
4. Photophobia or phonophobia, but not both
5. No other physical abnormality as a potential cause

Psychotherapy or relaxation methods, including meditation, hypnosis, and biofeedback, can be useful in many patients with tension-type headaches, particularly when underlying stressors or an anxiety or depressive disorder is present. Pharmacotherapy, however, is the mainstay of treatment for this type of headache.

Acute Treatment

Nonsteroidal Anti-inflammatory Drugs

NSAIDs and acetaminophen are the first-line treatments, and most individuals are helped by over-the-counter preparations. Acetaminophen is generally safe in recommended dosages, although there is some concern about renal toxic effects with chronic treatment. The NSAIDs have well-known toxic effects, including those involving the gastrointestinal, renal, and coagulation systems. A relatively new NSAID, nabumetone, is relatively selective for the COX-2 isozyme and is not excreted into the bile, making this potentially safer to the gastric mucosa. No data are available, however, on its efficacy in tension-type headaches.

Tricyclic Antidepressants

For patients who require daily analgesics for headaches, prophylaxis may often be achieved with a tricyclic antidepressant. Tricyclic antidepressants act by preventing presynaptic reuptake of norepinephrine and serotonin, although the exact mechanism by which they prevent headaches is incompletely understood. A good deal of evidence supports the efficacy of amitriptyline in this setting.[4] Side effects are prominent with this agent, including dry mouth, orthostasis, constipation, and sedation. Dosage should start at 10 to 25 mg at bedtime and gradually be escalated every 7 to 10 days until headaches are controlled or a dose of 100 to 200 mg/day has been reached. Other tricyclic agents, such as nortriptyline and desipramine, which have fewer anticholinergic and antihistaminergic side effects, and the newer selective serotonin reuptake inhibitors, such as fluoxetine, have been used, but no clinical trials are available that support their effectiveness.

Other Treatments

For particularly severe headaches, or headaches with some migraine features, migraine-type therapies can be useful. β-Blockers, calcium-channel blockers, and dihydroergotamine, especially, have been found to be particularly efficacious in this setting.[4]

Benzodiazepines and opioids should be avoided in most circumstances because of the chronicity of this condition and the attendant dangers of dependence in this patient population.

CLUSTER HEADACHE

Cluster headache is a severe unilateral orbital or periorbital headache, often stabbing in nature, which reaches its peak within 15 minutes and generally lasts less than 2 hours. Headaches occur one to six times per day and have a propensity to wake patients from sleep. As the name implies, the headaches tend to be clustered in 4- to 12-week cycles with pain-free intervals of 1 month to several years. Associated symptoms include lacrimation (84%), conjunctival injection (58%), ptosis (57%), nasal stuffiness (48%), rhinorrhea (43%), bradycardia (43%), nausea (40%), and general perspiration (26%).[6] Cluster headache is primarily a disease of males, with a male-to-female ratio of 5:1 to 6:1 and a mean age at onset of 30 years. Some association with cigarette smoking and alcohol use is often present. It is uncommon to find a positive family history for cluster headaches.

The two major types of cluster headache, the more common episodic type (which affects approximately 80% of patients) and the chronic type, are distinguished by the length of the remission period. Chronic cluster headache is defined by a lack of remission within a 1-year period.

However, in terms of pharmacologic treatment, these types may largely be considered a single entity.

Acute Treatment

Oxygen

Administration of 100% oxygen via face mask at a rate of 7 L/minute has been found to be effective in about three fourths of patients. However, headaches have a tendency to recur shortly after cessation of therapy.[7]

Sumatriptan

As acute treatment, sumatriptan should be administered subcutaneously because of its rapid onset. A randomized crossover study has demonstrated significant improvement in headache symptoms in 74% of patients given a single 6-mg subcutaneous dose.[8]

Glucocorticoids

Glucocorticoids are valuable agents, often providing headache relief within 48 hours of beginning therapy. Prednisone, at a dosage of 40 to 60 mg/day in a single daily dose, is tapered over a 3-week period. Maintenance therapy, as outlined below, should be started promptly, because headache is likely to recur during tapering of the steroid unless therapeutic levels of maintenance agents have been established.[7]

Prophylactic Treatment

Calcium-Channel Blockers

Prophylactic treatment is often initiated with verapamil, although some evidence has suggested efficacy of other calcium-channel blockers. It often takes at least a week to show clinical effect, leading some to suggest that the action of verapamil on serotonin receptors, rather than calcium channels, is operative here. Several reports indicate that verapamil is effective in 70% of patients.[7] Dosage begins at 80 mg, three to four times daily, and may require titration to 600 mg/day. Verapamil can be slowly tapered after the patient has been headache-free for several weeks.

Lithium

Several studies have shown lithium to be effective prophylaxis in approximately 70% of patients with cluster headaches.[7] A daily dose of 600 to 900 mg is required to achieve therapeutic plasma levels of 0.5 to 1.0 mEq/L.[7] Side effects, which generally occur at levels greater than 1.5 μmol/L, include nausea, polyuria, diarrhea, and tremor. Renal and thyroid function studies should be performed prior to initiation of therapy and, in addition to serum lithium levels, should be rechecked at regular intervals.

Other Treatments

Ergotamine is indicated at an oral dose of 2 mg at bedtime for attacks that occur at night. It may also be used for headaches that are resistant to verapamil or lithium.[7] Methysergide has a clinical efficacy comparable to that of verapamil or lithium. The recommended dose is 3 to 6 mg/day. Tachyphylaxis is common. The use of ergotamine is limited by retroperitoneal, pulmonary, and endomyocardial fibrosis, which mandate discontinuance of the drug for 2 or more months each year. Early evidence suggests roles for valproic acid, transdermal clonidine, and intranasal capsaicin. Optimal dosage schedules have not been established.

Alcohol and tobacco products should be avoided, especially if they are identified as cluster headache triggers.

INDOMETHACIN-SENSITIVE HEADACHE

There is a heterogeneous group of headache disorders that merits attention. Despite the rarity of the disorders included in this group, they are responsive (sometimes exquisitely so) to indomethacin. Chronic paroxysmal hemicrania shares many features with cluster headache, including severity, laterality, and autonomic features. But it is distinguished by its brevity, greater frequency, lack of remission, and female preponderance. Hemicrania continua headaches are moderate to severely painful, lateralized, and continuous, with superimposed jabbing pains or focal throbbing pains lasting up to 45 minutes and occurring up to five times per day. Three other descriptively named headache types—benign cough headache, benign exertional headache, and sexual headache—are not as absolutely responsive to indomethacin.

Indomethacin, an inhibitor of prostaglandin synthesis and phosphodiesterase, is rapidly absorbed after oral or rectal administration, with peak blood levels achieved within 1 to 2 hours and an elimination half-life of 5 to 10 hours. Gastrointestinal side effects, such as nausea and dyspepsia, which are prominent with this drug may be minimized by co-administration with food and/or H_2-blockers, slow dose escalation, or rectal administration. Central nervous system side effects include dizziness, fatigue, and somnolence. The initial dose is 25 mg, orally or rectally, twice daily, which may be increased by 50 mg every 3 or 4 days until symptoms have been relieved or a maximum of 250 mg/day has been reached.[9]

POST–DURAL PUNCTURE HEADACHE

Post–dural puncture headache, as a result of spinal anesthesia, diagnostic lumbar puncture, or myelography, is a frequent cause of secondary headache. It is seen more frequently in females, in the young, and in those with a history of motion sickness or previous post–dural puncture headache. It is also related to the size and bevel design of the spinal needle. The headache usually begins 1 to 3 days following the procedure, and it resolves within 5 days in the majority of patients. Symptoms consist of a postural headache that typically is partially or completely relieved on assuming a supine position. The headache may be bilateral, frontal, and/or occipital and may involve neck stiffness or soreness. Auditory or visual disturbances are rare, particularly cranial nerve III palsy. Effective prevention includes using the smallest effective spinal needle, keeping the bevel of the needle parallel to the long axis of the body to avoid cutting dural fibers, or using a noncutting needle tip (e.g., Sprotte or Whitacre). It is of note that enforced recumbency does not reduce the incidence of post–dural puncture headache. In fact, several reports suggest that early ambulation may actually decrease the incidence of this type of headache.[10]

Most of these headaches resolve spontaneously over several days. Symptomatic treatment (e.g., bed rest, copious fluid intake, and analgesics) is effective while spontaneous dural healing occurs. Caffeine, 0.5 mg intravenously over 1 to 2 hours or 500 mg orally, is an effective adjunct to this regimen.

For the patient with a severe headache, the patient who cannot wait for spontaneous resolution (e.g., the postpartum patient), or the patient in whom conservative therapy fails, epidural blood patch is a safe and effective treatment. Fifteen to 20 mL of aseptically drawn blood is injected into the epidural space at a rate of 1 mL every 3 seconds. If it is injected too quickly the patient will complain of an uncomfortable pressure sensation, which subsides within a minute of cessation of injection at that point. Frequently, additional blood can be injected at a very slow rate without further pressure. The patient should remain supine for approximately 30 minutes after the procedure. This is effective in approximately 90% of patients. A second patch may be effective in an additional 7%.[11] The patient should be advised to avoid strenuous activities for several days, particularly those that increase intra-abdominal pressure and may thereby cause dislodgement of the clot. Stool softeners should be prescribed, as should antitussives, if necessary. Some evidence suggests that epidural saline infusion is as effective as epidural blood patch. The more prolonged course necessitated by the infusion can be a major drawback, particularly in the outpatient setting.

Not all headaches after procedures that broach the dura are post–dural puncture headaches. The differential diagnosis in this setting includes meningitis, epidural abscess, and subarachnoid hemorrhage, as well as any preexisting primary headache disorder.

REFERENCES

1. Pfaffenrath V, Scherzer S: Analgesics and NSAIDs in the treatment of the acute migraine attack. Cephalalgia 15(suppl):14–20, 1995.
2. Tfelt-Hansen P: Drug treatment of migraine: Acute treatment and migraine prophylaxis. Curr Opin Neurol 9:211–213, 1996.
3. Ferrari M, Haan J: Acute treatment of migraine attacks. Curr Opin Neurol 8:237–242, 1995.
4. Kumar K, Cooney T: Headaches. Med Clin North Am 79:261–286, 1995.
5. Rasmussen BK, Jensen R, Schroll M, et al: Epidemiology of headache in a general population: A prevalence study. J Clin Epidemiol 44:1147–1151, 1991.
6. Manzoni CG, Terzano MG, Bono G, et al: Cluster headache: Clinical findings in 180 patients. Cephalalgia 3:21–30, 1983.
7. Lewis TA, Solomon GD: Advances in cluster headache management. Cleveland Clin J Med 63:237–244, 1996.
8. Ekbom K: Treatment of cluster headache: Clinical trials, design and results. Cephalalgia 15(suppl):33–36, 1995.
9. Raskin NH: Headache. New York, Churchill Livingstone, 1988.
10. Peterman SB: Postmyelography headache: A review. Radiology 200:765–770, 1996.
11. Leibold RA, Yealy DM, Coppola M, et al: Post-dural puncture headache: Characteristics, management, and prevention. Ann Emerg Med 22:1863–1870, 1993.

Chapter 46

Post–Dural Puncture Headache

Arti Patel, M.D.

In 1898, August Bier recorded one of the first accounts of a post–dural puncture headache. After undergoing a spinal injection of cocaine, he noticed a severe headache that was postural in nature. The headache was most prominent while he was in the upright or sitting position, and diminished in the recumbent position. This is the classic description of a post–dural puncture headache. Patients usually describe a severe, dull, nonthrobbing pain that is fronto-occipital in location and may be associated with nausea, vomiting, visual changes, tinnitus, or deafness.

The overall incidence of the post–dural puncture headache ranges from 1% to 30% and is related to many variables. The majority of cases resolve within 10 days, but after considerable inconvenience to the patient. Due to the postural nature of the headache, patients frequently miss days from work, extend their hospital stay, and avoid simple daily activities; in the case of the obstetric population, mothers are unable to participate in the care of their newborn babies.

PATHOPHYSIOLOGY

Leakage of cerebrospinal fluid (CSF) through the dural puncture appears to be the cause of post–dural puncture headache. As a needle is inserted through the skin it encounters several layers before reaching the subarachnoid space. The needle penetrates subcutaneous tissue, the supraspinous ligament, the interspinous ligament, and, finally, the ligamentum flavum, to reach the epidural space. If the needle is advanced further, it pierces the dura mater and arachnoid mater to enter the subarachnoid space, in which the CSF is contained.

CSF is produced at an average rate of 500 mL/day, and approximately 150 mL is circulating at any given time around the brain and spinal cord. Excess fluid may be excreted via arachnoid villi; however, the body cannot immediately compensate for loss of CSF.

A caudal shift of the brain occurs with a decreased amount of CSF, causing dural stretching and traction on pain-sensitive intracranial structures. The majority of pain-sensitive areas are supplied by branches of the first division of the fifth cranial nerve, so pain is experienced frontally. Occipital pain is thought to arise from the dura of the posterior fossa, which is supplied by the ninth and tenth cranial nerves. Tension on cranial nerve X may stimulate the chemoreceptors in the medulla to produce nausea. Traction on the first three cervical nerves may cause neck muscle stiffness.

Although the body cannot immediately produce an increased amount of CSF in response to leakage around a needle puncture, it can cause venous dilation in an attempt to compensate for loss of intracranial volume. This cranial vasodilation may be responsible for the sensation of pressure many patients experience. The postural nature of the headache is explained by the change in intracranial CSF pressure. When a patient is upright, the intracranial pressure decreases and the intracranial venous distention increases, worsening the headache. When the patient is supine, an equalization of intracranial cisternal and lumbar CSF pressures takes place, so no expansion of the venous system occurs, and the headache improves.

INCIDENCE AND RISK FACTORS

The overall incidence of post–dural puncture headache varies from less than 1% to 30%. Dural punctures with larger needles (e.g., 16- and 18-gauge epidural needles) are associated with an incidence of 70% to 80%. On average, symptoms develop 24 to 48 hours after the dural puncture. It is at this time that the rate of CSF loss exceeds the rate of production.

Post–dural puncture headaches are not life-threatening and are usually self-limited to 3 to 5 days. They seldom last longer than 1 week, with or without therapy, and 80% to 85% of cases are of less than 5 days' duration. Forty-nine percent of headaches are mild and 35% are moderate. The 15% that are rated as severe are extremely incapacitating and are associated with dehydration from nausea and vomiting.

Certain patient populations are at an increased risk

for development of post–dural puncture headache. Patients aged 20 to 40 years are most susceptible to post–dural puncture headache, whereas the lowest incidence occurs in pediatric, adolescent, and elderly patients. Women are more likely to be affected than men when risk is adjusted for age. This increased rate is present even when numbers are corrected for the obstetric population. Parturients constitute the highest-risk category for post–dural puncture headache, to which a number of factors contribute. Increases in CSF pressure from bearing down during vaginal delivery and postpartum decreases in intra-abdominal and peridural pressure may all contribute to increases in the incidence of post–dural puncture headache in this patient population. The lesser incidence of post–dural puncture headache in elderly persons is due to decreases in the elasticity of cranial structures, which occurs in the normal aging process, and in overall pain sensitivity.

PREVENTION

The prevention of headache after a dural puncture revolves around minimizing the postpuncture leakage of CSF. Traditional approaches have ranged from restricting activity to complete bed rest and have included application of abdominal binders to increase abdominal pressure, thereby decreasing leakage. These methods do little to prevent the occurrence of headache. In fact, the recumbent position may delay the onset and diagnosis of a headache and the discharge of a patient from the hospital. Patients should be instructed to lie in the supine position, mostly because this is the position in which they are most comfortable, not because it is a prophylactic measure against headache.

Other preventive measures relate to the needle size, shape, and bevel orientation. Most physicians agree that there is a direct correlation between needle size and risk of dural puncture. Vandam and Dripps[1] noted that the incidence ranges from 18% with a 16-gauge needle to 5% with a 26-gauge needle, whereas the overall risk of post–dural puncture headache was 11% in 11,000 cases of spinal anesthesia. The use of 29- and 30-gauge needles is associated with a less than 1% incidence of post–dural puncture headache; however these needles contribute to a higher rate of failure secondary to difficulty in their placement.

One study showed that it can take up to 61 seconds for CSF to appear at the hub of a 29-gauge needle.[2] For procedures such as myelography, a 25- or 26-gauge needle can be used, but physician acceptance of the smaller needles is hindered by the difficulty of injecting viscous contrast material through such a small orifice. Patients who have undergone previous back procedures may have scar tissue that is tough to penetrate with a small-gauge needle.

The size and shape of the dural puncture site is affected not only by the size but also the design of the needle tip. Blunt tip needles, such as Whitacre and Sprotte needles, are associated with lower post–dural puncture headache rates than are bevel-tip needles of the same size, such as a Quincke needle. Although the blunt tip needle produces a round hole and compresses dural fibers, the bevel tip needle has a tendency to cut dural fibers and to cause a more traumatic entry. In an in vitro study by Cruickshank and Hopkinson,[2] the median loss of volume in 5 minutes was statistically significantly less with a 22-gauge Whitacre needle than with a 22-gauge Quincke needle. This study was done on human postmortem thoracolumbar dura mater. The same study showed that there was a 21% reduction in the leakage of CSF if the Quincke bevel was parallel to the large axis of the vertebral column. Inserting the needle parallel to the dural fibers promotes separation rather than cutting of the fibers, thereby reducing the incidence of headache.

It has been suggested that an acute angle of insertion of a needle into the dura may produce a flap that can readily close on itself. This "tin lid" flap of dura can close holes made by even large spiral needles.

Some clinicians advocate the use of a prophylactic epidural saline infusion for patients with unintentional dural punctures who have an epidural catheter in place. It is believed that this reduces the incidence and severity of headache by preventing the leakage of CSF while a fibrin clot forms over the dural puncture site. Various studies have been done comparing controls to groups with intermittent boluses of saline as well as groups with a 24-hour continuous infusion of saline.[3,4] Although these studies have produced varying results on the efficacy of epidural saline in the prevention of post–dural puncture headache, none has been reproduced. Further studies need to be carried out before a final answer is found.

TREATMENT

Once a post–dural puncture headache is suspected, a number of treatment options are available, ranging from noninvasive pharmacologic approaches to invasive procedures. Because the natural history is one of spontaneous resolution, many authors recommend approximately 24 hours of conservative therapy. If the headache is severe, disabling, or accompanied by nausea, vomiting, visual disturbance, or tinnitus, the clinician must rule out tension headache, migraine headache, meningitis, and subarachnoid hemorrhage. If a classic history of postural headache persists and other causes are eliminated, several treatment options exist.

Conservative measures usually start with asking the patient to observe bed rest to avoid the discomfort associated with an upright position. Analgesics, such as acetaminophen and nonsteroidal anti-inflammatory drugs, may provide some benefit. Many postsurgical patients are already receiving mild opiates to treat postoperative pain.

Caffeine, a methylxanthine known to cause vasoconstriction, has been tried with some success. If one mechanism of headache production is cerebral vasodilation to compensate for CSF volume loss, then the vasoconstrictive properties of caffeine can cause a reduction of symptoms. Other effects of caffeine are a decrease in cerebral blood flow, an increase in cerebral vascular resistance, and an increase in CSF production by stimulation of sodium-potassium pumps. All of these contribute to decreasing the propagation of the headache.

Because caffeine is inexpensive, easy to obtain, and fairly risk free, it may be a reasonable first option in the treatment of post–dural puncture headache. Camann and colleagues[5] evaluated 40 postpartum patients with headache using a randomized, double-blind, placebo-controlled study. After receiving 300 mg of caffeine or placebo, orally, a visual analogue scale was used to evaluate the severity of symptoms. Although a 300% decrease in the visual analogue pain scale was noted at 4 hours in the caffeine group as compared to the placebo group, no difference was seen at 24 hours.

Intravenous (IV) caffeine has also been studied. The study by Sechzer and Abel[6,7] is most often cited as a randomized, double-blind, placebo-controlled study evaluating IV caffeine for the treatment of post–dural puncture headaches. Forty-one patients who suffered from headaches initially received placebo or IV caffeine (500 mg). All 41 patients subsequently received 500 mg of caffeine IV, regardless of initial treatment or outcome. Seventy-one percent of patients ultimately achieved relief. The investigators concluded that IV caffeine is a simple and effective method to treat post–dural puncture headache.

As noted, both oral and intravenous forms of caffeine have been successful in treating post–dural puncture headaches. Although the oral form is well absorbed, convenient, and readily available in caffeinated beverages, the specific amounts vary greatly, making it difficult to assess the exact quantity administered. However, IV caffeine, combined with sodium benzoate to enhance solubility, is easy to deliver, but it requires a trip to the physician's office or hospital for administration. The IV method may be most suitable for the postoperative inpatient, whereas the oral form may be well adapted for the outpatient with a mild to moderate headache.

Other pharmacologic parenteral agents used to treat post–dural puncture headaches include sumatriptan and adrenocorticotropic hormone. Both have therapeutic potential but need in-depth study before a conclusion about their efficacy in treating post–dural puncture headache can be made.

Intervention that involves penetration of the epidural space includes epidural saline, dextran patch, and epidural blood patch. The administration of these agents is thought to seal the tear created by the needle entry. The same risks that apply to any epidural needle placement are involved with these approaches. One must obtain a clear negative history of infection and coagulopathy prior to proceeding. The epidural placement of non-blood agents may be an alternative for several patient populations, including Jehovah's Witnesses, whose religion forbids blood product administration, and HIV-infected patients without CNS disease, in whom CNS introduction of blood may promote CNS spread of infection.

Epidural sodium chloride, 0.9%, given to treat post–dural puncture headache dates to 1950, when Rice and Dobbs[8] reported immediate relief of headache in 99.5% of cases with a 54% recurrence rate. Since then Usubi-

aga and co-workers[9] and Baysinger and colleagues[10] showed that intermittent injections of sodium chloride, 0.9%, in amounts of 10 to 30 mL relieved symptoms long term. The proposed mechanism of action of epidural sodium chloride, 0.9%, is that it causes an increase in epidural pressure, decreasing the outflow of CSF from that site. Another theory is that the sodium chloride provides transient tamponade until a fibrin clot can occur.

Epidural dextran works by the same mechanism of action as sodium chloride, 0.9%. Because of the large molecular weight of dextran, slower absorption from the epidural space provides a longer period of increased pressure. Successful studies have been conducted by Stevens and Peters-Asdourian,[11] and Barrios-Alarcon and colleagues.[12] The former performed the study in an HIV-positive patient and in another patient with possible systemic *Staphylococcus* infection. After an appropriate test to check for an anaphylactic reaction (20 mL of IV dextran), 20 mL of epidural dextran was administered. Both patients, whose headaches were initially refractory to bed rest, hydration, and caffeine, experienced long-lasting relief within 10 minutes of injection.

Most authors agree that the epidural blood patch is the most reliable cure for post–dural puncture headache. It is estimated that a 96% to 98%[13] success rate can be expected from a properly executed blood patch. The injection, first discovered by Gormley in 1960,[14] involves approximately 15 to 20 mL of autologous blood into the epidural space. Two persons are required to perform this procedure: one person gains access to the epidural space and the other obtains the blood in a sterile fashion. An intravenous line may be beneficial for hydration if the patient has experienced intractable nausea and vomiting.

Although the original reports recommended injection of 2 to 3 mL, failure rates were high. Fifteen to 20 mL seems to be the amount that has a higher cure rate. The blood should be injected at a rate of 1.0 mL over 3 seconds so as not to cause call lysis. The blood will not form a proper clot to seal the dural tear if it is injected too quickly. Patients may complain of increasing pressure and discomfort in the back, buttocks, or legs. If this is the case, the injection should be slowed or stopped.

It is suggested that the interspace below the original puncture be used, as blood tends to preferentially spread in a cephalad manner. Although blood spreads 9 to 10 spinal segments from a 20-mL injection, the majority of clot formation occurs 3 to 5 segments around the injection site. The blood patch should ideally be performed 24 hours after puncture to be more effective.[15] Careful examination for signs of superficial (on the skin) and systemic infection should be undertaken before proceeding. Last, the patient should remain supine and immobile for 30 minutes to 1 hour to allow the blood to form a clot.

Major complications from an epidural blood patch are rare. Many patients complain of mild low back pain for several days after the procedure. Other complications include bleeding, infection, arachnoiditis (if blood is injected into the subarachnoid space), and failure to relieve the headache. Two cases of facial nerve paralysis have been reported, both of which resolved spontaneously, and one case was reported of a patient who complained of intractable dizziness, vertigo, tinnitus, and ataxia.[16]

SUMMARY

Although post-dural puncture headaches are usually self-limiting and nonfatal, their postural nature prevents patients from performing activities of daily living. Preventive measures to help decrease the incidence of post-dural puncture headache include smaller needle size, shape of the needle, and, perhaps, direction of the needle bevel in relation to dural fibers. Patients aged 20 to 40 years have a higher incidence of post-dural puncture headache, but this should not preclude administration of a spinal or epidural injection to that age group.

Numerous pharmacologic and invasive procedures are available to treat post-dural puncture headache. More in-depth study of agents such as sumatriptan, epidural morphine sulfate, and adrenocorticotropic hormone may reveal new options. The epidural blood patch has the highest overall cure rate for post-dural puncture headache and is usually well tolerated by the patient.

REFERENCES

1. Vandam LD, Dripps RD: Long-term follow-up of patients who received 10,098 spinal anesthetics. JAMA 161:586–591, 1956.
2. Cruickshank RH, Hopkinson SM: Fluid flow through dural puncture sites: An in vitro comparison of needle point types. Anaesthesia 44:415–418, 1989.
3. Brownridge P: The management of headache following accidental dural puncture. Anaesth Intensive Care 11:4–15, 1983.
4. Crawford JS: The prevention of headache consequent upon dural puncture. Br J Anaesth 44:598–600, 1972.
5. Camann WR, Murray RS, Mushlin PS, et al: Effects of oral caffeine on post–dural puncture headache: A double-blind, placebo-controlled trial. Anesth Analg 70:181–184, 1990.
6. Sechzer P, Abel L: Post-spinal anesthesia headache treated with caffeine evaluation with demand method. Curr Ther Res 24:307–312, 1978.
7. Sechzer P: Post-spinal anesthesia headache treated with caffeine: II. Intracranial vascular distension: A key factor. Curr Ther Res 26:440–448, 1979.
8. Rice CG, Dobbs CH: The use of peridural and subarachnoid injections of saline solutions in the treatment of severe postspinal headache. Anesthesiology 11:17–23, 1950.
9. Usubiaga JE, Usubiaga LE, Brea LM, et al: Epidural and subarachnoid space pressures and relation to postspinal anesthesia headache. Anesth Analg 46:293–296, 1967.
10. Baysinger CL, Menk EJ, Harte E, et al: The successful treatment of dural puncture headache after failed epidural blood patch. Anesth Analg 65:1242–1244, 1986.
11. Stevens DS, Peters-Asdourian C: Treatment of post-dural puncture headache with epidural dextran patch. Reg Anesth 18:324–325, 1993.
12. Barrios-Alarcon J, Aldrete JA, Paragas-Tapia D: Relief of post-lumbar puncture headache with epidural dextran 40: A preliminary report. Reg Anesth 14:78–80, 1989.
13. Gielen M: Post-dural puncture headache: A review. Reg Anesth 14:101–106, 1989.
14. Gormley JB: Treatment of postspinal headache. Anesthesiology 21:565–566, 1960.
15. Abouleish EM, de la Vega S, Blendinger I, et al: Long-term follow-up of epidural blood patch. Anesth Analg 54:459–465, 1975.
16. Lowe DM, McCullough AM: Seventh nerve palsy after extradural blood patch. Br J Anaesth 65:721–722, 1990.

SUGGESTED READINGS

McSwiney M, Phillips J: Post–dural puncture headache. Acta Anaesthesiol Scand 39:990–995, 1995.
Morewood G: A rational approach to the cause, prevention and treatment of post–dural puncture headache. Can Med Assoc J 149:1087–1093, 1993.

Chapter 47

Spontaneous Intracranial Hypotension

Honorio T. Benzon, M.D.,
and Rimas Nemickas, M.D.

Spontaneous intracranial hypotension (SIH), also known as *low cerebrospinal fluid (CSF) pressure headache* is characterized by the signs and symptoms of post–dural puncture headache, but without a history of preceding lumbar puncture. The headache is postural and results from displacement or stretching of pain-sensitive structures in the cranial vault. Neck stiffness, nausea and vomiting, photophobia, general malaise, vertigo, tinnitus, and diplopia may be present.[1, 2] The vestibular and auditory symptoms are secondary to changes in the intralabyrinthine pressure secondary to alterations of the pressure gradient across the cochlear aqueduct.[1] The diplopia is due to lateral rectus palsy from downward displacement of the sixth cranial nerve.

MECHANISMS

Proposed mechanisms of SIH include reduced CSF production, increased CSF absorption, and leakage of CSF.[1-3] No evidence exists to support the first two theories. Leakage of CSF through a spontaneous dural tear or nerve root sleeve or a spontaneous rupture of an arachnoid cyst is the most plausible mechanism.[1, 4] Small defects may be present in the meninges, such as perineural or epidural cysts that are susceptible to rupture after minor trauma.[1] Alternatively, the root sleeve anatomy may be abnormal, predisposing to small tears or dehiscence of the dural sheath after exercise or a minor fall.[1]

DIAGNOSIS

Diagnostic lumbar puncture documents the low CSF pressure. CSF pressure less than 70 mm H_2O with the patient in the lateral decubitus position is sufficient for diagnosis,[3] although the usual finding is 30 to 40 mm H_2O. Analysis of the CSF shows elevated protein content (normal, 15 to 45 mg/dL) and increased red and white blood cell counts (normal, 0 to 10 cells). The increased protein is most probably due to alteration of the normal

hydrostatic and oncotic pressures across the venous sinus and arachnoid villi or the result of the passage of proteins into the CSF in the presence of a microscopic leak or a disruption of the meninges.[1]

Radionuclide cisternography may demonstrate the CSF leak. If no leak is shown, the CSF is presumed to have escaped through a microscopic dural tear. Often, the low CSF pressure prevents ascent of the tracer to the foramen magnum. Patients with SIH may have rapid appearance of the radioisotope tracer in the bladder and kidneys[2, 5] secondary to leakage of CSF through the dura and its uptake into the circulation via the epidural venous plexus.[1] Magnetic resonance imaging (MRI) usually shows meningeal enhancement; the enhancement is global and is usually thick, diffuse, and continuous.[6-8] The meningeal enhancement may be related to dural venous dilatation that accompanies reduced CSF volume. Follow-up MRI of patients who have had relief of the SIH showed resolution of the meningeal enhancement.[6, 7]

TREATMENT

The headache of SIH takes several weeks to months to resolve spontaneously. Treatments for SIH are essentially the same as those for post–dural puncture headache. These include bed rest, steroids, oral caffeine, continuous epidural saline infusion, and epidural blood patch.[1-5, 7, 9] Steroids favor fluid retention, decrease the inflammatory response to the presence of cells or proteins in the CSF, and decrease vascular leakage. Epidural injection of saline or blood increases the epidural and, therefore, the subarachnoid pressure. The increase in subarachnoid pressure normalizes the pressure gradient between the CSF, the intracranial vessels, and other structures. For epidural saline infusion to be effective, rates of 20 mL/hour for 48 hours have been recommended.[1, 5] The efficacy of epidural blood injections in SIH has been demonstrated in several case reports.[2-4, 9] Computed tomographic scan after epidural blood patch may show resuspension of the brain and decreased venous engorgement.[10] Fifteen milliliters of autologous blood has been recommended as the ideal volume, as this volume appears to spread bidirectionally—approximately six segments cephalad and three segments caudad.[11]

If epidural blood injection at the lumbar level does not relieve the patient's headache, then a repeat epidural injection at the thoracic level is recommended, because the leak may be located at a higher vertebral level.[4]

REFERENCES

1. Rando TA, Fishman RA: Spontaneous intracranial hypotension: Report of two cases and review of the literature. Neurology 42:481, 1992.
2. Marcelis J, Silverstein SD: Spontaneous low cerebrospinal fluid pressure headache. Headache 30:192, 1990.
3. Baker CC: Headache due to spontaneous low spinal fluid pressure. Minn Med 66:325, 1983.
4. Benzon HT, Nemickas R, Molloy RE, et al: Lumbar and thoracic epidural blood injections to treat spontaneous intracranial hypotension. Anesthesiology 85:920, 1996.
5. Gibson BE, Wedel DJ, Faust RJ, et al: Continuous epidural saline infusion for the treatment of low CSF pressure headache. Anesthesiology 68:789, 1988.
6. Fishman RA, Dillon WP: Dural enhancement and cerebral displacement secondary to intracranial hypotension. Neurology 43:609, 1993.
7. Pannullo SC, Reich JB, Krol G, et al: MRI changes in intracranial hypotension. Neurology 43:919, 1993.
8. Mokri B, Parisi JE, Scheithauer BW, et al: Meningeal biopsy in intracranial hypotension: Meningeal enhancement on MRI. Neurology 45:1801, 1995.
9. Gaukroger PB, Brownridge P: Epidural blood patch in the treatment of spontaneous low CSF pressure headache. Pain 29:119, 1987.
10. Weitz SR, Drasner K: Spontaneous intracranial hypotension: A series. Anesthesiology 85:923, 1996.
11. Szeinfeld M, Ihmeidan IH, Moser MM, et al: Epidural blood patch: Evaluation of the volume and spread of blood injected into the epidural space. Anesthesiology 64:820, 1986.

Chapter 48

Orofacial Pain

James C. Phero, D.M.D.,
and Gururau Sudarshan, M.D., F.R.C.A.

This chapter reviews the classic orofacial pain conditions and syndromes encountered by the clinician. The practitioner addressing the complexities of orofacial pain must be cautious to avoid the pitfall of symptom management in the absence of diagnosis. The orofacial pain categories in this chapter follow the system initiated by the International Association for the Study of Pain (IASP), with some additional material supported by the International Headache Society (IHS) and the American Academy of Orofacial Pain (AAOP) (Table 48–1).

OROFACIAL PAIN OF NEUROPATHIC ORIGIN

Neuropathic pain syndromes are painful conditions caused by a lesion or dysfunction of the nervous system. The term *deafferentation pain* is used when the lesion is in the central nervous system. Orofacial pain of neuropathic origin usually results from involvement of cranial nerves (trigeminal, facial, glossopharyngeal, vagus, hypoglossal), but it is possible for these syndromes to be caused by neoplastic, post-traumatic, or inflammatory lesions. Atypical facial pain is a global diagnosis that contains several distinct pain syndromes, typically including neuropathic and musculoskeletal components, that do not fit the category of *tic douloureux*.

Central Pain

A primary lesion of the central nervous system is an infrequent cause of orofacial pain. Central post-stroke pain (thalamic pain) is the most common cause and usually presents with typical features of neuropathic pain. It has been estimated to occur in 1% to 2% of all stroke patients. The thalamus appears to be the site of this lesion in more than half of these cases. Approximately 20% of these patients develop facial pain. Facial pain may also be a feature of neoplastic conditions affecting the brain, but it is seldom seen as the presenting symptom.

Trigeminal Neuralgia

Tic Douloureux

Tic douloureux is defined as a sudden, usually unilateral, severe, brief, stabbing, recurrent pain felt in the distribution of one or more branches of the fifth cranial nerve. Trigeminal root compression has been believed to be the primary cause of trigeminal neuralgia. Vascular loops compressing or contacting the trigeminal nerve at the root entry zone are observed in more than 80% of cases. The superior cerebellar artery and, in some patients, the inferior cerebellar artery are involved in this condition. Vascular anomaly, aneurysm, and bone architecture can also result in nerve compression. Multiple sclerosis may also contribute to trigeminal neuralgia

TABLE 48–1. OROFACIAL PAIN CATEGORIES

Orofacial pain of neuropathic origin
  Central pain
  Trigeminal neuralgia
    Tic douloureux
    Trigeminal neuralgia secondary to trauma
    Acute herpes zoster
    Postherpetic neuralgia
    Raeder's syndrome
  Geniculate neuralgia/Ramsay Hunt syndrome
  Nervus intermedius neuralgia/geniculate neuralgia
  Glossopharyngeal neuralgia
  Superior laryngeal neuralgia
  Hypoglossal/vagus neuralgia
  Tolosa-Hunt syndrome
  SUNCT syndrome
Non-neuropathic orofacial pain
  Extraoral pain
    Temporomandibular disorders
      Temporomandibular joint disorders
      Masticatory muscle disorders
    Carotidynia
    Sinusitis
  Intraoral pain
    Glossodynia
    Atypical odontalgia
    Burning mouth syndrome
    Cracked tooth syndrome
Treatment considerations

through segmental demyelination and microneuroma formation.

The paroxysmal pain attacks occur in one or more divisions of the trigeminal nerve, usually unilaterally. Trigeminal neuralgia is seldom bilateral. The pain is typically precipitated by light touch. The incidence in females is almost twice that in males. The age distribution is characterized by first occurrence in the 40s, reaching a peak in the 50s. Right branches are affected more frequently than left. Pain commonly occurs according to the distribution of the second and the third branches of the trigeminal nerve, with the first branch rarely involved. Pain is always transient, lasting from seconds to as long as a few minutes. The characteristic pain is expressed as lancinating, shooting, electric shock–like, and stabbing. Between episodes, sensations are essentially normal or a slight desensitization is present. No pain or numbness is observed in the affected area between periods of paroxysmal pain. A short refractory period follows each of the pain attacks. An episode of such attacks, however, can last for months. A break in these episodes usually occurs but these attacks can return months or years later.

Trigeminal neuralgia may respond to anticonvulsant medications such as carbamazepine (Tegretol) and gabapentin (Neurontin). Additionally, clonazepam (Klonopin), and baclofen (Lioresal) are of benefit. Barbiturates are contraindicated in management of these cases. If an adequate dose of carbamazepine is administered without side effects, the neuralgic pain can often be completely relieved. If pain attacks are relieved by this medication and no neurologic abnormalities are present, the condition is normally diagnosed as trigeminal neuralgia. Local anesthetic injected into the trigger zone often relieves the paroxysmal episodes. However, in advanced cases, patients gradually fail to respond to this treatment. This may be due to the change of the site or intensity of nerve root compression.

Trigeminal Neuralgia Secondary to Trauma

Paroxysmal pain in the affected trigeminal divisions may follow trauma, surgery, and peripheral lesions. Persistent burning, throbbing, or dull pain may also be observed. Peripheral neuropathy, classified as secondary trigeminal neuralgia, occurs relatively frequently after orthognathic surgery and fractures in the trigeminal distribution. Deafferentation and partial injury of peripheral nerves result in degeneration and regeneration. In cases in which this injury presents as neuritis, the pain is commonly characterized as burning. Hypoesthesia and dysesthesia are commonly observed in the affected nerve division. Allodynia and hyperalgesia are frequently observed.

Acute Herpes Zoster: Trigeminal Distribution

If the latent varicella zoster virus remains in the trigeminal and the geniculate ganglion and the immune activity of the host declines, the infection can involve the trigeminal nerve branches and facial nerve branches, respectively. Although most patients only recognize the dermal condition because the skin symptoms are most prominent, the virus also affects nerves, vessels, bones, and other structures. Practitioners must be aware that this is essentially a recurrent viral infection of the nerve. In postmortem studies, a marked loss of myelin in the peripheral nerve and sensory root is found in all patients with herpes zoster.

Trigeminal herpes zoster pain usually precedes dermal symptoms for a few days to a week, and sensory abnormality is observed in moderate and severe cases. Eruptions heal spontaneously within 3 weeks and may be associated with residual pigmentary changes in the moderate to severe cases. Induration of lymph nodes and high fever are often observed. The trigeminal nerve is involved in about 30% of all cases of herpes zoster. The first division of trigeminal nerve is affected most frequently in all dermatomal divisions. In 60% of cases of trigeminal herpes zoster, vesicular eruptions occur in the first division; the second division follows in frequency, with the third being the least frequent. Ramsay Hunt syndrome is observed in 2% or 3% of cases of herpes zoster of the head. One of the most common complications in herpes zoster ophthalmicus is distorted vision (20.5%), mostly owing to corneal opacity. In some severe cases, corneal ulcer results in loss of vision in the affected eye. Ophthalmoplegia, meningoencephalitis, and hemiplegia are also rarely observed. Alveolar bone can be destroyed and, in severe cases, teeth can be lost in the second and the third divisions. Some cases show symptoms of trigeminal herpes zoster and Ramsay Hunt syndrome without eruptions, or *zoster sine herpete*. These cases are very commonly misdiagnosed.

Diagnosis can be revealed by laboratory examinations. Elevated antibody level of varicella zoster virus should be observed for the diagnosis of trigeminal herpes zoster and Ramsay Hunt syndrome. Clinicians should remember that some patients with symptoms similar to those of trigeminal herpes zoster and Ramsay Hunt syndrome without vesicles can be infected by varicella zoster virus, and that a proper diagnosis can be revealed only by laboratory examination findings.

Postherpetic Neuralgia: Trigeminal Distribution

Postherpetic neuralgia is characterized by chronic pain with somatosensory abnormalities that persist in the affected trigeminal divisions after eruptions of acute trigeminal herpes zoster have healed. Postherpetic neuralgia is defined as pain that persists more than 4 months after the onset of rash. The essence of the pathology of postherpetic neuralgia is denervation of the affected nerve. Skin in the severely denervated area shows anesthesia. Atrophy of dorsal horn and pathologic changes in the sensory ganglion are found on the affected side but not on the unaffected side. Central sensitization and neuroplasticity are believed to be important contributory mechanisms to postherpetic neuralgia.

Postherpetic neuralgia is characterized by burning pain with hyperalgesia, allodynia, and dysesthesia in an area affected by a previous episode of herpes zoster.

The pain lasts far longer than the clinical appearance of the vesicles associated with herpes zoster. Hyperalgesia and allodynia may be observed. The diagnosis of post-herpetic neuralgia is assisted by a history of eruptions in the affected area and the presence of somatosensory abnormalities. Serum varicella zoster virus antibody level is not helpful for diagnosis in chronic cases.

Raeder's Syndrome

Raeder's syndrome is characterized by severe stabbing paroxysms in the first division of trigeminal nerve with sympathetic nervous system paralysis (Horner's syndrome). Sympatholysis is usually not accompanied by sudomotor dysfunction. The most common clinical presentation is severe, throbbing, supraorbital headache accompanied by ptosis and miosis in a middle-aged man. The headache is intermittent for several weeks or months.

Raeder's syndrome consists of two types. One type is related to a lesion in the middle cranial fossa, such as a neoplasm. The other type is related to benign conditions, such as unilateral vascular headache syndromes. Raeder's syndrome may be caused by any lesion affecting the postganglionic oculosympathetic fibers distal to the bifurcation of the common carotid artery. Parasellar neoplasms often involve multiple cranial nerves, and unilateral vascular headache syndromes may be elicited by lesions of the internal carotid artery. Raeder's syndrome can be distinguished from Horner's syndrome by observing facial sweating. The combination of magnetic resonance imaging (MRI) and MR angiography is a reliable noninvasive tool to investigate the differential diagnosis of pericarotid syndrome and paratrigeminal lesions.

Geniculate Neuralgia or Ramsay Hunt Syndrome

Geniculate neuralgia is due to an acute herpetic involvement of the afferent fibers that accompany the facial nerve, usually at the geniculate ganglion level. Lancinating pains are usually felt deep in the auditory meatus and are followed a few days later with typical vesicles around the concha and the mastoid area. Facial palsy is usually associated with this condition. Typical cases of Ramsay Hunt syndrome show the triad of auricular vesicles, ipsilateral peripheral facial palsy, and vestibular/cochlear symptoms. Redness, swelling, and vesicles usually follow the pain at the auricle, external auditory canal, postauricular region, occiput, or pharynx. Treatment is as for acute herpes zoster.

Nervus Intermedius Neuralgia/ Geniculate Neuralgia

This condition is noted for episodic, severe lancinating pain in the ear canal or posterior pharynx as the main presenting symptom. The etiology of nervus intermedius is unknown. There are no skin or mucous membrane lesions nor any sensory or motor deficits. It is uncommon before the fifth decade. Impingement of the nervus intermedius at the root entry zone has been demonstrated in those cases needing surgical treatment. Surgical decompression in these cases has resulted in long-term pain relief. The less intractable cases do respond to neuralgic medications such as carbamazepine.

Glossopharyngeal Neuralgia

Episodic, severe, stabbing, recurrent pains in the distribution of the glossopharyngeal nerve are the hallmark of this condition. The site of pain is confined to the tonsillar fossa. The trigger point is usually located in the faucial pillars. The pain may radiate to the external auditory meatus or to the neck. The symptoms may be associated with syncopal attacks. Vascular impingement of the nerve roots has been proposed as a central cause.

Treatment has been directed at peripheral as well as central nervous system causes. Microvascular compression is thought to be one of the primary causes of glossopharyngeal neuralgia. The posterior inferior cerebellar artery is the vessel that is most commonly responsible. However, vascular decompression does not yield the same relief as with trigeminal neuralgia, indicating the possibility of other sources. Invasion or compression by parapharyngeal and posterior fossa tumors, arteriovenous malformation, and choroid plexus are reported as other causes of glossopharyngeal neuralgia.

Superior Laryngeal Neuralgia

Neuralgia of the superior laryngeal nerve is felt as sudden, brief, recurrent, lancinating pain in the throat and laryngeal area. This pain can also be felt in the deep ear and angle of the jaw and is provoked by yawning, coughing, swallowing, and gargling. In some instances nerve-stimulating symptoms of vagus, such as salivation or hiccups, may be observed. Superior laryngeal neuralgia is more likely attributable to local lesions than to intracranial lesions. Differential diagnosis from glossopharyngeal neuralgia is often difficult because of similarity in clinical presentation. The trigger zone is often located in the larynx. A local anesthetic block of the superior laryngeal nerve is useful for the differential diagnosis. Tumors and infections should be investigated.

Hypoglossal/Vagus Neuralgia

Neuralgia of the vagus nerve and hypoglossal nerve are rare conditions that present with paroxysmal unilateral pain affecting the angle of the jaw, thyroid cartilage, piriform sinus, and posterior aspect of the tongue. Vagal neuralgia is often brought on by acts such as yawning, coughing, or swallowing. It can be difficult to differentiate this from glossopharyngeal neuralgia or carotidynia.

Tolosa-Hunt Syndrome

This condition refers to episodic unilateral pain in the ocular area associated with ipsilateral paresis of oculomotor nerves and the first branch of the trigeminal nerve. It is a condition that affects adults, usually in the fourth decade. Onset is gradual, with pain preceding the ophthalmoplegia. Trigger points are not present and there seems to be no predisposing or precipitating condition. Orbital phlebography can show the lesion in the majority of cases. The typical lesion is a narrowing or occlusion of ophthalmic venous channels around the area of the cavernous sinus. The exact pathology is unknown. The condition responds slowly but favorably to corticosteroids. The average duration of this condition is 8 to 12 weeks.

SUNCT Syndrome

SUNCT syndrome (short-lasting, unilateral, neuralgiform pain with conjunctival injection and tearing) is an idiopathic condition that is seen in adult males after the fifth decade and is associated with unilateral pain episodes lasting less than 2 minutes and affecting the orbit or periorbital area. Associated rhinorrhea, lacrimation, and conjunctival irritation are characteristic. The pain can be triggered by a variety of non-noxious stimuli and typically shows periodicity. No neurologic deficits are seen, and remissions may last for several months. The condition is resistant to classic forms of treatment.

NON-NEUROPATHIC OROFACIAL PAIN

Extraoral Pain

Temporomandibular Disorder

Temporomandibular disorder is a collective term that includes a number of clinical complaints involving the muscles of mastication, the temporomandibular joint (TMJ), and/or associated orofacial structures. Other commonly used terms are *Costen's syndrome*, *TMJ dysfunction*, and *craniomandibular disorders*. Temporomandibular disorders are a major cause of nondental pain in the orofacial region and are considered to be a subclassification of musculoskeletal disorders. In many temporomandibular disorder patients, the most common source of complaint is not the TMJ but the muscles of mastication. Therefore, the terms *TMJ dysfunction* or *TMJ disorder* are actually inappropriate for many of these complaints. It is for this reason that the American Dental Association (ADA) adopted the term *temporomandibular disorder*.

Signs and symptoms associated with temporomandibular disorders are a common source of pain complaints in the head and orofacial structures. These complaints can be associated with general joint problems and somatization. The primary signs and symptoms associated with temporomandibular disorders originate from the masticatory structures and are associated with jaw function. Pain during opening of the mouth or chewing are common. Some individuals report difficulty speaking or singing. Patients often report pain in the preauricular areas, face, and/or temples. TMJ sounds are frequently described as clicking, popping, grating, or crepitus. This condition can produce locking of the jaw during opening or closing. Patients frequently report painful jaw muscles. They may even report a sudden change in bite coincident with the onset of the painful condition. It is important to appreciate that pain associated with most TMJ disorders is increased with jaw function. Because

this is a condition of the musculoskeletal structures, functioning of these structures generally increases the pain. When a patient's pain complaint is not influenced by jaw function, other sources of orofacial pain should be suspected.

Temporomandibular disorders can be subdivided into two broad categories related to their primary source of pain and dysfunction. These classic subdivisions are TMJ intracapsular disorders and masticatory muscle disorders.

Temporomandibular Intracapsular Joint Disorders. The signs associated with functional disorders of the temporomandibular joints are probably the most common findings in a patient being examined for masticatory dysfunction. Many of these signs do not produce painful symptoms, and therefore the patient may not seek treatment. These disorders are classified in three categories: derangements of the condyle-disc complex, structural incompatibility of the articular surfaces, and inflammatory joint disorders. The first two categories have been collectively referred to as *disc-interference disorders*. The term *disc-interference disorder* was introduced to describe a category of functional disorders that arises from problems with the condyle-disc complex. Some of these problems are due to a derangement or alteration of the attachment of the disc to the condyle. Some problems are due to an incompatibility between the articular surfaces of the condyle, disc, and fossa. Other problems are due to the fact that relatively normal structures have been extended beyond their normal range of movement. With time, inflammatory disorders can arise from a localized protective response of the tissues that make up the TMJ. These disorders are often the result of chronic or progressive disc derangement disorders.

The two major symptoms of functional TMJ problems are joint pain and dysfunction. Joint pain can arise from healthy joint structures that are mechanically abused during function or from structures that have become inflamed. Pain originating from healthy structures is felt as sharp, sudden, and intense pain that is closely associated with joint movement. When the joint is rested, the pain resolves quickly. The patient often reports the pain as being localized to the preauricular area. If the joint structures have become inflamed, the pain is reported as constant, even at rest, yet accentuated by joint movement.

Dysfunction is common with functional disorders of the TMJ. Usually it presents as a disruption of the normal condyle-disc movement, with the production of joint sounds. The joint sounds may be a single event of short duration, known as a click. If this is loud, it may be referred to as a pop. Crepitation consists of multiple, rough, gravelly sounds, often described as grating and complicated. Dysfunction of the TMJ may also present as catching sensations during mouth opening. Sometimes the jaw can actually lock. Dysfunction of the TMJ is always directly related to jaw movement. A single click during opening of the mouth is often associated with an anteriorly displaced disc that is returned to a more normal position during the opening movement. This condition is referred to as disc displacement with reduction. When the patient closes the mouth, a second click is often felt, which represents the return of the disc to the anteriorly displaced position. For some patients the displacement of the disc progresses anteriorly, and the disc may not return to its normal relationship with the condyle during opening. This condition is referred to as disc displacement without reduction. When this occurs, the mouth often cannot be opened fully because the disc is blocking the translation of the condyle. For this reason the condition is often referred to as a closed lock.

Masticatory Muscle Disorders. Functional disorders of masticatory muscles are probably the most common temporomandibular disorder complaint of patients seeking treatment in the dental office. With regard to pain, these disorders are second only to odontalgia (tooth or periodontal pain) in terms of frequency. They are generally grouped into the large category *masticatory muscle disorders*.

The two major symptoms of functional TMJ problems are pain and dysfunction. The most common complaint of patients with masticatory muscle disorders is muscle pain, which may range from slight tenderness to extreme discomfort. Muscle pain, or myalgia, can arise from increased levels of muscular use. The symptoms are often associated with a feeling of muscle fatigue and tightness. Patients will commonly identify the location of the pain as broad, diffuse, and often bilateral. This complaint is quite different than the specific location of pain that is reported in intracapsular disorders. Although the exact origin of this type of muscle pain is debated, some authors suggest it is related to vasoconstriction of the relevant arteries and the accumulation of metabolic waste products in the muscle tissues. Within the ischemic area of the muscle, certain algogenic substances (e.g., bradykinins, prostaglandins) are released, causing muscle pain. However, the origins of muscle pain are far more complex than simple overuse and fatigue. Muscle pain associated with temporomandibular disorders does not seem to be strongly correlated with increased activity, such as spasm. It is now appreciated that muscle pain can be greatly influenced by central mechanisms.

The severity of muscle pain is directly related to the functional activity of the muscle involved. Therefore, patients often report that the pain affects functional activity. If the patient does not report an increase in pain associated with jaw function, the disorder is not likely related to a masticatory muscle problem, and other diagnoses should be considered. Dysfunction is a common clinical symptom associated with masticatory muscle disorders. Usually it is seen as a decrease in the range of mandibular movement. When muscle tissue has been compromised by overuse, any contraction or stretching increases the pain. To maintain comfort, the patient restricts movement within a range that does not increase pain levels. Clinically this is seen as an inability to open the mouth widely. The restriction may occur at any degree of opening, depending on where discomfort is felt. In some myalgic disorders the patient can slowly open wider, but the pain is still present and may even become worse.

Acute malocclusion is another type of dysfunction. Acute malocclusion refers to any sudden change in the occlusal position that has been created by a disorder. An acute malocclusion may result from a sudden change in the resting length of a muscle that controls jaw position. When this occurs, the patient describes a change in the occlusal contact of the teeth. The mandibular position and resultant alteration in occlusal relationships depend on the muscles involved. With functional shortening of the elevator muscles (clinically a less detectable acute malocclusion), the patient will generally complain of an inability to bite normally. It is important to remember that an acute malocclusion is the result of the muscle disorder and not the cause. Treatment should never be directed toward correcting the malocclusion. It should be aimed at eliminating the muscle disorder. When this condition is reduced, the occlusal condition returns to normal.

Carotidynia. Carotidynia is characterized by unilateral continuous aching or throbbing pain, usually starting in the ipsilateral anterior neck. The pathology of carotidynia is unknown. Some cases have been reported to be associated with migraine, aneurysm, and long intraluminal clots with incomplete vessel obstruction of the internal carotid artery. Tenderness of the carotid artery, especially around the bifurcation, is the most common feature. Palpation may aggravate head and neck pain. In cases of headache, the pain complaint may resemble that of migraine. Autonomic symptoms are not observed, although some associated symptoms with migraine, such as photophobia and nausea, may be present. Episodes are superimposed on the continuous pain. Pain is precipitated by swallowing, coughing, and rotating or extending the neck. A careful review of the history and physical examination findings can lead to the diagnosis. Laboratory studies enable exclusion of other causes. Migraine, giant cell arteritis, and glossopharyngeal neuralgia should be differentiated.

Sinusitis. Sinus pain is characterized as continuous aching or throbbing pain in the infraorbital, temporal, frontal, ear, upper molar, and/or premolar region due to inflammation of the sinuses. Pain is located unilaterally in the early stage; however, it extends to the opposite side of the face according to the involvement of the sinuses on the other side. Pain is essentially the result of inflammation, and it is exacerbated when the mucosa is swollen and the ostia of the sinuses are occluded. Acute inflammation of sinuses cause throbbing or wrenching headache; however, chronic sinusitis usually leads to dull or tender pain. Oppressive pain may be observed in the infraorbital region. Purulent discharge to the pharynx is a common finding. Rapid changes of atmospheric pressure, such as that induced by diving or traveling on airplanes, aggravates the pain. Diagnosis is not difficult if purulent discharge from the sinus ostia and radiographic opacity in ipsilateral and/or bilateral sinuses are observed. Laboratory examination shows an inflammatory pattern.

Intraoral Pain

Pain of the oral cavity has multiple causes, for example, inflammation of the dental pulp or periodontal tissue or trauma of hard and soft tissues.

Glossodynia, Atypical Odontalgia, and Burning Mouth Syndrome

These disorders are the oral analogues of atypical facial pain. The practitioner is uncertain as to the cause of pain in the tongue, teeth, periodontal tissues, or the whole mouth. It is important to remember that these are not conditions but syndromes, which should be diagnosed only after all other possible causes have been ruled out. These syndromes classically occur with more frequency after the fourth decade. Patients complain of continuous sore, throbbing, or burning pain in the tongue, teeth, periodontal tissues, or whole mouth. The intensity of pain is moderate. Variation of the pain is observed, and specific precipitating factors are rarely noted. No pathology or distinct somatosensory anomaly can be observed at the site of pain. Findings from thermal and mechanical (percussion) tests to the teeth in the affected area are equivocal. These syndromes often have a psychosomatic aspect.

Cracked Tooth Syndrome

This pain results from an incomplete (cracked tooth) or a complete tooth fracture (split tooth). A cracked tooth induces dental pulp sensitization and pulpitis, and deep periodontal pockets can give rise to severe pain. Cracked tooth syndrome is primarily seen in the molar and the premolar teeth. Vertical root fractures most frequently occur in endodontically treated posterior teeth in patients between 45 and 60 years of age. When an incomplete fracture involves the dentinal layer of a vital posterior tooth, it may cause pain. Caries, inappropriate dental restoration design, overloading of the tooth, atypical root canal anatomy, and external root resorption of the tooth may predispose to this syndrome.

Location of the dentinal crack is difficult and must be guided by a precise history, thermal pulp testing, and inspection of the dentinal walls within the suspect tooth. The number, extent, and direction of the fracture lines may be ascertained readily by using transillumination and magnification. This allows the clinician to distinguish between oblique and vertical cracks. Intra-alveolar root fractures can be detected only by radiogram. Fracture detection can be increased by taking x-rays from more than one angle. Radiolucent areas occur in the region of the root fracture more readily than in the periapical region, in a ratio of 7:1.

TREATMENT CONSIDERATIONS WITH EMPHASIS ON TRIGEMINAL NEURALGIA

Conservative Management: Pharmacotherapeutic Options

Conservative management in a multidisciplinary pain clinic seems to provide the most promising results in the majority of cases of trigeminal neuralgia. Surgical management should be considered for patients in whom conservative management has failed. Conservative management relies mainly on pharmacotherapy with the following agents.

Carbamazepine

Carbamazepine, a tricyclic imipramine, is the drug of choice in the management of trigeminal neuralgia. The drug, however, is not without troublesome side effects and therefore must be introduced at a low dose. In the elderly, it is customary to start with a 100-mg dose, which is increased gradually by 100-mg increments every 3 days until pain relief occurs or side effects supervene. Doses in the range of 800 to 1200 mg/day are usually therapeutic. Approximately 20% of patients treated with carbamazepine experience some side effects. The most common side effects, dizziness and diplopia, are neurologic, although nausea is also a frequent complaint. The most sinister side effects, however, are hematologic: anemia, thrombocytopenia, and agranulocytosis. The elderly are more susceptible to these side effects. Serious side effects are rare (2 to 6 cases per million population per year). Megaloblastic anemia is the most frequently observed hematologic side effect. Transient or persistent decreases in platelet or leukocyte counts are also frequently observed in patients receiving this drug. Allergic reactions in the form of a delayed-onset nonspecific rash are not uncommon. Routine periodic hematologic monitoring is recommended for patients taking carbamazepine. Monitoring of blood levels for therapeutic efficacy, however, is more controversial. Carbamazepine is a potent hepatic enzyme inducer and induces its own metabolism. This property of autoinduction along with its unique pharmacokinetics leads to inconsistent blood levels (i.e., correlation between the dose and serum level is poor). However, drug monitoring has been used to individualize therapy and to check for patient compliance at intervals of 6 months. A target level of 4 to 12 μg/mL has been suggested. The response of trigeminal neuralgia to carbamazepine is good in approximately 70% of patients. The majority report relief within the first 2 days. Unfortunately, tolerance to therapy seems to develop over time. In such cases, response can be optimized by adding or changing to second-line drugs.

Gabapentin

Gabapentin is a new anticonvulsant agent that is structurally related to the inhibitory central nervous system neurotransmitter γ-aminobutyric acid (GABA). This drug has no direct GABA-mimetic action, and the exact mechanism of action is as yet unknown. The drug has shown immense promise in the treatment of neuropathic pain, although its use has not been based on prospective double-blind trials. There have been several case reports of its success in management of a variety of neuropathic pain syndromes, including trigeminal neuralgia. The major advantage of this new drug over carbamazepine seems to be the lack of dangerous side effects. It is not metabolized in the body nor does it cause induction of hepatic enzymes. Monitoring of blood levels is not necessary. Dosing can start at 300 mg/day (in divided doses) and can be increased gradually to a dose of 1800 to 3600 mg/day, until pain relief occurs or side effects are seen. The drug is well tolerated, with a less than 10% incidence of troublesome side effects. Severe side effects are not seen. The most frequent adverse effects of gabapentin therapy are sleepiness, dizziness, and ataxia. Other anticonvulsants, including phenytoin sodium, valproic acid, oxcarbazepine, and lamotrigine, have also been shown to be effective in trigeminal neuralgia. They are used as adjuvants or second-line drugs in the management of trigeminal neuralgia.

Baclofen

Baclofen is a skeletal muscle relaxant that is also structurally related to GABA. In animal experiments, baclofen has been shown to resemble anticonvulsants in its ability to depress excitatory synaptic transmission in the spinal trigeminal nucleus. In double-blind studies in humans, it has been shown to be an effective adjuvant for management of trigeminal neuralgia. Gradual dosing is recommended to avoid side effects such as ataxia, lethargy, and nausea. It is customary to start at 10 mg/day, increasing to a target dose of 40 mg/day over 2 weeks. It has been shown that L-baclofen is better tolerated than the commonly available racemic mixture.

Clonazepam

Clonazepam is a benzodiazepine that is known to be effective in myoclonic epileptic states. It has been shown to be effective in patients with trigeminal neuralgia who have shown resistance to carbamazepine therapy. The level of pain control achieved, however, is not good enough for clonazepam to be considered a first-line drug. Side effects include somnolence, ataxia, and fatigue. Therapeutic effects are seen in the dose range of 1 to 4 mg/day.

Other agents that have been tried with some success include tocainide, mexiletine, and topical capsaicin.

Role of Psychology

As a general rule, psychological factors are more observable in atypical facial pain than in trigeminal pain. Nevertheless, all patients with trigeminal neuralgia could benefit from the assistance of a clinical psychologist who, by instructing them in the use of coping strategies, may help patients to feel control over the pain. Medical and surgical management are directed at controlling pain, whereas psychological treatment helps patients alter attitudes toward anxiety and fear.

Role of Acupuncture

Patients with trigeminal neuralgia frequently seek alternative forms of therapy. Often, these patients have experienced troublesome side effects from medical treatment or serious complications from surgery. Acupuncture is one of the alternative treatments frequently sought by patients with this condition. The natural remission of trigeminal neuralgia makes it difficult to evaluate and compare the efficacy of acupuncture with that of well-established medical and surgical treatments. Ge and co-workers have published a report of the use of acupuncture in patients with trigeminal neuralgia. They have claimed a high success rate, especially in patients who did not have long-standing disease. The lack of dangerous side effects seems to be its main advantage. We feel that acupuncture has a place for short-term management of pain in such patients. It should be used in patients who are intolerant to medical treatment. It may also be used as an adjuvant to optimize medical treatment.

Surgical Management

Surgical treatment should be sought only after a thorough trial of medical treatment has failed. Because surgery has no role in atypical facial pain states, diagnosis is absolutely vital. Several surgical strategies are available for management of trigeminal neuralgia, but only two methods have been shown to be consistently effective:

1. Gangliolysis
2. Microvascular decompression

Gangliolysis has replaced previously used neurodestructive procedures such as peripheral nerve avulsion, alcohol injections, subtemporal rhizotomy, posterior rhizotomy, and descending trigeminal tractotomy. This percutaneous procedure involves localization of the trigeminal nerve at the foramen ovale, under fluoroscopic guidance, and creation of a lesion with radiofrequency. In skilled hands, the procedure has a high success rate and a low complication rate. The most feared complication is anesthesia dolorosa (painful paresthesia).

Microvascular decompression has become an extremely popular operation among neurosurgeons for the treatment of trigeminal neuralgia. This is posterior fossa surgery and requires general anesthetic. An operating microscope is used to delineate the vascular impingement of the nerve root as it courses through Meckel's cave to the pons. The success rate of this procedure at 1 and 5 years is 85% and 80%, respectively, and the estimated half-life of the procedure is about 15 years. The mortality rate is 0.5%, and other troublesome complications occur in 10% to 15% cases. Recent advances in stereotactic surgery with the Leksell gamma knife have been extended to the management of trigeminal neuralgia, and initial results look promising.

BIBLIOGRAPHY

Bender IB, Freedland JB: Clinical considerations in the diagnosis and treatment of intra-alveolar root fractures. J Am Dent Assoc 107:595, 1983.

Cannon CR: Carotidynia: An unusual pain in the neck. Otolaryngol Head Neck Surg 110:387, 1994.

Costen JB: Syndrome of ear and sinus symptoms dependent upon functions of the temporomandibular joint. Ann Otol Rhinol Laryngol 3:1, 1934.

Dandy WE: Concerning the cause of trigeminal neuralgia. Am J Surg 24:447, 1934.

Desai BT, McHenry L Jr, Stanley JA: Raeder's syndrome. Ann Ophthalmol 7:1082, 1975.

Dornan TL, Espir ML, Gale EA, et al: Remittent painful ophthalmoplegia: The Tolosa-Hunt syndrome? A report of seven cases and review of the literature. J Neurol Neurosurg Psychiatry 42:270, 1979.

Fromm GH, Shibuya T, Nakata M, et al: Effects of D-baclofen and L-baclofen on the trigeminal nucleus. Neuropharmacology 29:249, 1990.

Ge S, Xu B, Zhang Y: Treatment of primary trigeminal neuralgia with acupuncture in 1500 cases. J Tradit Chin Med 11:3-6, 1991.

Graff-Radford SB: Headache problems that can present as toothache. Dent Clin North Am 35:155, 1991.

Grimson BS, Thompson HS: Raeder's syndrome: A clinical review. Surv Ophthalmol 24:199, 1980.

Lund JP, Widmer CG, Feine JS: Validity of diagnostic and monitoring tests used for temporomandibular disorders. J Dent Res 74:1133, 1995.

Lund JP, Widmer CG: Evaluation of the use of surface electromyography in the diagnosis, documentation, and treatment of dental patients. J Craniomandib Disord 3:125, 1989.

McCreary CP, Clark GT, Merril RL, et al: Psychological distress and diagnostic subgroups of temporomandibular disorder patients. Pain 44:29, 1991.

Okeson JP: Management of Temporomandibular Disorders and Occlusion, ed 4. St Louis, Mosby–Year Book, 1997.

Okeson JP: Orofacial Pain: Guidelines to Assessment, Diagnosis and Management, ed 3. Chicago, Quintessence Publishers, 1996.

Panagopoulos K, Chakraborty M, Deopujari CE, et al: Neurovascular decompression for cranial rhizopathies. Br J Neurosurg 1:235, 1987.

Rappaport ZH, Devor M: Trigeminal neuralgia: The role of self-sustaining discharge in the trigeminal ganglion. Pain 56:127, 1994.

Resnick DK, Jannetta PJ, Bissonnette D, et al: Microvascular decompression for glossopharyngeal neuralgia. Neurosurgery 36:64–68, 1995.

Sist T, Filadora V, Miner M, et al: Gabapentin for idiopathic trigeminal neuralgia: Report of two cases. Neurology 48:1467, 1997.

Testori T, Badino M, Castagnola M: Vertical root fractures in endodontically treated teeth: A clinical survey of 36 cases. J Endod 19:87, 1993.

Tomita H, Tanaka M, Kukimoto N, et al: An ELISA study on varicella-zoster virus infection in acute peripheral facial palsy. Acta Otolaryngol 446(suppl):10, 1988.

van Loveren H, Tew J Jr, Keller JT, et al: A 10-year experience in the treatment of trigeminal neuralgia: Comparison of percutaneous stereotaxic rhizotomy and posterior fossa exploration. J Neurosurg 57:757, 1982.

Xu BR, Ge SH: Observation on the effect of acupuncture treatment in 300 cases of primary trigeminal neuralgia. J Tradit Chin Med 1:51, 1981.

Yang J, Simonson TM, Ruprecht A: Magnetic resonance imaging used to assess patients with trigeminal neuralgia. Oral Surg Oral Med Oral Pathol Oral Radiol Endod 81:343, 1996.

Young RF, Vermeulen SS, Grimm P, et al: Gamma knife radiosurgery for treatment of trigeminal neuralgia: idiopathic and tumor related [comments]. Neurology 48:608, 1997.

Chapter 49

Low Back Pain: Differential Diagnosis and Physical Examination

Kenneth Chiou, M.D.

Studies have suggested that 80% of the population will suffer lower back pain of moderate to severe intensity at some point during their lifetime. Analysis of data also implicates that low back pain is the second leading cause of work absenteeism in this country and the most expensive disease entity in terms of loss of productivity and medical care. Fortunately, the majority of cases of low back pain (80% to 90%) resolve in about 6 weeks, with or without treatment.

Common causes of low back pain include sciatica, degenerative disc disease, ruptured disc, spinal stenosis, myofascial pain syndrome, and fibrositis. Up to 85% of patients cannot be given a definitive diagnosis, because back pain is a symptom rather than a disease. Many structures of the lumbar spine have been implicated as the source of low back pain, including (1) intervertebral ligaments, (2) outer ring of the annulus fibrosus, (3) facet joint and nerves, (4) paravertebral muscles, (5) fascia, and (6) spinal nerve roots.

Numerous causes of low back pain are generated by or referred to these structures. The following is a simple classification.

ETIOLOGY OF LOW BACK PAIN

1. Anatomic anomalies of the spine
   Kyphosis
   Scoliosis
   Facet asymmetry
   Spondylolithiasis
2. Metabolic/endocrine disease
   Osteoporosis
   Osteopenia
   Hyperthyroidism
   Hyperparathyroidism
   Cushing's syndrome
3. Infection of spine structure
   Osteomyelitis
   Discitis
   Epidural abscess
   Sacroiliitis

4. Inflammatory rheumatologic disease
   Ankylosing spondylitis
   Chronic inflammatory bowel disease
   Reiter's syndrome
   Psoriatic arthritis
   Rheumatoid arthritis
   Osteoarthritis
5. Malignant neoplasm (primary or metastatic)
   Multiple myeloma
   Metastatic disease
   Lymphoma/leukemia
   Primary osseous tumor
   Spinal cord tumor
6. Trauma of spinal structures
   Lumbar musculoligament strain
   Lumbar spine fracture
   Facet arthritis
7. Degenerative disease of spine
   Herniation of the nucleus pulposus
   Spinal stenosis
   Spondylosis
   Spondylolisthesis
8. Visceral pain (referred lower back pain)
   Prostatitis
   Pelvic inflammatory disease
   Ovarian cyst
   Endometriosis
   Pyelonephritis
   Nephrolithiasis
   Cholecystitis
   Pancreatitis
   Peptic ulcer disease
   Abdominal aortic vessel disease
9. Psychosocial
   Hysteria
   Malingering
   Somatization

Given this long list, careful diagnostic evaluation is essential in finding a specific cause. In the era of sophisticated imaging and laboratory studies, a detailed history and physical examination remain the key to low back pain diagnosis.

215

The initial back pain history generally centers around the onset, location, duration, and nature of the pain symptom as well as on diagnostic or therapeutic interventions that have been performed. After obtaining basic information, the possibility of vascular, malignant, or infectious causes is ruled out.

An expanding or ruptured abdominal aneurysm is a rare catastrophic cause of acute low back pain. The history of prior vascular surgery, severe hypertension, and anticoagulation therapy, together with abdominal pain and distention, should raise the suspicion of this diagnosis.

A previous history of malignancy (especially breast, lung, or prostate), weight loss, and pain unrelieved by position change would require further diagnostic studies to rule out malignant causes. Unexplained fever, history of intravenous drug abuse, urinary tract infection, and recent spine procedures may suggest spinal infections.

The next task is to identify patients at risk of disability secondary to spinal cord or cauda equina compression. Cauda equina syndrome is uncommon, but it requires immediate surgical therapy. Symptoms include urinary retention, sciatica, saddle distribution sensory loss, and decreased anal sphincter tone.

Finally, the possibilities of psychological and social stresses, reactive or systemic depression, and secondary gain factors should be carefully considered.

After completion of the medical history, the physical examination is the next step in the diagnostic process. Physical examination starts from inspection of the patient's affect, physical status, posture, and gait. As the patient walks into the examining room, the gait should be observed for evidence of foot drop, instability, or any gross leg-length discrepancy.

Two major pathologic gaits are gluteus medius gait and antalgic gait. Gluteus medius gait is caused by weakness of the gluteus medius muscle, and it causes the patient to shift the trunk to the affected side to maintain the center of gravity. Antalgic gait is often seen in painful hip conditions and is characterized by a shortened stance phase time on the involved hip to relieve painful pressure.

Next, the skin surface of the back should be inspected for special markings. For example, "pigmented spit" (café au lait spots) may indicate neurofibromatosis or collagen disease. A hairy patch (faun's beard) on the midback may indicate a congenital neural axis defect.

The patient is asked to walk on the toes and then on the heels to detect instability or foot drop and to evaluate gastrocnemius, soleus, and peroneal muscles.

The patient should also be asked to do a deep knee bend and then to squat as fully as possible and arise. This maneuver will point out possible associated hip, knee, foot, and ankle problems.

For a range-of-motion test, the examiner should be aware that the spine is more flexible in younger patients. Normally there is 80 degrees of flexion, 25 degrees of extension, 25 degrees of lateral rotation to the right and left, and 25 degrees of lateral bending to the right and left. Extension is more likely to cause pain in the patient with facet disease or spinal stenosis, and pain with flexion is more common with disc herniation.

For purposes of neurologic examination, the patient should sit on the examination table facing the examiner, with the legs hanging over the edge of the table. The chief flexor of the hip is the iliopsoas group of muscles and is innervated by L1–4 nerve roots. The primary adductor is the adductor longus, which is innervated by the obturator nerve (L2–4). The secondary adductors are many, including the adductors brevis and magnus. The adductors of the hip are mostly innervated by the obturator nerve (L2–4). The abductors of the hip are innervated by the superior gluteal nerve (L4–S1). The primary abductor is the gluteus medius, which is innervated by the superior gluteal nerve (L4–S1). The secondary abductor is the gluteus minimus.

The quadriceps muscles control knee extension and are innervated by femoral nerve (L2–L4). Knee flexion is controlled by the tibial nerve (L5–S1). The tibialis anterior muscle is chiefly responsible for ankle dorsiflexion and is innervated by the deep peroneal nerve (L4–S1).

The superficial peroneal nerve (L4–S1) can be tested by eversion of foot and the posterior tibial nerve (L5–S1) by plantar flexion of foot.

Sensation to light touch, temperature, and pin-prick are assessed and any deficit pattern is matched with the sensory dermatome.

The patellar reflex (knee jerk) is elicited when the quadriceps contracts in response to a tap on the patellar tendon. Its absence may correlate with femoral nerve (L2–L4) impairment.

The Achilles reflex (ankle jerk) is elicited by contractions of gastrocnemius-soleus muscles in response to a tap on the Achilles tendon. Its absence may correlate with S1 impairment.

After the history and physical examination are completed, enough information should be available to judge whether additional diagnostic procedures may be needed. In the majority of instances, the physician should be able to recognize the likelihood of a malignancy, infection, or severe spine disease requiring surgery. In addition, the physician should be able to judge whether this is an acute "strain" (likely to require short-term, simple pain control measures, such as ice, analgesic medication, and restricted activity) or a more chronic and complex problem with a possible protracted radiculopathy, fibromyalgia, or chronic pain syndrome.

SPECIAL TESTS FOR LOW BACK EXAMINATION

Many tests are used to reproduce nerve root irritation by increasing intrathecal pressure. These tests cannot be completely objective and cannot rule out malingering.

Milgram Test

The patient, in a supine position, is asked to raise both extended legs 2 in. above the table for 30 seconds. The test is positive if the leg pain is reproduced when a complaint of back pain is insignificant.

Naffziger Test

The test is performed by compressing the jugular veins for 10 seconds as the patient's face flushes. The patient is asked to cough to cause an increase in intrathecal pressure.

Valsalva Test

The patient is asked to bear down, as during a bowel movement or coughing. The test is positive if the maneuver causes posterior leg pain.

Brudzinski Test

The patient lies supine, with the head passively flexed toward the chest. The reproduction of leg pain yields a positive finding.

Kernig Test

With the patient in a supine position, the thigh is flexed 90 degrees with the knee flexed 90 degrees to the thigh. Leg pain is a result of nerve root irritation.

Sober Test

The Sober test is used to measure flexibility of the lumbar spine. The patient's back is marked in the midline at the level of the sacroiliac dimples, and another mark is made 15 cm above the first. As the patient flexes the lumbar spine, the distance between two points should increase by 5 cm. The abnormal test suggests the presence of spondyloarthropathy.

Straight Leg Raising Test

This test is designed to reproduce low back pain due to disc herniation by stretching the affected nerve root and the dura. This test is especially useful for testing the lower lumbar nerve roots (L4, L5, and S1). The patient, in a supine position, raises the affected leg with the knee fully extended. The degrees of leg elevation and pain reproduction are recorded. Studies show that minimal tension is applied to the sciatic roots before 30 degrees of elevation and that no additional tension is generated after 70 degrees of elevation. A positive straight leg raising test result is defined as one that reproduces sciatica between 30 and 70 degrees of leg elevation. In addition, the physician should determine if the pain originates in the sciatic nerve or is a result of hamstring tightness.

Crossed or Well Straight Leg Raising Test (Fajersztajn Test)

The straight leg raising test is performed on the asymptomatic leg, and the test is positive when radicular pain is elicited in the abnormal leg. The test is highly specific as a positive result, often indicating severe disc herniation.

Lasègue Test

Often mistaken for a straight leg test, this test is performed with the patient's hip flexed to 90 degrees at the same time as the knee is slowly extended until sciatic pain is elicited. The test is more difficult to interpret, as both hip and knee joints are moving simultaneously.

Femoral Stretch Test

This is useful for testing for entrapment of upper lumbar nerve roots (mostly L2 and L3). With the patient in a complete prone position with the hip on the table, the knees are flexed as the legs are stretched toward buttocks. Pain on the front thigh may indicate a femoral nerve problem.

TESTS FOR SACROILIAC JOINT OR HIP DYSFUNCTION

Pathology of the sacroiliac joint is relatively uncommon. Tenderness on palpation of the sacroiliac joint does not necessarily signify sacroiliac joint dysfunction. The tests for sacroiliac joint disease should be interpreted with care, as their sensitivities are moderate at best.

Pelvic Rock Test

With the patient lying supine on the table, the examiner should place both hands on the superior anterior iliac spine and compress the pelvis toward the midline. Pain can be produced in the sacroiliac joint if there is localized pathology.

Gaenslen's Test

The patient is supine with the left leg beyond the edge of the table. The examiner flexes the patient's right knee and hip and presses downward over the left thigh to hyperextend the left hip. Pain is present on the left sacroiliac joint in the presence of sacroiliac joint dysfunction. The maneuver is repeated on the right side with the right leg by hanging over the edge of the table.

Patrick Test

The patient lies supine on the table and places the foot of the painful side on the opposite knee. The examiner can stress the sacroiliac joint by placing one hand on the flexed knee joint and the other hand on the anterior superior iliac spine of opposite side. This test is also called the FABER test, as it designates *f*lexion, *ab*duction, and *e*xternal *r*otation of involved sacroiliac joint or hip. This test is used to detect pathology in the sacroiliac joint as well as in the hip.

Extension Test

The patient is prone and the examiner places one hand under the thigh above the knee on the affected side. With the other hand, he presses downward over the crest of the ilium to elicit the pain in the sacroiliac joint.

Beevor Test

The recumbent patient raises the head against resistance, coughs, or attempts to rise to a sitting position from recumbency with the hands folded on the chest or behind the head. If the abdominal muscles contract equally on both sides of the midline, the umbilicus will remain in the midline. When abdominal muscles are weakened on one side, the movements are performed with difficulty. Moreover, with paralysis of the abdominal muscles on one side, the umbilicus is pulled to the normal side. Paralysis of the upper half of one side of the abdominal muscles is associated with a downward movement of the umbilicus when the abdominal wall is tense, whereas upward movement of the umbilicus occurs with paralysis of the lower half. This is termed *Beevor's sign*. When both sides of the abdominal muscles are paralyzed, the umbilicus bulges during coughing.

TESTS FOR MALINGERING OR FUNCTIONAL DISORDER

A number of objective clinical tests (e.g., Waddell test) are capable of detecting nonorganic causes of low back pain. These tests should be preformed with objectivity and the results interpreted with care. The diagnosis of malingering should be assigned or accepted with great caution.

Waddell Test

1. Pain and tenderness that is either superficial or nonanatomic in distribution.
2. Reproduction of back pain by axial loading stimulation (pressure on the head of the standing patient) or rotation of the pelvis and shoulders in the same plane, avoiding spinal movement.
3. Discrepancies in straight leg raising tests performed in the sitting and supine positions.
4. Sensory disturbance of nondermatomal pattern or motor weakness that cannot be explained on a neurologic basis.
5. Overreaction during the examination process.

Hoover Test

When the patient is in a supine position, an attempt to raise one leg off the table will simultaneously result in downward movement of the other leg. The downward movement of the opposite leg is automatic and reveals feigned weakness of that leg.

Voluntary Release Test

In a flexion and extension examination, the patient with a nonorganic cause tends to produce intermittent jerky movements instead of a smooth contraction and release.

Sit-up Test

Patient with acute disc disease or severe paraspinal muscle spasm will have difficulty sitting up with flexion of the lumbar spine. Such a patient tends to roll to one side and push up laterally with the arms.

TESTS FOR UPPER MOTOR NEURON LESION

With upper motor neuron lesions, the patient may exhibit muscle spasticity, tonic contractions, and hyperreflexia. The following are the pathologic reflexes associated with upper motor lesions.

Babinski Reflex Test

Stimulation is applied to the plantar aspect of the foot with a dull object. The test is positive when the lateral four toes flex and fan while the big toe extends.

Chaddock Reflex Test

The lateral aspect of the foot below the lateral malleolus is stimulated with a dull object. The positive response is similar to that of the Babinski test.

Oppenheim Reflex Test

The stimulation is elicited by pressing down the anterior tibia with a dull object. The response is similar to a positive Babinski test result.

BIBLIOGRAPHY

Deyo RA, Rainville J, Kent DL: What can the history and physical examination tell us about low back pain? JAMA 1992;268:760-765.
Nachemson AL: The lumbar spine and orthopedic challenge. Spine 1976;11:59-71.
Praemer A, Furners S, Rice DP: Musculoskeletal Conditions in the United States. Park Ridge, IL, American Academy of Orthopaedic Surgeons, 1992, pp 23-33.
Swezey RL: Pathophysiology and treatment of intervertebral disk disease. Osteoarthritis 1993;19:741-756.
Vukmir RB: Low back pain: Review of diagnosis and therapy. American Journal of Emergency Medicine 1991;9:328-335.
Waddell G, McCulloch J, Kummel E, Venner RM: Nonorganic physical signs in low back pain. Spine 1980;5:117-125.

Chapter 50

Injection of Epidural Steroids

Robert E. Molloy, M.D.,
and Honorio T. Benzon, M.D.

Injections of epidural steroids have been used for more than 35 years, and their history has been reviewed in detail elsewhere.[1-5] Use of caudal steroid injection to treat sciatica in the United States was first reported by Goebert and colleagues in 1960.[6] Numerous other publications subsequently appeared describing the results of epidural steroid injections (ESI). The value of lumbar ESI performed near the level of nerve root involvement with smaller volumes of diluent has been suggested. The use of cervical ESI was summarized in three separate reports in 1986.[7-9]

DRUGS USED FOR EPIDURAL INJECTION

Most reports indicate that either methylprednisolone acetate or triamcinolone diacetate is used. The concentration of methylprednisolone is either 40 or 80 mg/mL; the therapeutic dose is 80 mg. The concentration of triamcinolone is 25 mg/mL, and the therapeutic dose is 50 mg. No study has compared the effectiveness of these two agents, and both have been reported to be effective, safe, and long-acting. Most anesthesiologists dilute steroid drugs with local anesthetic or normal saline solution, and they apparently achieve equivalent results.

The volume of injectate varies with the site of injection. The injection of 6 to 10 mL has been recommended at the lumbar level to bathe both the injured nerve root that is adjacent to the disc pathology and additional nearby roots that are also inflamed.[4] At the cervical level, large-volume injections have been employed but 4 to 6 mL should be adequate to bathe the cervical roots; 6 mL is the most commonly reported volume. When the caudal route is selected, a larger volume (approximately 20 to 25 mL) is selected to ensure adequate spread of injectate to the midlumbar level.

MECHANISM OF ACTION

The indication for ESI is nerve root irritation and inflammation. Nerve root edema has been observed surgically and demonstrated with computed tomographic scanning in patients with herniated discs.[10] Surgical disc samples from patients with disc herniation contain extremely high levels of phospholipase A2.[11] This enzyme liberates arachidonic acid from cell membranes. Degenerative disc disease and tears of the annulus fibrosus may result in leakage of this enzyme from the nucleus pulposus, producing chemical irritation of nerve roots. Steroids induce synthesis of a phospholipase A2 inhibitor, preventing release of substrate for prostaglandin synthesis. Therefore steroids can interfere with the inflammatory process at an earlier step than systemic, nonsteroidal anti-inflammatory drugs (NSAIDs) do. This may benefit the many patients with a chemical rather than a compressive radicular pain syndrome and negative radiologic studies.

In addition to their anti-inflammatory effect, steroids also block nociceptive input. Corticosteroids suppress ongoing discharge in chronic neuromas and prevent the development of ectopic neural discharges from experimental neuromas.[12] This suppression of neuroma discharge has been attributed to a direct membrane action of the steroid. Local application of methylprednisolone acetate was found to block transmission in C fibers but not in Aβ fibers. The effect was reversible, suggesting direct membrane action of the steroid.[13]

INDICATIONS

Many authors have attempted to identify which patients are most likely to benefit from ESI. White and colleagues[14] observed how 304 patients responded to ESI and correlated these findings with the cause of their back pain. Response to ESI was predicted by nerve root irritation, recent onset of symptoms, and absence of psychological overlay. ESI was therapeutic for patients with herniated disc and either nerve root irritation or compression. These latter two factors were also associated with efficacy in patients with spondylolisthesis or scoliosis. Relief was transient in patients with chronic lumbar degenerative disc disease or spinal stenosis. Many other studies have reported efficacy for patients with radicular pain syndromes or herniated nucleus pulposus. In a review, Benzon summarized the questionable benefit of ESI in patients with chronic low back pain, degenerative bony pathology, or previous back surgery.[4]

Hacobian and associates[15] retrospectively evaluated 50 patients with lumbar spinal stenosis, back pain, or pseudoclaudication who were treated with one to three ESI. Initial results included complete relief in 8%, partial relief in 52%, and failure in 40%. The duration of pain relief was longer than 6 months in 26%, 1 to 6 months in 33%, and less than 1 month in 40%. Overall, 60% of these patients improved, but only 15% had a prolonged response.

Three studies have investigated predictors of response to lumbar ESI. Abram and Hopwood[16] prospectively investigated factors contributing to treatment success in 212 patients. Three factors were strongly associated with favorable response to injection: (1) advanced educational background, (2) a primary diagnosis of radiculopathy, and (3) pain duration of less than 6 months. Three factors that correlated with treatment failure were (1) constant pain, (2) frequent sleep disruption, and (3) being unemployed due to pain. Subsequently, Hopwood and Abram[17] analyzed factors associated with failure of ESI in 209 patients. There was a threefold increase in treatment failure with prolonged pain of more than 24 months' duration and with nonradicular diagnosis. A twofold increase in poor outcome was related to lack of employment because of pain, smoking, and symptom duration of 6 to 24 months.

Sandrock and Warfield[18] suggest that the five most important factors influencing the outcome of ESI are accuracy of the diagnosis of nerve root inflammation, shorter duration of symptoms, no history of previous surgery, younger age of the patient, and location of the needle at the level of pathology.

EFFICACY

Has the efficacy of ESI been established? The extensive literature on this question leaves much to be desired. Most studies were purely anecdotal, retrospective, and not randomized, controlled, or blinded. Patient populations were poorly defined and not homogeneous: patients who were studied had both acute and chronic pain, some had had back surgery, and their back pain was secondary to various causes. Finally, treatment protocols were variable, and outcome criteria were not well established.

Investigators who reviewed the literature came to different conclusions. Although Kepes and Duncalf[1] concluded that the rationale of ESI was not proved, Benzon[2] noted it to be effective in acute lumbosacral radiculopathy. Review articles on the subject also were not in complete agreement. Spaccarelli[19] concluded that ESI

was efficacious in lower extremity radicular pain syndromes at intermediate-term follow-up (2 weeks to 3 months) but that no difference could be expected at long-term follow-up. Koes and associates[20] found no suggestion of efficacy for ESI in patients with *chronic* low back pain *without* sciatica. However, they stated that 6 of 12 studies showed ESI to be more effective than the control treatment for patients *with* sciatica, while the other 6 showed it to be no better and no worse than the reference treatment. They concluded that the efficacy of ESI has not been established. This does not contradict the earlier findings of Benzon[2] that ESI may be effective in patients with acute lumbosacral radiculopathy.

A consistent verdict on treatment efficacy has not been supported by the available controlled studies. An additional analysis of this literature was published by Watts and Silagy.[21] Efficacy was defined as pain relief (at least 75% improvement) in the short term (60 days) and in the long term (1 year). ESI increased the odds ratio of pain relief to 2.61 in the short term and to 1.87 for long-term relief of pain. Efficacy was independent of the route of administration (i.e., caudal or lumbar). This analysis provided quantitative evidence that epidural corticosteroids are effective in the management of lumbosacral radicular pain when injected by either the lumbar or the caudal route.

There have been three prospective, randomized, double-blind, placebo-controlled studies of patients with documented herniated disc and pain present for less than 1 year who received *lumbar* ESI (Table 50–1). Dilke and associates[22] showed significantly better pain relief and better rates of return to work with ESI than with interspinous ligament saline injections at 3 months' follow-up. Snoek and colleagues[23] reported greater subjective and objective improvements after ESI compared with placebo injection, but this difference did not reach statistical significance. Their study used undiluted steroid in a 2-mL volume and evaluated patients after 24 to 48 hours (compared with 6 days in the study by Dilke and colleagues[22]). Carette and co-workers[24] administered ESI up to three times and found that the differences in improvement between groups were not significant, except for improvements in the finger-to-floor distance ($P = 0.006$) and in sensory deficits ($P = 0.03$), which were greater in the methylprednisolone group. ESI did not offer significant functional benefit, nor did it reduce the need for surgery in these patients with pain and neurologic deficits due to significant disc herniation.

Bush and Hillier[25] employed *caudal* epidural steroid or normal saline injections in a randomized, double-blind, placebo-controlled study of clinically well-defined patients with radicular pain, paresthesias, and positive straight-leg raising. They found significantly better pain relief at both 4 weeks (visual analog scale 16.0 vs. 45.0) and 52 weeks (14.2 vs. 29.6) for ESI compared with placebo.

Prospective long-term follow-up studies after ESI are lacking. Persistent benefit after ESI was reported by Dilke and co-workers[22] after 3 months (36% complete and 55% partial relief); by Green and associates[26] (41%

TABLE 50–1. RESULTS OF WELL-CONTROLLED STUDIES ON LUMBAR EPIDURAL STEROID INJECTIONS FOR PATIENTS WITH ACUTE HERNIATED DISC

Study	Type of Study	Symptom Duration	Treatments Studied and Route	Success Rate (%), Steroid vs. Control
Dilke et al[22]	P, R, DB	≤1 yr	MP, 80 mg in 10 mL NS vs. 1 mL NS, lumbar	60% vs. 31% initial pain relief; less pain, less analgesic use, and less failed return to work at 3 mo
Snoek et al[23]	P, R, DB	1–3 wk	MP, 80 mg in 2 mL NS vs. 2 mL NS, lumbar	25% to 70% improvement in multiple outcome measures, not significantly different from 7% to 43% in placebo group
Carette et al[24]	P, R, DB	<1 yr	MP, 80 mg in 8 mL NS vs. 1 mL NS, lumbar	Less sensory deficit and leg pain; functional disability and incidence of surgery the same

P, prospective; R, randomized; DB, double-blind; MP, methylprednisolone; NS, normal saline.

sustained relief for at least 1 year); and by Bush and Hillier[25] at 52 weeks (earlier benefit was maintained or improved), all in patients with discogenic, radicular pain. Abram and Hopwood[16] also monitored patients who received ESI and demonstrated persistent improvement at 6 and 12 months in those who initially responded. They reported that the patients had significantly better pain reduction and better rates of return to work than patients who failed ESI. In a more heterogeneous group of patients, White and co-workers[14] reported persistent improvement after 6 months in 34% of patients with acute pain and in 12% of patients with chronic pain.

CERVICAL INJECTION

Reports on the use of cervical ESI to treat cervical radiculopathy and various other diagnoses began to appear in 1986.[7-9] There have been no blinded, controlled, randomized studies to assess the efficacy of this procedure (Table 50–2).[27-31]

Stav and colleagues[29] reported on 50 patients with chronic, refractory neck and arm pain who were treated with physical therapy and continued NSAIDs. All patients had degenerative disc disease, osteoarthritis of the cervical spine, or both, with or without radiculopathy. In addition, all had had pain for longer than 6 months. Cervical ESI proved to be superior to posterior neck intramuscular injections for short- and long-term pain relief, improved range of motion, decreased analgesic consumption, and recovery of the capacity to work. At 1 year follow-up, good to excellent results were found in 68% of the patients in the ESI group vs. 12% in the intramuscular injection group.

Ferrante and colleagues[32] attempted to find predictors of clinical outcome in a retrospective review of 100

TABLE 50–2. RESULTS OF PUBLISHED REPORTS ON CERVICAL EPIDURAL STEROID INJECTIONS*

Study	Study Design	No. of Patients	Population	Response
Shulman[7]	D	96	Chronic neck pain, 68% spondylosis and 22% radiculopathy	41% good to excellent
Purkis[8]	D	58	Head and neck pain for longer than 6 mo, heterogeneous	66% had more than 50% decrease in VAS at 3 wk
Rowlingson and Kirschenbaum[9]	D	25	Cervical radiculopathy, well-defined	24% excellent, 40% good results up to 6 mo
Warfield et al[27]	D	18	Cervical radiculopathy, pain and numbness	67% initial relief and 44% response at 6 mo
Cicala et al[28]	D	79	Neck and arm pain, heterogeneous group	84% initial relief, 41% excellent at 6 mo
Stav et al[29]	P, R, D	50	Chronic neck and arm pain for longer than 6 mo, degenerative disc and cervical spine disease	68% good to very good after cervical epidural vs. 12% after intramuscular neck injection at 1 yr follow-up
Castagnera et al[30]	P, R, C	24	Chronic cervical radicular pain for longer than 12 mo, no nerve compression	71% had at least 75% decrease in VAS at 3 mo
Bush and Hillier[31]	P, D	68	Cervical radiculopathy, with neurologic signs, for 1–12 mo	76% pain free and 24% improved (average 2, range 1–4 on a 10-point scale)

C, controlled; D, descriptive; P, prospective; R, randomized; VAS, visual analog scale.
* No well-controlled studies of cervical epidural steroid injections are available.
All studies are retrospective except for those of Stav et al.[29] and Castagnera et al.[30]
Adapted from Molloy RE, Benzon HT: The current status of epidural steroids. Curr Rev Pain 1:1, 1996.

patients who received cervical ESI. Radicular pain predicted a better outcome; radiologic diagnosis of a normal scan or of disc herniation predicted a poor outcome. The authors recommended selection of patients for cervical ESI by the presence of radicular pain and either physical or radiologic findings corresponding to the painful nerve root.

COMPLICATIONS

Complications of ESI may be classified as those related to epidural technique and those related to injected drugs. Technical side effects include back pain at the injection site and temporarily increased radicular pain and paresthesias without persistent morbidity. Acute anxiety, lightheadedness, diaphoresis, flushing, nausea, hypotension, and vasovagal syncope may occur, especially during procedures performed with the patient in the sitting position. Headache may occur after accidental dural puncture, the most common complication of epidural injection. In experienced hands, this complication should occur in fewer than 1% of attempted epidural injections. MacDonald[33] cited an incidence of 0.33% for 5685 lumbar epidural injections. Waldman[34] reported dural puncture in 0.25% of 790 cervical epidural injections. Nonpostural headache due to subarachnoid air injection has been reported; Katz and colleagues[35] reported immediate onset of headache attributed to injection of air into the subdural space.

Retinal hemorrhage had been associated with rapid, large-volume caudal steroid injection performed under general anesthesia.[36] Significant epidural hemorrhage appears to be rare in the absence of coagulopathy. Williams and associates[37] reported a case of acute paraplegia caused by epidural hematoma formation after a seventh cervical ESI in a patient who had used indomethacin regularly for 6 years.

Infectious complications of ESI include bacterial meningitis and epidural abscess. Meningitis is unlikely to develop unless unintentional dural puncture occurs. Dougherty and Fraser[38] reported two cases of bacterial meningitis after attempted ESI. One patient had accidental lumbar puncture before steroid injection; dural puncture was neither diagnosed nor ruled out with a local anesthetic test dose in the other case.

Epidural abscess was reported by Shealy[39] in 1966 after a series of four epidural injections of steroid in a patient who had coexistent local spinal metastatic disease. Cancer cells were identified in the purulent material, but no bacteria were cultured. Five other cases of epidural abscess were reported between 1984 and 1997; one after cervical, three after lumbar, and one after caudal ESI[40-44] (Table 50–3). Cultures grew *Staphylococcus aureus* in all five patients. Three patients had diabetes mellitus; two had multiple (i.e., three) injections; one had had a surgical infection with *S. aureus* 2 weeks before ESI; and one had breast cancer with spinal metastasis located in the sacrum. All patients presented 3 days to 3 weeks after injection with fever, spinal pain, radicular pain, or progressive neurologic deficit; this scenario should elicit a high index of suspicion for epidural abscess. Rapid diagnosis and therapy, including surgical drainage, appears necessary if one hopes to achieve patient recovery with intact neurologic function. Magnetic resonance imaging appears to be the procedure of choice for the diagnosis of epidural abscess.[41] The combination of diabetes and steroid immunosuppression may predispose to epidural abscess formation. An additional two patients developed a thoracic epidural abscess after repeated epidural injections of bupivacaine and steroid to treat neuropathic pain secondary to herpes zoster infection[45-48] (Table 50–3).

TABLE 50–3. REPORTED CASES OF EPIDURAL ABSCESS AFTER EPIDURAL STEROID INJECTION

Study	Injections	Findings	Outcome	Medical History
Shealy[39]	L, × 4, M	Squamous cell cancer and inflammatory cells	Foot drop, late death due to cancer	Cancer
Chan and Leung[40]	L, × 1, T	*Staphylococcus aureus*	T8 paraplegia, near-complete recovery	Diabetes
Goucke and Graziotti[41]	L, × 3, M	*Staphylococcus aureus*	Death	Diabetes, recent postoperative staphylococcal sepsis
Waldman[42]	C, × 3	*Staphylococcus aureus*	C6-level quadriparesis	None
Mamourian et al[43]	L, × 1	*Staphylococcus aureus*	Death	Cancer
Knight et al[44]	S, × 2, T + P	*Staphylococcus aureus*	Paraplegia	Diabetes
Bromage[45]	Th, × 6, M	Not stated	Quadriplegia	Postherpetic neuralgia
Strong[46]	Th, × 1, M + B × 10 via 2 catheters	*Staphylococcus aureus*	Complete recovery	Resolving acute herpes zoster; two separate epidural catheters for 1 and 3 days; prophylactic oral antibiotics × 10 days

L, lumbar; C, cervical; S, caudal; Th, thoracic; M, methylprednisolone acetate; T, triamcinolone diacetate; B, bupivacaine; P, procaine.
Adapted from Molloy RE, Benzon HT: The current status of epidural steroids. Curr Rev Pain 1:1, 1996.

Complications related to the drugs used for ESI include pharmacologic effects of steroids and possible neurotoxicity. Temporary development of Cushing's syndrome,[47] weight gain, fluid retention, hyperglycemia, hypertension, and congestive heart failure have all been reported after ESI. Kaposi's sarcoma was observed after intra-articular steroid injection, and it later recurred after ESI.[48] A single case of allergic reaction to ESI was reported by Simon and coworkers.[49] Very delayed onset of a cutaneous, respiratory, and gastrointestinal reaction was noted and was reproduced with subsequent exposure to triamcinolone. Adrenal suppression is a well known result of ESI. Plasma cortisol levels are decreased for up to 3 weeks after epidural injection of 80 mg of methylprednisolone acetate. Kay and colleagues[50] described the effects of three weekly epidural triamcinolone injections on the pituitary-adrenal axis in humans. Depressed levels of adrenocorticotropic hormone (ACTH) and cortisol, and abnormal cortisol response to synthetic ACTH, were noted for up to 1 month after ESI. Relative adrenal insufficiency should be considered when major surgical stress occurs within 1 month after ESI.

Neurotoxicity has been attributed to spinal injections of depot steroids or to their preservatives. Adhesive arachnoiditis has been reported after repeated intrathecal steroid injections in patients with multiple sclerosis. There are no case reports of arachnoiditis after ESI alone. Abram and O'Connor[51] reviewed the risk of complications from ESI. They were unable to find a single report of arachnoiditis in 64 series describing these injections in about 7000 patients. They did, however, collect many reports of spontaneous arachnoiditis without prior spinal injection. Aseptic meningitis has been reported three times after intrathecal steroid injection and once after ESI.[52] These patients had headache, fever, and other systemic symptoms, and their cerebrospinal fluid was characterized by low glucose with elevated protein and leukocytes.

Nelson has questioned both the efficacy and the safety of intraspinal methylprednisolone acetate.[53] He recommended against its intrathecal use because of potential polyethylene glycol toxicity. He also attempted to implicate epidural injection as dangerous because of hypothetical migration into the subarachnoid space as well as accidental subdural or intrathecal injection. He believes that this may occur often with attempted epidural injection, especially after previous injections or back surgery.

Relevant animal data on neurotoxicity after ESI are limited. MacKinnon and coworkers[54] investigated the effects of various steroids injected into or near rat sciatic nerves. Nerve injury occurred only after direct intrafascicular injection. Benzon and associates[55] examined the effect of polyethylene glycol exposure on the electrophysiology of sheathed and unsheathed rabbit nerves. They demonstrated no effect from the clinically relevant 3% or even a 10% concentration but reversible decrements in conduction at 20% and 30% and no conduction at 40%. Abram and colleagues[56] studied the effects of serial intrathecal steroid injections on the rat spinal cord, finding no demonstrable analgesia with formalin pain testing and no histologic changes 21 days after injection. They concluded that accidental intrathecal injection during attempted ESI has a low potential to cause harm.

Abram and O'Connor[51] made several recommendations to avoid complications of ESI. They suggested a meticulous aseptic technique, especially in diabetic patients, to prevent infectious sequelae. They indicated that high-dose or repeated injections (more than one to three) have no support in the literature. They also recommended use of a local anesthetic test dose to prevent accidental, undetected intrathecal steroid injection and possible neurotoxic effects. The purported benefit to the patient must be weighed against the more likely risk of hemodynamic consequences when

TABLE 50–4. EVALUATION CRITERIA: SELECTION OF PATIENTS FOR EPIDURAL STEROID INJECTION

	Positive Factors	Negative Predictive Factors	Increased Risk
History	Radicular pain Radicular numbness Short symptom duration Absence of significant psychological factors	Axial pain primarily Work-related injury Unemployed due to pain High number of past treatments, high number of drugs taken Compensation due to pain Litigation pending Previous back surgery Smoking history Very high pain ratings	Immunosuppression Diabetes Peptic ulcer disease Tuberculosis AIDS Bacterial infection
Examination	Dermatomal sensory loss Motor loss correlated to symptoms Positive straight leg raising	Myofascial pain prominent	
Laboratory results	Abnormal electromyographic findings related to symptoms Lumbar herniated disc Cervical spondylosis	Normal cervical spine imaging scans Cervical herniated disc	

Data from Rowlingson and Kirschenbaum[9]; White, Derby, and Wynne[14]; Abram and Hopwood[16]; Hopwood and Abram[17]; Ferrante et al.[52]; Abram and Anderson[60]; and Jamison, VadeBoncoeur, and Ferrante.[61]

contemplating local anesthetic vs. saline epidural injection.

CURRENT ROLE

The efficacy of ESI has not been conclusively demonstrated, and it is unlikely that a definitive study will be completed. Nevertheless, many studies have confirmed very good short- to intermediate-term success rates in selected patients. Reviews by Rowlingson,[57] Abram,[58] and Hammonds[59] state the case for continued use of this therapy as part of the overall management of patients with acute radicular pain, herniated disc, or new radiculopathy superimposed on chronic back pain or cervical spondylosis. The analysis by Watts and Silagy[21] and the review by Spaccarelli[19] support the efficacy of ESI in lumbosacral radicular pain syndromes. This conclusion is challenged but not disproved by Koes and associates.[20] The presence of nerve root irritation is required to justify use of ESI. However, this therapy may be less efficacious in patients with neurologic deficits and a large disc herniation than in those with acute radicular pain alone.[24] Thorough patient evaluation, consideration of benefits and risks, and informed patient consent are essential to active selection of patients for this treatment (Table 50–4). Reliable patient follow-up and comprehensive management of physical, occupational, and emotional rehabilitation are necessary to avoid a too narrowly focused, block-oriented approach to these patients.

The authors' technique for ESI has been described.[4] Methylprednisolone acetate, 80 mg, is employed as the steroid drug. The diluent usually is normal saline, with the total volume being 6 to 10 mL at the lumbar level, 6 mL at the cervical level, and 20 mL when the caudal approach is selected. The injection is not repeated if there is complete relief. If partial relief occurs a second injection is offered, but a third injection is only rarely used. Repeat injections are not offered when benefit is transient but may be considered after prolonged responses of 6 to 12 months or longer.

REFERENCES

1. Kepes ER, Duncalf D: Treatment of backache with spinal injections of local anesthetics, spinal and systemic steroids. Pain 22:33, 1985.
2. Benzon HT: Epidural steroid injections for low back pain and lumbosacral radiculopathy. Pain 24:277, 1986.
3. Haddox JD: Lumbar and cervical epidural steroid therapy. Anesthesiol Clin North Am 10:179, 1992.
4. Benzon HT: Epidural steroids. In Raj PP (ed): Practical Management of Pain, ed 2. St. Louis, Mosby–Year Book, 1992, p 818.
5. Molloy RE, Benzon HT: The current status of epidural steroids. Current Review of Pain 1:1, 1996.
6. Goebert HW, Jallo ST, Gardner WS: Sciatica: Treatment with epidural injections of procaine and hydrocortisone. Cleve Clin Q 27:191, 1960.
7. Shulman M: Treatment of neck pain with cervical epidural steroid injection. Reg Anesth 11:92, 1986.
8. Purkis IE: Cervical epidural steroids. Pain Clinic 1:3, 1986.
9. Rowlingson JC, Kirschenbaum LP: Epidural analgesic techniques in the management of cervical pain. Anesth Analg 65:938, 1986.
10. Takata K, Inoue S, Takahashi K, et al.: Swelling of the cauda equina in patients who have herniation of a lumbar disc: A possible pathogenesis of sciatica. J Bone Joint Surg Am 70:361, 1988.
11. Saal JS, Franson RC, Dobrow R, et al.: High levels of inflammatory phospholipase A2 activity in lumbar disc herniations. Spine 15:674, 1990.
12. Devor M, Govrin-Lippman R, Raber P: Corticosteroids suppress ectopic neural discharge originating in experimental neuromas. Pain 22:127, 1985.
13. Johansson A, Hao J, Sjolund B: Local corticosteroid application blocks transmission in normal nociceptive C-fibers. Acta Anaesthesiol Scand 34:335, 1990.
14. White AH, Derby R, Wynne G: Epidural injections for the diagnosis and treatment of low back pain. Spine 5:78, 1980.
15. Hacobian A, Kahn C, Picard L, et al.: Treatment of spinal stenosis with epidural steroid injections: An outcome study. Reg Anesth 20(suppl):128, 1995.
16. Abram SE, Hopwood MB: What factors contribute to outcome with lumbar epidural steroids? In Bond MR, Charlton JE, Woolf CJ (eds): Proceedings of the Sixth World Congress on Pain. Amsterdam, Elsevier Science Publishers BV, 1991, p 495.
17. Hopwood MB, Abram SE: Factors associated with failure of lumbar epidural steroids. Reg Anesth 18:238, 1993.
18. Sandrock NJG, Warfield CA: Epidural steroids and facet injections. In Warfield CA (ed): Principles and Practice of Pain Management. New York, McGraw-Hill, 1993, p 401.
19. Spaccarelli KC: Lumbar and caudal epidural corticosteroid injections. Mayo Clin Proc 71:169, 1996.
20. Koes BW, Scholten RJPM, Mens JMA, et al.: Efficacy of epidural steroid injections for low-back pain and sciatica: a systematic review of randomized clinical trials. Pain 63:279, 1995.
21. Watts RW, Silagy CA: A meta-analysis on the efficacy of epidural corticosteroids in the treatment of sciatica. Anaesth Intensive Care 23:564, 1995.
22. Dilke TFW, Burry HC, Grahame R: Extradural corticosteroid injection in management of lumbar nerve root compression. Br Med J 2:635, 1973.
23. Snoek W, Weber H, Jorgensen B: Double blind evaluation of extradural methylprednisolone for herniated lumbar discs. Acta Orthop Scand 48:635, 1977.
24. Carette S, Leclaire R, Marcoux S et al: Epidural corticosteroid injections for sciatica due to herniated nucleus pulposus. N Engl J Med 336:1634, 1997.
25. Bush K, Hillier S: A controlled study of caudal epidural injections of triamcinolone plus procaine for the management of intractable sciatica. Spine 16:572, 1991.
26. Green PWB, Burke AJ, Weiss CA, et al.: The role of epidural cortisone injection in treatment of discogenic low back pain. Clin Orthop 153:121, 1980.
27. Warfield CA, Biber MP, Crews DA, et al.: Epidural steroid injection as a treatment for cervical radiculitis. Clin J Pain 4:201, 1988.
28. Cicala RS, Thoni K, Angel JJ: Long-term results of cervical epidural steroid injections. Clin J Pain 5:143, 1989.
29. Stav A, Ovadia L, Sternberg A, et al.: Cervical epidural steroid injection for cervicobrachialgia. Acta Anaesthesiol Scand 37:562, 1993.
30. Castagnera L, Maurette P, Pointillart V, et al.: Long term results of cervical epidural steroid injection with and without morphine in chronic cervical radicular pain. Pain 58:239, 1994.
31. Bush K, Hillier S: Outcome of cervical radiculopathy treated with periradicular/epidural corticosteroid injections: A prospective study with independent clinical review. Eur Spine J 5:319, 1996.
32. Ferrante FM, Wilson SP, Iacobo C, et al.: Clinical classification as a predictor of therapeutic outcome after cervical epidural steroid injection. Spine 18:730, 1993.
33. MacDonald R: Dr. Doughty's technique for location of the epidural space. Anaesthesia 38:71, 1983.
34. Waldman SD: Complications of cervical epidural nerve blocks with steroids: A prospective study of 790 consecutive blocks. Reg Anesth 14:149, 1989.
35. Katz JA, Lukin R, Bridenbaugh PO, et al.: Subdural intracranial air: An unusual cause of headache after epidural steroid injection. Anesthesiology 74:615, 1991.
36. Ling C, Atkinson PL, Munton CGF: Bilateral retinal haemorrhages following epidural injection. Br J Ophthalmol 77:316, 1993.

37. Williams KN, Jackowski A, Evans PJD: Epidural haematoma requiring surgical decompression following repeated cervical epidural steroid injections for chronic pain. Pain 42:197, 1990.

38. Dougherty JH, Fraser RAR: Complications following intraspinal injections of steroids. J Neurosurg 48:1023, 1978.

39. Shealy CN: Dangers of spinal injection without proper diagnosis. JAMA 197:1104, 1966.

40. Chan ST, Leung S: Spinal epidural abscess following steroid injection for sciatica. Spine 14:106, 1989.

41. Goucke CR, Graziotti P: Extradural abscess following local anesthetic and steroid injection for chronic low back pain. Br J Anaesth 65:427, 1990.

42. Waldman SD: Cervical epidural abscess after cervical epidural nerve block with steroids. Anesth Analg 72:717, 1991.

43. Mamourian AC, Dickman CA, Drayer BP, et al.: Spinal epidural abscesses: Three cases following spinal epidural injection demonstrated with magnetic resonance imaging. Anesthesiology 78:204, 1993.

44. Knight JW, Cordingley JJ, Palazzo MGA: Epidural abscess following epidural steroid and local anaesthetic injection. Anaesthesia 52:576, 1997.

45. Bromage PR: Spinal extradural abscess: Pursuit of vigilance. Br J Anaesth 70:471, 1993.

46. Strong WE: Epidural abscess associated with epidural catheterization: A rare event? Report of two cases with markedly delayed presentation. Anesthesiology 74:943, 1991.

47. Tuel SM, Meythaler JM, Cross LL: Cushing's syndrome from epidural methylprednisolone. Pain 40:81, 1990.

48. Trattner A, Hodak E, David M, et al.: Kaposi's sarcoma with visceral involvement after intraarticular and epidural injections of corticosteroids. J Am Acad Dermatol 28:890, 1993.

49. Simon DL, Kunz RD, German JD, et al.: Allergic or pseudoallergic reaction following epidural steroid deposition and skin testing. Reg Anesth 14:253, 1989.

50. Kay J, Findling JW, Raff H: Epidural triamcinolone suppresses the pituitary-adrenal axis in human subjects. Anesth Analg 79:501, 1994.

51. Abram SE, O'Connor JC: Risk of complications following epidural steroid injections. Reg Anesth 21:149, 1996.

52. Gutknecht DR: Chemical meningitis following epidural injections of corticosteroids [letter]. Am J Med 82:570, 1987.

53. Nelson DA: Intraspinal therapy using methylprednisolone acetate: Twenty-three years of clinical controversy. Spine 18:278, 1993.

54. MacKinnon SE, Hudson AR, Gentilli R, et al.: Peripheral nerve injection injury with steroid agents. Plast Reconstr Surg 69:482, 1982.

55. Benzon HT, Gissen AJ, Strichartz GR, et al.: The effect of polyethylene glycol on mammalian nerve impulses. Anesth Analg 66:553, 1987.

56. Abram SE, Marsala M, Yaksh TL: Analgesic and neurotoxic effects of intrathecal corticosteroids in rats. Anesthesiology 81:1198, 1994.

57. Rowlingson TC: Epidural steroids: Do they have a place in pain management? APS Journal 3:20, 1994.

58. Abram SE: Risk versus benefit of epidural steroids: Let's remain objective. APS Journal 3:28, 1994.

59. Hammonds WD: Epidural steroid injections: An unproven therapy for pain. APS Journal 3:31, 1994.

60. Abram SE, Anderson RA: Using a pain questionnaire to predict response to steroid epidurals. Reg Anesth 5:11, 1980.

61. Jamison RN, VadeBoncoeur T, Ferrante FM: Low back pain patients unresponsive to an epidural steroid injection: Identifying predictive factors. Clin J Pain 7:311, 1991.

Chapter 51

 # Facet Arthropathy and Facet Joint Injections

Honorio T. Benzon, M.D.

ANATOMY

The zygapophyseal (facet) joints are true synovial joints which connect adjacent vertebrae posteriorly. The synovial membrane of the joint contains a rich supply of blood vessels and nerves. The capsule of the facet joint blends with the ligamentum flavum medially and superiorly, preventing the capsule from protruding into the spinal foramen or between the articular processes of the joint.

Each vertebra has a superior and an inferior articular process. The superior articular process of the facet joint originates from the vertebra below the joint, faces posteriorly, and forms the lateral border of the facet joint. The inferior articular process of the facet joint originates from the vertebra above the joint, faces anteriorly, and forms the medial border of the joint. A bony prominence on the superior articular process is called the *mammillary process*. A prominence on the transverse process, called the *accessory process*, is connected to the mammillary process by the mammillary-accessory ligament. This ligament forms a tunnel on the superomedial aspect of the transverse process.[1, 2]

The dorsal primary ramus of the spinal nerve gives off its medial and lateral branches at about the level of the intervertebral disc. The lateral branch passes into the longissimus and iliocostalis muscles of the back. The medial branch runs caudally and rostrally, lying against bone, through the tunnel formed by the mammillary-accessory ligament. The medial branch supplies the facet joint: it gives off a proximal zygapophyseal branch which ascends through the soft tissue to innervate the joint from its caudal aspect. It then continues distally as the medial descending branch to innervate the superior and medial aspects of the facet joint below.[2] It can be seen from this arrangement that the facet joint receives innervation from the spinal nerve (i.e., the medial branch of the dorsal primary ramus) that exits through its adjacent intervertebral foramen and from the spinal nerve above it.

LUMBAR FACET ARTHROPATHY

Certain features have been noted to occur in the computed tomographic scans of patients with facet arthropathies. These include facet joint asymmetries, joint space narrowing, subchondral sclerosis, erosions, and facet hypertrophy.[3] However, the presence of abnormal findings in the joint on radiographic or computed tomographic studies does not imply that they are the cause of the patient's back pain.

Symptoms of facet arthropathy[1, 4] include (1) hip and buttock pain; (2) cramping lower extremity pain, not lower than the knee; and (3) low back stiffness, especially in the morning.

Signs of lumbar facet arthropathy[1, 4] are (1) paraspinal tenderness, worse over the affected joint; (2) pain on spine hyperextension; (3) pain on the affected side on lateral rotation of the back; (4) hip, buttock, or back pain on straight leg raising; and (5) absence of signs of nerve root irritation.

In pure facet joint syndromes, there are no signs and symptoms of nerve root irritation. There are no paresthesias, no radicular leg pain, no neurologic deficits, no leg muscle weakness, and no pain on flexion of the back; there is very little limitation of straight leg raising.

Chronic facet joint disorders are more common in women than in men.[5] This is probably a result of the greater incidence of lumbar lordosis in women, which produces greater extension in their lumbar facet joints. Every degree of increased extension apparently leads to a 4% increase in peak articular pressure.[5]

LUMBAR FACET JOINT INJECTIONS
Indications

Indications for lumbar facet joint injection are as follows[4]: (1) lumbar facet joint pain, based on the previously described criteria, for 3 months; (2) lumbar

226

facet joint pain not controlled by adequate rest, use of nonsteroidal anti-inflammatory drugs, and physical therapy; (3) absence of radiologic evidence of disc herniation, spinal stenosis, or foraminal nerve root impingement.

Technique

Lau and associates[4] recommended injection of the ipsilateral L4–5 and L5–S1 facet joints for unilateral back pain (or on both sides for bilateral pain).

The technique is simple and can be done as an outpatient procedure.[1, 4] The procedure is done under fluoroscopy control. The table used is a fluoroscopy table which can be adjusted in height to accommodate the C-arm of the fluoroscope. The patient is placed prone with a pillow underneath the abdomen, or the patient is placed in a 30- to 45-degree oblique position. After the back is prepared and draped, the desired joint is visualized under fluoroscopy and a 22-gauge spinal needle is inserted into the joint (Fig. 51-1). One to two milliliters of a mixture of a local anesthetic agent, either lidocaine or bupivacaine, and 20 mg of methylprednisolone acetate (Depo-Medrol) is injected into each of the designated facet joints.

Response

Characteristics of patients who respond to facet joint injections are as follows[6, 7]: (1) acute onset of pain associated with movement; (2) pain in the low back and thigh; (3) absence of leg pain; (4) absence of pain or its aggravation with the Valsalva maneuver.

Although Fairbank and colleagues[6] noted that young adults responded better, the experience of Jackson and associates[7] was that older people had better response. The latter authors also noted that physical findings of

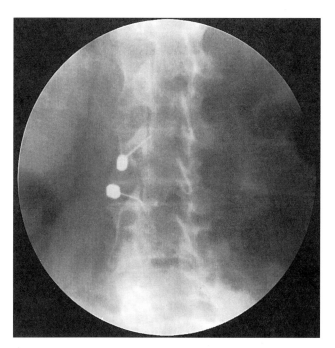

FIGURE 51–1. X-ray showing needles in the facet joints.

TABLE 51-1. HELBIG AND LEE SCORECARD FOR PROBABILITY OF PAIN RELIEF WITH FACET JOINT INJECTIONS

Back pain associated with groin or thigh pain	+ 30 points
Reproduction of pain with extension-rotation	+ 30 points
Well-localized paraspinal tenderness	+ 20 points
Significant corresponding radiographic changes	+ 20 points
Pain below the knee	− 10 points
TOTAL	100 points

From Helbig T, Lee CK: The lumbar facet syndrome. Spine 13:61, 1988.

normal gait, absence of muscle spasm, and pain on extension of the back correlated well with pain relief after facet joint injections.

Helbig and Lee[8] proposed a scorecard to predict the probability of pain relief from facet joint injections (Table 51-1). All patients with a score of 60 or higher had 100% prolonged response from a facet joint injection. A score of 40 points or higher predicted 78% prolonged response.[8]

Outcome Studies

Two outcome studies on the efficacy of facet joint injections have been published. Lilius and co-workers[9] studied 109 patients and compared results of three treatments: (1) cortisone (80 mg of methylprednisolone acetate) plus local anesthetic (6 mL of bupivacaine) injected into each of two facet joints; (2) cortisone plus local anesthetic injected pericapsularly around the two joints; and (3) 8 mL of saline injected into the two joints. Their selection criteria included back pain localized to one side, tenderness and muscle spasm over the facet joint, pain radiating to the posterior thigh, and negative straight leg raising. Although there was significant improvement in pain relief (36% had continued pain relief at 3 months), in work attendance, and in disability scores, improvement was independent of the type of treatment given.[9]

The selection criteria in Lilius' study[9] were good. However, some of the steroid and local anesthetic injected around the joint may have diffused into the joint. The injection of saline into the joint may have broken the joint capsule (the capacity of the joint is 1 to 2 mL) and thereby relieved the patient's pain.

Another study is that of Carette and colleagues.[10] In phase I, 2 mL of 1% lidocaine was injected into the L4–5 and L5–S1 facet joints of patients with back pain. Patients with more than 50% relief were enrolled in phase II. In phase II, methylprednisolone (20 mg of methylprednisolone acetate mixed with 1 mL of isotonic saline) was injected into the L4–5 and L5–S1 facet joints of patients in the treatment group, whereas the control group received placebo (2 mL of isotonic saline). Follow-up evaluations were performed at 1, 3, and 6 months after injection. Evaluation criteria included relief of pain, functional status, and improvement in movements of the spine. There were no differences between the two groups at 1 month or at 3 months, but at 6 months the methylprednisolone group had significantly better response: less pain, less physical disability, and greater improvement in spine movement. Forty-six percent of the patients in the methylprednisolone group reported improvement, compared with 15% in the placebo group ($P = 0.002$). However, these differences were reduced when concurrent interventions (epidural steroid injections, antidepressant medications, and physical therapy) were taken into account, to 31% in the methylprednisolone group vs. 13% in the placebo group ($P = 0.05$).

The study by Carette and colleagues[10] was poorly done. The authors did not have strict selection criteria; any patient with low back pain was eligible for inclusion in phase I of their study. Most important, they did not control for concurrent treatments of their patients; they should have restricted additional treatments during the study.

Although it appears from these two studies that injections of steroids into the lumbar facet joints of patients with lumbar facet arthropathy are not effective, no study to date has fulfilled the following criteria: prospective, randomized, controlled, with strict selection criteria, and strict adherence to guidelines (e.g., restriction of other treatments) during the administration of the study.

CERVICAL FACET ARTHROPATHY

Selection of the affected cervical facet joint is very difficult. Dory[11] and Wedel and Wilson[12] based selection primarily on the distribution of the pain (Table 51–2).

Technique

The technique for cervical facet arthropathy[12] is as follows. The patient is positioned prone on the fluoroscopy table with a cushion placed underneath the chest to allow forward flexion of the neck.[12] An anteroposterior fluoroscopic view of the appropriate facet joint is obtained; the head is turned slightly to the opposite side with the mouth open to avoid obstruction by the mandible or teeth. After the posterior neck is prepared and draped, a 22-gauge spinal needle is advanced under fluoroscopic control at a 45-degree angle to the skin into the joint capsule. A small amount (0.1 to 0.2 mL) of dye may be injected to confirm correct needle placement. Forty milligrams of triamcinolone diacetate in 0.5 mL of saline or local anesthetic (e.g., 0.5% bupivacaine)

is injected into each joint. Note that methylprednisolone is not recommended for cervical facet joint injections. Its unintentional injection into the vertebral artery and into the brain may have serious consequences (e.g., cerebral embolism) because it precipitates.

Although Dory[11] and Wedel and Wilson[12] recommended the prone position, cervical facet joint injections can also be performed with the patient in the supine position. The supine position allows for better management of the patient's airway.

Outcome Studies

Barnsley and co-workers[13] looked into the efficacy of cervical facet joint injections. Patients enrolled in their study had previously responded to facet nerve blocks. The therapeutic part of the study was conducted in a double-blind fashion, with either 1 mL (5.7 mg) of betamethasone or 1 mL of 0.5% bupivacaine injected into the affected joint. They found that patients' pain was substantially reduced initially but returned to its usual level after 1 to 2 days. The median time for return to 50% of the preinjection level of pain was the same in both groups (3 to 3.5 days). Their conclusion was that intra-articular betamethasone is not an effective treatment of cervical facet pain. This paper was accompanied by an editorial by Carette, who recommended the discontinuation of cervical facet joint injections for whiplash injuries.[14]

There was no real control (placebo) group in Barnsley's study.[15] The short duration of pain relief is disturbing. Because the patients had already responded to local anesthetic blockade of the facet nerves, rhizotomy of the involved facet nerves should probably have been done, rather than injection of steroid into the facet joint. Radiofrequency rhizotomy of the cervical facet nerves has been found to be an effective treatment for cervical zygapophyseal joint pain[15] (see Chapter 52).

REFERENCES

1. Lippit AB: The facet joint and its role in spine pain: Management with facet joint injections. Spine 9:746, 1984.
2. Bogduk N, Long DM: The anatomy of the so-called articular nerves and their relationship to facet denervation in the treatment of low back pain. J Neurosurg 51:171, 1979.
3. Bogduk N: Back pain: Zygapophyseal blocks and epidural steroids. *In* Cousins MJ, Bridenbaugh PO (eds): Neural Blockade in Clinical Anesthesia and Management of Pain, ed 2. New York, JB Lippincott, 1988, p 935.
4. Lau SW, Littlejohn GO, Miller MH: Clinical evaluation of intra-articular injections for lumbar facet joint pain. Med J Aust 143:563, 1985.
5. Lynch MC, Taylor JF: Facet joint injection for low back pain: A clinical study. J Bone J Surg Br 68:138, 1986.
6. Fairbank JCT, Park WM, McCall IW, et al: Apophyseal injection of a local anesthetic as a diagnostic aid in primary low-back syndromes. Spine 6:598, 1981.
7. Jackson RP, Jacobs RR, Montesano PX: Facet joint injection in low back pain: A prospective statistical study. Spine 13:966, 1988.
8. Helbig T, Lee CK: The lumbar facet syndrome. Spine 13:61, 1988.
9. Lilius G, Laasonen EM, Myllynen P, et al: Lumbar facet joint syndrome: A randomized clinical trial. J Bone J Surg Br 71:681, 1989.
10. Carette S, Marcoux S, Truchon R, et al: A controlled trial of

TABLE 51–2. DISTRIBUTION OF PAIN OF CERVICAL FACET JOINT ORIGIN

Joint	Distribution
C2–3	Occiput and cervical spine
C3–4	Neck
C4–5	Lateral aspect of the nape of the neck (Dory) shoulder (Wedel and Wilson)
C5–6	Arm (Wedel and Wilson)
C6–7, C7–8	Shoulder or upper dorsum as far down as the scapula (Dory)

Adapted from Dory DA: Arthrography of the cervical facet joints. Radiology 148:379, 1983; Wedel DJ, Wilson PR: Cervical facet arthrography. Reg Anesth 10:7, 1985.

corticosteroid injections into facet joints for chronic low back pain. N Engl J Med 325:1002, 1991.

11. Dory DA: Arthrography of the cervical facet joints. Radiology 148:379, 1983.

12. Wedel DJ, Wilson PR: Cervical facet arthrography. Reg Anesth 10:7, 1985.

13. Barnsley L, Lord SM, Wallis BJ, et al: Lack of effect of intraarticular steroids for chronic pain in the cervical zygapophyseal joints. N Engl J Med 330:1047, 1994.

14. Carette S: Whiplash injury and chronic neck pain. N Engl J Med 330:1083, 1994.

15. Lord SM, Barnsley L, Wallis BJ, et al: Percutaneous radio-frequency neurotomy for chronic cervical zygapophyseal joint pain. N Engl J Med 335:1721, 1996.

FURTHER READING

Dreyer SJ, Dreyfuss PH: Low back pain and the zygapophyseal (facet) joints. Arch Phys Med Rehabil 77:290, 1996.

Hogan QH, Abram SE: Neural blockade for diagnosis and prognosis: A review. Anesthesiology 86:205, 1997.

Chapter 52

Facet Nerve Blocks and Rhizotomy

Honorio T. Benzon, M.D.

ANATOMY

The anatomy of the lumbar dorsal ramus is different at vertebral levels L1 through L4 than at L5.[1] At the L1 through L4 levels, each dorsal ramus, after arising from the spinal nerve, passes dorsally and caudally to enter the back through a foramen in the intertransverse ligament. The dorsal primary ramus then divides into its medial and lateral branches, the lateral branch passing into the longissimus and iliocostalis muscles of the back. The medial branch runs caudally and dorsally, at the junction of the root of the transverse process with the superior articular process, through the tunnel formed by the mammillary-accessory ligament. As it passes under the ligament, it gives rise to the proximal zygapophyseal branch, which supplies the facet joint from its caudal aspect. The medial branch then continues caudomedially across the vertebral lamina. As it courses through the vertebral lamina, the medial branch gives off its distal zygapophyseal branch, which continues caudally to supply the rostral aspect of the facet joint below. Therefore, each facet joint receives a dual innervation: by the proximal zygapophyseal nerve from the medial branch of the dorsal primary ramus at its related vertebral level, and by the distal zygapophyseal nerve from the medial branch of the next rostral segment[1] (Fig. 52-1).

At the L5 level, the transverse process is replaced by the ala of the sacrum. The L5 dorsal ramus, after arising from the spinal nerve just outside the L5-S1 intervertebral foramen, passes dorsally over the ala, lying in a groove formed by the junction of the ala of the sacrum with the root of the superior articular process of the sacrum.[1] It divides into a medial and lateral branches. The medial branch hooks medially around the posterior lumbosacral joint, whereas the lateral branch courses caudally to communicate with the lateral branch of the S1 dorsal ramus.

TARGET POINTS

At the L1 through L4 levels, the appropriate target point is the dorsal surface of the root of the transverse process—that is, at the junction of the root of the transverse process with the root of the superior articular process of the facet joint (Fig. 52-2).

At the L5 level, the target point is where the nerve runs along the groove between the ala of the sacrum and the root of the superior articular process.[1]

DIAGNOSTIC MEDIAL BRANCH BLOCKS

The patient lies prone on a fluoroscopy table, and the desired target point is visualized on a posteroanterior screening. A 22-gauge spinal needle is introduced through a skin wheal lateral to the target point.[2, 3] With the use of fluoroscopic guidance, the needle is directed ventrally and medially toward the target point. The oblique lateral approach avoids the superior articular process.[2] Two to three milliliters of local anesthetic (e.g., 0.5% bupivacaine) is injected at each target point.

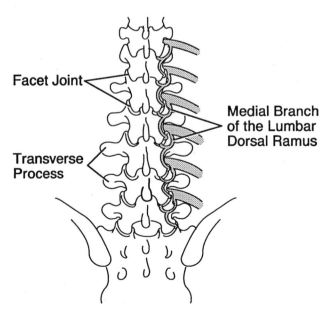

FIGURE 52-1. Innervation of the facet joint.

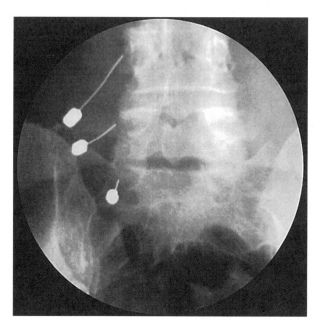

FIGURE 52–2. X-ray showing needles at the junction of the transverse process and the superior articular process of the facet joint. The lowest needle is at the groove between the ala of the sacrum and the root of the superior articular process. The needle positions are acceptable for diagnostic blocks with local anesthetic. For radiofrequency facet denervation, an oblique view should be obtained to confirm the needle position at the leading edge of the superior and medial border of the transverse process.

Subjective relief of pain of at least 50% is considered a positive response.[3, 4] The duration of pain relief should coincide with the anticipated duration of the local anesthetic used. Rashbaum[3] recommended a second injection, using a different local anesthetic, before RF denervation is considered.

North and colleagues[5] found that there was no association between the results of the nerve blocks and clinical findings (history, physical examination, and diagnostic imaging). Negative nerve blocks (i.e., lack of pain relief after the block) had a negative prognostic value, but isolated positive nerve blocks had limited specificity for localizing sources of pain. North's group found that blockade of the paraspinal lumbosacral nerve root and the medial branch of the posterior primary rami (distal or collateral to the area of pain) brought temporary relief to a majority of their patients, but so also did blockade of the sciatic nerve (distal to the site of pain). They concluded that uncontrolled local anesthetic blocks have a limited role in the diagnostic evaluation of sciatica caused by lumbosacral spine disease.[5, 6]

RADIOFREQUENCY FACET DENERVATION

The technique for RF denervation is the same as for medial branch blocks. Special equipment, manufactured by Radionics Inc. (Burlington, Mass.), is utilized. The length of the needle (called the SMK needle) depends on the vertebral level (e.g., 10 cm for a lumbar facet nerve, 5 cm for a cervical facet nerve). A lateral roent-genogram is recommended to confirm that the electrode tip is not too close to the primary spinal nerve root. If the electrode tip is too close, severe radicular pain in a characteristic dermatome distribution occurs with stimulation of less than 1 V, and muscle contractions (e.g., quadriceps muscle) occur at 1 to 2 V.[7]

Sensory and motor stimulation should be performed before the RF lesion is made. Sensory stimulation is created with a current of 1 V and a frequency of 50 Hz and should reproduce the patient's pain. The pain often radiates to the buttock and along the sciatic distribution but rarely distal to the knee.[7] Stimulation parameters for motor stimulation are 3 V and 2 Hz; there should be no palpable twitch of the quadriceps (or other appropriate muscle). After the proper responses to sensory and motor stimulation have been confirmed, the RF lesion is made with the thermistor temperature increased to 80°C and maintained for 90 seconds.

Bogduk and associates,[8] using egg whites and fresh meats as experimental models, determined the size and shape of the lesions made by the RF electrode. They noted that lesions did not extend distal to the tip of the electrode but extended radially around the electrode tip in an oblate spheroid shape, with a maximal radius of only 2 mm. Therefore, if the electrode is directed perpendicularly onto a nerve, the lesion generated may not encompass the whole nerve. Bogduk and associates recommended that the electrode be placed parallel to the target nerve so that the lesion generated encompasses the whole nerve.[8] It is for this reason that some experts recommend walking the tip of the cannula over the leading edge of the superior and medial border of the transverse process and then advancing the tip approximately 2 to 3 mm in an anterior fashion.

Results of Clinical Studies

Ogsbury and colleagues[9] performed RF rhizotomies in 75 patients, 25 (35%) of whom had continued relief of pain at 13 months' follow-up. Pain recurred after 6 months (average, 8.4 months) in 11 patients. Nine patients had a second rhizotomy, which produced long-term relief in three. In this study there were no selection criteria; all patients with low back or leg pain of spinal origin who had no relief after 10 days of bed rest or after physical therapy were included. However, the patients underwent a trial injection before the RF rhizotomy; the authors did not state whether the trial injection was a facet nerve block or a facet joint injection.

Mehta and Sluijter[10] observed 260 patients after RF rhizotomy. They considered their results to be good if the patient had considerable pain relief and increased mobility, fair if the improvement was less and there was occasional back pain or intermittent use of analgesic drugs, and poor if there was little or no pain relief. Their findings at the initial assessment, 1 month after the procedure, were good results in 116 patients (45%), fair in 54 (21%), and poor in 90 (35%). At 1-year follow-up of 162 patients, results were good in 44 (28%), fair in 36 (22%), and poor in 82 (50%). As with Ogsbury's study,[9] Mehta and Sluijter[10] used no diagnostic criteria; patients who were referred to their clinic and had no response to conservative management were included. However, diagnostic facet joint injections were performed before the RF procedure was used.

In contrast to the previous two studies, Rashbaum[3] limited his patients to those who had signs and symptoms of facet syndrome. In addition, his patients had relief greater than 70% after a diagnostic medial branch block, and the duration of relief coincided with the duration of the local anesthetic used. Eighty-two percent of 100 patients who underwent RF rhizotomy in this study had relief of their pain at 3 to 6 months, and 68% had sustained relief at 3 years.[3]

North and colleagues[4] published their clinical experience in 1994. They performed diagnostic medial branch posterior primary ramus blocks in 82 patients, 56 of whom had prior low back surgery. Forty-two of the 82 patients who had relief greater than 50% proceeded to RF denervation. Of those, 45% had at least 50% relief at long-term follow-up (mean, 3.2 years).[4] Although this study was retrospective, it was limited to patients with lumbar facet syndrome.

The better results of the latter two studies[3, 4] compared with the former two,[9, 10] show the importance of patient selection. Only patients with signs and symptoms of facet syndrome and those who show a favorable response to diagnostic medial branch blocks (preferably two or more diagnostic blocks) should undergo the RF facet rhizotomy.

CERVICAL MEDIAL BRANCH BLOCKS

The medial branches of the dorsal rami of C4 through C7 arise from their parent nerves in the cervical intertransverse spaces and then wrap around the waists of their respective articular pillars. Each medial branch is related to the articular pillar of the vertebra with the same segmental number as the nerve. Near the posterior surface of the articular pillar, each medial branch sends articular branches to the facet joints above and below its course before proceeding into the multifidus muscle.

Diagnostic blocks of the cervical facet nerve are recommended before RF lesioning of the nerve is performed. To denervate the C3–4, C4–5, and C5–6 facet joints, the patient is placed in a supine position and an oblique approach is used. A 50-mm SMK (Sluijter-Mehta) cannula is passed from an area posterior to the spine and moved upward in anterior fashion until it aligns with the waist of the facet joint column, below the associated transverse process at the posterior and inferior border of the associated foraminal opening. It is recommended that radiographic views from two different angles be taken to confirm correct needle placement. Oblique and posteroanterior views should be taken to confirm that the cannula is lying next to the midportion or waist of the facet joint line. Stimulation is performed, similar to the stimulation of the lumbar facet nerves, as previously described. There should be reproduction of the patient's pain with sensory stimulation and absence of motor fasciculation with motor stimulation. Once these criteria are met, 0.5 mL of 2% lidocaine is injected and RF denervation is performed (80°C for 90 seconds).

For nerves lower than C5-6, the patient is placed prone and the approach is similar to that for denervation of the lumbar facet nerves. A posterior approach is taken; the needle is passed onto the superior medial aspect of the transverse process and walked off the leading edge (2 mm) in an anterior fashion. Patients with short, thick necks may also require a posterior approach for denervation of the C5-6 facet nerves. An oblique or lateral view is taken to confirm that the needle tip is not too close to the foraminal opening.

Like Rashbaum,[3] Lord and co-workers[11] used a double-anesthetic blockade technique before proceeding with RF facet rhizotomy. They performed diagnostic medial branch blocks three times: once with placebo, once with lidocaine, and once with bupivacaine. The duration of the patient's pain relief was demonstrated to coincide with the duration of the local anesthetic used before RF rhizotomy was performed.[11]

The most common side effect of RF rhizotomy is burning pain in the dermatome of the treated nerve root. This disappears within 6 weeks after rhizotomy; follow-up electromyography shows no signs of denervation.[12] A possible side effect of upper cervical medial branch blocks, especially at C3, is ataxia or dizziness.[13]

Results of Clinical Studies

Previous studies of RF rhizotomy of the cervical medial branch were open series (i.e., not randomized and without a control group). Lord and colleagues[13] tabulated the results of these studies and found that 37% to 89% of the patients had more than 40% relief of their pain (Table 52-1).[13] The poor success rates were attrib-

TABLE 52–1. RESULTS OF OPEN STUDIES OF RADIOFREQUENCY NEUROTOMY FOR CERVICAL FACET JOINT PAIN

Author and Reference No.	No. of Patients	Mean Duration of Follow-up (mo)	Percent of Patients With >40% Relief
Schaerer[14]	50	15	50
Schaerer[15]	81	20	71
Sluijter and Koetsveld-Baart[16]	100	16–31 (range)	61
Sluijter[17]	58	12	79
Hildebrand and Argyrakis[18]	35	14	37–66
Schaerer[19]	466	2–128 (range)	75
Vervest and Stolker[20]	46	2	89

Adapted from Lord SM, Barnsley L, Bogduk N: Percutaneous radiofrequency neurotomy in the treatment of cervical zygapophyseal joint pain: A caution. Neurosurgery 36:732, 1995.

uted to inadequate patient selection, inaccurate anatomy, and technical errors. The authors noted that in their own series C3 neurotomy had a high failure rate and consequently recommended that RF rhizotomy of this nerve be abandoned.

In a randomized double-blind trial, Lord and co-workers[11] performed RF neurotomy in patients with mechanical neck pain caused by an automobile accident. The source of pain had been identified with the use of double-blind, placebo-controlled local anesthesia (i.e., no relief with placebo and complete relief with the local anesthetic). Twenty-four patients were studied, and 12 underwent RF rhizotomy. The median time that elapsed before pain returned to at least 50% of the pretreatment level was 263 days in the RF group and 8 days in the control group (RF current not turned on). It appears from this study that RF rhizotomy of the involved cervical facet nerves is an appropriate treatment for cervical zygapophyseal joint pain.

REFERENCES

1. Bogduk N, Long DM: The anatomy of the so-called articular nerves and their relationship to facet denervation in the treatment of low back pain. J Neurosurg 51:172, 1979.
2. Bogduk N: Back pain: Zygapophyseal blocks and epidural steroids. In Cousins MJ, Bridenbaugh PO (eds): Neural Blockade in Clinical Anesthesia and Management of Pain, ed 2. New York, JB Lippincott, 1988, p 935.
3. Rashbaum RF: Radiofrequency facet denervation: A treatment alternative in refractory low back pain with or without leg pain. Orthop Clin North Am 14:569, 1983.
4. North RB, Han M, Zahurak M, Kidd DH: Radiofrequency lumbar facet denervation: Analysis of prognostic factors. Pain 57:77, 1994.
5. North RB, Kidd DH, Zahurak M, et al.: Specificity of diagnostic nerve blocks: A prospective, randomized study of sciatica due to lumbosacral spine disease. Pain 65:77, 1996.
6. North RB: Treatment of spinal pain syndromes. N Engl J Med 335:1763, 1996.
7. Shealy CN: Facet denervation in the management of back and sciatic pain. Clin Orthop 115:157, 1976.
8. Bogduk N, Macintosh J, Marsland A: Technical limitations to the efficacy of radiofrequency neurotomy for spinal pain. Neurosurgery 20:529, 1987.
9. Ogsbury JS, Simon RH, Lehman RAW: Facet denervation in the treatment of low back syndrome. Pain 3:257, 1977.
10. Mehta M, Sluijter ME: The treatment of chronic back pain: A preliminary survey of the effect of radiofrequency denervation of the posterior vertebral joints. Anaesthesia 34:768, 1979.
11. Lord SM, Barnsley L, Wallis BJ, et al.: Percutaneous radio-frequency neurotomy for cervical zygapophyseal-joint pain. N Engl J Med 335:1721, 1996.
12. van Kleef M, Spaans F, Dingemans W, et al.: Effects and side effects of a percutaneous thermal lesion of the dorsal root ganglion in patients with cervical pain syndrome. Pain 52:49, 1993.
13. Lord SM, Barnsley L, Bogduk N: Percutaneous radiofrequency neurotomy in the treatment of cervical zygapophyseal joint pain: A caution. Neurosurgery 36:732, 1995.
14. Schaerer JP: Radiofrequency facet rhizotomy in the treatment of persistent headache and neck pain. Int Surg 63:53, 1978.
15. Schaerer JP: Radiofrequency facet denervation in the treatment of persistent headache associated with chronic neck pain. J Neurol Orthop Surg 1:127, 1980.
16. Sluijter ME, Koetsveld-Baart CC: Interruption of pain pathways in the treatment of the cervical syndrome. Anaesthesia 35:302, 1980.
17. Sluijter ME: Treatment of chronic back pain and neck pain by percutaneous thermal lesions. In Lipton S, Miles J (eds): Persistent Pain: Modern Methods of treatment. London, Academic Press, 1993, p 141.
18. Hildebrand J, Argyrakis A: Percutaneous nerve block of the cervical facets: A relatively new method in the treatment of chronic headache and neck pain. Manual Med 2:48, 1986.
19. Schaerer JP: Treatment of prolonged neck pain by radiofrequency facet rhizotomy. J Neurol Orthop Surg 9:74, 1988.
20. Vervest ACM, Stolker RJ: The treatment of cervical pain syndromes with radiofrequency procedures. Pain Clinic 4:103, 1991.

Chapter 53

Sacroiliac Joint Dysfunction

Dwight Ligham, M.D.,
and Lloyd Saberski, M.D.

The two most common causes of lost work days cited by Pope and colleagues[1] and by Weinstein and Wiesel[2] are back pain and the common cold. One may expect an 80% incidence of back pain over a lifetime. The diagnosis of a specific pain generator in patients with back pain is relevant because treatment and prognosis differ significantly according to the origin of the pain.

The sacroiliac joints are symmetrically located in the pelvis and function to join the sacrum to the iliac bones. They are synovial joints with rough articular surfaces. They are not designed for mobility but for stability. The weight of the upper body must be transferred through the sacroiliac joints to the lower extremities. The joints are stabilized by major ligaments between the spine, the sacrum, and the iliac bones laterally and posteriorly and the pubic symphysis anteriorly.[3, 4] This anatomic design allows for expansion of the pelvis in childbirth to facilitate passage of the fetal head. The effect of pregnancy hormones on relaxation of maternal ligaments is well described.[5] A monolithic pelvis would not function well in childbirth. However, this anatomic design to maximize flexibility presents its own set of problems to the patient with pain referable to this site.

The L3-5 and S1-4 nerve roots and their peripheral nerves pass over the posterior aspect of the sacroiliac joint. The sacroiliac joints are innervated by the posterior primary divisions of the S1-3 nerve roots.[6] Inflammation at the sacroiliac joint may account for the commonly seen pattern of pain referral into the ipsilateral leg and groin. One may argue that this pattern results from direct irritation of peripheral nerves as they cross the joint and are involved by the inflammatory process at the joint. Additionally, there may be pain referral along the sacroiliac supporting ligaments resulting in diffuse back pain axially and across the sacrum and iliac crests. This makes the distinction of sacroiliac pain from radicular pain difficult. The referral of pain may be to any location in the lumbar and sacral back or in the ipsilateral leg.[7] Cervical and thoracic pain from a functional scoliosis is not uncommon.

Patients presenting with back pain of sacroiliac origin usually describe a history of pain onset after falling, lifting and turning, pushing and turning, or bracing with a leg in an automobile collision. This mechanism has been described as "rotation coupled with an axial load."[7] Many times a history of exacerbations and remissions over many years is described once this injury is established.

Pain is exacerbated with bending and with prolonged sitting or standing. Many times it is worse in the morning and improves with daily activities. Extension exercises may be helpful. Riding in a car may be difficult. Pregnancy, with increased weight and hormone-induced ligament laxity, usually exacerbates this syndrome.

The physical examination must include range of motion of the spine at the pelvis, including flexion, extension, and lateral bending. The back is examined for points of tenderness at the lumbosacral junctions, over the iliac crests, at the iliolumbar ligaments, and in the buttocks, hips, and trochanteric bursa.

The pelvis is examined for obliquity, as are the scapulae. The spine is evaluated for scoliosis, which may be functional secondary to pelvic obliquity. A full neurologic examination is performed. There should be neither motor weakness nor reflex asymmetries from sacroiliac dysfunction.[7]

The straight leg raising test is performed. It usually is positive for low back pain secondary to distraction of the sacroiliac joint. There may also be leg pain, but usually the straight leg raising maneuver is ambivalent and augmentation with foot dorsiflexion is negative.

One must suspect radicular pain in the presence of radiating limb pain on straight leg raising and pain exacerbation with foot dorsiflexion. The Patrick test, Gaenslen's maneuver, and pelvic compression maneuvers may be positive for lumbosacral junction pain. In the presence of neurologic abnormalities or a positive straight leg raising test, a lumbosacral radiograph is indicated to evaluate vertebral foramina, oblique views to evaluate facets, flexion-extension views to rule out dynamic spondylolisthesis, and a magnetic resonance imaging (MRI) study of the lumbosacral spine to rule out spinal cord or nerve root compression.

A constellation of findings, including pelvic and scapular obliquity, functional or anatomic scoliosis, and pain at the lumbosacral junctions, iliolumbar ligament, and hip and trochanteric bursa, are usually present in varying degrees in patients with sacroiliac dysfunction. Unequal height of the iliac crests or scapulae when compared side to side with the patient erect constitutes an obliquity.

This constellation of signs and symptoms becomes important when one considers the force vector distribution across the spine and pelvis. The distribution of weight across the pelvis and sacroiliac joints is normally symmetrical and equal. A pelvic obliquity results in asymmetrical distribution of force across the sacroiliac joints. The force vectors that normally are vertical in direction become oblique, applying nonphysiologic tangential force to the sacroiliac joints and proximal femur (i.e., hip and trochanteric bursa).[8] A cycle of pain and inflammation results. Excessive weight load, manifested as obesity, pregnancy, or vocationally required lifting and carrying, exacerbates this problem.

The diagnosis of sacroiliac dysfunction is made with a fluoroscopically guided injection of local anesthetic into the sacroiliac joint. For this procedure, the patient is placed in the prone position on the fluoroscopy table. The fluoroscopy tube is rotated laterally to a plane parallel to the ipsilateral iliac wing. This projection allows the operator to look "through" the sacroiliac joint. A 22-gauge, 3.5-in. spinal needle is seated in the joint. An arthrogram may be performed, using a radiographic contrast agent to ensure needle placement within the joint. A small volume of local anesthetic is used to minimize the effect of the procedure on neighboring structures; 3 to 5 mL of bipuvicaine 0.5% solution is recommended. A long-acting steroid such as triamcinolone may be injected at this time. Patients with sacroiliac dysfunction obtain significant albeit temporary relief of low back pain from the local anesthetic injection. Short-term pain relief from this injection however, is diagnostic of sacroiliac joint dysfunction. The patient should understand that this injection will have no effect on hip, trochanteric bursa pain, or piriformis or gluteal muscle pain, if present.

The differential diagnosis of lumbosacral junction pain includes sacroiliac dysfunction as well as sacroiliac joint fractures (stress or osteoporotic), infection, collagen vascular disease (ankylosing spondylosis, psoriatic arthritis, Reiter's disease), osteoarthritis, metabolic abnormalities (gout, pseudogout, ochronosis, acromegaly), tumors (rarely primary), and surgical causes (bone harvest or pelvic tumor resection). Pain referral to the lumbosacral junction can result from lumbar radiculopathy, facet joint disease, discogenic disease, hip pathology, or muscle dysfunction (multifidus, gluteal, and/or piriformis).

Radiographic imaging of the sacroiliac joint is usually nonspecific and nondiagnostic. Diagnostic studies are indicated in the presence of neurologic localizing signs or unexpected findings on the physical examination. MRI is best for soft tissue imaging. Computed tomography can identify bony abnormalities. Bone scanning is sensitive for inflammatory conditions such as infection, neoplasm, and metabolic disease.

The goals of treatment for sacroiliac dysfunction are to correct abnormal force vectors across the spine and pelvis and to break the cycle of inflammation at the lumbosacral junction.

Equalization of force across the pelvis is most easily accomplished by means of a shoe lift worn in the shoe of the leg with the lower iliac crest. Lifts of graduated sizes are tested in the office to identify the size that best corrects pelvic and scapular obliquities and scoliosis. Many times this simple device corrects the pelvic obliquity, the functional scoliosis, and the scapular obliquity. Correction of these abnormal mechanical forces is a prerequisite to healing. Over time the obliquity may resolve with healing making the lift unnecessary.

The cycle of inflammation is broken with the injection of a long-acting steroid. Two approaches can be used: The sacroiliac joint itself may be injected at the time of fluoroscopy, or a caudal epidural steroid injection may be performed at a later time. The authors prefer the latter approach, because the injectate flows from the sacral hiatus through the sacral foramina to affect both the joint and the involved soft tissue. This technique effectively covers a greater area than the single-joint injection does.

Osteopathic and chiropractic therapy in conjunction with the steroid treatment may be most effective in hastening healing and pain relief.

Pharmacologic therapy for pain relief is limited in sacroiliac dysfunction syndrome. Even the most potent narcotics fail to effect significant relief. For this reason, potent opioids are not advocated for analgesia. Nonsteroidal anti-inflammatory drugs may be helpful to decrease inflammation, but their analgesic effects are limited.

Other modalities found to be helpful include cold or warm therapy, a sacroiliac belt for support, and transcutaneous electrical nerve stimulation. Exercises to strengthen pelvic support musculature are important; hip adduction and abduction, isometric exercises, and stretching techniques may be helpful.

With improvement in pain, function should be encouraged through a physiatrist-supervised work hardening program. Pain referable to sacroiliac dysfunction is prone to exacerbation and reinjury. For this reason, patient education in biomechanics is important for continued wellness. In many cases, job retraining is necessary to avoid recurrent injury.

For patients who do not respond to conservative therapy, proliferative therapy has been advocated for strengthening the ligamentous supports of the pelvis. This is accomplished through a series of injections at ligamentous sacroiliac attachments over several sessions. The injectate's active ingredient is an irritant used to encourage fibroblast proliferation, which results in the deposition of collagen. In animal models, this technique has been shown to increase the diameter of treated ligaments. The result is stronger and shorter ligaments supporting the pelvis.[9]

REFERENCES

1. Pope MH, Anderson GBJ, Frymeyer JW, et al: Occupational Low Back Pain: Assessment, Treatment, and Prevention. St. Louis, Mosby-Year Book, 1991, pp 132-147.
2. Weinstein JN, Wiesel SW: The Lumbar Spine. Philadelphia, WB Saunders, 1990, pp 846-859.
3. Anderson JE: Grant's Atlas of Anatomy. Baltimore, Williams & Wilkins, 1983, pp 3-4, 5, 6.
4. Hendler N, Kozikowski JG, et al: Diagnosis and management of sacroiliac joint disease. Journal of the Neuromusculoskeletal System 3:169, 1995.
5. Chestnut DH: Obstetric Anesthesia. St. Louis, Mosby-Year Book, 1994, p 28.
6. Bonica JJ: The Management of Pain. Baltimore, Williams & Wilkins, 1990, p 1284.
7. Dreyfuss P, Cole AJ, Pauza K: Sacroiliac joint injection techniques. Phys Med Rehabil Clin North Am 6:785-813, 1995.
8. Travell JG, Simons DG: Myofacial Pain and Dysfunction: The Trigger Point Manual, Vol 2. Baltimore, Williams & Wilkins, 1983, pp 45-54.
9. Reeves RD: Techniques of Prolotherapy: Physiatric Procedures in Clinical Practice. Philadelphia, Hanley & Belfus, 1995, pp 57-70.

Chapter 54

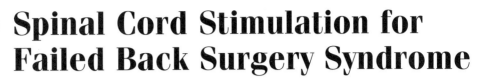

Spinal Cord Stimulation for Failed Back Surgery Syndrome

Sherwin E. Hua, M.D.,
and Robert M. Levy, M.D., Ph.D.

FAILED BACK SURGERY SYNDROME

Failed back surgery syndrome (FBSS), also called post-laminectomy syndrome, is defined as the persistence of back or leg pain, or both, after one or more reparative spine surgeries. It is estimated that approximately 20% to 40% of the 200,000 patients who undergo lumbosacral spine surgery each year in the United States experience persistent or recurrent pain.[1] The postsurgical pain often contributes to a decrement in the patient's lifestyle, functional capacity, and productivity as well as to an increase in the intake of pain medications and the development of psychosocial problems such as depression. Because patients with FBSS are varied with respect to their pathophysiology, clinical complaints, and psychological status, it is difficult to evaluate the outcome of specific therapeutic interventions. The management of patients with FBSS involves initially a rigorous and systematic evaluation of pain complaints. Depending on the results of this evaluation, pain therapy is tailored to the individual patient with a multidisciplinary approach initially involving physical therapy, pharmacotherapy, and psychological modalities. Should this initial management fail to adequately control the patient's pain, then neuroaugmentative procedures such as epidural spinal cord stimulation (SCS) should be considered.

CAUSES OF FBSS

One of the major reasons for the failure of lumbar surgery is improper patient selection. Although many patients have abnormal radiographic findings suggestive of disc herniation and spondylosis, these findings are common in the asymptomatic general population and do not necessarily warrant surgery. Therefore, radiographic findings in patients with back or limb pain are nonspecific unless they are correlated with the clinical complaints and physical examination. Even more ill conceived is surgery in the absence of any significant pathology on neuroradiologic evaluation. Nevertheless, many patients undergo lumbar spine surgery with inadequate indications; this leads to FBSS in many cases.

Timing of surgery also contributes to the large number of FBSS patients. Although a period of conservative therapy including bed rest, physical therapy, and use of nonsteroidal anti-inflammatory agents (NSAIDs) is recommended for patients without acute or progressive neurologic deficit, patients are often taken to surgery without a period of conservative therapy. Early lumbar surgery in the absence of acute or progressive neurologic deficit is correlated with an increased incidence of FBSS.

The specific causes of continued pain in patients with previous lumbar surgery are diverse. FBSS is broadly defined, and this diagnosis covers a complex and heterogeneous group of patients with different medical, surgical, and psychosocial histories. Despite this diversity, the decision to pursue spine surgery in the absence of clear clinical and neuroradiologic indications is a universal predictor for increased rates of FBSS. When spine surgery is contemplated to repair a straightforward and clearly demonstrated problem, such as a herniated lumbar disc producing a radiculopathy in the appropriate nerve root distribution, the results are excellent. When surgery is contemplated to prevent progressive neurologic decompensation, as for relief of documented spinal cord or nerve root compression or spinal instability or for repair of postoperative complications such as pseudomeningocele, the results are similarly excellent. On the other hand, surgery for stable and chronic problems such as pain in the absence of neurologic deterioration, including attempts to treat postsurgical epidural scarring or arachnoid fibrosis, is seldom successful and often leads to FBSS. With the availability of multidisciplinary pain therapy and effective interventional pain techniques, such surgeries are currently ill conceived.

FBSS may arise as a result of well conceived but technically inadequate prior surgery. Foraminal or lateral recess stenosis may be inadequately decompressed, especially when an obvious disc herniation is treated simultaneously. In these cases, repeat surgery and bony decompression may be an effective therapy, although a recent prospective randomized trial suggests that even in this setting SCS may be superior to reoperation. Similarly, previous surgery may be ineffective at relieving pain because of retained disc fragments or a recurrent disc herniation. Less often, the initial operation was performed at the wrong level or a new herniated disc or further degenerative disease developed at another level of the spine. In all these circumstances, reevaluation and consideration of repeat spine surgery are indicated.

Aside from those with problems that require surgical intervention, many patients with FBSS can be managed conservatively. Myofascial pain syndrome is a frequent cause of chronic back or leg pain, especially after lumbar surgery. Appropriate treatment includes use of physical therapy, trigger point injections, NSAIDs, and other pharmacotherapeutic agents, including tricyclic antidepressants or anticonvulsants. Psychological therapies such as biofeedback may also be effective. If such treatment fails, neuroaugmentation procedures such as SCS may be indicated.

SCS can be particularly effective in the setting of FBSS when there is demonstrated arachnoiditis. Arachnoiditis, or arachnoid fibrosis, is especially common in patients with histories of multiple surgeries or myelograms. Arachnoid adhesions can bind to and compress nerve roots, causing radiculopathic symptoms. SCS can also effectively treat FBSS secondary to epidural fibrosis or neuropathic pain secondary to nerve root injury.

DIAGNOSIS AND EVALUATION OF FBSS

Patients with FBSS must be thoroughly evaluated to look for correctable causes of pain. During history taking, it is important to carefully characterize the pain with respect to its nature, frequency, and location (radicular or axial). The presence of associated paresthesias or motor deficits and any changes in the pain since the spine surgery are important clinical issues. Postoperative pain that is identical to that before surgery suggests that the procedure was either inadequate or ill conceived. Changes in the nature or distribution of the pain suggest a new problem or one that has recurred since the operation. Worsening of pain in the setting of deteriorating neurologic function suggests nerve root or spinal cord compression that must be evaluated quickly. The history should also explore for associated symptoms or past medical history that can point to an altogether different source of pain mimicking radicular pain. Rheumatoid arthritis, ankylosing spondylitis, peripheral vascular disease, peripheral neuropathies, osteoporosis, and tumors can all cause symptoms of back and limb pain.

It is important to investigate a patient's psychosocial history in the setting of FBSS. Patients with psychiatric illnesses and severe personality disorders are usually excluded from surgical procedures, but some patients with subtle psychosocial disorders often do undergo surgery. These psychological and personality traits can influence the subjective impression of pain. Other patients may demonstrate addiction and drug-seeking behavior. A thorough social history that includes alcohol and drug use is important in the evaluation of these patients; behavioral therapy and drug detoxification may be the next step in chronic pain therapy. However, the existence of psychosocial comorbidities should not automatically exclude a patient from surgical or invasive procedures. Depression and drug dependency are sometimes the result rather than the cause of medical attention-seeking for pain. Alleviation of the pain by surgery or other means may improve the patient's functional capabilities and lifestyle, thereby reducing depression and dependence on pain medication. Additionally, any pending legal claims, settlements, or workers' compensation issues should be brought to light. The physician should be aware of patients who have such psychological, social, and legal issues and should take these factors into consideration when deciding the best treatment strategy for the pain. Although they are not absolute contraindications to repeat spine surgery or neuroaugmentative procedures, these issues tend to decrease the likelihood that further intervention will be successful in controlling the pain.

Included in the history should be an accurate evaluation of the patient's current and past medications and their dosages. The duration, impact, and side effects of each agent should be considered. Inadequate dosing of a particular medication does not necessarily indicate failure of that agent, because the patient may respond to the medication if it is given in sufficient dosages for sufficient periods.

The baseline functional capacity of the patient should be assessed before a treatment program is initiated. The patient's occupational history and current job requirements are important as a baseline measure of functional capacity. Any improvements in the ability to work or in the type of work the patient can do may be a good reflection of treatment efficacy. Similarly, a baseline description of activities of daily living (e.g., walking, household chores, sleep habits) is also useful for future comparison. Standard questionnaires that measure such functional capacities are often used in outcome assessment studies, and these assessment panels may be useful in the physician's office as well.

A thorough physical examination, focusing on the musculoskeletal and neurologic systems, is then mandatory. Neurologic tests of sensation, motor strength, and tendon reflexes can suggest ongoing nerve root compression or damage. Overlap of abnormal findings on examination with reported painful sensations in a radicular distribution suggest possible disc herniation, retained disc fragment, lateral recess syndrome, or permanent nerve root injury. Evaluation of gait can also give the physician a sense of the patient's functional capacity. Other important features of the physical examination include asymmetries or deformities of the spine. Scoliosis can arise from inadequate lumbar fixation or from prolonged muscular compensation for pain or weakness. Additionally, palpation of the paraspinal muscles for trigger points can indicate possible myofascial causes of the patient's pain. Myofascial pain syndrome can be managed conservatively with medications, physical therapy, and trigger point injections.

Appropriate neuroimaging studies are then necessary for the evaluation of spinal anatomy. Plain x-ray studies with the patient in flexion and in extension are important for the evaluation of spinal stability. Any significant spinal instability must be evaluated for surgery. Next, high-resolution magnetic resonance imaging is excellent for providing detailed anatomic examination of the spine as for assessment of the discs and nerve roots. Gadolinium contrast allows the physician to differentiate among scarring, disc, tumors, and other masses. For those who have had complicated spine surgery and reconstructions, three-dimensional computed tomography can help visualize the extent of the anatomic abnormalities and the surgical anatomy. Last, myelography and postmyelography computed tomographic scanning may visualize nerve roots and herniated discs or masses that are not clearly evident on magnetic resonance imaging.

MANAGEMENT STRATEGIES AND TREATMENT OPTIONS FOR FBSS

If the diagnostic steps outlined previously confirm a specific pathologic diagnosis, steps necessary to correct the problem should be taken. Most often, however, a specific diagnosis is elusive. When this is the case, multidisciplinary pain evaluation and treatment is indicated. Conservative therapy should be initiated, usually including physical therapy and pharmacotherapy. Initial pharmacotherapy often includes NSAIDs, tricyclic antidepressants, and/or anticonvulsants. If these are ineffective, narcotic analgesics may be considered. Aggressive physical therapy is often useful in patients with chronic low back pain, especially that of muscular origin. Abnormal muscular contraction commonly accompanies low back pain and may arise from compensatory use of different muscle groups. Additionally, myofascial pain can develop, requiring trigger point injections and specific physiatric myofascial techniques.

If conservative therapy proves ineffective, the patient should be evaluated for further invasive procedures; currently, neuroaugmentative procedures such as SCS are favored. Formal psychological testing is usually a prerequisite for further invasive procedures. Patients with gross personality disorders or frank psychiatric illness are referred for psychiatric counseling and behavioral therapy. Patients with drug habituation problems are referred to appropriate centers for behavioral therapy and detoxification. Once psychosocial comorbidities have been adequately treated, interventional procedures may be considered.

Surgeries for pain control include both neuroablative and neuroaugmentative procedures. The most commonly used neuroaugmentative procedures are SCS and intraspinal drug administration; these procedures leave the nervous system intact and are reversible. In contrast, neuroablative procedures destroy pain pathways permanently. Common neuroablative procedures include neurectomy, rhizotomy, and dorsal root ganglionectomy. Of these, dorsal root ganglionectomy has been tried most frequently for pain related to FBSS. However, the success rate of this procedure is poor, with only 23% of patients experiencing moderate pain control after 5 years.[2] Furthermore, such destructive techniques may compromise the effectiveness of neuromodulatory procedures by destroying the neural substrates necessary for stimulation-induced pain relief.

SPINAL CORD STIMULATION FOR FBSS

Repeat spine surgery, neuroablative procedures, and neuroaugmentative pain procedures represent the three major categories of invasive techniques used to manage medically intractable pain from FBSS. Neuroaugmentative procedures such as SCS are favored because, in contrast to repeat spine surgery and ablative procedures, they are more effective and do not cause permanent neurologic changes.

It is believed that SCS blocks the transmission of pain at the level of the spinal cord dorsal horn by the spinal gate mechanism first proposed by Melzack and Wall.[3] Electrical stimulation over the dorsal columns selectively recruits larger Aα and Aβ fibers. Retrograde activation of collaterals from these large-fiber afferents to the target cells, which give rise to the spinothalamic tract results in competitive inhibition of nociceptive inputs and blockade of nociceptive transmission.

In a retrospective analysis of the effectiveness of SCS implantation in patients with FBSS, roughly 50% reported successful pain relief after 5 years.[4] Success is often difficult to measure, but a 50% reduction in pain is typically used as the criterion for success. In this study, success also required a positive response to the question, "Would you go through it all again for the result you have obtained?" In addition to pain relief, patients tended to decrease or discontinue use of narcotic analgesics, and some of the patients were able to return to work after SCS implantation. Improvements in lifestyle and activities of daily living also were noted. In comparison, 32% of patients in a similar study by the same group reported a successful outcome after repeat spine surgery for FBSS.[5] These studies were biased against SCS, however, because patients were first screened as candidates for repeat spine surgery and only those who were not thought to be candidates for reoperation were offered SCS as a therapeutic option. Success rates of 50% to 60% with follow-up of up to 15 years have been reported for SCS in patients with FBSS.

In order to directly compare SCS and reoperation in patients with FBSS, a randomized, prospective study was initiated.[6] The outcome measure was the frequency of crossover to the other procedure, which was an option given to patients at the 6-month postoperative follow-up. Preliminary results showed that SCS was at least equally if not more effective for FBSS than was reoperation. More long-term evaluation indicated that SCS was clearly superior to repeat spinal operation for patients with FBSS and also appeared to be more cost-effective.[7] Therefore, SCS should be considered, not as a procedure of last resort after surgical options are exhausted, but at the time of failure of medical management and before other surgical interventions for FBSS.

Repeat spine surgery should be reserved for cases of gross spinal instability or significant nerve root or spinal cord compression in the setting of a neurologic deficit.

PATIENT SELECTION AND SURGICAL PROCEDURE FOR SPINAL CORD STIMULATION

A more detailed account of SCS is provided in Chapter 24; a brief description of the process of SCS implantation in the context of the FBSS is provided here. FBSS is the most common indication for SCS and is one of the most effective uses of SCS.[8] Careful patient selection is the most important predictor of success for SCS. In particular, it is important to demonstrate an objective basis for the complaint of pain (e.g., postlaminectomy syndrome, postsurgical epidural scarring, arachnoiditis). Furthermore, patients should undergo a psychiatric or psychological evaluation so that those with frank psychiatric disorders, untreated severe depression, drug dependency issues, or secondary gain issues are excluded until adequately treated. Patients with a significant predominance of leg over back symptoms are good candidates for SCS; with presently available technology, long-term coverage of low back pain with SCS is difficult at best.

Implantation of an SCS system is preceded by a trial of SCS using a temporary electrode to predict efficacy. This temporary electrode is placed percutaneously in the fluoroscopy suite or operating room with a procedure that involves physiologic mapping of the spinal segment to locate the optimal site for stimulation. The goal in electrode placement is to achieve stimulation paresthesias that overlap completely the distribution of pain. This overlap has been reported to be an important prognostic indicator for the success of SCS implantation. The trial period lasts up to several days, and a reduction in the patient's pain by 50% is a usual criterion determining the success of the trial. Most studies have reported successful results with the trial electrode in more than 90% of patients with FBSS. Patients with a successful trial proceed to implantation of the permanent system.

Because proper location of the electrode is critical to the effectiveness of SCS, electrode design and localization technique are important factors for overall success. Placement of the electrode is determined during implantation by stimulation of the electrode poles and recording of patient responses. Optimal electrode localization is that in which stimulation of multiple electrode poles produces paresthesias that completely overlap the distribution of the pain. After placement, slight shifts of electrode position may occur over time as the patient changes posture or flexes and extends the spine. For this reason, the design of the electrode to compensate for subtle migration is vital to the long-term effectiveness of SCS. Over the 30 years that SCS has been used, electrode design has improved considerably; the addition of multiple contacts along a single electrode in particular has resulted in improved long-term results.[9]

Currently available electrodes have a multipolar configuration allowing for stimulation between one or more cathodes and anodes. Modern electrodes typically have four or eight contacts and allow both cathode and anode leads at each contact, leading to a multitude of possible electrode configurations. This flexibility allows compensation for minor shifts in electrode position.

There are two electrode designs in general use, the percutaneous and the laminectomy (plate-type) electrode. Both types have multiple contacts. Plate-type electrodes require a small laminotomy for their insertion, whereas percutaneous electrodes are inserted through the barrel of a Tuohy-type needle. Laminectomy electrodes provide added stability and can be sutured to the dura for increased resistance to electrode migration. In general, trial stimulation is accomplished with the use of percutaneous electrodes because of their easy insertion. Permanent stimulation can be accomplished with either percutaneous or plate-type electrodes. Should a percutaneous electrode prove to be too sensitive to movement, with significant fluctuations in perceived stimulation intensity or distribution, then it may be replaced with a plate-type electrode. If a prior laminectomy has been performed at the desired level of stimulation, a plate-type electrode usually is necessitated by epidural scarring, which prevents the accurate placement of a percutaneous electrode.

Power to the electrode can be supplied by either an external or an internal power source. An internal lithium battery pulse generator allows maximum convenience; all components are internal, and stimulation parameters can be altered by telemetry through the skin. Once the battery is exhausted, however, replacement by open surgery is necessary. An external radiofrequency pulse generator uses an alkaline battery that can easily be replaced. The patient uses the stimulator by attaching an antenna to the external power source and placing the antenna over an implanted inductive coil. Because the antenna and the battery-powered transmitter are worn outside the body, this system can significantly limit freedom of movement and make activities such as swimming inconvenient.

Overall, SCS is a safe procedure with a low risk of complications. Although isolated cases of spinal cord injury during implantation have been reported, major morbidity and mortality are extremely rare. Superficial infection has been reported in 12% of patients; infection requires removal of the entire system and introduction of antibiotic therapy. Other reported complications include cerebrospinal fluid leak, hardware failure, and muscle spasms. Up to 48% of patients are reported to require some secondary procedure such as electrode revision, but this is becoming less common with advances in electrode and signal generator design.[4]

CONCLUSION

FBSS remains a complex and difficult problem to manage. A multidisciplinary approach, composed of a broad and systematic diagnostic evaluation coupled with an individualized treatment plan, is necessary to adequately treat this difficult problem. Once more conservative measures such as pharmacotherapy, physical therapy, and psychological techniques have failed, SCS may be indicated for the treatment of FBSS, especially when there is an overwhelming predominance of leg pain over back pain. SCS clearly is superior to other interventional procedures for FBSS, including dorsal root ganglionectomy and repeat spine surgery. Good to excellent pain relief can be expected in about 60% of patients, and this success appears to be long-lived, with follow-up of more than 15 years. Therefore, in patients with medically refractory pain and FBSS, SCS should be considered as a significant therapeutic option because of its safety, efficacy, and reversibility.

REFERENCES

1. Wilkinson HA: The Failed Back Syndrome: Etiology and Therapy, ed 2. New York, Harper & Row, 1991.

2. North RB, Kidd DH, Campbell JN, et al: Dorsal root ganglionectomy for failed back surgery syndrome: A 5-year follow-up study. J Neurosurg 74:236–242, 1991.

3. Melzack P, Wall PD: Pain mechanisms: A new theory. Science 150:971–978, 1965.

4. North RB, Ewend MG, Lawton MT, et al: Failed back surgery syndrome: 5-Year follow-up after spinal cord stimulator implantation. Neurosurgery 28:692–699, 1991.

5. North RB, Campbell JN, James CS, et al: Failed back surgery syndrome: 5-Year follow-up in 102 patients undergoing repeated operation. Neurosurgery 28:685–690, 1991.

6. North RB, Kidd DH, Lee MS, et al: 1994. A prospective, randomized study of spinal cord stimulation versus reoperation for failed back surgery syndrome: Initial results. Stereotact Funct Neurosurg 62:267–272, 1994.

7. North RB: Personal communication, October 1997.

8. North RB, Kidd DH, Zahurak M, et al: Spinal cord stimulation for chronic, intractable pain: Experience over two decades. Neurosurgery 32:384–394 [discussion, 32:394–395], 1993.

9. North RB, Ewend MG, Lawton MT, et al: Spinal cord stimulation for chronic, intractable pain: Superiority of "multi-channel" devices [see comments]. Pain 44:119–130, 1991.

Chapter 55

Epidural Endoscopy

Lloyd R. Saberski, M.D.

The presumption with an epidural steroid injection is that it is important for the material injected to reach the nerve root causing patient discomfort.[1] However, standard technique using loss of resistance as an indicator does not guarantee accurate placement and may present a hazard itself.[2] The injectate takes the pathway of least resistance, which is generally away from the target. Even with fluoroscopic imaging, the physician can be misled as to flow of nonionic contrast material, since only two planes of reference are provided at a time. Epidural endoscopy provides a three-dimensional, real-time, color view of local anatomy and pathology and allows for exact targeting of the injectate. Therefore, epidural endoscopy, also known as epiduroscopy, is a technique that facilitates a directed vision of epidural steroid injection.

PLACEMENT OF THE INTRODUCER

The first obstacle that the clinician must surmount after making the decision to perform epiduroscopy is to gain access to the epidural space. It is relatively easy for the skilled clinician to enter the epidural space at almost any level of the spine, but the technique becomes more involved for epiduroscopy, because a system that allows for the fiberoptic catheter, irrigation with normal saline solution, a steering mechanism, and perhaps future instrumentation must be introduced. Direct visualization of the lumbosacral epidural space through the sacral hiatus is an adaptation of the Seldinger technique that is familiar to most clinicians.[3]

The technique of epiduroscopy involves the following steps.

1. Place the patient prone with a pillow under the abdomen. The feet are internally rotated to provide better exposure of the sacral hiatus. Identify the sacral hiatus anatomically by palpation for the sacral cornua and the canal. The cornua lie on either side of midline just above the natal crease. A midline position is confirmed by posteroanterior (PA) fluoroscopy.

2. With a 25-gauge or smaller needle, place 3 mL of local anesthetic onto each side of the floor of the sacral canal. This should provide adequate cutaneous anesthesia. Pass the local anesthetic needle cephalad to confirm canal location.

3. Insert a 17-gauge Tuohy needle into the sacral hiatus and advance it cephalad. The loss-of-resistance technique can be used to identify entry into the canal. A lateral fluoroscopic projection should show the needle in the canal. If the needle is noted to be dorsal to the canal, remove the needle and reposition it.

4. Inject a nonionic contrast agent, 5 to 15 mL, and follow with PA fluoroscopy to show a caudal epidurogram. This often outlines nerve roots and scar adhesions.

5. Thread the flexible end of the guidewire through the Tuohy needle. The guidewire should thread cephalad. Follow this procedure with PA fluoroscopy. Repositioning and flushing of the Tuohy needle with normal saline solution may be necessary to facilitate passage toward the target lesion. After confirming the position of the wire with PA and lateral fluoroscopy, remove the Tuohy needle.

6. Carefully introduce the dilator and sheath over the wire. Using a no. 11 scalpel, widen the aperture to allow for easier passage of the introducer. If significant bleeding occurs, use firm pressure with gauze or additional local anesthetic with epinephrine, or both. A rotary movement as the dilator goes through the soft tissues facilitates passage. As the dilator and sheath are passed cephalad, the wire should be tested frequently to see that it moves freely. If the guidewire cannot be moved easily, then there is a kink. PA and lateral fluoroscopy can help determine what has happened. If a kink is present, it is best to remove the dilator and sheath and slide the Tuohy needle back over the guidewire so the wire can be removed and inspected. If the wire is kinked, a new wire should be used.

7. After the dilator and sheath are inserted, remove the dilator, leaving the introducer sheath.

8. Flush the side arm of the introducer sheath with 5 to 10 mL of normal saline solution. Place the fiberoptic cable through the steering handle; orient the image projected on the monitor to be true both up and down

and right and left. Focus the fiberoptic cable on a sterile ruler or other recognizable structure.

9. Insert the steering handle containing the fiberoptic cable through the introducer. Turn on the camera and start the video recorder. Flush 5 mL normal saline solution through the side arm, and advance the steering handle into the caudal epidural space. To keep the epidural space distended, it is necessary to keep constant pressure on the saline syringe or to attach the side arm to a normal saline bag pressurized to 50 to 75 mm Hg. Higher pressures are thought to be safe for brief periods. (The pressures generated by a bolus from a 10-mL syringe can easily be higher than 300 mm Hg when injected rapidly.[4]) The author's practice is to sustain pressure for 2 to 3 minutes at a time and then reduce to resting pressure. This should prevent compromise of perfusion. Keep accurate accounting of the fluid injected. In general, the amount used is approximately 60 mL per procedure. Most procedures last 20 minutes after the fiberoptic cable is placed.

EPIDURAL IMAGES

In order to follow the epidural anatomy in a given case, it is important to maintain orientation. This is achieved by simultaneous use of fluoroscopy and often by placement of lumbar epidural needles guided into position with fluoroscopy. With each epiduroscopy it is best to proceed with specific objectives in mind regarding areas to be examined, as opposed to general exploration of the canal, epidural space, and contents.[5] This shortens patient exposure to a pressurized epidural space. Prolonged exposure to elevated epidural pressures has not been proved to be without hazard.

POTENTIAL COMPLICATIONS

In order for epiduroscopy to be performed, it is necessary to distend the epidural space with normal saline solution. This allows the fiberoptic cable to achieve its required focal length and reveals intricate epidural structure that could not otherwise be seen. A possible complication of this technique is the generation of excessive epidural pressures[6] which could effect local or distant perfusion, or both. The epidural pressures generated can be transmitted cephalad through cerebrospinal fluid and perhaps effect perfusion at remote levels.[3] For these reasons it is essential that the procedure be performed on a lightly sedated, well informed patient and that pressures generated by the flush system be monitored carefully. After each 2- to 3-minute period of epidural viewing, it is advisable to turn off the normal saline flush so that epidural pressure can equilibrate with atmospheric pressure. In the author's experience after approximately 1000 cases, no long-term neurologic catastrophe has been reported as a complication of this technique. However, a single episode of macular hemorrhage occurred; the patient made an uneventful recovery.

It is not uncommon for patients to have postoperative discomfort. As a rule this is well handled with 50 μg of epidural fentanyl and oral opioid when necessary.

CONCLUSIONS

It appears that the epidural space can be accessed safely with flexible fiberoptic catheters via the sacral hiatus, yielding three-dimensional color images of the contents.[7-9] In addition, the steerable handle and gentle rotatory movements allow the fiberoptic catheter to be steered toward structures of interest. The technique allows for examination of specific nerve roots and injection of a steroid, normal saline solution, or local anesthetic preparations onto epidural adhesions and roots. Further study is needed to see whether this technique holds advantages over currently practiced fluoroscopic techniques. There is reason to believe that directed-vision epidural injections will play a significant future role in management of patients with radiculopathy. However, the applications of epiduroscopy may not be limited directed injection of epidural steroids. There is potential to perform closed procedures, including removal of extradural or intradural scar tissue, drainage of cysts, biopsies, and retrieval of foreign bodies.[4] Even more exciting is the possibility of interfering with the immunobiology that is responsible for inflammatory disc disease. The fiberoptic scope is introduced from a site remote from suspected pathologic lesions. This provides the opportunity to examine native tissues that have not been altered by surgical incision or puncture. This aspect of the procedure may be significant, since bleeding into the surgical site can be associated with generation of scar and adhesion. When scarring occurs, there is potential loss of glide between adjacent tissue planes. This perhaps is associated with forms of persistent postoperative back pain. We can conclude that, as the technology grows, so will the ability to provide new, safe, and effective therapies.

REFERENCES

1. Saberski LR, Thimineur MA: New Horizons in Pain Management: Epidural Steroid Injections and Procedures. Curr Rev Anesth 17:lesson 19, 1996.
2. Saberski LR, Kondamuri S, Osinubi OO: Identification of the epidural space: Is loss of resistance to air a safe technique? Reg Anesth 22:3-15, 1997.
3. Saberski LR, Kitahata LM: Direct visualization of the lumbosacral epidural space through the sacral hiatus. Anesth Analg 80:839-840, 1995.
4. Saberski LR, Garfunkel D: Unpublished data, 1990.
5. Saberski LR, Kitahata LM: Protocol for epidural endoscopy. Conn Med 60:71-73, 1996.
6. Serpell MG, Coombs DW, Colburn RW, et al.: Intrathecal pressure recordings due to saline instillation in the epidural space. Abstract 1535. Abstracts of the Seventh World Congress on Pain, Paris, August 1993.
7. Saberski LR, Kitahata LM: Persistent radiculopathy diagnosed and treated with epidural endoscopy. J Anesth 10:292-295, 1996.
8. Saberski LR, Brull S: Epidural endoscopy-aided drug delivery: A case report. Yale J Biol Med 68:17-18, 1995.
9. Saberski LR, Brull S: Fiberoptic visualization of the spinal cord: A historical review and report of current methods. Yale J Biol Med 68:7-16, 1995.

Chapter 56

Terminology and Pathophysiology of Complex Regional Pain Syndromes

Anthony Guarino, M.D., and
Srinivasa N. Raja, M.D.

Weir Mitchell first used the term *causalgia* to describe the classic chronic pain syndrome observed in Unionist soldiers after injuries in the American Civil War. It was almost half a century after the original description of the syndrome before the sympathetic nervous system was implicated in causalgic pain by the French surgeon, Leriche. The term *reflex sympathetic dystrophy* (RSD) was first introduced by Evans in the middle of the 20th century. Over subsequent years, the terms RSD and causalgia were used and defined in many different and confusing ways. A variety of terms have been applied to these syndromes, which have similar clinical features (Table 56–1), resulting in an ambiguous literature and a lack of progress in our understanding of the basic pathophysiology of the disease. Additionally, in many people with the diagnosis of RSD a sympathetic component is not evident by the clinical presentation, diagnostic testing, or therapeutic response to neural blockade.

In 1994 and 1995, a group of experts in the field came to the consensus that the terms RSD and causalgia had lost their usefulness as clinical designations and had become a "grab-bag" diagnosis for patients with varying degrees of neuropathic pain and/or resistance to traditional therapeutic strategies.[1] A new nomenclature was

TABLE 56–1. TERMS USED FOR RSD AND CAUSALGIA SYNDROMES

Acute atrophy of the bone
Algoneurodystrophy
Causalgia
Chronic traumatic edema
Post-traumatic dystrophy
Post-traumatic spreading neuralgia
Postinfarctional sclerodactyly
Post-traumatic osteoporosis
Reflex neurovascular dystrophy
Reflex sympathetic dystrophy
Shoulder-hand syndrome
Sudeck's atrophy
Sympathalgia
Traumatic angiospasm
Traumatic vasospasm

suggested and subsequently adapted by the International Association for the Study of Pain in their *Classification of Chronic Pain.*[2]

DEFINITION OF CRPS

The new umbrella term that was introduced to encompass all chronic pain states previously diagnosed as RSD or causalgia-like syndromes was complex regional pain syndrome (CRPS). *Complex* indicates the varied and dynamic nature of the clinical presentation, not only within a single patient over time but also between patients with apparently similar disorders. *Regional* denotes the distribution of the symptoms, which typically is nondermatomal and often with signs and symptoms beyond the region of the original injury. *Pain* is out of proportion to the inciting events. *Syndrome* describes the constellation of symptoms and signs that can be characterized as a distinct entity. Because the contribution of the sympathetic nervous system in CRPS is not constant across patients, the term "sympathetic" is avoided in the definition. CRPS, then, describes a variety of chronic pain states that usually occur after a traumatic event, typically are regional and distal in the distribution of pain and sensory changes, exceed in duration and in magnitude the clinical course of the inciting event, have a variable clinical course over time, and often result in significant impairment of motor function.

CRPS type I (RSD) is defined as a syndrome that develops after an initiating noxious event. Ongoing spontaneous pain often is associated with hyperalgesia to cutaneous stimuli. The symptoms are not limited to the territory of a single peripheral nerve, and they are disproportionate to the inciting event. There is or has been evidence of edema, skin blood flow abnormality, or abnormal sudomotor activity in the painful region since the inciting event. The diagnosis is excluded by the existence of conditions that would otherwise account for the degree of pain and dysfunction that is found. *CRPS type II (causalgia)* differs from CRPS type I by the presence of a known nerve injury.

In certain patients with CRPS, pain depends on sympathetic activity in the affected areas. The term *sympathetically maintained pain* (SMP) describes that aspect of the pain that is relieved by blockade of the efferent sympathetic nervous system. In contrast, *sympathetically independent pain* (SIP) refers to that aspect of the pain that is not alleviated by sympathetic blockade. Clinically, a patient with CRPS may present with SMP, SIP, or a mixture of both in a chronic pain syndrome.[3] Therefore, CRPS may or may not have components of SMP. There is no definitive way to diagnose SMP on the basis of signs, symptoms, or clinical history. Two patients may have similar clinical presentations and yet one patient could have SMP and the other may not. To differentiate the sympathetic component, a selective sympathetic block (described in subsequent chapters) can be performed. The SMP/SIP terminology is an operational definition by which the chronic pain syndrome is categorized according to the response to selective sympathetic blockade. Defining a sympathetic component to the CRPS is useful from a clinical perspective, since treatment is accordingly influenced.

Many components contribute to the overall clinical picture of CRPS: sympathetic, sensory, autonomic, inflammatory, motor, and psychological phenomena (Fig. 56-1). Individual patients can have varying degrees of each of these aspects, which together constitute each person's unique pain experience.[4] In addition, clinical observations indicate that CRPS is a dynamic entity. The different components contributing to a patient's pain can vary with time; the sympathetic efferents may contribute the majority of a patient's pain on one day and on another occasion only a small proportion of the overall pain. A patient can have CRPS without any sympathetic contribution to the pain.

The sensory symptoms and signs in CRPS are spontaneous pain, hyperpathia, allodynia, and hyperalgesia.[5, 6] *Hyperpathia* refers to pain elicited by a noxious stimulus that is delayed in onset but outlasts the stimulus duration and spreads beyond the site of the stimulus. *Allodynia* refers to pain resulting from a normally innocuous stimulus, such as a cold breeze or touching or brushing of the skin. *Hyperalgesia* refers to increased pain to a noxious stimulus. Other associated clinical phenomena include changes in skin color, skin temperature, sweating, motor function, and structure of superficial and deep tissues (trophic changes). The syndrome occurs predominantly in the extremities and typically does not follow a dermatomal or peripheral nerve distribution. Patients with CRPS may have associated psychological and psychiatric disturbances. It is generally agreed that these are consequences rather than causes of the disorder in most cases.

RSD was earlier considered to progress through different stages. The stages were described based on the duration of the disease, certain clinical characteristics, or both. The consensus of the panel that introduced the new terminology was that staging or grading of CRPS based on clinical presentation had little utility from a descriptive, diagnostic, or treatment standpoint.

NEURAL MECHANISMS UNDERLYING CRPS: A HYPOTHESIS

The exact pathophysiology of CRPS is unclear. However, clinical and experimental studies in animal models of neuropathic pain have shed considerable light on the plastic changes in the peripheral and central nervous systems that may contribute to the mechanisms of persistent pain.[7] A schema of the mechanisms hypothetically leading to CRPS is shown in Figure 56-2. An initial injury activates nociceptors and results in signals along nociceptive pathways from the periphery to the spinal cord. The input of signals in nociceptive neurons to the spinal cord leads to alterations in spinal modulatory mechanisms, resulting in sensitization of central pain-signaling neurons. The sensitized dorsal horn neurons are then activated by low-threshold mechanoreceptive afferents, leading to the clinical phenomenon of allodynia.[8]

An important question is what maintains the state of central hyperexcitability (i.e., sensitization). Unlike the inflammatory pain states, in which the hyperalgesia subsides after local healing of tissues, the pain persists in CRPS. It is postulated that the persistence of the central state of hyperexcitability is dependent on continued input from the periphery along the nociceptive pathways. Nociceptive input may result from several possible mechanisms: ectopic activity that develops in neuro-

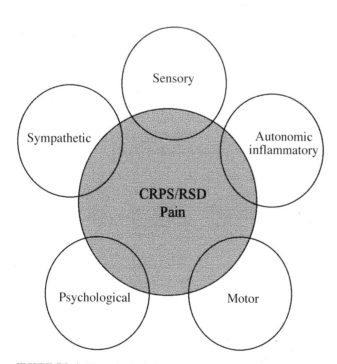

FIGURE 56–1. The principal clinical components of CRPS/RSD. The magnitude of each component as depicted in the figure should not be construed as reflecting quantitative relationships. The multidisciplinary approach to the management of RSD should therefore take into consideration all elements of the syndrome. (From Boas RA: Complex regional pain syndromes: Symptoms, signs, and differential diagnosis. *In* Jänig W, Stanton-Hicks M (eds): Reflex Sympathetic Dystrophy: A Reappraisal. Seattle, IASP Press, 1996, p 88.)

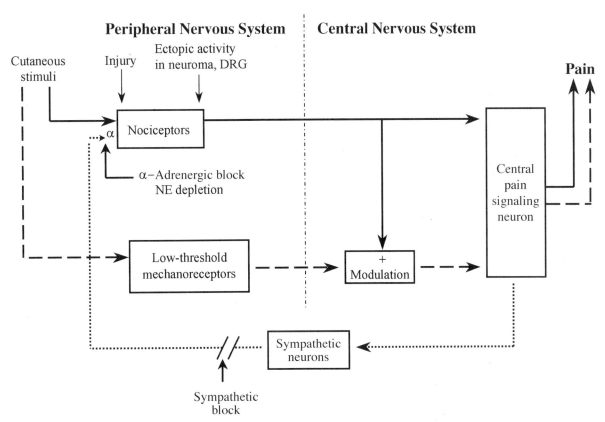

FIGURE 56–2. Model for sympathetically maintained pain. In SMP, nociceptors develop adrenergic sensitivity such that the release of norepinephrine by the sympathetic efferent fibers produces activity in the nociceptors. This activity maintains the central nervous system in a sensitized state. Pain to light touch is signaled by activity in low-threshold mechanoreceptors in the presence of an enhanced efficacy of the central pain-signaling neurons. Local anesthetic blockade of the sympathetic neurons or a peripheral adrenergic block (phentolamine infusion) will eliminate this ongoing activity in the nociceptors and thus lead to reversal of the central sensitized state. PNS, peripheral nervous system; CNS, central nervous system; *dashed lines*, hyperalgesia; *solid lines*, ongoing pain.

mas at the site of a nerve injury, ectopic generators in the dorsal root ganglia, or coupling between sensory and sympathetic fibers.

Sympathetic-sensory interactions leading to increased activity in nociceptive neurons may result from development of α-adrenergic receptor sensitivity in nociceptors such that the nociceptors are activated by the norepinephrine released by tonic activity in sympathetic efferent fibers. Abnormalities in sweating and vasomotor tone led some earlier investigators to postulate an increased sympathetic efferent activity in SMP. However, several experimental and clinical studies have confirmed that there is no evidence for an increase in sympathetic drive. In fact, the regional release of norepinephrine in the affected limb may be less than in the unaffected extremity.

A potential goal in the therapy may be identification of the site where the nociceptive input is generated and intervention to block the signals from reaching the central nervous system, thereby interrupting the vicious cycle. Such a maneuver allows the central pain-signaling neurons to reset themselves to a state of normal excitability. Considerable research is being conducted to determine the pharmacologic mechanisms for the sensitization of central neurons in an attempt to interrupt or reverse this process.

REFERENCES

1. Stanton-Hicks M, Jänig W, Hassenbusch S, et al.: Reflex sympathetic dystrophy: Changing concepts and taxonomy. Pain 63:127–133, 1995.
2. Merskey H, Bogduk N: Classification of Chronic Pain, Description of Chronic Pain Syndromes and Definition of Pain Terms. Seattle, IASP Press, 1994, pp 40–43.
3. Wesselmann U, Raja SN: Reflex sympathetic dystrophy/causalgia. Anesthesiol Clin North Am 15:407–427, 1997.
4. Baron R, Blumberg H, Jänig W: Clinical characteristics of patients with complex regional pain syndrome in Germany with special emphasis on vasomotor function. *In* Jänig W, Stanton-Hicks M (eds): Reflex Sympathetic Dystrophy: A Reappraisal, Progress in Pain Research and Management, vol 6. Seattle, IASP Press, 1996, pp 25–48.
5. Low PA, Wilson PR, Sandroni P, et al.: Clinical Characteristics of Patients with Reflex Sympathetic Dystrophy (Sympathetically Maintained Pain) in the USA. *In* Jänig W, Stanton-Hicks M (eds): Reflex Sympathetic Dystrophy: A Reappraisal, Progress in Pain Research and Management, vol 6. Seattle, IASP Press, 1996, pp 49–66.
6. Raj P: Complex regional pain syndromes (reflex sympathetic dystrophy and causalgia). Pain Digest 6:298–316, 1996.
7. Jänig W: The Puzzle of "Reflex Sympathetic Dystrophy": Mechanisms, Hypotheses, Open Questions. *In* Jänig W, Stanton-Hicks M (eds): Reflex Sympathetic Dystrophy: A Reappraisal, Progress in Pain Research and Management. Seattle, IASP Press, 1996, pp 1–24.
8. Campbell JN: Complex Regional Pain Syndrome and the Sympathetic Nervous System. *In* Campbell JN (ed): Pain 1996: An Updated Review (Refresher Course Syllabus). Seattle, IASP Press, 1996.

Chapter 57

● # Diagnosis of Complex Regional Pain Syndrome

Anthony Guarino, M.D., and Srinivasa N. Raja, M.D.

The diagnosis of complex regional pain syndrome (CRPS) is predominantly based on the characteristic clinical features. CRPS type II (causalgia) differs from CRPS type I (reflex sympathetic dystrophy, or RSD) in that the former is the result of a nerve injury. In this chapter, the clinical features of CRPS are further expounded and tests that help in the differential diagnosis of CRPS are discussed.

Epidemiologic studies show that the peak incidence of CRPS is at about 50 years of age. Until the mid-1980s it was thought that CRPS does not occur in children or adolescents. However, more recent observations indicate that CRPS does occur in children, although it is uncertain whether the course of the disease is similar in the pediatric population and in adults.

Several predisposing factors have been considered as potential factors for the development of CRPS, including genetic predisposition, disuse, and psychological factors. Women with certain HLA profiles seemed to be predisposed to development of refractory RSD. Other studies report a familial tendency. Using a rat model of experimental neuropathy, Devor and Rabor[1] demonstrated genetic traits to autotomy, a behavior considered to be indicative of pain. These observations raise the possibility of a genetic predisposition to CRPS. Clinical reports have postulated that lack of movement and activation of an extremity can play a role in the development of CRPS. There is no good evidence that CRPS is a psychogenic condition. It is likely that anxiety, stress, and chemical dependence may increase the pain.

CLINICAL CHARACTERISTICS OF CRPS

Spontaneous Pain

CRPS typically is experienced as spontaneous pain in an extremity. This pain usually occurs after tissue injury in an extremity, but it is characteristically disproportionate in severity, duration, and extent to that expected from the clinical course of the initial injury. CRPS has been reported after central nervous system injuries and after visceral or psychological disorders. Case reports suggest that, although it is uncommon, a similar regional pain syndrome can occur in the trunk and face. The common descriptors used by the patients are a burning pain, a constant ache, throbbing, deep pressure, or shooting pain. Blumberg and Jänig[2] describe an orthostatic component to the pain, with pain decreasing when the limb is elevated and increasing when it is lowered. Patients therefore prefer to keep the affected extremity elevated above the heart.

Allodynia and Hyperalgesia

Most patients (70% to 80%) have altered cutaneous sensibility that manifests as allodynia or hyperalgesia. Patients often exhibit guarding behavior to prevent contact with external objects. Alternatively, patients may wrap the part to avoid the effects of a cold breeze. It is not uncommon for patients to present in summer wearing gloves or in winter wearing shorts.

One striking clinical feature of sympathetically maintained pain (SMP, see previous chapters) is hyperalgesia to cold stimuli. Frost and colleagues[3] observed in patients with chronic pain syndromes due to traumatic nerve or soft tissue injury that the hyperalgesia to mechanical stimuli was similar between patients with SMP and those with sympathetically independent pain (SIP). However, all patients with SMP had hyperalgesia to cooling stimuli, whereas fewer than 40% of SIP patients had hyperalgesia to cooling. Therefore, hyperalgesia to cooling stimuli is a sensitive but not specific test for SMP. These observations were confirmed with quantitative sensory testing by Wahren and associates[4] who also found lower thresholds for heat pain in SMP patients. Quantitative thermal sensory testing may help to predict which patients have SMP and can achieve pain relief with sympatholytic procedures.

Tissue Swelling and Edema

Patients usually describe swelling of the extremity, although at the time of the visit to the clinic this often is not evident. Another potential reason for the swelling may be dependent edema secondary to disuse of the extremity. The swelling may lead to the characteristic shiny appearance of the skin in some patients.

Temperature and Color Changes

A history of temperature and color changes in the affected extremity is obtained from almost all patients. Although traditionally the limb is described as warmer in the early stages of the disease and colder in the later stages, these observations have not been consistent. Patients often describe the limb as mottled with dark, bluish or pale white discoloration. Sometimes the limb is described as being hot and red. Studies indicate that the temperature differences in CRPS are dynamic and are influenced by environmental conditions.

Sudomotor and Vasomotor Symptoms

Sweating abnormalities have been reported frequently in patients with CRPS. Most commonly sweating is increased in the affected region, but sometimes the skin in the affected region is dry and scaly. The presence of a cold or warm limb is considered to be a sign of altered vascular regulation.

Motor Changes

Distal tremors, dystonia, weakness, reduced movement, and joint stiffness are sometimes observed in patients with CRPS. These motor disturbances can result in marked functional limitation. It is unclear whether the motor symptoms are part of the clinical presentation of the disease or result from protection of the painful limb as a consequence of disuse.

Trophic Changes

Alterations in skin, nail, and hair growth often are observed in patients with severe allodynia to mechanical stimulation. Osteoporosis may be evident in patients with severe pain and guarding. The demineralization of small bones, particularly in a periarticular distribution, is considered to be characteristic of this disease. Atrophic shiny skin, muscle wasting, and joint stiffness are observed in a subset of patients.

With current knowledge it is difficult to predict which patient with CRPS has SMP or SIP, based on the clinical presentation alone. Some patients with SMP present with pronounced abnormalities in sudomotor and vasomotor function of the affected painful area. Other patients may have minimal signs of sympathetic dysfunction and still have SMP. Therefore, it is important that selective blockade of sympathetic function be carried out to determine the component of the pain syndrome that is sympathetically mediated.

DIAGNOSTIC TESTS

SMP by definition is eliminated by blockade of sympathetic efferent innervation of the painful area. There-fore, the sympathetic component should be assessed by blockade of the sympathetic ganglia supplying the area of pain. It is the efferent sympathetic fibers, and not the afferent, that account for SMP, as evidenced by aggravation or rekindling of pain with exogenous administration of norepinephrine intradermally. Areas of SMP have been shown to have a normal or decreased sympathetic outflow, indicating that the pain is not a result of increased sympathetic activity.

Local Anesthetic Sympathetic Blocks

The traditional sympatholytic test is sympathetic ganglion block with a local anesthetic. Local anesthetic is administered ipsilaterally in the region of the stellate ganglion or of the lumbar paravertebral sympathetic ganglion for upper or lower extremity pains, respectively. However, the results of local anesthetic sympathetic blockade need to be interpreted with caution. First, it is important to know whether the sympathetic blockade is complete, especially in patients who do not experience significant pain relief. The efficacy of sympathetic blockade can be objectively assessed by evaluating the effects on sympathetic sudomotor and vasoconstrictor function on skin blood flow, skin temperature, and skin resistance. Second, in patients who do have pain relief from local anesthetic sympathetic blockade, it is important to do a careful sensory examination, since local anesthetic can spread directly to nearby nerve roots, resulting in a somatic nerve block that may have significant effects on the patient's pain. Third, depending on the total dose of local anesthetic used, pain relief may result from systemic uptake of the local anesthetic. Fourth, the invasive procedure may have a significant placebo effect. And fifth, local anesthetic sympathetic blockade may result in interruption of signals not only in sympathetic efferent fibers but also in autonomic afferent fibers traveling in the sympathetic chain. However, this is a less likely possibility based on anatomic factors.

Regional Intravenous Blockade

Wahren and colleagues[4] used regional intravenous blockade with guanethidine for the diagnosis of SMP. Patients who had prolonged pain relief lasting 2 weeks to 6 months were classified as having SMP. Patients who had no pain relief, or minor pain relief lasting less than 5 days, were classified as having SIP. The effects of guanethidine are assumed to be related to its action on the noradrenergic system. Guanethidine is taken up by the noradrenergic varicosities of postganglionic sympathetic axons and depletes norepinephrine from its stores. This can lead to short-term excitation of nociceptors, which often is observed as increased pain during the test. Guanethidine then prevents further release of noradrenaline from depleted postganglionic axons for up to 1 or 2 days. However, guanethidine is not available for this use in the United States.

TABLE 57–1. ALGORITHM FOR DIAGNOSIS OF CRPS

Pain

The diagnosis of CRPS cannot be made in the absence of pain; it is a pain syndrome. However, the characteristics of the pain may vary in terms of the initiating event and other factors. The pain is often described as burning, and it may be spontaneous or evoked in the context of hyperalgesia or allodynia. Spontaneous and evoked pain may occur together.

History

Develops after an initiating noxious event or immobilization.
Unilateral-extremity onset (rarely may spread to another extremity).
Symptom onset usually within 1 mo.

Exclusion Criteria

Identifiable major nerve lesion (CRPS II).
Existence of anatomic, physiologic, or psychological conditions that would otherwise account for the degree of pain and dysfunction.

Symptoms (Patient Record)

Pain (spontaneous or evoked)
    Burning.
    Aching, throbbing.
Hyperalgesia or allodynia (at some time in the disease course) to mechanical stimuli (light touch or deep pressure), to thermal stimulation, or to joint motion.
Associated symptoms (minor).
    Swelling.
    Temperature or color asymmetry and instability.
    Sweating asymmetry and instability.
    Trophic changes (hair, nails, skin).

Signs (Observed)

Hyperalgesia or allodynia (light touch, deep pressure, joint movement, cold).
Edema (if unilateral and other causes excluded).
Vasomotor changes (color, temperature instability, asymmetry).
Sudomotor changes.
Trophic changes (skin, joint, nail, hair).
Impaired motor function (may include components of dystonia and tremor).

Criteria Required for Diagnosis of CRPS I

History of Pain

Plus allodynia, hyperalgesia, or hyperesthesia.
At least two other signs from the above list.

Characteristics of Spontaneous Pain

Sympathetically maintained pain (SMP).
Sympathetically independent pain (SIP).
Combined SMP and SIP.

Criteria for Diagnosis of Sympathetic Dysfunction

Noninvasive Tests

Surface temperature asymmetry by ≥1°C, either spontaneous or in response to provocative testing.
Resting or evoked sudomotor asymmetry.

Invasive Tests

Sympathetic ganglion block (if equivocal, up to three tests may be required); usually considered adequate only if there is demonstrated inhibition of sympathetic-mediated vasoconstriction of the involved extremity.
Systemic α-adrenergic antagonists, placebo-controlled.
Neuraxial blockade above the lesion may provide useful information.

Tests of Unknown Pathophysiologic Significance

Three-phase bone scan.
Radiographic patchy demineralization.
Tourniquet ischemia test.
Measurements of cutaneous blood flow with laser Doppler, percutaneous oxygen partial pressure differences, and computer-assisted sensory examination are interesting but evolving technologies that require further study.
Somatosensory-evoked potential measurement is not of demonstrated utility.
Regional sympathetic blockade is not recommended for diagnostic use due to multiple physiologic actions that confound interpretation.

From Wilson PR, Low PA, Bedder MD, et al.: Diagnostic algorithm for complex regional pain syndrome. *In* Jänig W, Stanton-Hicks M (eds): Reflex Sympathetic Dystrophy: A Reappraisal. Progress in Pain Research and Management, vol 6. Seattle, IASP Press, 1996.

Quantitative Sensory and Autonomic Testing

Since pain induced by cooling stimuli is a characteristic feature of SMP, quantitative sensory testing is helpful to aid in the diagnosis of SMP. Low suggested assessment of the vasomotor and sudomotor function in patients with CRPS to quantify autonomic dysfunction and to predict the response to sympathetic blockade.[5]

Skin Blood Flow Measurements

Kurvers and colleagues[6] observed disturbances in total skin blood flow in patients with CRPS. At the early stages, it is increased, whereas it is decreased in later stages. Assessment of this parameter therefore may provide an additional criterion to monitor CRPS.

Ischemia Test

It has been observed that interruption of the circulation in the distal part of the affected extremity by a cuff with a pressure above the systolic blood pressure reduces pain in the affected extremity. Blumberg and Jänig[2] suggested use of this observation as an additional diagnostic tool. The mechanisms of pain relief achieved by this test are unclear, but it is not considered to be the result of blockade of cutaneous A or C fibers. It has been hypothesized that the effects may be related to microvascular conditions in the deep somatic tissues of the extremities and that there is a decrease in activity in small-diameter deep somatic sensory fibers due to decreased vascular filling. A positive test is reported to have a high predictive value for pain relief associated with other sympatholytic procedures.

Phentolamine Infusion Test

This test was introduced independently by two groups of investigators as an additional test for SMP that could minimize expectation bias and placebo responses (see next chapter).

DIFFERENTIAL DIAGNOSIS

Many other disease processes may appear as CRPS, including unrecognized local pathology (e.g., fracture, strain, sprain), traumatic vasospasm, cellulitis, Raynaud's disease, thromboangiitis obliterans, and thrombosis.

Other neuropathic pain states, such as entrapment syndromes, occupational overuse syndromes, and diabetic neuropathy, may share some clinical features of CRPS. It is important to confirm a diagnosis before pursuing treatments that could potentially harm the patient.

Wilson and associates[7] present a diagnostic algorithm (Table 57-1) that provides a useful, practical guide to clinicians. At present such an algorithm remains expert opinion and needs validation with scientific data. The algorithm takes into account the symptoms reported by the patient, the signs observed by the clinician, and the results of additional diagnostic tests.

REFERENCES

1. Devor M, Rabor P: Heritability of symptoms in an experimental model of neuropathic pain. Pain 42:51-67, 1990.
2. Blumberg H, Jänig W: Clinical manifestations of reflex sympathetic dystrophy and sympathetically maintained pain. In Wall PD, Melzack R (eds): Textbook of Pain. London, Churchill Livingstone, 1994, pp 685-697.
3. Frost SA, Raja SN, Campbell JN, et al.: Does hyperalgesia to cooling stimuli characterize patients with sympathetically maintained pain (reflex sympathetic dystrophy)? In Dubner R, Gebhart GF, Bond MR (eds): Proceedings of the Fifth World Congress on Pain. Amsterdam, Elsevier, 1988, pp 151-156.
4. Wahren LK, Torebjörk E, Nystrom B: Quantitative sensory testing before and after regional guanethidine block in patients with neuralgia in the hands. Pain 46:23-30, 1991.
5. Low PA: Laboratory Evaluation of Autonomic Failure. In Low PA (ed): Clinical Autonomic Disorders: Evaluation and Management. Boston, Little, Brown, 1992, pp 169-196.
6. Kurvers HAJM, Jacobs MJHM, Beuk RJ, et al.: Reflex sympathetic dystrophy: Evolution of microcirculatory disturbances in time. Pain 60:333-340, 1995.
7. Wilson PR, Low PA, Bedder MD, et al.: Diagnostic algorithm for complex regional pain syndrome. In Jänig W, Stanton-Hicks M (eds): Reflex Sympathetic Dystrophy: A Reappraisal. Progress in Pain Research and Management. Seattle, IASP Press, 1996, 93-105.

FURTHER READING

Boas RA: Complex regional pain syndromes: Symptoms, signs, and differential diagnosis. In Jänig W, Stanton-Hicks M (eds): Reflex Sympathetic Dystrophy: A Reappraisal. Seattle, IASP Press, 1996, pp 79-92.
Campbell JN, Raja SN, Selig DK, et al.: Diagnosis and management of sympathetically maintained pain. In Fields HL, Liebeskind JC (eds): Pain Research and Management, vol 1. Seattle, IASP Press, 1994.
Gracely RH, Price DD, Roberts WJ, et al.: Quantitative sensory testing in patients with complex regional pain syndrome (CRPS) I and II. In Jänig W, Stanton-Hicks M (eds): Reflex Sympathetic Dystrophy: A Reappraisal, Progress in Pain Research and Management, Seattle, IASP Press, 1996, 151.
Wesselmann U, Raja SN: Reflex sympathetic dystrophy/causalgia. Anesthesiol Clin North Am 15:407-427, 1997.

C h a p t e r   5 8

● Phentolamine Infusion Test

Srinivasa N. Raja, M.D.

The traditional test to determine whether there is a sympathetically maintained component to the pain in patients with complex regional pain syndromes such as causalgia or reflex sympathetic dystrophy is a local anesthetic sympathetic ganglion block. In the hands of an experienced anesthesiologist, the risks associated with diagnostic nerve blocks are minimal. However, as discussed in Chapter 57, the results of these blocks need to be interpreted with caution. Because the prognosis and treatment of pain states depend on accurate diagnosis, incorrect interpretation of the results of a nerve block may result in inappropriate therapy.[1] Diagnosing sympathetically maintained pain and subjecting a patient to multiple therapeutic sympathetic blocks based on a single diagnostic sympathetic ganglion block, without taking into consideration potential false-positive test results, can be detrimental to the overall management of the patient.

Two principal factors that result in false-positive responses to diagnostic nerve blocks (i.e., decreased test specificity) are placebo effects and expectation bias. In reviewing the importance of placebo effects in pain treatment and research, Turner and coworkers[2] showed that placebos can closely mimic active medications in their effects. There is considerable misconception among practitioners concerning the nature of the placebo response. As stated by Wall,[3] the placebo effect is often perceived by researchers as a "tiresome and expensive artefact" which interferes with the demonstration of the "true effect" of a manipulation or therapy. Anxiety, expectation, and learning play important roles in the placebo response. Positive expectations of both the physician and the patient can lead to positive outcomes, and negative expectations can negatively influence the outcome of the diagnostic tests. Some studies have suggested a relatively high incidence of placebo response in patients with chronic neuropathic pain.[4, 5] Standardization of instructions given to the patient before a diagnostic test is performed can help minimize the influence of expectation bias.

Certainly, the complexity of placebo responses in patients presenting with chronic pain syndromes should be further explored and rational algorithms should be established to minimize the potential pitfall of placebo responses in this patient population that is often desperately seeking relief. Invasive procedures such as sympathetic ganglion blocks are difficult to perform in a placebo-controlled fashion. An important observation in patients with complex regional pain syndrome is that placebo effects often last only a short time.[6] This information is useful when effects of sympatholytic procedures, which usually are expected to last for several days, are assessed. Long-term follow-up of patients after sympatholytic procedures is therefore necessary to interpret the results of interventional strategies to alleviate pain.

Currently, attempts are being made to develop more specific diagnostic tests for certain pain syndromes that are based on pathophysiologic mechanisms. The specificity of diagnostic nerve blocks will be greatly improved if selective agents can be developed that act specifically on the nerve fibers of interest. Basic research into the membrane receptors involved in neuropathic pain has already pointed to some possibilities. For example, the development of specific sodium channel blockers may be useful in the diagnosis of neuropathic pain in which the ectopic neural activity is thought to be caused by an accumulation of sodium channels. Similarly, the development of more selective adrenergic antagonists may prove to be useful in the diagnosis of sympathetically maintained pain (SMP).

The phentolamine test was introduced by two groups of investigators as an additional test to evaluate for SMP.[7, 8] Phentolamine, a mixed α_1- and α_2-adrenergic antagonist, is infused via a peripheral vein. The rationale for this test is that excitation of nociceptive sensory neurons through norepinephrine released from postganglionic axons is prevented by blockade of α-adrenergic receptors. If pain is reduced during the phentolamine infusion, the sympathetic nervous system is likely to be involved in the generation of pain. Arner[7] demonstrated that patients who obtained pain relief with a phentolamine infusion were likely to respond to treatment with intravenous guanethidine. Similarly, Raja and colleagues[8] showed a high correlation of pain relief achieved with intravenous phentolamine infusion and local anesthetic sympathetic blockade. The efficacy of phentolamine in blocking adrenoceptor function is dose-dependent.[9] In another study, the efficacies of stellate ganglion blocks and intravenous phentolamine infusions were compared in patients with chronic pain syndromes of the upper extremities.[10] The phentolamine infusion appeared to be a less sensitive but more specific test for SMP than the local anesthetic sympathetic block. However, the investigators used a dose that was lower than our recent recommendations based on optimal dosing for α-adreno-ceptor blockade. Major advantages of intravenous phentolamine administration were minimal risk or discomfort for the patient, lack of invasive injections, ease of obtaining repetitive pain assessments, and placebo control.[11]

The protocol used at the Pain Treatment Center at the Johns Hopkins Hospital is outlined in Table 58-1. Phentolamine (1 mg/kg) is infused over 10 minutes at a time unknown to the patient. Drug infusions are done in a single-blinded fashion (behind a screen, out of view of the patient, so that there are no clues as to the time of drug administration). Skin temperature measurements

Phentolamine Test: Changes in Skin Temperature

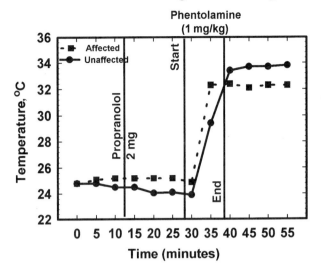

Phentolamine Test: Pain Ratings

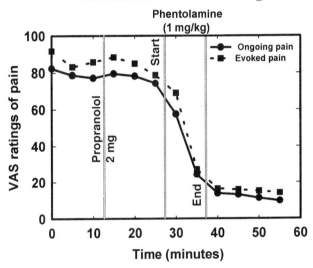

FIGURE 58-1. Phentolamine test: The typical increase in skin temperature and the decrease in pain ratings after the intravenous infusion of phentolamine (1 mg/kg) in a patient with complex regional pain syndrome type 1 (RSD) with a sympathetically maintained pain state. Pain ratings were obtained at 5-minute intervals and the patient was blinded to the time of drug infusion.

TABLE 58-1. PROTOCOL FOR PHENTOLAMINE INFUSION

Patient preparation	Informed written consent is obtained.
	A standardized set of directions is read to the patient; the patient is told that pain may increase, decrease, or stay the same, and that the results will help guide future treatments.
	The patient is placed in supine position.
	Electrocardiography, blood pressure, heart rate, and skin temperature are monitored.
	An intravenous line is established.
	A baseline pain level is established (pain score must be above 4 on a 10-point visual analog scale).
Saline pretreatment	Lactated Ringer's solution is administered at 600 mL/hr throughout the test.
	Sensory testing is done every 5 min for at least 30 min or until a stable pain rating is achieved*; if pain level is not stable, the test is deferred.
Phentolamine infusion	Propranolol 1-2 mg is administered intravenously.
	An infusion of phentolamine (1 mg/kg) is given over a 10-min period in single-blinded fashion (no clues provided to the patient on time of initiation of drug infusion).
	Sensory testing is continued every 5 min during phentolamine infusion.
Post-phentolamine testing	Sensory testing is continued for 15-30 min.
	Electrocardiography, blood pressure, heart rate, and skin temperature monitoring are continued for 30 min or longer, depending on stability of vital signs and presence or absence of orthostatic hypotension.

*Sensory testing is done for ongoing pain at rest and for stimulus-evoked pain (mechanical, cold) if applicable.

provide an objective measure of blockade of vasoconstrictor function. A typical response to phentolamine infusion in a patient with a significant component of SMP is shown in Figure 58-1. Possible side effects of the test are hypotension and tachycardia. The safety of intravenous phentolamine infusion from the cardiovascular perspective has been established.[11]

A potentially useful role of diagnostic blocks is in guiding therapy. However, very little information is available to help identify which diagnostic block will predict success of subsequent therapy with specific pharmacologic agents or interventional strategies. Preliminary studies to determine the prognostic value of infusion tests have only recently been conducted in the pain field.[12] Carefully conducted studies to document the prognostic value of diagnostic tests used in patients with chronic pain are required.

REFERENCES

1. Hogan QH, Abram SE: Neural blockade for diagnosis and prognosis: A review. Anesthesiology 86:216-241, 1997.
2. Turner JA, Deyo RA, Loeser JD, et al: The importance of placebo effects in pain treatment and research. JAMA. 271:1609-1614, 1994.
3. Wall PD: The placebo effect: An unpopular topic. Pain 51:1-3, 1992.
4. Verdugo RJ, Ochoa JL: Sympathetically maintained pain: I. Phentolamine block questions the concept. Neurology 44:1003-1010, 1994.
5. Verdugo RJ, Campero M, Ochoa JL: Phentolamine sympathetic block in painful neuropathies: II. Further questioning of the concept of sympathetically maintained pain. Neurology 44:1010-1014, 1994.
6. Price DD, Gracely RH, Bennett GJ: The challenge and the problem of placebo in assessment of sympathetically maintained pain. In Jänig W, Stanton-Hicks M (eds): Reflex Sympathetic Dystrophy: A Reappraisal, Progress in Pain Research and Management. Seattle, IASP Press, 1996, pp 173-191.
7. Arner S: Intravenous phentolamine test: Diagnostic and prognostic use in reflex sympathetic dystrophy. Pain 46:17-22, 1991.
8. Raja SN, Treede RD, Davis KD, et al: Systemic alpha-adrenergic blockade with phentolamine: A diagnostic test for sympathetically maintained pain. Anesthesiology 74:691-698, 1991.
9. Raja SN, Turnquist JL, Meleka S, et al: Monitoring adequacy of α-adrenoceptor blockade following systemic phentolamine administration. Pain 64:197-204, 1996.
10. Dellemijn PLI, Fields HL, Allen RR, et al: The interpretation of pain relief and sensory changes following sympathetic blockade. Brain 117:1475-1487, 1994.
11. Shir Y, Cameron LB, Raja SN, et al: The safety of intravenous phentolamine administration in patients with neuropathic pain. Anesth Analg 76:1008-1011, 1993.
12. Galer BS, Harle J, Rowbotham MC: Response to lidocaine infusion predicts subsequent response to oral mexiletine: A prospective study. J Pain Symptom Manage 12:161-167, 1996.

Chapter 59

Anesthesiologic Treatments for Complex Regional Pain Syndrome

David J. Lee, M.D.,
and Honorio T. Benzon, M.D.

DEFINITION

Complex regional pain syndrome (CRPS), or reflex sympathetic dystrophy (RSD), is a chronic pain syndrome with sympathetic manifestations that classically afflicts individuals who have suffered trauma to a limb. Three criteria are basic to the definition: (1) diffuse pain in an anatomic area not corresponding to the distribution of a peripheral nerve; (2) diminished function of the affected area and stiffness of involved joints; and (3) characteristic skin and soft tissue changes, ranging from swelling, hyperhidrosis, and warmth in early stages to atrophy, stiffness, and coldness as the syndrome progresses; vasomotor instability usually is present.

The International Pain Nomenclature Group has proposed for RSD the substitute CRPS:

A term describing a variety of painful conditions following injury that appears regionally having a distal predominance of abnormal findings, exceeding in both magnitude and duration the expected clinical course of the inciting event often resulting in significant impairment of motor function, and showing variable progression over time.[1]

CRPS is divided into type I (RSD) and type II (causalgia). Because the term CRPS is not used consistently at the present time, CRPS and RSD are used interchangeably in this chapter.

ETIOLOGY

The physiologic cause of CRPS is not known. Trauma secondary to accidental injury is the most common cause of CRPS. It has been reported after minor injury to a peripheral nerve, iatrogenic complication of surgical or medical therapy, myocardial infarction, cerebral vascular accident, soft tissue injury, and malignancy.[2]

CLINICAL MANIFESTATIONS

The course of CRPS varies depending on the severity of the disorder and whether proper treatment is insti-tuted. Without treatment, three clinical stages are classically described, corresponding to the physical changes accompanying progression of the disease from acute inflammatory onset (stage I, early) through dystrophy (stage II, intermediate), and finally to atrophy or disuse stiffness (stage III, late).

In stage I (acute), the pain is constant, usually aching or burning, and frequently is disproportionate to the injury. In stage II (dystrophic) the skin becomes indurated, cool, pale, and occasionally cyanotic. Stage III (atrophic) is marked by wasting, atrophy of the skin and subcutaneous tissue, fixed joint contractures, and osteoporosis.

DIAGNOSIS

A diagnosis of CRPS is based on the following criteria[3]:

1. History of recent or remote accidental or iatrogenic trauma or disease
2. Presence of persistent pain that is burning, aching, and/or throbbing in character
3. Presence of one or more of the following:
   Vasomotor and/or sudomotor disturbances
   Trophic changes, edema of the limb, sensitivity to cold, muscle weakness or atrophy
4. Relief of pain and modification of signs after regional sympathetic blockade

A single reliable, sensitive, and specific diagnostic test for CRPS is currently not available. Sensory/sympathetic testing, thermography, bone radiography, and three-phase bone scanning are used by some clinicians. Temperature increases after sympathetic blockade depend on the stage of CRPS; greater increases are noted in patients with lower preblock temperatures.[4, 5] Three-phase bone scanning has a high degree of accuracy in diagnosis of late-stage CRPS, but its benefit in prevention and treatment is yet to be established.[6]

PROGNOSIS

Some mild, early cases subside spontaneously in a few weeks, and some moderately severe cases have a self-limited course and heal spontaneously within a year, but in most instances, CRPS without proper treatment progresses through the various phases. Patients develop irreversible trophic changes and psychological/emotional disturbances, so that there is mental as well as physical invalidism. Such severe prognosis emphasizes the great importance of prevention and early proper treatment of this syndrome. One of the most important features of CRPS is that sympathetic interruption promptly relieves the burning pain, allodynia, and hyperpathia. If sympathetic interruption is done early, it cures the condition.

TREATMENT

Patients who develop CRPS should receive early, specific, and aggressive treatment, which consists initially of a series of regional sympathetic blocks and oral sympatholytics. If these produce complete but only temporary relief of pain, permanent sympathectomy should be considered. Whether this should be achieved chemically or surgically depends on the particular patient's physical condition, the severity of the disease, and the patient's attitude toward both techniques. Other therapies that have been reported as effective include a vigorous physical therapy and exercise program, transcutaneous nerve stimulation, systemic steroids, and spinal cord stimulation. Intense psychological support and encouragement to undertake a vigorous program of physical therapy and exercise of the limb is an integral part of treatment.[3]

During the early stages of CRPS, regional sympathetic blockade achieved with a local anesthetic or with an intravenous regional sympathetic block constitutes the primary and most effective treatment and offers the best chance for complete relief. In carrying out this treatment, care must be exercised to avoid blocking somatic nerves, because blockade of these nerves would provide a false-positive result. It is essential that the procedure produce complete denervation of the entire limb. The upper extremity derives outflow from T2 and T3 and not primarily from the stellate ganglion. A ganglionectomy as high as the T10 level may be required in some patients with CRPS of the lower extremity.

Regional sympathetic blockade for CRPS includes stellate ganglion block and paravertebral sympathetic block. The adequacy of the sympathetic blockade should be monitored (see Chapter 107). Repeat sympathetic blocks are recommended if there is progressive prolongation of pain relief after each block. An unanswered question on sympathetic blockade remains: If there is slight prolongation of pain relief after each block, how many sympathetic blocks should be done before proceeding to permanent sympathectomy?

The advent of intravenous regional sympathetic blockade and the use of oral sympatholytic drugs may replace both chemical and surgical regional sympathectomy.

The advantages of intravenous regional sympathetic blockade include the following: it can be carried out by physicians who do not have experience in regional anesthesia, it can be used in patients who are receiving anticoagulants, it eliminates the risk of the complications of regional anesthesia, and it produces sympathetic block that lasts for many hours or days. Disadvantages of this technique are that it cannot be used for CRPS involving the head, neck, or trunk and that, unless the technique is properly executed, complications result from the drug's entering the circulation after release of the tourniquet.[3]

Guanethidine displaces norepinephrine from its storage sites in the postganglionic sympathetic nerve endings, preventing its reuptake and subsequently its normal release in response to nerve stimulation. The resulting sympathetic block lasts for 48 to 72 hours. In 1974, Hannington-Kiff introduced the technique of regional sympathetic blockade using guanethidine.[7] Intravenous regional blockade with guanethidine has diagnostic and therapeutic value in CRPS. Its efficacy ranges from 71% to 89%.[7-10] Duration of pain relief is increased with consecutive blocks. Regional intravenous guanethidine blocks and stellate ganglion blocks have been compared in a randomized trial. An intravenous guanethidine block carried out every 4 days up to a total of four blocks is comparable to a stellate ganglion block done every day up to a total of eight blocks.[11] Both intravenous regional guanethidine and reserpine have been reported to be effective alternatives in treatment of CRPS. Reserpine depletes storage of norepinephrine at the postganglionic sympathetic nerve endings, inhibiting its synthesis and subsequently its release. No difference was found in the therapeutic efficacy between reserpine and guanethidine.[12] However, guanethidine is available only on a specific "rescue" protocol, and parenteral reserpine is no longer available in this country. The use of intravenous regional bretylium for the treatment of CRPS has been described. Bretylium accumulates in postganglionic sympathetic neurons and inhibits conduction of nerve impulses by preventing norepinephrine release. Intravenous regional bretylium in combination with lidocaine blockade provides significant short-term pain relief when compared with lidocaine for treatment of CRPS.[13]

Several lines of evidence suggest that peripheral α-adrenergic receptors play a critical role in CRPS. Stimulation of the peripheral but not the central cut end of the sympathetic chain reproduces pain in patients with CRPS after sympathectomy.[14] Local administration of norepinephrine rekindles the pain and hyperalgesia that were relieved by sympathetic block or sympathectomy in patients with CRPS but does not cause pain or hyperalgesia in normal subjects.[15] Local anesthetic blockade of the appropriate sympathetic ganglion or intravenous regional blockade rapidly abolishes CRPS.[16] The β-adrenergic antagonist propranolol has little effect on CRPS.[17, 18] Systemic α-adrenergic blockade with phentolamine achieves pain relief similar to that obtained by local anesthetic sympathetic blockade.[19]

Oral α-adrenergic antagonists have been shown to be of benefit in the diagnosis and treatment of CRPS.[20]

Prazosin is an oral antihypertensive agent that selectively blocks α_1-adrenergic receptors, with few side effects. It may prove to be effective in the treatment of CRPS. Phenoxybenzamine is an oral postsynaptic α_1-blocker and presynaptic α_2-blocking agent. It is an effective, simple, and safe treatment of CRPS.[21] Terazosin is an oral α_1-antagonist with a 12-hour elimination half-life. Its duration of action may extend beyond 18 hours. The prolonged α_1-blocking action of terazosin appears to be effective for the treatment of CRPS on a once-daily dosing regimen.[22]

Clonidine activates presynaptic α_2-autoreceptors, resulting in a reduction of norepinephrine release. This effectively decreases activation of the postsynaptic α_1-receptors. Clonidine is available for transdermal administration. It relieves hyperalgesia in patients with CRPS.[23] Clonidine may affect both peripheral and central α_2-receptors. Intraspinally administered clonidine may diminish pain in patients with CRPS by reducing sympathetic nervous system activity or decreasing transmission of pain information at the level of the spinal cord. Extensive analgesia may be obtained by epidural administration of clonidine.[24] The role for chronic epidural infusion of clonidine has not been established.

Gabapentin, a recently released anticonvulsant, is effective in pain control and possibly in early reversal of CRPS.[25] It is hypothesized that a gabapentin-induced increase in serotonin (5-hydroxytryptamine, or 5-HT) or a serotoninergic-like activity of gabapentin at a novel gabapentin-specific receptor site in the central nervous system and via the raphe-spinal descending control system inhibits pain sensation and causes an early reversal of at least some of the soft tissue and skin changes characteristic of CRPS.

Sympathectomy can be achieved by surgical ablation, chemical phenol, or radiofrequency sympatholysis. A single technique of radiofrequency sympatholysis does not appear to be applicable to all patients with CRPS; individualized patient management is necessary.[26]

Electrical stimulation is thought to produce analgesia by activation of the endogenous opiate pain suppression system, by activation of synaptic gating mechanisms at the spinal cord level or elsewhere in the neuraxis, and by the collision of stimulus-produced nerve activity with abnormal activity in peripheral nerves. Since the successful introduction of percutaneous spinal cord stimulation (SCS) by Shealy and colleagues in 1967,[27] significant advances have been made. The exact physiologic mechanisms of pain relief by this method in cases of CRPS are unclear. The theoretical basis for SCS is blockade of sympathetic fibers in the spinal cord dorsum.[28] Two technical problems are commonly encountered in patients with CRPS: (1) The disease spreads to several areas of the body; (2) Severe pain and tissue edema often occur in the area of any surgical procedure.[29] The method described by Racz and associates[30] raises the success rate with previously used techniques for upper- and lower-extremity involvement from 53% to 55% and from 32% to 33% respectively, and to more than 90% for both areas. The exact role of SCS in the management of CRPS is still unclear. The study by Barolat and colleagues[29] produced no evidence that stimulation reverses the course of disease, but patient population in their study had severe disease (stage II and III). Pain-alleviating effects of epidural SCS vary significantly by disease and site of pain.[31]

REFERENCES

1. Stanton-Hicks M, Janig W, Hassenbusch S, et al: Reflex sympathetic dystrophy: Changing concepts and taxonomy. Pain 63:127, 1995.
2. Stanton-Hicks M: Upper and lower extremity pain. *In* Raj PP (ed): Practical Management of Pain, ed 2. St Louis, Mosby–Year Book, 1992, pp 312.
3. Bonica JJ: Causalgia and other reflex sympathetic dystrophies. *In* Bonica JJ: The Management of Pain, ed 2. Philadelphia, Lea & Febiger, 1990, p 220.
4. Benzon HT, Avram MJ: Temperature increases after complete sympathetic blockade. Reg Anesth 11:27, 1986.
5. Malmqvist EL, Bengstsson M, Sorensen J: Efficacy of stellate ganglion block: A clinical study with bupivacaine. Reg Anesth 17:253, 1992.
6. Mackinnon SE, Holder LE: The use of three-phase radionuclide bone scanning in the diagnosis of reflex sympathetic dystrophy. J Hand Surg Am 9:556, 1984.
7. Hannington-Kiff JG: Intravenous regional block with guanethidine. Lancet 1:1010, 1974.
8. Holland AJC, Davies KH, Wallace DH: Sympathetic blockade of isolated limbs by intravenous guanethidine. Can Anaesth Soc J 24:597, 1977.
9. Driessen JJ, Van Der Weken C, Nicoli JPA, et al: Critical effects of regional intravenous guanethidine (Ismelin) in reflex sympathetic dystrophy. Acta Anaesthesiol Scand 27:505, 1983.
10. Eulry F, Lechevalier D, Pats B, et al: Regional intravenous guanethidine blocks in algodystrophy. Clin Rheumatol 10:377, 1991.
11. Bonelli S, Conoscente F, Movilia PG, et al: Regional intravenous guanethidine vs stellate ganglion block in reflex sympathetic dystrophies: A randomized trial. Pain 16:297, 1983.
12. Rocco AG, Kaul AF, Reisman RM, et al: A comparison of regional intravenous guanethidine and reserpine in reflex sympathetic dystrophy: A controlled, randomized, double-blind crossover study. Clin J Pain 5:205, 1989.
13. Hord AH, Rooks MD, Stephens BO, et al: Intravenous regional bretylium and lidocaine for treatment of reflex sympathetic dystrophy: A randomized, double-blind study. Anesth Analg 74:818, 1992.
14. Walker AE, Nulsen F: Electrical stimulation of the upper thoracic portion of the sympathetic chain in man. Arch Neurol Psychiatry 59:559, 1948.
15. Wallin G, Torebjork E, Hallin R: Preliminary observation on the pathophysiology of hyperalgesia in the causalgic pain syndrome. *In* Zotlerman Y (ed): Sensory Functions of the Skin in Primates. Pergamon Press, NY, 1976, p 489.
16. Treede RD, Raja SN, Davis KD, et al.: Evidence that peripheral alpha-adrenergic receptors mediate sympathetically maintained pain. *In* Bond CR, Charlton JE, Woolf CJ (eds): Proceedings of the 7th World Congress on Pain: Pain Research and Clinical Management. Amsterdam, 1991, p 377.
17. Simpson G: Propranolol for causalgia and Sudeck atrophy. JAMA 227:327, 1974.
18. Scadding JW, Wall PD, Wynn-Parry CB, et al: Clinical trial of propranolol in post-traumatic neuralgia. Pain 14:283, 1982.
19. Raja SN, Treede RD, Davis KD, et al: Systemic alpha-adrenergic blockade with phentolamine: A diagnostic test for sympathetically maintained pain. Anesthesiology 74:691, 1991.
20. Abram SE, Lightfoot RW: Treatment of long-standing causalgia with prazosin. Reg Anesth 6:79, 1981.
21. Ghostine SY, Comair YG, Turner DM, et al: Phenoxybenzamine in the treatment of causalgia: Report of 40 cases. J Neurosurg 60:1263, 1984.
22. Stevens DS, Robins VF, Price HM: Treatment of sympathetically maintained pain with terazosin. Reg Anesth 18:318, 1993.
23. Davis KD, Treede RD, Raja SN, et al: Topical application of

clonidine relieves hyperalgesia in patients with sympathetically maintained pain. Pain 47:309, 1991.

24. Rauck RL, Eisenach JC, Jackson K, et al: Epidural clonidine treatment for refractory reflex sympathetic dystrophy. Anesthesiology 79:1163, 1993.

25. Mellick GA, Mellick LB: Reflex sympathetic dystrophy treated with gabapentin. Arch Phys Med Rehabil 78:98, 1997.

26. Rocco AG: Radiofrequency lumbar sympatholysis: The evolution of a technique for managing sympathetically maintained pain. Reg Anesth 20:3, 1995.

27. Shealy CN, Mortimer JT, Reswick J: Electrical inhibition of pain by stimulation of the dorsal column: Preliminary clinical reports. Anesth Analg 46:489, 1967.

28. Linderoth B, Fedorcsak I, Meyerson BA: Peripheral vasodilatation after spinal cord stimulation: Animal studies of putative effector mechanisms. Neurosurgery 28:187, 1991.

29. Barolat G, Schwartzman R, Woo R: Epidural spinal cord stimulation in the management of reflex sympathetic dystrophy. Stereotact Funct Neurosurg 53:29, 1989.

30. Racz G, Lewis R, Laros G, et al: Electrical stimulation analgesia. *In* Raj PP (ed): Practical Management of Pain, ed 2. St Louis, Mosby–Year Book, 1992, p 922.

31. Shimoji S, Hokari T, Kano T, et al: Management of intractable pain with percutaneous epidural spinal cord stimulation: Differences in pain-relieving effects among diseases and sites of pain. Anesth Analg 77:110, 1993.

Chapter 60

Myofascial Pain Syndrome

Paul M. Park, M.D., and Robert E. Molloy, M.D.

Myofascial pain syndrome (MPS) is a soft tissue disorder that can cause chronic pain and disability. It can present with symptoms suggestive of other musculoskeletal conditions such as fibromyalgia syndrome (see Chapter 61), muscle strains, and sprains. However, MPS is now understood to be a distinct entity with its own set of diagnostic criteria.

There have been reports in the medical literature since the early 1800s of patients with pain due to tender areas within muscle groups. The current concepts and terminology used to refer to this disorder were developed primarily by the work of Travell and Simons since 1942 and later published in a book entitled *Myofascial Pain and Dysfunction: The Trigger Point Manual.*[1] However, the reader should be aware that a study in 1992 brought into question these concepts of MPS.[2]

DIAGNOSIS

The diagnosis is made by history and examination, because there are no specific diagnostic laboratory tests for this syndrome. Patients may complain of localized or diffuse muscle pain and tenderness, referred pain, paresthesias, vertigo, headache, visual disturbances, or discoordination. These symptoms are suggestive of a large group of disorders. The key to determining whether a clinical presentation qualifies as MPS is the presence of trigger points (TPs) on examination. TPs are painful regions and taut bands of muscle that cause reproducible referred pain in a nondermatomal distribution with the application of pressure. They may be located in muscle, joints, ligaments, or skin. Skeletal muscle TPs are emphasized in the medical literature and in clinical practice. On examination, the painful areas have been described as feeling like rope. A positive "jump" sign occurs when the TP is palpated and the patient "jumps" away from the pain. TPs can be found by palpating taut bands of muscle and eliciting a local twitch response. A local twitch response is described as a transient involuntary shortening of the fibrous muscular bands where the TP is located. TPs are classified

as active or latent.[3, 4] Active TPs cause ongoing pain and restrict the motion of the muscle. Patients with active TPs complain of spontaneous pain that is dull, constrictive, fairly well discriminated, varying in intensity, sudden or gradual in onset, continuous or intermittent, and present at rest or only on movement. Latent TPs are silent with respect to spontaneous symptomatology and cause muscle tightness, shortening, and dysfunction without the presence of persistent pain.

According to Simons,[5] the diagnosis of MPS requires the fulfillment of five major criteria and at least one of three minor criteria.

Major Criteria
1. Localized spontaneous pain
2. Spontaneous pain or altered sensations in the expected referred pain area for a given TP
3. A taut, palpable band in an accessible muscle
4. Exquisite, localized tenderness in a precise point along the taut band
5. Some degree of reduced range of movement when measurable

Minor Criteria
1. Reproduction of spontaneously perceived pain and altered sensations by pressure on the TP
2. Elicitation of a local twitch response of muscular fibers by transverse "snapping" palpation or by needle insertion into the TP
3. Pain relieved by muscle stretching or injection of the TP

Because the clinical presentation of MPS can be similar to that of other disorders, the investigator should have a differential diagnosis which includes musculoskeletal, neurologic, and psychogenic conditions, infections, neoplasms, and visceral diseases (Table 60–1).

PATHOPHYSIOLOGY

Pathophysiologic explanations for the development of TPs and myofascial pain are hypothetical. Histopathologic findings from muscle biopsies have been inconsis-

TABLE 60–1. DIFFERENTIAL DIAGNOSIS IN MYOFASCIAL PAIN SYNDROME

Musculoskeletal conditions	Neoplasms
Arthritis	Infections
Tendinitis	Cellulitis
Bursitis	Infectious myositis
Myopathy	Poststreptococcal arthralgia
Polymyalgia	Rocky Mountain spotted
Neurological conditions	fever
Radiculopathy	Lyme disease
Neuropathy	Colorado tick fever
Psychogenic conditions	
Somatoform disorder	
Conversion disorder	
Histrionic disorder	
Secondary gain	

Modified from Goldman LB, Rosenberg NL: Myofascial pain syndromes and fibromyalgia. Semin Neurol 11:274, 1991.

tent. The most prevalent explanations use ideas suggested by Melzack[6] and by Simons and Travell.[7] Presumably, there is an initiating event such as trauma or prolonged tension from bad posture which results in disruption of the sarcoplasmic reticulum. This may cause release of calcium, which stimulates a local contractile cycle and thus increases the consumption of adenosine triphosphate (ATP). This cycle may exceed the supply of oxygen available for aerobic metabolism, causing local ischemia. This would subsequently cause an increase in anaerobic metabolism and production of anaerobic byproducts such as histamine, serotonin, prostaglandins, and kinins. These neurotransmitters may modulate pain by stimulating group III and group IV free nerve endings, mediating a referred pain syndrome via lamina I or lamina V dorsal horn cells.

The formation of fibrous bands may also be explained by this mechanism. Ongoing local ischemia at the muscle site may cause myocyte death. This would lead to an ingrowth of fibroblasts and collagen and the subsequent formation of fibrous bands.

TREATMENT

Four different treatment modalities have been described: (1) the spray and stretch technique, (2) ischemic compression massage, (3) TP injections, and (4) physical therapy.[4] The *spray and stretch* technique involves passive stretching of the affected muscle groups in conjunction with the use of a vapocoolant spray (e.g., ethyl chloride, fluoromethane) to facilitate muscle relaxation. This therapy often results in immediate short-term relief.

Ischemic compression massage involves applying a localized force of about 20 to 30 pounds to tissue surrounding the TP and then releasing it. The resultant reactive hyperemia may improve perfusion of the TP with oxygen and nutrients and allow formation of ATP, which is needed by the muscle fibers to relax. This therapy by itself may be inadequate, but it can be useful when applied in conjunction with other modalities.

TP injections are a mainstay in the treatment for MPS.

Presumably the mechanism for this therapy relies more on disruption of fibrous bands that have formed within the muscles by the mechanical action of the needle injection rather than the pharmacologic action of the injected solution. A study comparing TP injections with a dry needle versus 0.5% lidocaine showed that the elicitation of a local twitch response during injection was the best indicator of a successful procedure.[8] Although the success of this method does not seem to rely on the presence of a pharmacologic agent, use of an injection medium may facilitate the separation of fibrous bands as a result of the hydrostatic pressure created. Application of a local anesthetic will also cause relaxation of the muscle. TP injections of botulinum toxin were more successful than saline injections, and the improvement in symptoms lasted 5 to 6 weeks without apparent adverse reactions.[9] Botulinum toxin inhibits muscle contraction by inhibiting the release of acetylcholine from peripheral nerves. When the procedure is performed, the patient should be positioned so that the muscle group targeted is relaxed. If the needle injection elicits the usual pain symptoms and a strong local twitch response, then it is a successful procedure. Treatment success may be enhanced and post-treatment soreness decreased by application of pressure after the injection to decrease bleeding at the injection site. Use of the spray and stretch technique, ischemic compression, and application of warm packs in conjunction with TP injections may also increase the chance of success.

Physical therapy is also an essential treatment in MPS. As stated previously, passive stretching aids in muscle relaxation and in regaining normal length and elasticity. It is also important to implement a reconditioning program to restore muscle strength and maintain normal range of motion and flexibility. An aerobic conditioning program may prevent cardiovascular deconditioning and allows the patient to take an active role in treatment.

Application of all the above techniques should help improve if not resolve the myofascial pain, usually in 4 to 8 weeks.[4] However, several factors are associated with treatment failure, including unemployment, constant pain, severe pain and long duration, no relief from analgesics, limited social activity, and limited coping skills.[10]

REFERENCES

1. Travell JG, Simons DG: Myofascial Pain and Dysfunction: The Trigger Point Manual. Baltimore, Williams & Wilkins, 1983.
2. Wolfe F, Simons DG, Friction J, et al: The fibromyalgia and myofascial pain syndromes: A preliminary study of tender points and trigger points in persons with fibromyalgia, myofascial pain syndrome, and no disease. J Rheumatol 19:944, 1992.
3. Vecchiet L, Giamberardino MA, Saggini R: Myofascial pain syndromes: Clinical and pathophysiological aspects. Clin J Pain 7(suppl 11):S16, 1991.
4. Goldman LB, Rosenberg NL: Myofascial pain syndrome and fibromyalgia. Semin Neurol 11:274, 1991.
5. Simons DG: Muscular pain syndromes. *In* Friction JR, Awad E (eds): Advances in Pain Research and Therapy, vol 17. New York, Raven Press, 1990, p 1.
6. Melzack R: Myofascial trigger points: Relation to acupuncture and mechanisms of pain. Arch Phys Med Rehabil 62:114,1981.

7. Simons DG, Travell J: Myofascial trigger points: A possible explanation [letter]. Pain 10:106, 1981.

8. Hong C-Z: Lidocaine injection versus dry needling to myofascial trigger point: The importance of the local twitch response. Am J Phys Med Rehabil 73:256, 1994.

9. Cheshire WP, Abashian SW, Mann JD: Botulinum toxin in the treatment of myofascial pain syndrome. Pain 59:65, 1994.

10. Goldenberg DL: Fibromyalgia, chronic fatigue syndrome, and myofascial pain. Curr Opin Rheumatol 8:113, 1996.

Chapter 61

Fibromyalgia

Paul M. Park, M.D., and Robert E. Molloy, M.D.

Fibromyalgia is a pain syndrome characterized by chronic diffuse musculoskeletal pain and abnormal soft tissue tenderness. It was first described in the early 1800s and it has been known by many names, including fibrositis, muscle-tension pain syndrome, muscular rheumatism, and tension myalgia.[1, 2] It is a common disorder affecting 3 to 6 million people in the United States, and it occurs in all socioeconomic, ethnic, and racial groups.[3] The estimated prevalence in the general population is 0.7% to 3.2%, and women are much more likely to be affected than men.[3, 4] The syndrome is most frequently seen in women between 20 and 50 years of age, but it is also common in the elderly.

DIAGNOSIS

The diagnosis of fibromyalgia is based on clinical findings. The American College of Rheumatology established the diagnostic criteria for fibromyalgia in 1990, with a predicted sensitivity of 88% and a specificity of 81%[5]. The criteria are

1. Chronic widespread muscular pain of at least 3 months' duration above and below the diaphragm on both sides of the body
2. Painful tender points in at least 11 out of 18 characteristic locations (Fig. 61-1), including the right and left occiput, lateral epicondyle, lower cervical area, upper gluteal border, trapezius, greater trochanter, supraspinatus, medial knee, and second rib.

Tender points exist even in people without fibromyalgia. They are areas that are normally more sensitive to palpation than the surrounding areas. In patients with fibromyalgia the tender points become very sensitive because the pain threshold is decreased in general throughout the body. This abnormal tenderness at predesignated locations in the body is the most common physical finding.

The diagnosis of fibromyalgia requires a careful history and physical examination, because there are no specific diagnostic tests for this syndrome. However, it is not a diagnosis of exclusion, because fibromyalgia can coexist with other disorders. Disorders that can mimic fibromyalgia include myofascial pain syndrome, rheumatoid arthritis, osteoarthritis, chronic fatigue syndrome, rheumatic diseases (systemic lupus erythematosus, Sjögren's syndrome, ankylosing spondylitis), myopathies, disc herniation, polymyalgia rheumatica, anemia, and malignancy. Judicious use of laboratory tests to rule out other disorders helps in the diagnosis. The investigator may consider ordering a full blood examination, erythrocyte sedimentation rate, thyroid function tests, and determinations of antinuclear antibody, rheumatoid factor, and creatine kinase.

Fibromyalgia symptomatology is variable and most commonly includes widespread musculoskeletal pain and fatigue. The musculoskeletal pain is predominantly axial (neck, middle and lower back) and diffuse, but it may affect any region. The terms patients use to describe the pain range from sharp, aching, or cramping to dull or burning. The pain may be more severe in one area than another, or at times it may be felt all over. The musculoskeletal pain has a variable course, and changes in severity are caused by such factors as time, changing weather, physical activity, psychological stress, and poor sleep. Fatigue is also important and is often the most disabling symptom in fibromyalgia. Other associated symptoms include headaches, paresthesias, subjective swelling, morning muscle stiffness, abdominal pain, and sleep disturbance. Most patients with fibromyalgia have some degree of disability that may affect routine household chores or recreational activity, but some have profound disability to the point of being unable to work.

PATHOPHYSIOLOGY

The cause of fibromyalgia remains unclear. Several studies have failed to show abnormalities in the tissues where the pain is located. Histomorphometric studies, biochemical studies, and tests of strength and tension

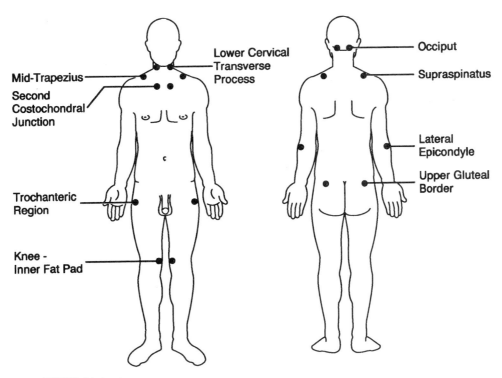

FIGURE 61–1. Characteristic locations of painful tender points for patients with fibromyalgia.

have shown only changes consistent with disuse or deconditioning.

There is a strong association between fibromyalgia and sleep disturbance. Normal sleep involves four non-dream stages (non-REM sleep) alternating with a dream stage (REM sleep). Stage IV of non-REM sleep is represented on electroencephalography by delta waves, indicating deepest sleep. Alpha waves are seen in lightly sleeping people. There is electroencephalographic evidence in people with fibromyalgia of reduced deep non-REM sleep, with interruption of the delta waves by alpha waves. Deprivation of stage IV sleep in normal control subjects has produced fibromyalgia symptoms and musculoskeletal pain in the classic tender point distribution.[3, 6] Therefore, chronic nonrestorative sleep has been suggested as a possible cause.

Other theories involve neurotransmitter imbalance. People with fibromyalgia have been found to have increased levels of substance P in the cerebrospinal fluid, suggesting that this may be a disorder of pain modulation. Decreased levels of tryptophan were also noted in people with fibromyalgia. This is significant because tryptophan is a precursor of serotonin, which is involved in the inhibitory descending pain pathway and in enhancing stage IV sleep.[3] However, it is unclear whether these abnormalities represent causes or effects.

It has been suggested that the symptoms of fibromyalgia result from depression and somatization disorders. However, most patients with fibromyalgia are not clinically depressed. The prevalence of depression is higher in people with fibromyalgia than in normal controls or age-matched controls with other illnesses, but depression in fibromyalgia is frequently a consequence of the chronic pain.[3]

TREATMENT

Physicians have used a combined approach in the treatment of fibromyalgia, which includes the following methods:

- Diagnosis and reassurance
- Avoidance of aggravating factors
- Pharmacologic options
- Physical modalities
- Exercise
- Patient's active role in treatment

Once an accurate diagnosis has been made, the first step is a comprehensive explanation of the disorder. Many patients have been to multiple physicians without an explanation for their chronic symptoms, and they may expect a pessimistic explanation for their pain and suffering. Patients should be reassured that the pain is not caused by disorders such as cancer or inflammation.

An important strategy is to break the cycle of pain and fatigue. It becomes more difficult to break the cycle as the duration of pain increases. One important step is to correct the sleep disturbance. Low-dose amitriptyline and cyclobenzaprine have been shown to increase stage IV sleep and decrease pain and tender points.[7] The dose for amitriptyline is lower than that used for depression, and it may work via its normalizing effects at the sleep center or by pain gating at the spinal cord level. Cyclobenzaprine is a tricyclic muscle relaxant. Nonsteroidal anti-inflammatory drugs may also be helpful. In unpublished investigational field trials, oral mexiletine has been shown to be beneficial in patients with fibromyalgia and chronic pain refractory to other medical treatments.[3] Mexiletine works by reducing muscle membrane depolarization through blocking of ion transport channels. The benefit of using fluoxetine, a selective serotonin reuptake inhibitor, is under study, and it has shown modest potential. Narcotic analgesics should be avoided, based on current information. Physical modalities such as massage, heat, stretching, sprays, topical anesthetics, and injection of painful areas with lidocaine or corticosteroids can be helpful.

It is important that the patient become involved in his or her own treatment and develop a sense of control and an understanding of the disorder. This helps alleviate some of the patients' fears and frustrations. Aerobic exercise has been shown to reduce pain, improve sleep, and restore fitness. Avoidance of aggravating factors such as a cold environment or excessive visual and auditory stimulation is helpful. Awareness that these interventions can be controlled by the patients underscores the fact that they, and not the doctor or the drugs, are an important reason for improvement in symptoms.

The outlook for patients seems promising. Many patients have fewer symptoms after correction of their sleep disturbance. A study of 44 fibromyalgia patients enrolled in a regimen of regular physical exercise showed that after 2 years 47% no longer fulfilled the American College of Rheumatology criteria for fibromyalgia and 24% were in remission.[3]

REFERENCES

1. Littlejohn GO: Rheumatology: II. Fibromyalgia syndrome. Med J Aust 165:387, 1996.
2. Doherty M, Jones A: ABC of rheumatology: Fibromyalgia syndrome. Br Med J 310:386, 1995.
3. Parziale JR, Chen JJ: Fibromyalgia. Med Health RI 79:188, 1996.
4. Goldenberg DL: Fibromyalgia, chronic fatigue syndrome, and myofascial pain. Curr Opin Rheumatol 8:113, 1996.
5. Wolfe F, Smythe HA, Yunus MB: Report of the Multicenter Criteria Committee: The American College of Rheumatology 1990 criteria for classification of fibromyalgia. Arthritis Rheum 33:160, 1990.
6. Moldofsky H, Scarisbrick P: Induction of neurasthenic musculoskeletal pain syndrome by selective sleep deprivation. Psychosom Med 38:35, 1976.
7. Goldenberg DL: Management of fibromyalgia syndrome. Rheum Dis Clin North Am 15:499, 1989.

Chapter 62

Acute Herpes Zoster

Richard V. Gregg, M.D.

Acute herpes zoster (AHZ), or shingles, represents a reinfection of one or more nerve roots by a latent varicella-zoster (chickenpox) viral particle. Any patient with this problem must have a history of chickenpox, and titers drawn in the acute phase demonstrate an elevation in antibodies to varicella-zoster. The skin eruptions involve a variable part or all of the nerve distribution. It is possible that some patients actually have no skin lesions; this is known as zoster sine herpete, but there is not a large amount of proof for this disease process.

PATHOLOGY

The outbreak begins in either the dorsal root ganglion cells or satellite cells of the dorsal root ganglion. The virus particles travel or are transmitted to the nerve endings, both distal and proximal to the dorsal root ganglion. In some cases, the motor nerve also appears to be affected. It has been documented from patients who died during or long after an acute shingles outbreak that at times the dorsal root entry zone and even dorsal columns and trigeminal brain-stem area demonstrate inflammatory changes.[1] It is not certain whether these changes occur secondary to nerve damage or are related to the primary infection. It is also uncertain what pathologic changes cause AHZ pain or postherpetic neuralgia (PHN); these changes are evident from patients both with and without a history of PHN.

The skin eruptions begin as erythema followed by blisters or pustules that break down and crust over. These can become secondarily infected and may take weeks or months to heal. Affected skin is often scarred and depigmented. Outbreaks of the trigeminal V1 distribution can involve the cornea and, rarely, the retina. This should be considered an ophthalmologic emergency, and immediate consultation should be obtained.

EPIDEMIOLOGY

The annual incidence of shingles has been stated to be between 1.3 to 4.8 cases per 1000 population. The incidence increases significantly with age, so that 10% of the population have had at least one episode of shingles by age 65 and 50% by age 85. Second infections, or outbreaks, are approximately equal in incidence or percentage to the first outbreaks, apparently indicating that the initial outbreak does not transfer further immunity regarding shingles. One article documented that approximately one half of second outbreaks occur in the same distribution as the first AHZ outbreak.[2]

AHZ infections often are preceded by some other infection, trauma, stress, chemotherapy, or cancer, whether diagnosed or not yet known. Leukemia and lymphoma stimulate an especially high prevalence of shingles outbreaks. Other causes for immunosuppression, such as prolonged use of prednisone or use of immunosuppressants after transplantation, also markedly increase the incidence of AHZ. There may be some variation between races regarding the incidence of AHZ, with the white race having a fairly high incidence relative to others.

Although the reason is not known, there is a significant distribution tendency to these outbreaks. Thoracic spinal roots are most commonly affected (50%), and the trigeminal cranial nerve is the next most common site. Within the trigeminal distribution, V1 is more common than V2, which is more common than V3, and occasionally multiple branches of the trigeminal nerve are involved. The order then follows with cervical spinal roots, lumbar spinal roots, and sacral spinal roots, with involvement of other cranial nerves being quite uncommon.[2]

Patients' descriptions of pain and sensitivity during AHZ outbreaks are quite variable. Frequently, pain precedes the outbreak of lesions, leading to assessments for other causes of neuralgic pain. Some patients experience pain at the same time as or even after development of the skin eruptions. The severity of pain complaints ranges from no pain or just itching to severe or horrible pain. Frequently there are both constant and intermittent or lancinating qualities to the pain, and surface sensitivity often develops after the skin lesions begin to mature or become inflamed. Frequently patients' sleep patterns are disturbed, and they particularly note pain or discomfort when contact is made on the area of the outbreak during sleep.

TREATMENT

Treatment of AHZ is generally aimed at aiding early healing, decreasing the acute pain, and decreasing the incidence of PHN. Prevention of PHN is discussed in Chapter 63. Patients younger than 50 years of age rarely develop prolonged pain after AHZ, and therefore it may be reasonable to consider symptomatic treatment only in that population. In patients older than 50 years of age, acute pain is often worse and PHN is more likely. Therefore, more aggressive treatment often is recommended.

Antiviral agents are the mainstay of treatment for AHZ. A number of them are currently on the market, including acyclovir, famciclovir, and valaciclovir; several others are in various stages of testing. There are fairly well performed placebo-controlled studies documenting faster healing and decreased intensity and duration of AHZ pain with each of these agents. It is possible that some of them are better than others, but more studies need to be performed to clarify that issue. These antiviral agents are fairly expensive, so mild, uncomplicated cases in patients younger than 50 years of age may not warrant their use. It should also be noted that, even though these agents do appear to have significant effects, there are many patients who still have pain even with their use.

Standard analgesics, such as nonsteroidal anti-inflammatory drugs or opiates, may be useful in helping patients get through acute episodes. Not all patients find benefit with these medications, but if they are helpful their use is reasonable in AHZ. Frequently an adjunct medication, something to help with sleep, is requested. A tricyclic antidepressant may help with sleep and pain if a sufficient dose for control of neuralgia can be achieved. If these measures are inadequate and the pain continues to be severe, other neuralgic medications, as mentioned in Chapter 63, are reasonable considerations early in the course.

Systemic corticosteroids have also been recommended in AHZ. Several moderately controlled studies demonstrate some efficacy, but the most recent study, which was well controlled, did not demonstrate significant benefit. It would appear that the steroids do improve healing and reduce pain. It is unclear whether they decrease the duration of AHZ pain, because the most recent studies investigated combined use of steroids and antivirals. Because use of systemic steroids does carry some significant risks, particularly in the elderly and in certain other medical populations, the benefits must be weighed against those risks.

Nerve blocks are touted throughout anesthesia and pain literature as beneficial for acute pain and prevention of PHN. Unfortunately, most of the studies examining this therapy are poorly controlled or fairly anecdotal. It is difficult to control, in a blinded fashion, against a treatment that causes numbness, acute relief of pain, and frequently a drop in blood pressure. However, one study documented reduction in the severity of pain while acknowledging these difficulties in blinding.[3] That study examined epidural injection, which blocks both somatic and sympathetic nerves. There are also studies examining only sympathetic blockade (e.g., stellate ganglion blocks). These also have demonstrated reduced pain, although again with difficulties regarding blinding and controls.

Frequently steroids are added to the nerve blocks for treatment of the pain of AHZ. This is probably the least studied of the treatments, although some abstracts have been published. Local anesthetic and steroid have been injected from the periphery, including just beneath the lesions at the skin, to the peripheral nerves that are affected, up to and including the epidural space. Those published reports regarding these treatments state that they are helpful for pain, but again the documentation is poor regarding controls or blinding. There is inflammation noted at all of the sites, which is a potential justification for the use of steroids. It may be considered that, because the dorsal root ganglion is the source of the infection or damage, the use of epidural steroids would be most logical, but logic and results do not necessarily coincide. In extremely severe cases (e.g., patients who are suicidal because of the pain), a continuous infusion may be warranted for as long as 1 or 2 weeks to try to maintain pain relief on a consistent basis. It is certainly not tested whether this provides any improvement regarding longer-term pain relief, but it at least provides some acute control in the most difficult cases.

REFERENCES

1. Watson CPN, Deck JH, Morshead C, et al.: Post-herpetic neuralgia: Further post-mortem studies of cases with and without pain. Pain 44:105, 1991.
2. Hope-Simpson RE: The nature of herpes zoster: A long-term study and a new hypothesis. Proc R Soc Med 58:9, 1965.
3. Tenicela R, Lovasik D, Eaglstein W: Treatment of herpes zoster with sympathetic block. Clin J Pain 1:63, 1985.

FURTHER READINGS

Watson CPN (ed): Herpes Zoster and Post-herpetic Neuralgia: Pain Research and Clinical Management, vol 8. Amsterdam, Elsevier, 1993.
Weller TH: Varicella and herpes zoster: Changing concepts of the natural history, control and importance of a not-so-benign virus. N Engl J Med 309:1362, 1434, 1983.

Chapter 63

Postherpetic Neuralgia

Harsha V. Sharma, M.D., and
Richard V. Gregg, M.D.

Postherpetic neuralgia (PHN) is probably the most dreaded complication of infection with the varicella-zoster virus (VZV). The most accepted definition of PHN is pain in the area or areas afflicted with acute herpes zoster (AHZ) that lasts for longer than 4 to 6 weeks after termination of the acute phase of infection.[1]

INCIDENCE AND EPIDEMIOLOGY

PHN develops in about 10% of all patients with AHZ.[2] Patients with prodromal pain or severe AHZ pain are more likely to have PHN. Age-adjusted male and female incidence ratios are not different. The most consistent predictor of susceptibility to PHN and of a protracted course is old age. Persons with AHZ who are older than 60 years of age have a 30% to 50% chance of developing PHN. On the other hand, those younger than 50 years of age have only a 5% chance of developing PHN. No racial or geographic differences in prevalence of PHN have been described. No difference has been noted in the incidence of PHN among various dermatomes afflicted by AHZ.[3]

NATURAL HISTORY

The natural history is the most commonly ignored factor when the efficacy of a therapeutic measure is being evaluated over a period of time. A proportion of patients with PHN improve without any intervention. Only about 35% to 50% of patients with PHN continue to complain of pain at 3 months after diagnosis. At the end of 1 year, only 22% to 33% of the original number still have pain.[4]

CLINICAL FEATURES AND DIAGNOSIS

Duration

PHN commonly manifests as constant pain with superimposed intermittent aggravation. This may last from months to many years (longer than 1 year in 22% of patients, longer than 5 years in 2%).

Intensity and Quality

PHN pain is commonly a background, spontaneous, severe, aching or burning pain. Superimposed on this are subjective reports of intermittent paresthesias and dysesthesias, both spontaneous and evoked. Descriptors often used include nagging, flickering, sharp, gnawing, shooting, tiring, tender, itching, and stabbing.

Aggravating Factors

The most often reported aggravating factors are psychosocial stressors, environmental temperature changes, and local mechanical stimulation (touch sensitivity).

Psychological Factors

Anxiety and depression may not be overt, although reports of suicidal ideation and/or attempts exist. Overt pain behavior is rare. Patients tend to be obsessive, narcissistic, and independent personalities who show a concerned preoccupation with their pain. In addition, they are often openly critical of those who have been unable to help them with the relief of their pain in the past. The patients remain extroverted and, despite their pain, continue to interact socially at workplaces and otherwise. A clear-cut association exists between life stressors and acute exacerbation of PHN pain.[5] There also seems to be a high incidence of narcotic tolerance and dependence as well as sleep disturbances.

Associated Findings

Although Rosenak's work 60 years ago revealed the role of sympathetic blockade in terminating AHZ, no evidence exists to definitively link the sympathetic nervous system (sympathetically mediated pain) to PHN pain.[1]

267

Examination

Signs of peripheral sensory neuropathy (both small and large fiber size) are present in all cases and should be sought. Signs such as hypalgesia (reduced pin-prick sensation) and hypesthesia (cold, heat, light touch, vibration sense, and two-point discrimination) are easily checked. Signs of phenomena that may result from a combination of peripheral and central neurologic dysfunction (see later discussion) include hyperalgesia, dysesthesias, hyperpathia, and allodynia. Allodynia is present in 80% to 90% of patients and is usually of the dynamic type and to cold stimuli.

Secondary myofascial pain often is present as a result of altered body mechanics and guarding.

Skin scarring and pigmentary changes are likely to be present.

PATHOPHYSIOLOGY

Electrophysiologic Studies

Electrophysiologic studies reveal sensory axonopathy. Electromyographic studies may reveal motor axonal damage. Comparison of AHZ patients with and without PHN revealed no significant differences in these measurements.[6]

Postmortem Studies

Widespread degenerative and inflammatory changes throughout the involved spinal and peripheral sensory units were found in a few PHN patients who underwent postmortem studies, although these pathologic findings have not been reproduced in subsequent studies. Atrophy of the dorsal horn and loss of both axons and myelin in the affected sensory roots, dorsal root ganglia, and peripheral nerves have been described. The pathologic findings in the peripheral nerves are of greatest interest. They revealed an abnormality in the ratio of small-diameter, unmyelinated axons to large-diameter, myelinated axons (see later discussion). The question remains as to which of these pathologic changes is the primary reason for pain in PHN.[7]

Role of the Sympathetic Nervous System

Sympathetic nervous system stimulation, hypothetically accomplished by the VZV, its toxin, or inflammation, may result in vasoconstrictive compromise of blood flow (vasa nervosum) to the involved nerves. This in turn results in hypoxic and ischemic damage to the nerve that is worsened by endoneurial edema, a result of endothelial damage. Smaller fibers are more resistant to such insults, which may result in the aforementioned reversal of the normal axon type ratio.[7, 8] Noordenbos referred to this as "fiber dissociation."

Hypotheses of Pathogenesis

The *spontaneous constant pain* of PHN may be explained by the gate control theory proposed by Wall and Melzack in 1965. As a result of the fiber dissociation that occurs in the afflicted nerve, there is a relative loss of the inhibitory action of the large-diameter axons on entry of noxious impulses into the spinal cord via the smaller-diameter fibers. Non-noxious stimuli may also be misinterpreted in the central nervous system (CNS) as pain.[8] This may be an example of deafferentation-induced CNS reorganization.

Hypesthesia and hypalgesia result from the peripheral axonal damage and loss. The degree of these abnormalities is variable depending on the severity of damage.

Both central and peripheral mechanisms have been employed to explain the *allodynia, hyperalgesia, paresthesias, and dysesthesias*. The previously mentioned deafferentation-induced CNS reorganization may result in incorrect (e.g., painful) interpretation of normally non-noxious stimuli; hyperalgesia and allodynia occur. In all likelihood such deafferentation is not complete in most patients. The remaining completely normal or partially damaged nerve axons may develop sites anywhere along their course (sensory root, dorsal ganglion, peripheral extensions, terminal nociceptors) that show spontaneous electrical impulse-generating activity. Such activity may occur in a number of axons and may have the ability to summate through ephaptic connections.[9]

TREATMENT

A reasonable treatment plan should start with a correct diagnosis followed by a sequential trial with available interventions as deemed necessary. Start with noninvasive, safer, less costly modalities, keeping the more invasive, more expensive approaches, which may also carry a greater risk profile with their use, for later trials if then required. Such a treatment paradigm should be acceptable to most patients and to the economically sensitive care provider.

Pharmacologic Therapies

As an introduction, it should be noted that medications for neuralgia are a rapidly changing field in medicine; PHN has both peripheral and central pathology, and medications for either source, if effective, are reasonable for trial.

Antidepressants and Neuroleptics

Tricyclics (TCAs) are the most studied antidepressants. The efficacy of amitriptyline in established PHN has been confirmed with double-blind crossover studies. The timing of treatment commencement may be important: the earlier the better. The usefulness of TCAs seems to be unrelated to their antidepressant activity. Side effects can be problematic, especially in the older patient; drowsiness, confusion, dry mouth, urinary retention, constipation, blurred vision, and postural hypotension may be seen. Low starting doses with gradual increments to an effective dose, accomplished over weeks, may be the most optimal method of treatment. Other TCAs with fewer anticholinergic effects, such as nortriptyline, may be better tolerated. Good starting doses, administered at night, are 10 mg in patients older than 65 years of age and 25 mg for younger patients. Elderly patients seem to have a longer elimination half-life for TCAs and may need longer to achieve steady levels in the blood. Other types of antidepressants, such as selective serotonin reuptake inhibitors, have also been used with varied reports of success. Although of unproven efficacy, neuroleptics occasionally are combined with antidepressants by some clinicians. Their side effects profile warrants caution in the elderly population.[4, 10, 11]

Analgesics

Simple analgesics like acetaminophen and nonsteroidal anti-inflammatory drugs are relatively safe and worth a try. Narcotic analgesics have a greater side effect profile, may result in the development of tolerance and dependence, and are best tried in the more refractory cases. Many believe that pain in PHN is not very responsive to narcotics. Their use in nonmalignant chronic pain states is receiving a wider acceptance currently.

Anticonvulsants

The proven efficacy of anticonvulsants in other neuropathic pain states with a paroxysmal, lancinating feature (present in some PHN patients) has led to their empirical use in this pain syndrome. Studies employing carbamazepine, phenytoin, and valproic acid have results that are either unimpressive or difficult to interpret. Possible side effects, some quite serious, must be kept in mind when using such medications.[4] Gabapentin is a newer, safer, and promising but unproven option.

Baclofen

There is scant evidence to support the usefulness of baclofen in the treatment of facial PHN. It may have some role in the management of spinal PHN.

Local or Systemic Corticosteroids

Because evidence for inflammatory changes has been seen at the level of the dorsal root ganglion and in peripheral nerve in postmortem studies of some patients with long-standing PHN, the use of local or systemic corticosteroids may seem reasonable, although few studies have shown effectiveness. The risk-benefit ratio is even poorer than for acute shingle pain.

Anesthetics

Local and Topical Anesthetics

Agents such as ethyl chloride spray, EMLA cream, and 5% lidocaine ointment have been used and may be of temporary benefit to some patients. Local infiltration and specific nerve blocks with local anesthetics also provide transient relief which may occasionally outlast the duration of action of these agents. In well established cases their efficacy can be very disappointing.

Epidural Local and Steroid Injections

Controversy exists regarding the efficacy of these blocks in established PHN. Two studies reported that as many as 90% of patients with PHN of greater than 6 months' duration were pain free at the end of 1 year after three weekly epidural injections with methyl prednisolone (60 mg to 120 mg) and 0.5% bupivacaine (5 mL in cervical or thoracic or 7 mL in lumbar injections); the patients received this intervention early on, within 10 weeks of the diagnosis of PHN.[12, 13] Unfortunately, most well controlled studies do not demonstrate such good results.

Sympathetic Blocks

The role of the sympathetic nervous system in a number of chronic pain states remains a mystery. Although evidence exists to support the use of sympathetic blocks to prevent the occurrence of PHN, studies both support and dispute their utility in established PHN. This seems to hold true for both trigeminal and spinal PHN cases.[1, 4, 11]

Neuroaugmentation Therapies

Transcutaneous Electrical Nerve Stimulation

Continuous application of the transcutaneous electrical nerve stimulation (TENS) unit, as opposed to intermittent use, may be of benefit to some patients.[4]

Spinal Cord Stimulation

A few studies have looked at the efficacy of spinal cord stimulation in PHN. The numbers of patients studied have been small, but overall this therapy seems to have a success rate of approximately 60% in carefully selected (psychologically screened) patients.[14]

Surgical Therapies

Surgical approaches range from superficial procedures such as undermining or excising the affected skin to more serious procedures, including neuroablation, that may involve either the peripheral nervous system (cryoprobe nerve lesions, sympathectomy, trigeminal tractotomy, subperineural doxorubicin [Adriamycin]), the spinal cord (dorsal root entry zone lesions, dorsal rhizotomy, cordotomy), or the brain (cingulotomy, frontal lobotomy). Such ablative options carry a risk of being poorly efficacious, having a significant morbidity, and perhaps causing a new source of pain.[1]

Behavioral Medicine Interventions

Behavioral medicine interventions need to be individualized. Some focus should be placed on teaching patients with PHN techniques to identify and better manage social and interpersonal stressors that may cause painful exacerbation.[5]

Other Therapies

Patients who use *topical capsaicin* may show a favorable response of 55% to 75%. The burning sensation may be ameliorated with prior application of lidocaine ointment. Patients should be encouraged to apply the capsaicin four to five times daily for at least 4 weeks before considering it a failure.[4]

Acupuncture is considered to be ineffective in patients with PHN.[4]

PREVENTION

Antivirals

Many newer antiviral agents with activity against VZV are being studied. These include acyclovir, famciclovir, valaciclovir, penciclovir, and sorivudine. Although their efficacy in shortening the acute phase of the disease (i.e., pain and rash) and attenuating the possibility of cutaneous scarring is evident, controversy exists in crediting these agents with actually preventing the occurrence of PHN. Several studies demonstrate a shorter duration of PHN with these agents compared with placebo. In addition, there is some evidence that patients with the complication of PHN who receive antivirals early in the acute phase of AHZ infections have a better, and 50% quicker, response to antidepressants.[10]

Corticosteroids

Evidence exists to support the use of systemic steroids to prevent PHN, but caution should be exercised in their use in the immunocompromised patient. The use of steroids in immunocompromised patients may result in the dissemination of AHZ. The most recent, well designed study[15] did not show any benefit with the use of steroids. No studies have looked at the preventive role of epidurally administered steroids.[4]

Amantadine

There are some data to support the use of amantadine, especially in patients in whom there are contraindications for the use of steroids. Common side effects result from the CNS effects and may include visual hallucinations, seizures, nightmares, or mania. In addition, toxicity may occur in patients with end-stage renal disease, causing psychosis, cardiovascular problems, and even coma.[4] Therefore, this drug should be prescribed with caution in such patients.

Sympathetic Blockade

Studies[7, 8, 10] have indicated that, when a sympathetic block is placed within 2 months of the onset of AHZ, the pain is decreased and there is a decrease in the development of PHN. Sympathectomies are accomplished via a local anesthetic stellate injection, thoracic or lumbar epidural injections, or peripheral nerve blocks, depending on the afflicted area. It is believed that such blocks result in an improvement in the blood supply to the affected nerves and thereby reduce the nerve damage that may otherwise have occurred. This may explain the critical nature of timing the intervention.[8]

REFERENCES

1. Hogan QH: The sympathetic nervous system in post-herpetic neuralgia. Reg Anesth 18:271, 1993.
2. Ragozzino MW, Melton LJ III, Kurland LT, et al.: Population based study of herpes zoster and its sequelae. Medicine 61:310, 1982.
3. Burgoon CF, Burgoon JS, Baldridge GD: The natural history of herpes zoster. JAMA 164:265, 1957.
4. Watson CPN: Post herpetic neuralgia. Neurol Clin 7:231, 1989.
5. Pilowsky I: Psychological aspects of post-herpetic neuralgia: Some clinical observations. Br J Med Psychol 50:283, 1977.
6. Mondelli M, Romano C, Della Porta P, et al.: Electrophysiological findings in peripheral fibers of subjects with and without post-herpetic neuralgia. Electroencephalogr Clin Neurophysiol 101:185, 1996.
7. Watson CPN, Deck JH, Morshead C, et al.: Post-herpetic neuralgia: Further post-mortem studies of cases with and without pain. Pain 44:105, 1991.
8. Winnie AP, Hartwell PW: Relationship between time of treatment of acute herpes zoster with sympathetic blockade and prevention of post-herpetic neuralgia: Clinical support for a new theory of the mechanism by which sympathetic blockade provides therapeutic benefit. Reg Anesth 18:277, 1993.
9. Schon F, Mayer ML, Kelly JS: Pathogenesis of post-herpetic neuralgia. Lancet 2:366, 1987.
10. Bowsher D: Post-herpetic neuralgia in older patients. Drugs Aging 5:411, 1994.
11. Robertson DRC, George CF: Treatment of post herpetic neuralgia in the elderly. Br Med Bull 46:113, 1990.
12. Forrest JB: The response to epidural steroid injections in chronic dorsal root pain. Can Anaesth Soc J 27:40, 1980.
13. Schreuder M: Pain relief in herpes zoster. S Afr Med J 63:820, 1983.
14. Meglio M, Ciolo B, Rossi GF: Spinal cord stimulation in management of chronic pain: A 9-year experience. J Neurosurg 70:519, 1989.
15. Benoldi D, Minizzi S, Zucchi A, et al: Prevention of post-herpetic neuralgia. Evaluation of treatment with oral prednisone, oral acyclovir, and radiotherapy. Pharmacol Ther 30:288, 1990.

FURTHER READING

Noordenbos W: Pain. Amsterdam, Elsevier, 1959, p 182.
Rosenak S: Procaine injection treatment of herpes zoster. Lancet 2:1056, 1938.

Chapter 64

Phantom Pain

Paul M. Park, M.D.,
and Honorio T. Benzon, M.D.

PHANTOM SENSATION

Phantom sensation is the persistent perception that a body part exists after it has been removed by amputation or trauma. Phantom sensations are common after surgery. The incidence is 90% during the first 6 months after surgery, with one third of patients noticing it within 24 hours after surgery.[1] Excision of a body part is not essential for phantom sensation. Phantom sensation of the arm has been reported after avulsion of the brachial plexus without amputation of the limb.[2] These sensations are common for distal parts of excised extremities, but phantom sensations may also be felt in other body parts, such as tongue, bladder, rectum, breast, and genitalia, after excision.[2, 3] Phantom sensation can have various manifestations, including paresthesia, tingling, touch, pressure, itching, heat, cold, and wetness.[2, 3] Sometimes the representation of the missing body part is distorted, as with the perception that the hand or foot is twisted. At the start of the phenomenon, the sensation usually feels so real that the patient may actually reach for objects or attempt to ambulate with a phantom limb.[2] However, after a certain period, phantom sensations of the distal extremities change and become less distinct, so that, for example, the patient may feel a hand but not the arm. The phenomenon called *telescoping* refers to the progressive shortening of the phantom body part so that the patient has the sense that the distal part of the limb is becoming more proximal.[1] Complete paraplegic and quadriplegic patients also have phantom sensation.[2, 3]

PHANTOM PAIN

Phantom pain is the perception of a painful, unpleasant sensation in the distribution of a missing body part. About two thirds of patients who undergo amputation are reported to have phantom limb pain in the first 6 months after surgery, and 60% of patients still have significant phantom pain 2 years after surgery.[4] The overall incidence of phantom pain several years after surgery has been reported to be as high as 85%.[3, 4] The pain can vary in character, duration, frequency, and intensity. It can produce a sharp, dull, burning, squeezing, or electrical sensation.[3] In a prospective study by Jensen and colleagues[4] on 58 patients undergoing limb amputation, phantom pain changed in presentation within the first 6 months after amputation. The characteristic of the phantom pain changed from a mainly exteroceptive (knifelike or sticking) type of pain, localized in the entire limb or at least involving proximal parts of the lost limb, to a mainly proprioceptive (squeezing or burning) type of pain localized in the distal parts of the amputated limb.[4] Forty-seven percent of patients had phantom pain within 24 hours after the amputation, and 83% within the first 4 days. The study also showed that the frequency, duration, and severity of the phantom pain decreased during the first 6 months, and then the characteristics of the phantom pain did not change significantly thereafter. Sometimes, phantom pain resolves spontaneously, with or without treatment. However, it seems that phantom pain persisting 6 months after the amputation is difficult to treat.[3]

The incidence of phantom pain seems to be independent of the patient's age, sex, previous health status, or cause of amputation.[3, 4] One factor that increases the incidence of phantom pain after amputation is the persistence of pain in the limb before amputation.[1, 4, 5] In a prospective study of 56 patients who had amputation of a lower limb, Nikolajsen and colleagues[5] noted that the presence of preamputation pain significantly increased the incidence of stump pain and phantom pain after 1 week and the incidence of phantom pain after 3 months. Approximately 42% of the patients reported that their phantom pain resembled the pain they had experienced at the time of amputation.

STUMP PAIN

Stump pain is somatic pain arising from the residual body part after amputation. Common causes of stump pain are an improperly fitted prosthesis, neuroma formation, arthritis, sympathetically maintained pain, referred pain, and ischemic pain.[3] Stump pain must be differentiated from phantom pain, because the most common reason for stump pain is an ill-fitting prosthesis, which can cause pressure on the skin, leading to ulcers and infection.[3] This problem can be resolved by careful evaluation and proper fitting of the prosthesis.

THEORETICAL MECHANISMS

The proposed mechanisms for phantom sensation and phantom pain are unclear and controversial. They may not even be explained by the same mechanism, because the relief of one is not always associated with relief of the other.[3] It has been reported that phantom sensation disappears after a parietal cortical lesion but phantom pain remains.[5] The mechanism for phantom phenomena has been ascribed to peripheral, spinal cord, and supraspinal mechanisms. There is evidence to support peripheral mechanisms. Peripheral nerve damage during an amputation initiates axonal regeneration, creating an area of hyperexcitability known as a neuroma, which may generate pain spontaneously. The demonstration of spontaneous neuronal activity in the proximal end of cut nerves,[6] the presence of stump pathology in some patients with phantom pain, and the relief of phantom pain after the injection of local anesthetic into the painful stump have all been considered as supportive evidence of peripheral mechanisms of phantom pain.[1] However, there is evidence against a purely peripheral mechanism for phantom phenomena. Total spinal anesthesia, cordotomy, and cordectomy have all failed to relieve phantom pain.[7, 8]

There is reason to think that a spinal cord mechanism explains phantom phenomena. Peripheral nerve injury leads to removal of afferent input to the dorsal column of the spinal cord, causing structural, neurochemical, and physiologic changes to the neurons. This concept is referred to as *plasticity*, and these changes create areas that initiate spontaneous pain sensations which are transmitted centrally. Peripheral sensory input at the level of the spinal cord also has inhibitory effects on the transmission of pain centrally. The changes in the dorsal horn and the loss of afferent input lead to decreased impulses from the brain-stem reticular areas that normally have inhibitory effects on sensory transmission.[7] Therefore, the absence of inhibitory effects of sensory input from the missing peripheral body part causes increased autonomous activity of the dorsal horn neurons, in effect becoming "sensory epileptic discharges."[3, 4] The spinal cord mechanism is supported by the fact that anticonvulsants and lesions placed in the substantia gelatinosa are effective in treating phantom pain.[7]

The proposed supraspinal mechanism to explain phantom pain is the neuromatrix theory of Melzack.[2, 9] The neuromatrix consists of a network of neurons which extends throughout the brain. The repeated cyclical processing of peripheral nerve impulses in the neuromatrix imparts a characteristic pattern, a neurosigna-

ture, according to Melzack. Therefore, a person may have the sensation that a body part is present even in the absence of peripheral input. In the absence of modulating input from the limbs, the neuromatrix produces abnormal signature patterns which are interpreted as painful sensation.[2, 9] In phantom limb pain, the pattern produced is transduced in the neural hub as a hot or burning sensation. The cramping muscle pain may be caused by messages from the action-neuromodule to move the muscles of the absent limb.[2]

TREATMENT

Bach and associates[10] showed that epidural bupivacaine, with or without morphine, when given for 72 hours before amputation, decreased the incidence of phantom limb pain.[10] The incidences of phantom pain at 1 week, 6 months, and 1 year in the epidural group were 27%, 0%, and 0%, respectively. These incidences were significantly less than the corresponding incidences of 64%, 38%, and 27% in the control group.[10]

Surgical interventions have not been shown to be of significant benefit in phantom pain.[3] Spinal cord stimulation has been recommended to replace the loss of afferent input to the dorsal column and enhance the descending inhibition of pain transmission. However, the results with dorsal column stimulation have not been uniform.[11, 12] The same results have been found with dorsal root entry zone (DREZ) lesions. Although the procedure showed promise as treatment for avulsion injuries, its long-term effect on phantom pain has been fair, at best.[13]

Various physical modalities such as ultrasound, vibration, transcutaneous electrical nerve stimulation (TENS), and acupuncture offer temporary relief with no significant long-term benefits.[3, 14] These therapies rely on the gate-control theory of pain transmission, which proposes that stimulation of large nerve fibers closes the gate and inhibits the transmission of pain centrally.

Numerous medical treatments have been proposed. The most commonly used medications are the anticonvulsants and the antidepressants.[3, 7] Other drugs include β-blockers, neuroleptic agents, intravenous calcitonin, mexiletine, and capsaicin. Combined treatment with anticonvulsants and antidepressants is the usual regimen, treating both the lancinating pain and the burning pain components of phantom limb pain.[7] Clonazepam is probably the anticonvulsant of choice, but valproic acid or carbamazepine can be used. For cramping pain, stump movement disorders, or flexor spasticity, baclofen or clonazepam may be effective.[7] Opioids are not effective for phantom pain.

Psychological interventions for phantom pain include hypnosis, biofeedback, cognitive and behavioral therapies, and support groups.[15, 16] These interventions may facilitate adaptation to a change in body image, adaptation to chronic pain, and relief of grief and anger.[17]

Psychological preparation, treatment of the patient's pain, and educational efforts during the preamputation and postamputation periods can be very helpful. These include psychological preparation of the patient for amputation, preparation for change in body image, introduction to the use of a prosthesis, care and treatment of the stump, and explanation of the rehabilitation process.[3]

REFERENCES

1. Jensen TS, Krebs B, Nielsen J, et al: Phantom limb, phantom pain and stump pain in amputees during the first 6 months following limb amputation. Pain 17:243, 1983.
2. Melzack R: Phantom limbs. Reg Anesth 14:208,1989.
3. Davis RW: Phantom sensation, phantom pain, and stump pain. Arch Phys Med Rehabil 74:79, 1993.
4. Jensen TS, Krebs B, Nielsen J, et al: Immediate and long term phantom pain in amputees: Incidence, clinical characteristics and relationship to preamputation pain. Pain 21:267–278, 1985.
5. Nikolajsen L, Ilkjaer S, Kroner K, et al: The influence of preamputation pain on postamputation stump and phantom pain. Pain 72:393, 1997.
6. Carlen PL, Wall PD, Nadvorna H, et al: Phantom limbs and related phenomena in recent traumatic amputations. Neurology 28:211, 1978.
7. Iacono RP, Linford J, Sandyk R: Pain management after lower extremity amputation. Neurosurgery 20:496–500, 1987.
8. Murphy JP, Anandaciva S: Phantom limb pain and spinal anesthesia. Anaesthesia 39:188, 1984.
9. Melzack R: Phantom limbs and the concept of a neuromatrix. Trends Neurosci 13:88, 1990.
10. Bach S, Noreng MF, Tjellden NU: Phantom limb in amputees during the first 12 months following amputation, after preoperative lumbar epidural blockade. Pain 33:297, 1988.
11. Wester K: Dorsal column stimulation in pain treatment. Acta Neurol Scand 75:151, 1987.
12. Kumar K, Nath R, Wyant GM: Treatment of chronic pain by epidural spinal cord stimulation: A 10-year experience. J Neurosurg 75:402, 1991.
13. Saris SC, Iacono RP, Nashold BS: Dorsal root entry zone lesions for post-amputation pain. J Neurosurg 62:72, 1985.
14. Lundgerg T: Relief of pain from a phantom limb by peripheral stimulation. J Neurol 232:79, 1985.
15. Sherman RA, Sherman CJ, Bruno GM: Psychological factors influencing chronic phantom limb pain: An analysis of the literature. Pain 28:285,1987.
16. Siegel EF: Control of phantom pain by hypnosis. Am J Clin Hypn 21:285, 1979.
17. Arena JG, Sherman RA, Bruno GM, et al: The relationship between situational stress and phantom limb pain: Cross lagged correlation data from six month pain logs. J Psychosom Res 34:71, 1990.

Chapter 6 5

Central Pain States

Vernon B. Williams, M.D.,
and Marco Pappagallo, M.D.

Central pain is the result of lesions or diseases affecting the pain pathways within the central nervous system (CNS)—that is, the spinal cord, brain, or both. The discussion of central pain has in some cases been expanded to include pain experienced via a prolonged or excessive activation of central pain mechanisms. This expanded consideration would include instances in which the primary lesion resides in the periphery but secondarily activates central pain mechanisms. The recognition of central pain as a concept and clinical entity is important in that, although the condition is extremely difficult to treat in many cases, the very presence of a diagnosis is often helpful in providing appropriate prognostic counseling to patients. The diagnosis is also of value for communicating to other treating physicians, preventing unnecessary diagnostic testing, and providing a framework for study of the efficacy of treatment strategies. The most important considerations before designing a treatment strategy for patients with central pain are the cause, the pathophysiology, and the clinical presentation of the pain state.

CAUSES OF CENTRAL PAIN

Any pathologic process affecting the CNS may result in central pain, particularly if the lesion affects some portion of the spinothalamic or thalamocortical tracts. Traumatic injury is a leading cause of central pain originating in the spinal cord. Mass lesions of any type, including neoplastic processes and chronic abscesses, can rarely cause central pain. Demyelinating lesions can result in central pain. For example, approximately 20% of patients with multiple sclerosis have central pain. Chronic degenerative diseases of the CNS have been studied less systematically in terms of their likelihood of causing central pain, but anecdotally there is significant prevalence of central pain in these disorders. For instance, some reports have suggested that sensory complications including pain are present in almost 10% of patients with Parkinson's disease. Epilepsy disorders can manifest as painful seizures. These are most frequently associated with findings of structural lesions on imaging or at autopsy. Although trauma, neoplasm, demyelinating disease, and degenerative diseases of the CNS can all lead to central pain, stroke appears to be the most common cause. About 1% to 2% of the 2,000,000 stroke patients in the United States (prevalence) has central pain. The thalamus is one location for a lesion leading to a classic central pain syndrome. In contrast to most pathologic processes affecting the nervous system, there has been an almost alarming inability to predict development of central pain based on the specific location of a particular lesion. However, Nasreddine and Saver (1997) reported a right thalamic predominance in the development of central pain after thalamic stroke. Overall, supratentorial lesions are more likely than brainstem lesions to cause central pain.

PATHOPHYSIOLOGIC MECHANISMS

The pathophysiology underlying central pain syndrome is poorly understood. It is believed that irritation or damage to the central pain pathways (i.e., spinothalamic tract, thalamus, or projections from the thalamus to the cortex) can lead to physiologic changes that ultimately result in central pain. The pathophysiologic mechanisms involved in causing and maintaining central pain are supposed to be related to the following:

- Disinhibition of nociceptive input (i.e., the injury causes loss of negative feedback control over painful impulses).
- Denervation supersensitivity (i.e., loss of innervation releases abnormally excessive activity of central pain signaling neurons such as those seen in the thalamus or dorsal horn).
- Maladaptive reorganization (i.e., CNS plasticity allows abnormal reorganization after injury and altered processing of nociceptive and/or innocuous input to the forebrain).

These mechanisms may work in concert, leaving the normal pain pathways in a state of disarray and causing central pain syndrome clinically. The complex neurochemistry of these mechanisms may involve a variety of endogenous neurotransmitters, including serotonin, norepinephrine, γ-aminobutyric acid (GABA), and excitatory amino acids.

CLINICAL PRESENTATIONS

Patients with central pain frequently describe aching, burning pain with associated symptoms that begins days to weeks (occasionally longer) after a CNS lesion. The discomfort is constant but may wax and wane; it is poorly localized and often has both a deep and a superficial component. In addition, there can be sharp or shooting pains of extreme intensity. Cold temperature, anxiety, and fear may exacerbate symptoms.

Some patients with central pain are among the most striking seen in clinical practice. For example, patients with the Dejerine-Roussy syndrome (the classic clinical central pain syndrome seen after thalamic injury) have characteristic features that include a rapidly regressing hemiparesis and a sensory deficit to touch, pain, and temperature. Allodynia, hyperalgesia, and spontaneous, severe paroxysmal pain on the hemiparetic side are often seen as well. Patients with central pain of all kinds may have some or all of these features, depending on the location of the underlying lesion. Organic signs on sensory examination of patients with thalamic lesions also include the so-called thalamic midline split for sensory loss and pain. In central pain of any cause there may be a delayed pain sensation after a skin stimulus (delayed hyperalgesia), supporting a polysynaptic response. Allodynia and other sensory phenomena are also commonly found on examination. For example, patients may exhibit *mitempfindung* ("with sympathy"), a phenomenon in which stimulation in one area of the body results in a simultaneous sense of the provoked sensation in another part of the body, or *alloesthesia*, in which sensory stimulus on one side of the body is perceived on the other side. Although some disturbance of sensory function is almost always present on physical examination, there are many patients with very few or only subtle clinical findings. Identification of these changes may require a very detailed neurologic examination. Quantitative sensory testing may reveal side-to-side asymmetries in thresholds to cooling, warmth, and heat pain.

TREATMENT OPTIONS

The most important aspect of treating patients with central pain is to define and continuously review the goals of treatment. Complete cessation of pain is rare, and this fact should be emphasized to patients. Therefore, the goal should be to reduce pain and improve function as much as possible without creating intolerable side effects. In addition, it is of paramount importance to consider the multiple components of the central pain syndrome and include treatment strategies for each of the components. In short, the patient's anxiety, fear, depression, even suicidal ideation should be treated as well as the pain itself.

A variety of medications and surgical treatments have been used for central pain. The pharmacologic approach is based on a strategy of stepwise *combination therapy* (Fig. 65–1). It is likely that more than one single drug class will be required to achieve satisfactory analgesia. The complexity of treatment is related to the complexity of the unbalanced neurochemistry involved in maintaining central pain. Tricyclic antidepressants are supposed to increase the CNS levels of serotonin and norepinephrine, and they occasionally have been effective in relieving central pain. Anti-epileptic drugs (AEDs) may be of value in central pain. Carbamazepine

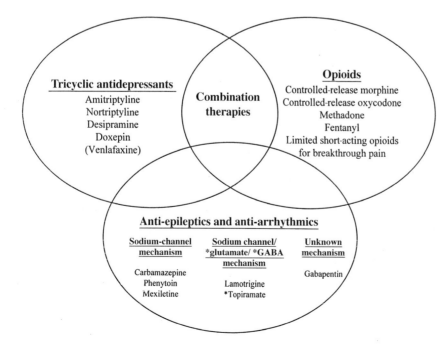

FIGURE 65–1. General principles of pharmacologic management of central pain:

1. Most patients will require combination therapy with agents from several drug classes and different mechanisms.
2. Although a stepwise approach is generally used to add individual agents, *it is not unreasonable to initiate treatment with combination therapy* given the extreme refractory nature of central pain.
3. Augmentive agents (dextromethorphan for opioids; selective serotonin reuptake inhibitors for tricyclic antidepressants) boost the effect and serum concentration of the primary agents and are often of value, but they must be added carefully, with attention given to adverse reactions as well as signs and symptoms of toxic effects.
4. Patients may benefit from a short inpatient trial with IV patient-controlled analgesia (PCA) for determination of response to opioids and rapid titration to effective dose.

has been the AED of choice for several years, but gabapentin, an agent more recently approved by the U.S. Food and Drug Administration, seems to be promising for the treatment of neuropathic pain, including central pain. Lamotrigine and topiramate are other AEDs of interest. They each possess sodium channel blocking activity. Topiramate has non-NMDA, glutamate receptor antagonist effects and seems to act on the GABA-A receptors as well. Opioids represent the mainstay of therapy for some chronic pain conditions, and a large anecdotal experience supports their usefulness for neuropathic pain and central pain as well. A careful titration of long-acting agents (e.g., controlled-release morphine sulfate, oxycodone, fentanyl, methadone) can be carried out in selected patients. Opioid analgesia can be augmented or tolerance to opioid analgesia can be decreased by the concurrent use of N-methyl-D-aspartate (NMDA) receptor antagonists, in particular dextromethorphan, which can be given on a dosage schedule of three to four times per day. Dextromethorphan is a low-affinity NMDA antagonist, and the daily oral dose may range according to a ratio of 1:1 mg with morphine (or morphine equianalgesic doses for other opioids). Titration must be carefully conducted to avoid drowsiness and ataxia. Among the surgical techniques, the dorsal root entry zone (DREZ) lesion procedure for brachial plexus avulsions and the neuromodulatory procedures (spinal cord stimulation, deep brain stimulation) have provided relief and are used at some centers.

The treatment of concomitant depression in patients with central pain is very important. The degree of suffering and functional disability caused by unrelenting pain or by the underlying disease can lead to suicidal ideation and attempt. Depression must be anticipated, investigated, and aggressively treated. Selective serotonin reuptake inhibitors (SSRIs) can augment the antidepressant effects of the tricyclic antidepressant medications when used for pain treatment. Care must be taken in that the SSRIs can increase the serum levels of the tricyclic agents and of dextromethorphan. Finally, physical therapy and behavioral therapy, including biofeedback, are of benefit in helping some patients take an active role in the therapeutic process and assisting with the development of coping strategies to more productively deal with their pain.

BIBLIOGRAPHY

Casey K: Pain and Central Nervous System Disease: The Central Pain Syndromes. New York, Raven, 1991.

Casey K: Central Pain: An Update. Presented at American Academy of Neurology 49th Annual Meeting Pain Symposium, Boston, April 1997.

Dejerine J, Roussy G: Le syndrome thalamique. Rev Neurol 14:521–532, 1906.

Gonzales G. Central pain: Diagnosis and treatment strategies. Neurology 45(suppl 9):S11–S16, 1995.

Merskey H, Bogduk N (eds): Classification of Chronic Pain: Description of Chronic Pain Syndromes and Definitions of Pain Terms, ed 2. Seattle, IASP Press, 1994.

Nasreddine ZS, Saver JL: Pain after thalamic stroke: Right diencephalic predominance and clinical features in 180 patients. Neurology 48:1196–1199, 1997.

Chapter 66

Pelvic Pain

Sunil J. Panchal, M.D.

Chronic pelvic pain (CPP) is a common problem for women and may lead to a significant impairment in the ability to lead a productive life. It has been estimated that approximately 10% of visits to gynecologists are related to complaints of CPP.[1] Numerous causes are theorized for this condition, impeding the development of a widely accepted specific definition at this time. However, CPP is distinguished from acute pelvic pain by the nature of the progression of complaints. Acute pelvic pain develops over the course of days with a rapid onset and usually is caused by infection, torsion, or rupture of visceral structures. The events causing acute pelvic pain can also result in CPP.

Causes for CPP include endometriosis, dysmenorrhea, dyspareunia, mononeuropathies, myofascial pain, vulvitis, cystitis, and sympathetically maintained pain. Many patients have no known or suspected organic pathology for their discomfort; this results in a diagnosis of pelvic pain of unknown etiology. Other terms include pelvic congestion, pelvic fibrosis, pelvic neurodystonia, pelvalgia, and irritable uterus syndrome. Confounding factors include a high incidence of physical and/or sexual abuse (30% to 50%) in this patient population, underscoring the need for a multidisciplinary approach.[2]

EPIDEMIOLOGY

The estimated percentage of new referrals to gynecology clinics for CPP is approximately 10%. These patients are estimated to undergo up to 20% of hysterectomies and 40% of laparoscopies in the general population.[3, 4] Thirty to fifty percent of patients with CPP are classified as having "chronic pelvic pain without obvious pathology." This difficulty in determining a diagnosis is underscored by the high incidence of hysterectomy without pelvic pain relief (about 25%).[5] Laparoscopy of patients with CPP reveals endometriosis in one third of patients, adhesions in one third, and no apparent pathology in the remaining third, but laparoscopy also reveals significant pathology in other women who do not complain of pain.[6] This makes diagnosis difficult in the CPP population.

ASSOCIATION OF PELVIC PAIN AND ABUSE

An accurate history of sexual or physical abuse is often difficult to obtain, and this fact has resulted in controversy regarding studies finding a high correlation of such histories with CPP. Some studies report a 50% or higher incidence of abuse in patients with CPP.

Comparison of patients with a history of abuse vs. nonabused control subjects reveals a higher incidence of unexplained gastrointestinal and pelvic symptoms, psychiatric diagnoses, and surgical procedures. Therefore, the physician should always be concerned about a history of abuse in patients who do not respond well to pharmacologic interventions or diagnostic blockade.

ETIOLOGY

Pain in the pelvic region can originate from the following structures:

1. Pelvic viscera: uterus, ovaries, bladder, urethra, rectum, sigmoid, or descending colon
2. Somatic structures: skin, vulva, clitoris, vaginal canal
3. Musculoskeletal and ligamentous structures
4. Spinal lesions or gastrointestinal or urologic conditions (referred pain)

Acute pelvic pain may originate from ectopic pregnancy, ruptured ovarian cyst, pelvic abscess, ureteral stone, urinary tract infection, or cystitis. CPP may be caused by ectopic endometrial tissue, infection, neoplasm, trauma, postsurgical changes, or somatization disorder.

HISTORY

The taking of a history from a patient with pelvic pain should be thorough and detailed and should include the following:

- Pattern of onset
- Inciting event
- Quality (e.g., burning, aching, dull, sharp, cramping)
- Severity
- Duration and progression of complaints
- Constant or intermittent nature
- Exacerbating factors (e.g., position, eating, urination, defecation, Valsalva maneuver)
- Alleviating factors
- Efficacy and toxicity of previous medications
- Association with menstrual cycle
- Incontinence
- Pregnancy
- Sexual activity
- Sudden weight loss or gain
- Breast or endocrinologic difficulties
- Family history of ovarian, uterine, or breast cancer

A comprehensive assessment often demonstrates associations that make diagnosis simpler for the physician. These associations are discussed under specific syndromes later in this chapter.

PHYSICAL EXAMINATION

A thorough physical examination is critical. A complete neurologic examination should be performed to identify any cause of neural injury, possibly from the central nervous system, or injury to peripheral innervation. Allodynia, hyperesthesia, or hyperalgesia may indicate injury to the pudendal nerve, intercostal nerve, ilioinguinal nerve, iliohypogastric nerve, genitofemoral nerve, or a nerve root (T10-L2, S2-4). Examination of surgical scars may indicate nerve entrapment or a possible neuroma formation. Abdominal examination is useful to localize the source of pain and to determine whether there are any objective signs of an acute process (i.e., rebound tenderness). Finally, a bimanual pelvic examination in the presence of a nurse should be performed. Cervical tenderness may indicate infection. The existence of anatomic abnormalities of the uterus or adnexa and the presence of any trigger points in the musculature must be determined. All findings should be discussed with the referring gynecologist to assess any progression of complaints.

DIAGNOSTIC STUDIES

Diagnostic studies are tools to assist in making a diagnosis and should always be used as an adjunct to the history and physical examination, not as a substitute. Infection, bleeding, and inflammatory processes should be assessed by checking a complete blood count, urinalysis, urine and cervical cultures, and erythrocyte sedi-

mentation rate. A determination of the level of the β-subunit of human chorionic gonadotropin should be performed in fertile women for the possibility of ectopic pregnancy. Computed tomography or ultrasound help in evaluating a possible mass lesion, free fluid, or free air (e.g., hemorrhage, perforated viscus).

Diagnostic neural blockade is an invaluable tool if used appropriately. Diagnostic blockade indicates whether a particular neural structure is a pathway for nociception for the patient's complaints. Blockade of the pudendal nerve, intercostal nerves, ilioinguinal nerves, iliohypogastric nerve, genitofemoral nerve, spinal nerve root, or trigger point should provide relief if pain originates from the somatic structures. Blockade of visceral afferent fibers can be achieved by superior hypogastric nerve block or ganglion impar block, resulting in relief for pain originating from the uterus, bladder, ovaries, testicles, sigmoid colon, descending colon, or rectum. The physician utilizing diagnostic blocks must always perform a neurologic examination after the intervention to determine whether the targeted nerve was successfully blocked and whether there was any inadvertent blockade of other neural structures before arriving at a conclusion. Differential epidural and intrathecal blocks cannot selectively block specific fiber classes (Aβ vs. Aδ vs. C fibers) and should no longer be used for diagnosis.[7] A neuraxial sensory block may help to differentiate a central pain syndrome, however. Diagnostic laparoscopy is a safe, effective, and well accepted tool to detect or confirm endometriosis, adhesions, ovarian cyst, ectopic pregnancy, and uterine malformations. As previously discussed, findings during laparoscopy do not necessarily correlate with presence or absence of pelvic pain.

GENERAL CONCEPTS OF VISCERAL PAIN APPLIED TO PELVIC PAIN

Visceral pain refers to pain mediated by the soft organs in the thorax, abdomen, and pelvis. It is usually described as dull and vague in location and radiates away from the affected organ. It frequently is associated with hyperalgesia (or spasm) of the overlying somatic tissues. Its poor localization is probably caused by the small number of visceral afferents, which subserve a wide anatomic area and then converge in the spinal cord at the same site at which somatic structures converge. Only 2% to 15% of afferents in the spinal cord (7% in the thoracic region) arise from the viscera.[8] These visceral afferents synapse on second-order neurons at the same level of the spinal cord as somatic afferents. Specifically, visceral afferents terminate in laminae I and V of the dorsal horn, with significant ramification occurring in lamina I both rostrally and caudally, therefore achieving wide receptive fields.[9] This *viscerosomatic convergence* (visceral innervation that converges terminally in the spinal cord at the same level as overlying somatic structures) is what makes it difficult for the patient to accurately distinguish between visceral and somatic origins for the pain and explains the commonly described phenomena of referred pain to the mandible or left upper extremity during myocardial ischemia and referred pain to the shoulder from diaphragmatic irritation. Accordingly, it is difficult to accurately diagnose visceral pain problems on the basis of the pain complaint. In a review of 64 patients with abdominal pain, only 15% had an accurate diagnosis.[10]

Visceral pain can be induced by

1. Abnormal distention and contraction of the hollow visceral walls
2. Rapid stretching of the capsules of hollow visceral organs
3. Formation and accumulation of algogenic substances
4. Ischemia of visceral musculature
5. Direct action of chemical stimuli on compromised mucosa
6. Traction or compression of ligaments, vessels, or mesenteries[11]

Notably, the viscera generally are not sensitive to heat or cutting stimuli.

Anatomically, the majority of visceral afferents run with sympathetic fibers via the celiac and other plexi; travel through the sympathetic chain on their way to the dorsal root ganglion, where the cell bodies for these fibers reside; and terminate in the dorsal horn laminae I and V. Vagal afferent neurons project viscerotopically to the nucleus of the solitary tract in the medulla oblongata. Functionally, there exist three general classes of visceral afferents. There are low-threshold mechanosensitive afferents that respond to distention and contraction and other stimuli; specific chemosensitive afferents (probably vagal); and high-threshold mechanosensitive afferents.[9] This separation of function was investigated in the cat model, with identification of ischemia-sensitive C-fiber afferents. Graded distention of the gastrointestinal tract demonstrated that ischemia-insensitive C fibers had a low threshold in response to distention (13 ± 5 mm Hg) with a plateau of discharge frequency. This contrasted sharply with ischemia-sensitive C fibers, which had a high threshold (86 ± 12 mm Hg) and a larger peak response to distention in the noxious range (60 to 180 mm Hg).[12]

Visceral afferents can be sensitized, and hyperalgesia may ensue. This has been demonstrated experimentally in rats by applying intracolonic acetic acid to create visceral inflammation, with subsequent sensitization recorded in both low- and high-threshold mechanosensitive afferents.[13] This phenomenon has also been observed in patients with irritable bowel syndrome, who reported pain at significantly lower volumes of colonic balloon distention than did control subjects.[14] Therefore, visceral afferents may undergo a change in function similar to those of somatic nociceptors.[15]

ENDOMETRIOSIS

Endometriosis is defined as the presence of endometrial tissue outside the uterus. It has a prevalence of approximately 7% among women of reproductive age. Ectopic sites include the peritoneum, uterosacral ligaments, fallopian tubes, round and broad ligaments, and, most commonly, the ovaries.[16] This ectopic spread may be caused by retrograde menstruation or by lymphatic or hematogenic spread. Pain may result from prostaglandin release, distention, nerve irritation, or tissue irritation by menstrual products. Pain is typically cyclical, increasing during menstruation and subsiding a few days after its completion. Patients complain of pelvic pain, dysmenorrhea, and dyspareunia, which often resolve with menopause or oophorectomy. Diagnosis requires visualization of lesions during laparoscopy or laparotomy.

Therapy options take into consideration evidence correlating pain and size of endometrial implants with plasma estrogen levels. After considering the patient's age and reproductive desires, the options include hormonal manipulation (usually a 6-month trial, with a response rate of approximately two thirds) and surgery (controversial). Hormonal manipulation may consist of reduction of estrogen (leuprolide acetate; Lupron), reduction of pituitary gonadotropin production (danazol), or use of low-dose oral contraceptives. Surgical options are removal of endometrial implants (resection, laser, thermal probes), total abdominal hysterectomy for severe endometriosis (ovaries may be preserved if they are disease free), and presacral neurectomy.

INFECTION

Infection is often a cause of CPP and may predispose patients to infertility. Infection of the uterus is called endometritis; it is associated with events facilitating entrance of bacteria via the cervix, such as dilation and curettage, term pregnancy, or spontaneous abortion. Infection by normal vaginal flora or a sexually transmitted organism usually results in crampy suprapubic pain and uterine tenderness. Other findings include foul-smelling discharge, bleeding, urinary frequency, low-grade fever, and leukocytosis. Gram staining and cultures should be performed, followed by appropriate antibiotic treatment. Urinalysis may help distinguish this condition from cystitis.

Pelvic inflammatory disease (PID) is an infection involving the pelvic organs and nearby supportive structures. PID is associated with loss of cervical integrity, multiple sexual partners, sex with an infected person, and use of intrauterine devices (IUDs), especially the Dalkon shield. *Neisseria gonorrhoeae* and *Chlamydia trachomatis* are the most common causative organisms. Gonorrhea produces severe postmenstrual pain, whereas chlamydia is usually asymptomatic. Findings include dyspareunia, dysuria, generalized abdominal and pelvic pain, rebound tenderness, pain with cervical manipulation, nausea, and diarrhea. Cultures and antibiotic treatment are essential. Approximately 50% of patients with PID develop CPP, and 30% become infertile.

OTHER CAUSES OF UTERINE PAIN

Primary dysmenorrhea is pain associated with menstruation that has no other identifiable cause. It is present in 50% of adult women and is severe in 15% of women. Patients have increased levels of prostaglandins in endometrium and menstrual products. Treatment includes nonsteroidal anti-inflammatory drugs (NSAIDs), oral contraceptives to reduce menstrual flow, and calcium-channel blockers or β_2-agonists to reduce uterine contractility.

Secondary dysmenorrhea is pain associated with menstruation that is caused by fibroids, adenomyosis, or an IUD. It commonly occurs in patients in their late 30s or 40s. Patients may have heavy, irregular bleeding and anemia. Sharp, sudden exacerbation may indicate fibroid degeneration and ischemia. Fibroid resection or removal of the IUD may be successful. Hysterectomy is appropriate for heavy bleeding, severe pain, or ureteral compression, but in more than 25% of cases this fails to relieve pain.

PELVIC CONGESTION

Observations of absent venodilation with exacerbation of pain from administered vasoactive compounds supports a theory of pelvic venous congestion as a cause of CPP.[17] It has been proposed that venous stasis and reflux in dilated ovarian varices causes pelvic pain, especially with prolonged standing. Further observations include reduced pain in patients with venographic evidence of diminished congestion from hormonal therapy.[15]

Proponents of this theory claim associated findings that include uterine enlargement, thickened endometrium, and polycystic ovaries and have advocated ovarian vein ligation, bilateral venous embolization, and hysterectomy. To date, this diagnosis remains controversial because the literature lacks good documentation.

PELVIC ADHESIONS

The idea that adhesions are a cause for unexplained pelvic pain remains controversial. Laparoscopies in patients with CPP demonstrate a prevalence of 30% to 50%, with prior pelvic surgery as a predictor of presence of adhesions.[19] Because adhesions are found during laparoscopy in many patients without CPP, the correlation is tenuous. One randomized trial suggested successful outcome in women with CPP who underwent adhesiolysis for dense, vascularized adhesions, especially if they involved the gastrointestinal tract, but this treatment was not very effective for moderate adhesions.[20]

OVARIAN REMNANT SYNDROME

Ovarian remnant should be included in the differential diagnosis for patients with CPP after bilateral oophorectomy. Increased levels of follicle-stimulating hormone and luteinizing hormone in women of reproductive age are suggestive of this syndrome. An adnexal mass that is palpable or imaged by ultrasound is supportive as

well. Surgical resection is the recommended treatment.[21]

CANCER PAIN

Carcinoma of pelvic structures may elicit pain due to distention of a hollow viscus, pressure or traction of sensitive tissues, obstruction, inflammation, necrosis, or direct invasion of neural elements. Pain is often diffuse and may radiate to the lower back or rectum.

Treatment of pain from pelvic neoplasms includes surgical resection or debulking when technically feasible, chemotherapy, or radiation therapy. This is supplemented with systemic pharmacologic agents such as NSAIDs, tricyclic antidepressants, and opioids. Anticonvulsants are added for neuropathic symptoms.

If inadequate analgesia or intolerance of side effects occurs, intraspinal drug delivery or neurolytic techniques may be attempted. If life expectancy is 3 months or less, an externalized epidural catheter is appropriate after evaluation for spinal metastases. Longer life expectancy would indicate use of an implanted intrathecal pump. Drugs approved for use in implanted pumps by the U.S. Food and Drug Administration include only morphine and baclofen, but reports exist of successful use of other opioids, local anesthetics, and clonidine in various combinations.

NEURAL BLOCKS AND CONSIDERATION FOR NEUROLYSIS

General principles for neural blocks include the diagnostic value of local anesthetic injection, and many physicians have observed improved pain in response to a series of local anesthetic injections (with or without steroids) in patients with chronic neuropathic nonmalignant pain. The mechanism of this seeming reversal of adverse neuroplastic changes is unknown. Once the nociceptive pathways have been identified, neurolysis may be of long-term benefit. Complications from neurolysis include possible neuroma formation, deafferentation pain, permanent motor or sensory deficits, orthostatic hypotension, diarrhea, sexual dysfunction, and bowel or bladder incontinence. Risk of neuroma formation varies with choice of technique. Neuroma formation is more likely with surgical or radiofrequency ablation than with alcohol, phenol, or cryolysis, because cutting or burning destroys the neural sheath.[22] Neuritis is another risk, but it occurs rarely with neurolysis of sympathetic nerves or visceral afferents.

Peripheral Nerve Blocks

These blocks are valuable for neuropathic pain or neuroma of somatic nerves of the pelvic skin, muscles, and bone. Neurolysis should be cautiously considered for severe nonmalignant pain that is refractory to conservative measures.

Superior Hypogastric Nerve Block (Presacral Nerve)

Surgical presacral neurectomy has a long history of success for relief of pain of pelvic visceral structures by an open approach, and more recently via the laparoscope.

A percutaneous technique to block the superior hypogastric plexus has been described for treatment of pelvic cancer pain. The plexus is located anterior to the L5 vertebral body and sacrum at the bifurcation of the common iliac vessels. The visceral afferents that travel through this plexus have their cell bodies located in the dorsal root ganglia from T10 to L2. Blockade of the superior hypogastric plexus has been reported to decrease pelvic pain by 70% in patients with cervical, prostate, or testicular cancer.[23] No complications were reported. This can be performed by a bilateral posterior approach with fluoroscopy or by a single-needle anterior approach with computed tomography guidance.

Ganglion Impar (Ganglion of Walther) Block

The ganglion impar is the termination of the paired paravertebral sympathetic chains. This terminal end is a single ganglion located anterior to the sacrococcygeal junction. Blockade of this structure has been introduced within the last decade to manage intractable perineal cancer pain involving the sympathetic nervous system.

Sympathetically mediated perineal pain usually is poorly localized and has components of burning and urgency. Ganglion impar block and neurolysis has been reported to achieve 70% to 100% pain relief for perineal pain caused by cancer of the cervix, colon, bladder, rectum, or endometrium.[24] The procedure is performed with the patient in the lateral decubitus position with a single, bent needle inserted just superior to the anus and advanced to the sacrococcygeal ligament. The position is confirmed with injection of contrast medium under fluoroscopy. Local anesthetic or neurolytic solution is then injected, usually with a volume of 4 to 6 mL. No complications have been reported to date.

Intrathecal and Epidural Block and Neurolysis

Intractable pelvic cancer pain with somatic involvement may be alleviated by destruction of the appropriate somatic sensory fibers. Intrathecal neurolysis is preferred for unilateral pain and carries a reduced risk of motor fiber destruction. In patients who have undergone a urinary diversion and colostomy, epidural or saddle block neurolysis is an effective means of achieving effective pain relief, but the risk of incontinence or lower extremity paresis is high.

Neurosurgical Ablative Techniques

Percutaneous cordotomy provides unilateral relief only. *Bilateral cordotomy* is rarely performed and carries a significant risk of fatal sleep apnea (Ondine's curse). *Midline myeletomy* is very invasive; it may be successful for bilateral pain, but the results are unpredictable.

CONCLUSION

Pelvic pain has often been difficult to diagnose and treat, resulting in frustrated patients with little support from family and friends. A thorough multidisciplinary assessment is critical, with appropriate use of diagnostic studies and nerve blocks. Application of visceral pain studies involving the gastrointestinal tract supports concepts of sensitization of the pelvic viscera. This further supports use of tricyclic antidepressants, anticonvulsants, and opioids in patients with otherwise undetectable pathology. Nerve blocks, spinal cord stimulators, and implantable pumps are also appropriate in carefully selected candidates. Neurolytic techniques have been reported for general diagnoses of CPP, but most experts advocate restriction of these procedures for pain of oncologic origin.

REFERENCES

1. Reiter RC, Gambone JC: Demographic and historic variable in women with idiopathic chronic pelvic pain. Obstet Gynecol 75:428–432, 1990.
2. Toomey TC, Hernandez JT, Gitelman OF, et al: Relationship of sexual and physical abuse to pain and psychological assessment variables in chronic pelvic pain patients. Pain 53:105–109, 1993.
3. Lee NC, Dicker RC, Rubin GL, et al: Confirmation of the preoperative diagnosis of hysterectomy. Am J Obstet Gynecol 150:283–287, 1984.
4. Peterson HB, Hulka JF, Phillips JM: American Association of Gynecologic Laparoscopists' 1988 membership survey on operative laparoscopy. J Reprod Med 35:587–589, 1990.
5. Stovall TG, Ling FW, Crawford DA: Hysterectomy for chronic pelvic pain of presumed uterine etiology. Obstet Gynecol 75:676–679, 1990.
6. Stout AL, Steege JF, Dodson WC, et al: Relationship of laparoscopic findings to self-report of pelvic pain. Am J Obstet Gynecol 164:73–79, 1991.
7. Hogan QH, Abrams SE: Neural blockade for diagnosis and prognosis: A review. Anesthesiology 86:216–241, 1997.
8. Cervero F, Connel LA: Distribution of the somatic and visceral primary afferents of the thoracic spinal cord of the cat. J Comp Neurol 230:88–98, 1984.
9. Jänig W: Neurobiology of visceral afferent neurons: Neuroanatomy, functions, organ regulations and sensations [review]. Biol Psychol 42:29–51, 1996.
10. Sarfeh IS: Abdominal pain of unknown etiology. Am J Surg 132:22–25, 1976.
11. Docherty RH: Visceral pain. In Raj P (ed): Pain Medicine: A Comprehensive Review. St. Louis, Mosby–Year Book 1996, 430–438.
12. Pan HL, Longhurst JC: Ischaemia-sensitive sympathetic afferents innervating the gastrointestinal tract function as nociceptors in cats. J Physiol (Lond) 492:841–850, 1996.
13. Sengupta JN, Su X, Gebhart GF: Kappa, but not mu or delta, opioids attenuate responses to distension of afferent fibers innervating the rat colon. Gastroenterology 111:968–980, 1996.
14. Ritchie J: Pain from distension of the pelvic colon by inflating a balloon in the irritable colon syndrome. Gut 14:125–132, 1973.
15. Panchal SJ, Staats PS: Visceral pain: From physiology to clinical practice. Journal of Back and Musculoskeletal Rehabilitation 9:233–246, 1997.

16. Johnson JG: Gynecologic pain: Locating its source. Pain Management May/June: 143-152, 1990.

17. Stones RW, Thomas DC, Beard RW: Suprasensitivity to calcitonin gene-related peptide but not vasoactive intestinal peptide in women with chronic pelvic pain. Clin Auton Res 2:343-348, 1992.

18. Reginald PW, Adams J, Franks S, et al: Medroxyprogesterone acetate in the treatment of pelvic pain due to venous congestion. Br J Obstet Gynaecol 96:1148-1152, 1989.

19. Stovall TG, Elder RF, Ling FW: Predictors of pelvic adhesions. J Reprod Med 34:345-348, 1989.

20. Peters AAN, Trimbos-Kemper GCM, Admiraal C, et al: A randomized clinical trial on the benefit of adhesiolysis in patients with intraperitoneal adhesions and chronic pelvic pain. Br J Obstet Gynaecol 99:59-62, 1992.

21. Webb MJ: Ovarian remnant syndrome. Aust NZ J Obstet Gynaecol 29:433-435, 1989.

22. Panchal SJ: The rationale and efficacy of zygapophyseal blocks and denervation techniques for low back pain. Submitted to Journal of Back and Musculoskeletal Rehabilitation.

23. Plancarte R, Ahescha C, Patt RB, et al: Superior hypogastric plexus block for pelvic cancer pain. Anethesiology 73:236, 1990.

24. Kames LD, Rapkin AJ, Naliboff BD, et al: Effectiveness of an interdisciplinary pain management program for the treatment of chronic pelvic pain. Pain 41:41-46, 1990.

Chapter 67

 # Sickle Cell Anemia

David R. Walega, M.D.,
and Honorio T. Benzon, M.D.

Sickle cell anemia is a genetic disorder of hemoglobin synthesis that follows classic mendelian inheritance. Normal hemoglobin A (HbA) is formed by two alpha chains and two beta chains. Hemoglobin S (HbS) differs from normal adult HbA by the substitution of valine for glutamic acid at the sixth position on the beta chain. This replacement leads to interaction between hydrophilic regions on adjacent hemoglobin molecules. Patchy aggregation of HbS occurs under deoxygenated conditions (i.e., partial pressure of oxygen <40 mm Hg). Repeated deoxygenation and prolonged hypoxia result in cellular membrane damage, cellular dehydration, and formation of sickled cells.[1] The incidence of sickle cell anemia in the black American population is 0.15%.[2]

The natural history of sickle cell anemia is characterized by frequent and unpredictable painful vasoocclusive crises, caused by sludging of red blood cells in the microcirculation, with resultant tissue hypoxia and infarction.[3] Nociceptors are then activated by hypoxia, acidosis, and the release of chemical mediators of inflammation, such as potassium, adenosine triphosphate, bradykinins, prostaglandins, and substance P. Although the pain of sickle cell crisis may be triggered by bacterial or viral infection, dehydration, hypothermia, hypoxemia, or acidosis, there is often no clear etiologic factor.[2] The frequency of sickle cell crisis is variable, ranging from less than one crisis per year to several crises each month.[4] The pain can be either acute or chronic and may be somatic, visceral, or neuropathic in nature.

Acute pain can occur at multiple sites. Abdominal pain can mimic other surgical causes of acute abdomen, including appendicitis, perforated viscus, cholecystitis, and splenic infarction. Acute chest syndrome is not uncommon, yet pneumonia and pulmonary embolus should be ruled out. After childhood, the majority of sickle cell patients have no splenic function as a result of frequent thromboses and autoinfarction. These patients are immunocompromised and are especially susceptible to encapsulated gram-positive organisms. Acute arthritis with synovial effusion can also occur and should be differentiated from crystal-induced or septic arthritis by joint fluid examination. Bone pain is a frequent complaint. Male patients can present with painful priapism.[5]

Chronic pain is common in the sickle cell patient. Chronic hemolysis can lead to pigment gallstone formation and chronic cholecystitis. Aseptic necrosis of the humeral or femoral head and compression fractures from chronic vertebral bone infarction may occur. Chronic painful leg ulcers are also common.[5]

Because of the variability in frequency and pain in sickle cell patients, this disease remains a challenge to manage clinically. In the normal patient, acute pain is often accompanied by signs of sympathetic nervous system activation, such as tachycardia, hypertension, diaphoresis, and pupillary dilatation.[5] These signs are helpful in objectively assessing or substantiating a patient's subjective level of pain. However, when pain becomes chronic, as in sickle cell anemia, objective autonomic signs are often absent. Common pain behaviors were studied in sickle cell patients and included guarding, bracing, rubbing, grimacing, and sighing. Of these, guarding was the most frequently observed behavior, and it was highly correlated with the physician's rating of the patient's pain.[6]

Medication is the mainstay of treatment, especially during the acute painful episode. Medications include nonsteroidal anti-inflammatory drugs (NSAIDs), acetaminophen, opioids, and tricyclic antidepressants. The World Health Organization ladder for the treatment of cancer-related pain is applicable to management of the acute episode. Acetaminophen or NSAIDs are used for mild pain, and a weak opioid is added for moderate pain. A strong opioid is administered, usually by the parenteral route, for severe pain. The type of drug administered and the route of administration are the same as for opioid use in acute pain problems.

Most painful episodes in children and adolescents are treated at home.[7] The fact that almost 90% of painful episodes are treated at home[7] necessitates the development of programs designed to help children and families to manage their pain. One advantage of home treatment programs is that the patient remains in familiar surroundings and has support from relatives, facilitating early return to activities of daily living.

Sickle cell crises may be treated aggressively in the emergency department with a regimen of continuous opioid infusion.[8] Morphine, in initial doses of 2 to 12 mg/hour, is infused. If the pain is not relieved, the hourly dose is increased by 10% to 20% every few hours; the rate is also adjusted every 3 hours depending on the patient's degree of pain. Patients who report significant relief within 4 to 6 hours are discharged, if they desire, with a 1- to 2-week supply of oral sustained-release morphine. Patients who do not obtain satisfactory relief are admitted to the hospital.[8]

Patients with moderate to severe pain are hospitalized for intravenous hydration, administration of parenteral opioids, and treatment of any underlying cause. Parenteral administration is necessary if the patient is obstructed, vomiting, or cannot take oral medications.

The choice of opioid and route of administration vary from institution to institution. The primary goal in the treatment of pain with opioids is to provide a constant level of analgesia and avoid the extremes of pain and sedation. Meperidine appears to be the most frequently used opioid despite its considerable potential for side effects and weak analgesic action in comparison with other choices.[9] The pharmacokinetics of meperidine have been shown to be abnormal in sickle cell patients. In one study, sickle cell patients were found to have lower peak plasma concentrations, compared with control (postoperative) patients.[10] A diurnal variation in meperidine clearance was noted in another study of meperidine pharmacokinetics in sickle cell patients, with faster clearance observed in the evening.[11] At present, there is no explanation for the different pharmacokinetic profiles in sickle cell patients.

Normeperidine is a renally excreted, active metabolite of meperidine with a half-life of 18 hours. It can accumulate in patients with borderline or compromised renal function who are given frequent or high doses of meperidine. Normeperidine toxicity manifests as tremors, agitation, multifocal myoclonus, and seizures.[12] The risk of seizures and dysphoria is the main reason that meperidine is no longer recommended for the treatment of sickle cell pain. Other opioids, such as morphine or hydromorphine, are at least as effective.

The opioid requirements of patients with acute sickle cell crisis are high,[8] because the vasoocclusive episodes are quite painful. In addition, these patients develop tolerance to opioids easily because of previous opioid use. Regardless of their requirements, rapid titration to effect is necessary.

Intermittent intravenous/intramuscular injection is the most popular route of delivery. The use of patient-controlled analgesia (PCA) is increasingly popular. PCA has several advantages over other methods of opiate delivery. First, in an era of cost containment and managed care, PCA is a much more effective use of nursing resources. Second, PCA offers a better pharmacokinetic profile, because it avoids high peaks and low troughs of plasma concentrations.[13] Third, patients feel more in control of their care, which may add a psychological benefit to their therapy. No study has shown an increase

in addiction potential in sickle cell patients who are treated with PCA. On the contrary, many studies showed a lower total dose of opioid with PCA compared with intermittent intravenous/intramuscular dosing.[5, 13] Finally, PCA can also be used in the pediatric patient.

It is recommended that patients be given a 2-week supply of a controlled-release opioid and an immediate-release opioid as a rescue drug at discharge from the hopsital.[8] This regimen, preceded by an initial treatment with a continuous opioid infusion, has been shown to decrease the number of emergency room visits, the number of admissions, and the duration of hospital stays for the inpatient treatment of sickle cell crisis.[8]

The management of frequent or daily severe pain with chronic opioid therapy is controversial. Some clinicians report improved quality of life of these patients, while others are concerned about treatment of the pain symptom with lack of recognition of other factors such as anxiety and depression. The use of tricyclic antidepressants and multidisciplinary management of the patient's physical, psychological, and social problems may be helpful in these instances.

The use of epidural analgesia in the management of severe vasooclusive sickle cell crisis has been described.[14] Children who were previously unresponsive to conventional therapy, including intravenous meperidine, had immediate and continuous relief after an epidural infusion. After an initial injection of 0.25% bupivacaine, lidocaine (5 mg/mL, 1.5 mg/kg/hour), or bupivacaine (0.625 to 1.0 mg/mL, 0.2 to 0.4 mg/kg/hour), with or without fentanyl, was infused. The infusion lasted 1.5 to 5 days.[14]

Behavior modification techniques such as biofeedback, self-hypnosis, and relaxation techniques may be useful in the treatment of chronic sickle cell pain in both adults and pediatric patients. Transcutaneous nerve stimulation and acupuncture have been used with varying results. Physical approaches include heat, positioning, and the use of splinting for a painful extremity.

Important areas of future investigation include novel routes of analgesic administration,[15] new parenteral NSAIDs, and use of agonist-antagonist opioids in pain crisis. The combination of hydroxyurea and erythropoietin has been employed increasingly to increase fetal hemoglobin levels.[16] The incidence and severity of sickle cell pain crisis in this population of patients also needs further investigation.

The management of the pain in sickle cell disease involves symptomatic treatment of the acute crisis and identification and treatment of any underlying cause. With resolution of the acute crisis, the management should be directed toward any applicable psychological, social, and cultural factors involved.

REFERENCES

1. Hebbel RP: Beyond hemoglobin polymerization: The red cell membrane and sickle disease pathophysiology. Blood 77:214, 1991.
2. Platt O, Dover G: Sickle cell disease. Nathan D, Oski F (eds): Hematology of Infancy and Childhood, ed 4. Philadelphia, WB Saunders, 1993, p 732.

3. Beutler E: Disorders of hemoglobin. Fauci A, Braunwald E, Issel-bacher K, et al (eds): Harrison's Principles of Internal Medicine, ed 14. New York, McGraw-Hill, 1998, p 645.

4. Vichinsky EP, Lubin BH: Sickle cell anemia and related hemoglo-binopathies. Pediatr Clin North Am 27:429, 1980.

5. Payne R: Pain management in sickle cell disease: Rationale and techniques. Ann NY Acad Sci 565:189, 1989.

6. Gil KM, Phillips G, Abrams MR, et al: Observation of pain behaviors during episodes of sickle cell disease pain. Clin J Pain 10:128, 1994.

7. Shapiro BS, Dinges DF, Orne EC, et al: Home management of sickle cell–related pain in children and adolescents: Natural history and impact on school attendance. Pain 61:139, 1995.

8. Brookoff D, Polomano R: Treating sickle cell pain like cancer pain. Ann Intern Med 116:363, 1992.

9. Inturrisi CE, Foley KM: Narcotic analgesics in the management of pain. Kuhar MR, Pasternak GW (eds): Analgesics: Neurochemical, Behavioral, and Clinical Perspectives. New York, Raven Press, 1984, p 257.

10. Abbuhl S, Jacobson S, Murphy JG, et al: Serum concentration of meperidine in patients with sickle cell crisis. Ann Emerg Med 15:433, 1986.

11. Ritschel WA, Bykadi G, Ford DJ, et al: Pilot study on disposition and pain relief after I.M. injection of meperidine during the day or night. Int J Clin Pharmacol Ther Toxicol 21:218, 1983.

12. Kaiko RF, Foley KM, Grabinski PY, et al: Central nervous system excitatory effects in cancer patients. Ann Neurol 13:180, 1983.

13. Gonzalez GR, Bahal N, Hansen LA, et al: Intermittent injection vs patient-controlled analgesia for sickle cell crisis pain. Arch Intern Med 151:1373, 1991.

14. Yaster M, Tobin JR, Billet C, et al: Epidural analgesia in the management of severe vaso-occlusive sickle cell crisis. Pediatrics 93:310, 1994.

15. Christensen ML, Wang WC, Harris S, et al: Transdermal fentanyl administration in children and adolescents with sickle cell pain crisis. J Pediatr Hematol Oncol 18:372, 1996.

16. Juneja HS, Shulman E: Pathophysiology and management of sickle cell pain crisis. Lancet 346:1408, 1995.

Chapter 68

Diabetic and Other Peripheral Neuropathies

James P. Rathmell, M.D.,
and Jeffrey A. Katz, M.D.

DEFINITIONS

The term *neuropathy* describes a disturbance of nerve function or structure. Neuropathies arise from many different etiologies and can be painful (e.g., diabetic neuropathy) or painless (e.g., neuropathy of chronic renal failure). Single or multiple peripheral nerves, as well as cranial nerves, may be involved. Painful neuropathies fall under the broader descriptive category of *neuropathic pain,* or pain arising from abnormalities within the central or peripheral nervous systems. This chapter presents a brief overview of the evaluation of patients with painful peripheral neuropathy, describes an approach to the differential diagnosis of these disorders, and outlines the therapeutic modalities that may be useful in treating patients with neuropathic pain.

CLASSIFICATION

Neuropathic Pains

Because of the many etiologies and manifestations of neuropathic pain, it is helpful to categorize the types broadly according to the site of initial injury (Table 68-1).[1] Injury to the nervous system that results in chronic pain can occur anywhere from the peripheral nerve terminal to the cerebral cortex. Despite the differing locations and the myriad of underlying causes for injury, patients with neuropathic pain often share similar symptoms (Table 68-2).[2]

Peripheral Neuropathies

There are numerous potential causes for painful polyneuropathy. They include metabolic derangement, drug toxicity, paraneoplastic processes, vasculitis, and genetic disturbances. It is important to diagnose the underlying etiology in the hope of reversing nerve dysfunction or preventing further nerve damage. A classification of painful neuropathies based on their etiology is shown in Table 68-3.[3]

THE PATHOPHYSIOLOGY OF DAMAGED PERIPHERAL NERVES

Devor[4] has written an in-depth discussion of the pathophysiology of damaged peripheral nerves. Pain is normally felt when impulses reach the brain along fine myelinated (Aδ) and unmyelinated (C) nociceptive afferent nerve fibers. "Normal" ("nociceptive") pain results when activity is aroused by intense stimuli in healthy nociceptive afferents. Pathophysiologic ("neuropathic") pain results when the baseline sensitivity of the somatosensory system is altered. Such changes in sensitivity may arise through a number of changes in the nervous system. Peripheral nociceptors can become sensitized, resulting in non-noxious stimuli eliciting pain (e.g., via release of local mediators like bradykinin and histamine). Indeed, such sensitization serves a protective role following trauma. The injured area becomes sensi-

TABLE 68-1. NEUROPATHIC PAIN SYNDROMES

Peripheral

Painful peripheral polyneuropathies
Focal entrapment/traumatic neuropathies
Postsurgical syndromes
    Phantom pain and stump pain following amputation
    Post-thoracotomy syndrome

Central

Traumatic brachial plexus avulsion
Traumatic spinal cord injury
Ischemic cerebrovascular injury
Syringomyelia
Arachnoiditis

Mixed

Complex regional pain syndromes
    Type I (reflex sympathetic dystrophy)
    Type II (causalgia)
Meningoradiculopathies
Epidural spinal cord compression
Acute herpetic and postherpetic neuralgia

Adapted from Elliott KJ: Taxonomy and mechanisms of neuropathic pain. Semin Neurol 14:195-205, 1994.

TABLE 68–2. THE ABNORMAL SENSATIONS OF NEUROPATHIC PAIN

Spontaneous pain: Burning, shooting, lancinating
Paresthesias: Abnormal nonpainful sensations that may be spontaneous or evoked (tingling)
Dysesthesias: Abnormal pain that may be spontaneous or evoked (unpleasant tingling)
Hyperalgesia: An exaggerated painful response to a normally noxious stimulus
Hyperpathia: An exaggerated painful response evoked by a noxious or non-noxious stimulus
Allodynia: A painful response to a normally non-noxious stimulus (e.g., light touch is perceived as burning pain)

Adapted from Mersky H (ed): Classification of chronic pain: Description of chronic pain syndromes and definition of pain terms. Pain Suppl 3:S1, 1986.

tive to even light touch, leading the organism to protect the area until healing ensues. Such sensitization can persist in neuropathic pain states becoming manifest as allodynia and hyperpathia. Neuropathic pain may also arise when abnormal (ectopic) impulses are generated along the course of peripheral nerves (e.g., at sites of injury such as those found in neuroma formation). Finally, pathophysiologic pain may arise from increased gain in central processing circuits ("central sensitization") leading to spontaneous pain or pain triggered by non-nociceptive input. Recent studies of animal nerve injury models support the idea that in situations where injured and intact fibers coexist in a nerve, both the injured and noninjured fibers are capable of sustaining spontaneous and evoked pain.[5]

The two major pathologic processes in peripheral neuropathy are axonal degeneration and segmental demyelination. Both processes are usually present, although in varying proportions in different disease states. Along with morphologic changes in peripheral nerves, abnormal spontaneous neural discharge has been observed in animal models of diabetic neuropathy and heavy metal intoxication. The relationship of morphologic and electrophysiologic changes in peripheral nerves to painful symptoms remains poorly understood.

TABLE 68–3. ETIOLOGIES OF PAINFUL PERIPHERAL POLYNEUROPATHY

Metabolic	Genetic
Diabetes mellitus	Fabry's disease
Amyloidosis	Hereditary sensory neuropathy
Multiple myeloma	**Infectious**
Hypothyroidism	
Nutritional	Acquired immunodeficiency syndrome
Beriberi	Acute inflammatory polyneuropathy
Alcoholic	
Pellagra	
Toxic	
Isoniazid	
Cisplatin	
Arsenic	
Thallium	

Adapted from Lewis MS, Hill CS, Warfield CA: Medical diseases causing pain. *In* Raj PP (ed): The Practical Management of Pain. St. Louis, Mosby-Year Book, 1992, pp 329–342.

EVALUATION OF THE PATIENT WITH NEUROPATHIC PAIN

When a patient presents with signs and symptoms suggestive of neuropathic pain—most notably allodynia—the first useful distinction to be made is the pattern of involvement. Focal lesions of peripheral nerves (mononeuropathies) result from processes that produce localized damage and include nerve entrapment; mechanical injuries; thermal, electrical, or radiation injuries; vascular lesions; and neoplastic or infectious processes. In contrast, polyneuropathies result in a bilaterally symmetrical disturbance in function as a result of agents that act diffusely on the peripheral nervous system—toxic substances, deficiency states, metabolic disorders, and immune reactions. The diagnosis of painful polyneuropathy is most often made by history and standard neurologic examination. In some cases, ancillary studies may be needed to document the disease process.

History

Pain is often the presenting symptom for polyneuropathy, and the characteristics are those of neuropathic pain (see Table 68–2).[2] Sensory symptoms often accompany pain in polyneuropathy. Paresthesias ("tingling" or "pins and needles" sensations) are common, as are demonstrable sensory deficits. The location of the pain and other symptoms is frequently the most important piece of historical information.

Neurologic Examination

In the patient suspected of having polyneuropathy, the clinician should focus on sensory evaluation. Strength and deep tendon reflexes are preserved in many patients with polyneuropathy. In addition to testing vibration, proprioception, and light touch, the sensory examination should include several special stimuli including light-touch rubbing, ice, single pin-prick, and multiple pin-prick. Lightly stroking the affected area with a finger assesses for allodynia (pain provoked by non-noxious stimuli). Ice application tests for both temperature sensation and abnormal sensations such as pain and lingering after-sensations. Single pin-prick testing may elicit a sensory deficit or hyperpathia (an exaggerated response to a normally painful stimulus). Repeated pin-prick testing may elicit summation (pain growing more intense with subsequent stimuli) or lingering after sensations, both common findings in polyneuropathy.

Electrodiagnostic Testing

Patients suspected of having polyneuropathy should be considered for electromyography and nerve conduction studies. These tests are best used to demonstrate large-fiber involvement and may help differentiate between demyelinating neuropathies (reductions in nerve conduction velocities) and axonal neuropathies (reductions in the amplitude of evoked responses). Electrodiagnostic studies may be completely normal in patients with painful polyneuropathy resulting from small nerve fiber dysfunction.

DIFFERENTIAL DIAGNOSIS

After assembling the historical information, neurologic examination, and results of electrodiagnostic studies, the underlying etiology will most often already be apparent. Several recent reviews present detailed discussions of diagnosis and management of the patient with painful polyneuropathy.[3, 6] A brief description of the clinical features and useful supportive tests for the most common painful polyneuropathies follows.

Metabolic Causes of Peripheral Polyneuropathy

Painful polyneuropathy is most often caused by a metabolic disorder, the most common being diabetes mellitus. The reported frequency of neuropathy in patients with diabetes mellitus ranges from 4% to 8% at the time of initial presentation and rises to 15% to 50% after 20 to 25 years of follow-up.[7] Neuropathy occurs with both insulin-dependent and non–insulin-dependent diabetes and may be more common in the latter.[8] There is strong evidence that good glycemic control can prevent the appearance and worsening of polyneuropathy in patients with both insulin-dependent[9] and non–insulin-dependent diabetes mellitus.[4]

A practical clinical classification scheme for diabetic neuropathy that divides the neuropathies according to the pattern of distribution of involved nerves is shown in Table 68–4.[5] The most common form of diabetic neuropathy is distal symmetrical polyneuropathy. It is predominantly a sensory disturbance. Patients present with gradual onset of paresthesia and pain in the legs and feet. Symptoms begin in the toes and gradually ascend over months to years to involve more proximal levels. The fingertips and hands become involved later, usually when symptoms in the lower extremities have ascended to the knee level. Allodynia (e.g., pain in the feet brought on by even the light pressure of contact with bed sheets) and burning pain are common and are

TABLE 68–4. CLASSIFICATION OF NEUROPATHIES ASSOCIATED WITH DIABETES MELLITUS

Generalized Polyneuropathies
Distal symmetrical polyneuropathy
Acute painful diabetic neuropathy
Autonomic polyneuropathy

Multiple Mononeuropathies
Proximal lower extremity motor neuropathy
Truncal neuropathy

Mononeuropathies
Cranial mononeuropathy
Compression mononeuropathy

Adapted from Ross MA: Neuropathies associated with diabetes. Contemp Clin Neurol 77:111–124, 1993.

often worse at night. Examination reveals graded distal sensory loss predominantly affecting vibration and position sensation. Reflexes may be diminished or absent. Electrophysiologic testing reveals decreases in the amplitude of evoked responses to a greater degree than reduction in nerve conduction velocities as the neuropathy progresses.[6] This reflects primarily axonal damage rather than demyelination. Severe sensory loss may allow repeated trauma to go unnoticed, resulting in development of foot ulcers and diabetic neuroarthropathy (Charcot's joints).

The syndrome of acute painful diabetic neuropathy also may occur.[3, 5] This uncommon disorder involves the rapid onset of severe pain in the distal lower extremities characterized by constant burning in the feet, dysesthesias, allodynia, and lancinating leg pains. Examination reveals little or no sensory loss, with preserved reflexes. Electrophysiologic testing reveals decreased amplitude or absent sensory potentials but may be normal. This type of neuropathy often remits within a year after blood sugars are controlled.

Autonomic neuropathy manifest by abnormalities in tests of autonomic function occurs in 20% to 40% of diabetics.[5] Symptomatic autonomic neuropathy most often occurs as a component of distal symmetrical polyneuropathy. Autonomic nervous system abnormalities include postural hypotension, impaired heart rate control (resting tachycardia and fixed heart rate), esophageal dysmotility, gastroparesis, and erectile dysfunction.

Lower extremity proximal motor neuropathy is an uncommon painful disorder associated with diabetes.[5] It is characterized by acute or subacute onset of moderate to marked weakness and wasting of the pelvifemoral muscles accompanied by back, hip, and thigh pain with preserved sensation in the regions of pain. The condition may be painless or accompanied by pain described as a constant, severe, deep ache. Complete recovery occurs in 60% of patients over 12 to 24 months.

Diabetic truncal neuropathy involves acute or gradual onset of unilateral pain in the chest or abdomen and may mimic myocardial infarction, intra-abdominal pathology, or spinal disorders.[10] Examination reveals marked allodynia and hyperpathia in the distribution of pain. Truncal neuropathy occurs most often in long-standing diabetics and in those older than 50 years. Electromyography typically reveals denervation in the abdominal or intercostal musculature.

Cranial mononeuropathies involving the oculomotor, abducens, trochlear, and facial nerves may occur in diabetic patients.[5] The most common of these is oculomotor neuropathy, which is manifest as ophthalmoplegia and ptosis. The eye is deviated laterally and has impaired movement vertically and medially. Pain occurs in 50% of patients and may precede ophthalmoplegia by several days.

Entrapment neuropathies are believed to occur more frequently in patients with diabetes mellitus.[5] Carpal tunnel syndrome is believed to occur more than twice as frequently as in the nondiabetic population. This association must be kept in mind when evaluating the diabetic patient with an isolated peripheral mononeuropathy.

The cause of diabetic neuropathy has not been determined with certainty.[11] Current hypotheses focus on the possibilities of metabolic and ischemic nerve injury. Pathologic examination of nerves taken from diabetic patients has revealed evidence of microvascular disease supporting the ischemic nerve theory. Metabolic abnormalities include accumulation of sorbitol in diabetic nerve, as excess glucose is converted to sorbitol by the enzyme aldose reductase. Therapeutic strategies aimed at reducing sorbitol accumulation (aldose-reductase inhibitors) have demonstrated only minor improvements in neuropathy.

Metabolic causes of painful peripheral neuropathy other than diabetes mellitus are uncommon. Amyloidosis is a disease caused by extracellular deposition of amyloid, a fibrous protein. Amyloidosis can be primary, familial, or associated with other conditions such as multiple myeloma, chronic infectious or inflammatory states, aging, and long-term hemodialysis. The biochemical composition of the amyloid protein varies with the associated disease state. Painful peripheral neuropathy in amyloidosis is characterized by deep aching and occasional shooting pains, distal sensory loss, and autonomic and motor involvement.[12] As the neuropathy progresses, all modalities are affected, reflexes are lost, and there is motor involvement. Treatment of neuropathy associated with amyloidosis is aimed at the underlying condition when such is identifiable.

Multiple myeloma is caused by malignant plasma cell growth. Painful neuropathy can appear in myeloma with or without amyloid deposition. The neuropathy is extremely variable in severity and rate of progression, ranging from a mild, predominantly sensory neuropathy to a complete tetraplegia.[10] Pain in myeloma often declines with successful treatment using chemotherapy, radiation therapy (especially for isolated plasmacytomas), or plasmapheresis.

Patients with untreated hypothyroidism may also develop painful sensorimotor neuropathy.[10] This uncommon disorder may present with longstanding pain in either the hands or the feet accompanied by weakness in the distal limb musculature. The neuropathy often resolves with successful replacement of thyroid hormone.

Nutritional Causes of Peripheral Polyneuropathy

Thiamine deficiency is seen in alcoholics, chronic dialysis patients, and people on restrictive diets. Thiamine deficiency appears to lead to beriberi, which consists of heart failure, vasodilatation, and peripheral neuropathy. The neuropathy is characterized by hand, foot, and calf pains with allodynia, decreased sensation, and motor involvement.[13] Administration of thiamine may reduce the symptoms of neuropathy, including pain. The incidence of neuropathy in chronic alcoholism is about 9%.[10] Alcoholic neuropathy is characterized by motor and sensory deficits, often accompanied by pain.[10] The pain consists of aching in the legs or feet, with intermittent lancinating pains. The upper limbs are rarely involved. Burning of the soles and allodynia also may occur. Alcoholic neuropathy occurs only after chronic and severe alcohol abuse and is invariably accompanied by severe nutritional deficiency. Pathologically, alcoholic neuropathy cannot be distinguished from beriberi, and both likely result from thiamine deficiency. Treatment consists of abstinence and thiamine supplementation.

Pellagra is caused by niacin deficiency and is rarely seen in the United States.[10] Signs and symptoms include dermatitis, gastrointestinal complaints, neurasthenia, and spinal cord dysfunction. Pellagra is associated with a mixed, painful polyneuropathy similar to that seen with beriberi. A predominant feature of the sensorimotor neuropathy is spontaneous pain in the feet and lower legs, with tenderness of the calf muscles and cutaneous hyperesthesia of the feet. Treatment of pellagra with niacin often results in resolution of all symptoms except the peripheral neuropathy.

Toxic Causes of Peripheral Polyneuropathy

Isoniazid is a frequently used antituberculous drug. Chronic administration in individuals with slow metabolism of the drug (slow acetylators) is associated with the development of painful neuropathy.[3, 10] Initial symptoms of distal numbness and tingling paresthesia are later accompanied by pain, which may be felt as a deep ache or burning. The calf muscles are painful and tender, and symptoms are often aggravated by walking. Symptoms may be particularly troublesome at night. Prophylactic coadministration of pyridoxine (vitamin B_6) prevents development of neuropathy. Once neuropathy develops, administration of pyridoxine does not have an effect on recovery.

Cisplatin is a chemotherapeutic agent used to treat solid tumors and can lead to a painful, dose-dependent peripheral neuropathy.[14] The earliest manifestations of neuropathy are decreased vibration sense in the toes and loss of ankle jerk reflexes. At larger doses, paresthesias may appear and progress to severe dysesthesias. The neuropathy is reversible, but recovery may take more than a year after discontinuation of cisplatin.

Arsenic is now ingested only rarely in suicide or homicide attempts. It is associated with a painful subacute sensorimotor peripheral neuropathy.[15] Acute ingestion is followed by gastrointestinal symptoms, psychosis, delirium, stupor, and renal failure. Cardiovascular collapse may occur. If the patient survives the initial insult, signs of chronic exposure including skin and nail changes and pancytopenia may appear. Five to ten days after arsenic ingestion, symptoms of neuropathy, including aching, burning, tingling, and numbness, may appear. Treatment begins with removing further exposure. Recovery from neuropathy may take years. British antilewisite (dimercaprol) may reverse other symptoms of acute arsenic poisoning but has little effect on recovery from neuropathy.

Thallium is used as an insecticide and rodenticide and in small doses in myocardial perfusion imaging. In many ways, thallium poisoning resembles arsenic toxicity. During the first day, gastrointestinal symptoms and cardiovascular collapse may occur. Within the following week, confusion, psychosis, choreoathetosis, convulsions, and coma may ensue. Alopecia, the hallmark of thallium poisoning, develops weeks after exposure. Nail changes may also occur late. Painful neuropathy may appear within 48 hours of ingestion. Initially, leg and arm pains and distal paresthesias occur.[3] In severe cases, cranial nerves and the muscles of respiration may be involved. Treatment should include intravenous hydration and diuresis to promote urinary excretion of thallium. Early use of charcoal hemoperfusion may be of benefit. Neurologic function should improve over time but may be incomplete.

Genetic Causes of Peripheral Polyneuropathy

Fabry's disease is an X-linked recessive disease caused by accumulation of ceramide trihexose in the absence of α-galactosidase A. These patients typically present as boys or young men with a painful neuropathy characterized by tender feet and burning in the calves.[16] Abdominal pain also may occur. Other manifestations include multiple angiokeratomas, anhidrosis, renal failure, corneal and lenticular opacities, hypertension, stroke, and myocardial infarction. No specific therapy exists for Fabry's disease. Peripheral neuropathy has been treated with some success using phenytoin and carbamazepine.

Dominantly inherited hereditary sensory neuropathy is insidious in onset and typically appears in the second decade of life or later.[3] Decreased sensation in the feet and distal legs occurs, leaving patients prone to ulcer formation often leading to cellulitis and osteomyelitis. Associated peroneal muscle atrophy and hearing loss may be present. Patients often experience intermittent lancinating pains in the shoulder, thigh, leg, and foot. There is no specific treatment for this disorder.

Infectious and Inflammatory Causes of Peripheral Polyneuropathy

As many as 30% of patients with acquired immunodeficiency syndrome or acquired immunodeficiency syndrome–related complex may develop painful neuropathy.[17] Patients report pain in the soles with accompanying paresthesias in the feet. Allodynia may be so severe as to interfere with walking. Electromyographic testing often reveals evidence of denervation. Treatment consists of zidovudine, tricyclic antidepressants (TCAs), and anticonvulsants.

Acute inflammatory polyneuropathy (AIP, or Guillain-Barré syndrome) is characterized by areflexic motor paralysis.[18] It is often preceded by viral infections with relationships to cytomegalovirus, Epstein-Barr virus, and smallpox vaccine. Guillain-Barré syndrome also may follow surgery. The onset of symptoms develops over several weeks. Pain is a common early symptom; weakness, usually in the legs, may progress to respiratory failure requiring mechanical ventilation. Sensory symptoms include paresthesias, often in the presence of decreased sensation in a glove-stocking distribution. Autonomic dysfunction is also common, evidenced by tachycardia and orthostatic hypotension. Pain may occur in as many as 72% of patients. The pain is principally an ache, strain, or deep burning sensation in the thigh or buttocks and can be quite severe. Although pain in AIP may be severe, it is usually transient. Pain is usually worse at night. Nerve conduction studies and lumbar puncture aid the diagnosis. General therapy for AIP is supportive, along with plasmapheresis. Glucocorticoids and other immunosuppressants have not been clearly shown to be helpful. Pain may respond to oral narcotics, quinine, and other drugs typically useful for treating neuropathic pain. Epidural narcotics have also been used successfully in relieving pain associated with Guillain-Barré syndrome.[19]

Neuroma

Although not considered classically to be a neuropathy, neuromas are a not infrequent cause of pain from peripheral nerve injury. Typically resulting from the complete disruption of a peripheral nerve, the ends of the axons continue to grow. However, anatomic separation of the ends prevents proper realignment. The proximal end may continue to grow around itself in an unorganized bulbous collection of unmyelinated fibers, producing a neuroma. Neuromas are far more thermosensitive and mechanosensitive than normal nerve endings and can produce spontaneous discharges as well. Furthermore, abnormal afferent impulses can result in the dorsal root ganglia following injury to the peripheral nerve.[20]

TREATMENT OF NEUROPATHIC PAIN

There are a wide variety of medications and proposed algorithms used in the treatment of neuropathic pain, reflecting the lack of any one highly effective regimen. Proper randomized, double-blind, placebo-controlled studies are largely lacking, and given the inconsistency and variability of most neuropathic conditions, the conclusions from a study of one group of patients with neuropathy will likely not apply to another. Nonetheless, some data exist for certain conditions.

Antidepressants

The most widely used medications in treating neuropathic pain are the TCAs.[4] The onset of pain relief occurs more rapidly than the usual 2-week delay in the onset of antidepressant effects. Within hours after administration, synaptic levels of monoamine neurotransmitters are elevated; analgesic action of TCAs appears to be related to these elevated monoamine levels.[21]

The tertiary amine compounds (amitriptyline, imipramine, doxepin) have the greatest effect on serotonergic systems, variable effects on norepinephrine systems, and strong anticholinergic activity. Amitriptyline, nortriptyline, and desipramine have all been established as effective analgesics for diabetic neuropathy, independent of the effect on depression.[22] The selective serotonin reuptake inhibitors have fewer side effects; paroxetine appears to be effective in diabetic neuropathy, whereas fluoxetine proved no better than placebo.[19] The secondary amines (nortriptyline, desipramine) are less sedating than amitriptyline and have proven to be equally effective in treating diabetic neuropathy. The effectiveness of second-generation antidepressants (trazadone) remains unproven.

Although the pharmacology of antidepressants is reviewed elsewhere in this book, some effects are of particular relevance to the patient with peripheral neuropathy. Orthostatic hypotension is among the most bothersome symptoms in the elderly, but the autonomic dysfunction present in diabetics could amplify this effect. TCAs are best avoided in patients with heart block, left bundle branch block, congestive heart failure, or recent myocardial infarction, all of which occur in significant frequency in patients with diabetes.

Anticonvulsants

Anticonvulsants, including newer agents such as gabapentin, have become a common part of the pharmacotherapy for neuropathic pain.[4] Animal data demonstrate that both carbamazepine and phenytoin suppress spontaneous ectopic discharges in experimental neuromas.[23, 24] Carbamazepine and phenytoin have demonstrated significant analgesic efficacy in painful diabetic neuropathy in controlled trials. Other anticonvulsants, including clonazepam and valproic acid, have been used to treat neuropathic pain successfully but have been less rigorously studied. The newer anticonvulsants gabapentin and lamotrigine have shown early promise as analgesic agents in treating neuropathic pain.[25] Dose-response relationships have not been clearly demonstrated for anticonvulsants with reference to pain; however, clinical experience points to significant interpatient variability. The pharmacology of these agents is reviewed in detail elsewhere.

Local Anesthetics and Antiarrhythmics

In animal models, systemic local anesthetics have been recognized as suppressing ectopic impulses, both at sites of experimental nerve injury and in the axotomized dorsal root ganglion cells.[26] Intravenous infusion of lidocaine has proven useful in treating pains arising from peripheral nerve injuries and diabetic polyneuropathy.[20] Most protocols use a brief intravenous infusion of lidocaine, which, when effective, produces analgesia lasting for several hours. Mexiletine, an orally administered congener of lidocaine, can be an effective analgesic in a variety of neuropathic pain syndromes.[20] There have been few controlled trials to examine the relationship between analgesia with lidocaine and that with mexiletine.[27] Nonetheless, brief analgesia with intravenous lidocaine is often viewed as predictive of subsequent response to oral mexiletine. Mexiletine is contraindicated in patients with second- or third-degree heart block. Hypotension and bradycardia may occur with overdosage. The most common adverse effect is upper gastrointestinal distress. This side effect can be minimized by taking the drug with food and escalating the dosage slowly. Less-common side effects include dizziness, tremor, nervousness, and headache.

Sympatholytic Agents

Sympatholytic agents are being studied for the treatment of a variety of neuropathic pains. Methods used for treatment include intravenous phentolamine infusion, oral phenoxybenzamine, oral terazosin, and oral and transdermal clonidine. These agents are used most often for the diagnosis of sympathetically maintained pain; many patients with peripheral neuropathies present with signs and symptoms of sympathetically maintained pain (e.g., allodynia, burning dysesthesias, vasomotor instability). Such patients may respond to sympatholytic agents.

Analgesic response to intravenous phentolamine infusion may be predictive of response to regional sympathetic ganglion blockade[28] and oral or transdermal sympatholytic agents.[4] Tachycardia and orthostatic hypotension may occur following intravenous phentolamine but are rarely problematic in previously normotensive individuals. The more common side effects include nasal congestion, flushing, and dizziness. Peak pain relief after phentolamine may be delayed for 24 to 48 hours and last for several days. For those patients reporting long-lasting pain relief after intravenous phentolamine, repeated infusions can be used as the primary therapy.

The α_2-adrenergic agonist clonidine has been reported as a useful analgesic in treating neuropathic pain.[20] Clonidine can also be administered orally or using a topical transcutaneous delivery patch. Drowsiness is the major side effect of clonidine. When discontinuing clonidine therapy, the dosage should be slowly tapered to avoid rebound hypertension.

Prazosin, terazosin, and phenoxybenzamine are oral α-adrenergic antagonists that have shown anecdotal evidence of analgesic efficacy in neuropathic pain.[4] Prazosin and terazosin are relatively selective for α_1-adrenergic blockade. Terazosin offers the advantage of once-daily dosing. All of the α-adrenergic antagonists are associated with orthostatic hypotension, particularly after the drug is first started. Other side effects include drowsiness, nasal congestion, tachycardia, miosis, and inhibition of ejaculation.

Corticosteroids

Corticosteroids, both systemically and by peripheral application, have been used, based on empirical response. When injected perineurally (but not systemically), corticosteroids reduce the spontaneous ectopic discharge rate seen following nerve injury and in neuromas, probably by a membrane-stabilizing effect.[29] They also have been found to have a short-lasting suppressive effect on transmission in normal C fibers, but more recent studies on peripheral nerve injury models in the rat confirm that local application of steroid on the area of injured nerve may produce an analgesic effect by suppression of peripheral ectopic sites.[30]

Chronic Opioid Therapy

Use of opioids for the long-term treatment of noncancer pain remains controversial.[31] Opioids are among the most universally effective analgesic agents known, but fear of addiction and tolerance limits their usefulness. Historically, neuropathic pain has been considered "opioid resistant," and evidence exists to support that contention.[32] However, data also exist supporting the concept that opioids are capable of relieving noncancer neuropathic pain.[33] Several case series have been published regarding the chronic use of opioids for noncancer pain, including pain from peripheral neuropathy; although these studies report successful treatments, the data remain empirical, without controls or blinding. In those who have failed trials of nonopioid analgesics, opioid therapy may be a reasonable alternative. A small series of patients with neuropathic pain who responded to intrathecal morphine has been reported[34]; it is unclear where in the treatment process this option should be considered. The use of opioids in chronic benign pain, including neuropathic pain, is reviewed in detail elsewhere.[35]

Other Treatment Options

Various book chapters and review articles mention other options for approaching patients with pain from peripheral neuropathies, including sympathetic nerve blocks, neurolytic sympathetic blocks, spinal cord stimulation, transcutaneous electrical nerve stimulation, and deep brain stimulation. As the information in such sources is anecdotal, it is not possible to draw conclusions beyond that these are possible options worth further study.[36, 37]

REFERENCES

1. Elliott KJ: Taxonomy and mechanisms of neuropathic pain. Semin Neurol 14:195-205, 1994.
2. Mersky H (ed): Classification of chronic pain syndromes and definition of pain terms. Pain Suppl 3:S1, 1996.
3. Lewis MS, Hill CS, Warfield CA: Medical diseases causing pain. In Raj PP (ed): The Practical Management of Pain, 2nd ed. St. Louis, Mosby-Year Book, 1992, pp 329-342.
4. Devor M: The pathophysiology of damaged peripheral nerves. In Wall PD, Melzack R (eds): Textbook of Pain. New York, Churchill Livingstone, 1992, pp 79-100.
5. Yoon Y, Na H, Chung J: Contributions of injured and intact afferents to neuropathic pain in an experimental rat model. Pain 64:27-36, 1996.
6. Galer BS: Painful polyneuropathy: Diagnosis, pathophysiology, and management. Semin Neurol 14:237-246, 1994.
7. Ross MA: Neuropathies associated with diabetes. Contemp Clin Neurol 77:11-124, 1993.
8. Partenen J, Niskanen L, Lehtinen J, et al.: Natural history of peripheral neuropathy in patients with non-insulin-dependent diabetes mellitus. N Engl J Med 333:89-94, 1995.
9. The Diabetes Control and Complications Trial Research Group: The effect of intensive treatment of diabetes on the development and progression of long-term complications in insulin-dependent diabetes mellitus. N Engl J Med 329:977-986, 1993.
10. Harati Y, Niakin E: Diabetic thoracoabdominal neuropathy: A cause for chest and abdominal discomfort. Arch Intern Med 146:1493-1494, 1986.
11. Thomas PK: Diabetic neuropathy: Models, mechanisms, and mayhem. Can J Neurol Sci 19:1, 1992.
12. Scadding JW: Peripheral neuropathies. In Wall PD, Melzack R (eds): Textbook of Pain. New York, Churchill Livingstone, 1992, pp 667-683.
13. Victor M: Polyneuropathy due to nutritional deficiency and alcoholism. In Wilson JD, Braunwald E, Isselbacher KJ, et al. (eds): Harrison's Principles of Internal Medicine, 12th ed. New York, McGraw-Hill, 1991, pp 2045-2054.
14. Mollman JE: Cisplatin neurotoxicity. N Engl J Med 22:126-127, 1990.
15. Windebank AJ: Metal neuropathy. In Dyck PJ, Thomas PK, Griffin JH, et al. (eds): Peripheral Neuropathy, 3rd ed. Philadelphia, WB Saunders, 1993, pp 1549-1570.
16. Brady RO: Fabry disease. In Dyck PJ, Thomas PK, Griffin JH, et al. (eds): Peripheral Neuropathy, 3rd ed. Philadelphia, WB Saunders, 1993, pp 1169-1178.
17. Cornblath DR, McArthur JC, Parry GJG, Griffin JW: Peripheral neuropathies in human immunodeficiency virus infection. In Dyck PJ, Thomas PK, Griffin JH, et al. (eds): Peripheral Neuropathy, 3rd ed. Philadelphia, WB Saunders, 1993, pp 1343-1353.
18. Arnason BGW, Solevin B: Acute inflammatory demyelinating polyradiculopathy. In Dyck PJ, Thomas PK, Griffin JH, et al. (eds): Peripheral Neuropathy, 3rd ed. Philadelphia, WB Saunders, 1993, pp 1437-1497.
19. Connelly M, Shagrin J, Warfield C: Epidural opioids for the management of pain in a patient with Guillain-Barré syndrome. Anesthesiology 72:381-383, 1990.
20. Hartrick C: Pain due to trauma including sports injuries. In Raj PP (ed): Practical Management of Pain, 2nd ed. St. Louis, Mosby-Year Book, 1992, p 425.
21. Hammond DL: Pharmacology of central pain-modulating networks (biogenic amines and non-opioid analgesics). Adv Pain Res Ther 9:499, 1985.
22. Calissi PT, Jaber LA: Peripheral diabetic neuropathy: Current concepts in treatment. Ann Pharmacother 29:769-777, 1995.
23. Yaari Y, Devor M: Phenytoin suppresses spontaneous ectopic discharge in rat sciatic nerve neuromas. Neurosci Lett 58:117-122, 1985.
24. Burchiel K: Carbamazepine inhibits spontaneous activity in experimental neuromas. Exp Neurol 102:249-253, 1988.
25. Galer BS: Neuropathic pain of peripheral origin: Advances in pharmacologic treatment. Neurology 45(suppl 9):S17-S25, 1995.
26. Devor M, Wall P, Catalan N: Systemic lidocaine silences ectopic neuroma and DRG discharge without blocking nerve conduction. Pain 48:261-268, 1992.
27. Galer B, Harle J, Rowbotham M: Response to intravenous lidocaine infusion predicts subsequent response to oral mexiletine: A prospective study. J Pain Symptom Management 12:161-167, 1996.
28. Raja SN, Treede RD, Davis KD, Campbell JN: Systemic alpha-adrenergic blockade with phentolamine: A diagnostic test for sympathetically maintained pain. Anesthesiology 74:691-698, 1991.
29. Devor M, Govrin-Lippman R, Raber P: Corticosteroids suppress ectopic neural discharge originating in experimental neuromas. Pain 22:127-137, 1985.
30. Johansson A, Bennett G: Effect of local methylprednisolone on pain in a nerve injury model. Reg Anesth 22:59-65, 1997.
31. Portenoy RK: Chronic opioid therapy for chronic nonmalignant pain: From models to practice. Am Pain Soc J 1:285-288, 1992.
32. Arner S, Meyerson B: Lack of analgesic effect of opioids on neuropathic and idiopathic forms of pain. Pain 33:11-23, 1988.
33. Dellemijn P, Vanneste J: Randomised double-blind active-placebo-controlled crossover trial of intravenous fentanyl in neuropathic pain. Lancet 349:753-758, 1997.
34. Penn RD, Paice JA: Chronic intrathecal morphine for intractable pain. J Neurosurg 67:182-186, 1987.
35. Rathmell JP, Jamison RN: Opioid therapy for chronic noncancer pain. Curr Opin Anesthesiol 9:436-442, 1996.
36. Tasker R, Filho O: Deep brain stimulation for neuropathic pain. Stereotactic Funct Neurosurg 65:122-124, 1995.
37. Kumar K, Toth C, Nath R: Spinal cord stimulation for chronic pain in peripheral neuropathy. Surg Neurol 46:363-369, 1996.

Chapter 69

Entrapment Neuropathies

Vernon B. Williams, M.D.,
and Marco Pappagallo, M.D.

Entrapment neuropathy is a type of neuropathy in which anatomic structures cause focal, chronic compression of a peripheral nerve. Many authorities reserve the term *entrapment* for a specific subtype of compression in which nerve dysfunction is a result of compression by anatomic structures, as opposed to compression from, for example, a tumor or chronic inflammatory process. Alternatively, nerves that course more superficially are at risk for external compression on the basis of posture or positioning. In general, nerves may be compressed chronically by external or internal forces, ultimately resulting in symptoms indicative of dysfunction.

Although a peripheral nerve can be compressed anywhere along its course, there are characteristic locations at which certain nerves are particularly vulnerable and focal compression results in sensory and/or motor signs and symptoms. There are several well-described entrapment neuropathy syndromes of the upper and lower extremities. Some of them frequently cause pain and paresthesias and warrant a more detailed discussion.

GENERAL PRINCIPLES

Presenting Signs and Symptoms

Patients with entrapment neuropathies frequently present with complaints typical of nerve dysfunction. They may describe pain in an extremity as being sharp, stinging, burning, or shooting in character. Paresthesias, such as tingling, or sensation of numbness in the extremity are noted. These symptoms are often, but not always, present in an identifiable peripheral nerve distribution. Patients may also complain of weakness in the extremity. It is important to note the onset and progression of symptoms, which could be subacute or chronic. An acute onset is less consistent with symptoms usually seen in an entrapment neuropathy. Signs on physical examination include sensory abnormality, with or without motor deficit, in an identifiable peripheral nerve distribution. Lower motor neuron signs, such as muscle atrophy, fasciculations, or depressed deep tendon re-

flexes, may be present. Presence of upper motor neuron signs (e.g., hyperreflexia, increased tone) should prompt a search to rule out an alternative cause for the patient's symptoms, perhaps localized to the brain or spinal cord. Finally, there are patients who have typical symptoms in several peripheral nerve distributions at once, or repeatedly over time. They may be more susceptible because of body habitus, activity, or occupation or because of hereditary predisposition to pressure palsies, a condition in which an abnormality of myelin resulting in nerve hypertrophy increases the susceptibility to compression.

Basic Diagnostic Procedures

A thorough neurologic examination is paramount for correct diagnosis of an entrapment neuropathy and to prevent misdiagnosis and inappropriate management. Certain entrapment syndromes have specific diagnostic signs found on physical examination; these are discussed in subsequent sections. Electrophysiologic testing (e.g., electromyographic/nerve conduction velocity testing, searching for focal slowing or conduction block) and diagnostic peripheral nerve blockade are most helpful in confirming clinical suspicion and objectively documenting the pathologic location of the entrapment neuropathy. Serologic testing may be of benefit to rule out predisposing or underlying conditions contributing to a focal neuropathy. Metabolic conditions including amyloidosis, diabetes mellitus, chronic renal insufficiency requiring hemodyalisis, hyperparathyroidism, hypothyroidism, gout, acromegaly, and pregnancy can have similar presentations. Inflammatory or immunologic processes such as rheumatoid arthritis, systemic lupus erythematosus, polymyalgia rheumatica, and scleroderma may also contribute to an entrapment neuropathy. Finally, diagnostic imaging techniques such as computed tomography or magnetic resonance imaging may reveal abnormal fibrous structures, abnormal tendons, vascular lesions, ganglion cysts, infection, bone, or soft tissue tumors forming a compressive lesion that contributes to a patient's signs and symptoms. These basic

TABLE 69–1. COMMON SYNDROMES OF THE UPPER EXTREMITY

Entrapped Structure	Name of Syndrome and Key Anatomic Structures	Symptoms	Physical Findings	Key Points
Median nerve	Carpal tunnel syndrome	Tingling/burning pain in first two fingers and thumb. (Pain may be referred to elbow.) Worse at night. May "shake hands out" in morning to help symptoms.	Sensory deficit in distal palm and motor deficit in the LOAF muscles.	If bilateral, consider workup (diagnostic procedures) described in text. Check for Tinel's and Phalen's signs. Distinguish from overuse syndromes in which pain is caused by tendinitis/ fibrositis.
	Anterior interosseus syndrome: origin of FDS, accessory head of FPL	Pain over proximal forearm, weakness.	No sensory deficit. No thenar weakness. Weakness of FDP I and II and FPL.	May be related to vigorous exercise. Weakness often more prominent than pain. Often cannot do a circle sign with thumb and index finger.
	Pronator syndrome: muscle hypertrophy, fibrous band from ulnar head of pronator teres to sublimis bridge	Forearm pain, hand paresthesias, weakness.	Forearm tenderness, sensory deficit in median nerve distribution. May present with thenar weakness.	Symptoms worse with forearm pronation or deep palpation of pronator muscle. May have Tinel's sign over area of entrapment. Electromyographic abnormalities spare pronator teres and may spare FDP I and II and FPL.
Radial nerve	Posterior interosseus syndrome; arcade of Frohse, supinator muscle	Usually painless, finger weakness early, wrist drop late.	Weakness of finger and wrist extension, no sensory deficit. Tenderness on deep palpation.	Compression may be related to mass lesion (tumor, lipoma), bursitis, or synovitis.
Ulnar nerve	Guyon's canal	Numbness in little finger and medial aspect of hand.	Weakness of hypothenar and interosseus muscles, sensory deficit in ulnar distribution. May have Tinel's sign.	Dorsal ulnar cutaneous nerve spared. If deep terminal branch of ulnar is affected, the syndrome is pure motor. If superficial terminal branch of ulnar is affected, the syndrome is pure sensory at distal palm. May be caused by scarring after injury, lipoma, ganglion, and so on.
	Cubital tunnel (nerve passes between heads of flexor carpi ulnaris)	Pain near elbow, spreading proximally and/or distally, paresthesias in fourth and fifth digits and medial hand, weakness.	Weakness of ulnar musculature, atrophy, claw-hand deformity. May have Tinel's sign.	Similar symptoms from external compression in ulnar groove at medial epicondyle, particularly in anesthetized or unconscious patients, or with certain elbow positions if the groove is shallow. Consider and rule out brachial plexus or radicular lesions of C8–T1.
C8–T1 roots/ lower brachial plexus trunk	Thoracic outlet syndrome: fibrous band from C7 transverse process to first rib; cervical rib; large C7 transverse process	Pain and/or paresthesias in medial arm and hand, but also neck, shoulder and chest.	Weakness in the thenar musculature. May have Tinel's sign over brachial plexus at supraclavicular fossa. Pain worse with downward or upward arm traction, relieved with shoulder elevation and neck turning toward symptomatic arm.	Imaging in addition to electrophysiologic studies are key in diagnosis (rule out cervicogenic pathology). Female predominance (droopy shoulders with long, thin neck).

LOAF muscles, first and second lumbricals, opponens pollicis, abductor pollicis brevis, and flexor pollicis brevis; FPL, flexor pollicis longus and brevis; FDS, flexor digitorum sublimis; FDP, flexor digitorum profundus.

TABLE 69–2. COMMON SYNDROMES OF THE LOWER EXTREMITY

Entrapped Structure	Name of Syndrome and Key Anatomic Structures	Symptoms	Physical Findings	Key Points
Lateral femoral cutaneous nerve	Meralgia paresthetica: iliacus muscle, inguinal ligament	Burning or shooting pain and paresthesias in anterolateral thigh.	Sensory deficit or hyperesthesia in affected area.	May be caused by intrinsic compression or extrinsic, such as obesity, wearing belts or girdles. May be aggravated by walking or other physical maneuvers.
Femoral nerve	Psoas muscle, inguinal ligament	Inguinal pain, burning pain and paresthesias in anterior thigh or anteromedial leg.	Quadriceps weakness with or without iliopsoas weakness, depressed patellar reflex, sensory deficit.	Hip adductors should have normal strength. May be caused by pelvic or inguinal compression. No iliopsoas weakness with inguinal compression. Hematoma, tumor, and history of lithotomy position are potential causes.
Peroneal nerve (common, deep, and superficial)	Head of fibula, anterior compartment, lateral compartment, interosseus membrane	Variable (paresthesias in foot, weakness, pain in anterior or lateral leg).	Variable (foot drop with weak dorsiflexion and eversion, sensory deficit in anterolateral leg and dorsum of foot).	Common peroneal syndrome often seen in "crossed leg palsy." Compartment syndromes (anterior or posterior) are more likely to be associated with pain and tenderness. Surgery may be indicated.
Tibial nerve	Tarsal tunnel, flexor retinaculum	Pain and paresthesias in sole of foot.	Weakness and atrophy of abductor digiti minimi, tenderness with palpation of flexor retinaculum.	May be aggravated by ambulation. Some patients have worsening at night.
Digital nerves	Morton's neuroma	Toe pain and numbness.	Tenderness with hyperextension of toe or palpation of deep transverse metatarsal ligament.	May be caused by trauma.

TABLE 69–3. ELECTROMYOGRAPHY AND NERVE CONDUCTION STUDIES IN ENTRAPMENT NEUROPATHIES*

Electromyography		Nerve Conduction Studies	
Analyzes spontaneous muscle activity Evaluates motor units after voluntary activation Presence of abnormality dependent on axonal involvement Abnormalities should be restricted to muscles innervated by the entrapped nerve and distal to the area of entrapment		Both sensory and motor nerves can be tested Sensory conduction studies usually more sensitive than motor Stimulation above and below the area of entrapment can help confirm localization and document nerve dysfunction	

Abnormal spontaneous activity
  Fibrillation potentials
  Positive sharp waves
	Examples
	Positive sharp waves
	
	Fibrillation potentials
		Abnormal conduction velocity/ latency
		  Slowed conduction across the site of entrapment
			Examples
			Normal
			
			Prolonged latency/slow

Neurogenic motor unit potentials
  Large amplitude
  Polyphasic
	Examples
	Normal
	
	Neurogenic
		Decreased amplitude/conduction block
		  Indicates axonal involvement
			Examples
			Normal
			
			Conduction block

*An EMG/NCS study is an electrodiagnostic study that tests motor and large-diameter sensory nerve fiber function. Used properly (as an *adjunct* to physical examination and clinical localization of lower motor neuron disorders), the study can help confirm clinical impressions, help distinguish between pathologic processes, and help determine extent of damage and prognosis for recovery. Knowledge of muscle innervation, nervous system anatomy, and anatomic relationships between nerves and surrounding structures is key in using EMG/NCS as a tool in patients with entrapment neuropathies.

diagnostic tests can be very important because patients with systemic polyneuropathy or a radicular lesion often are more vulnerable to compression or entrapment.

General Treatment Strategies

There are conservative and invasive treatment modalities for the entrapment neuropathies. In general, conservative management, including oral medications for symptomatic pain control, evaluation by rehabilitation specialists for splinting and/or padding of susceptible nerves and joints, and instruction on behavior modification to prevent and reduce extremity postures or positions that may exacerbate compression are first-line treatments. Frequently prescribed medications include nonsteroidal anti-inflammatory drugs and antiepileptic medications such as carbamazepine and gabapentin. More aggressive treatment is indicated if symptoms progress despite attempts at conservative therapy or if neurologic dysfunction (particularly motor dysfunction) is present. These interventions range from steroid injection to open surgical decompression.

SPECIFIC SYNDROMES

See Tables 69-1 for upper-extremity and 69-2 for lower-extremity syndromes.

ELECTROMYOGRAPHY AND NERVE CONDUCTION STUDIES IN ENTRAPMENT NEUROPATHY

See Table 69-3.

BIBLIOGRAPHY

Brazis PW, Masdeu JC, Biller J: Localization in Clinical Neurology, ed 3. Boston, Little, Brown, 1996.

Johnson R, Griffin J: Current Therapy in Neurologic Disease. St. Louis, Mosby-Year Book, 1997.

Shuman S, Osterman L, Bora FW: Compression neuropathies. Semin Neurol 7:1-8, 1987.

Stewart JD: Focal Peripheral Neuropathies. New York, Raven Press, 1993.

Chapter 70

Chronic Pain Management in Children

Santhanam Suresh, M.D.

Pain has become a recognized entity in children in the last decade. Management of pain from operative and other procedures is now routine in most centers in the United States, but chronic pain in children is still ignored to a great extent. Recurrent or persistent pain is seen in 5% to 10% of all unselected children. School absenteeism and inability to participate in normal activities as a child lead to fear, anxiety, depression, and anger in almost all cases.

There are several chronic pain syndromes that are frequently experienced by children (Table 70-1). Adult pain problems like neck and back pain are rarely seen in children. School absenteeism is analogous to work absenteeism in adults and should be addressed immediately. Modeling of illness behavior often exists. It is very important to break this family cycle of disability. There are significant differences in the diagnosis and management of chronic pain in children compared with adults.

COMPLEX REGIONAL PAIN SYNDROMES

Neuropathic conditions are those that are associated with injury, dysfunction, or altered excitability of portions of the peripheral or central nervous system. Complex regional pain syndromes (CRPS) are divided into two types: CRPS I or reflex sympathetic dystrophy (RSD), and CRPS II or causalgia.

TABLE 70–1. COMMON DIAGNOSES
IN PEDIATRIC PAIN CLINICS

Headache
Chest pain
Recurrent abdominal pain
Back pain
Neuropathic pain
    Complex regional pain syndromes I and II
    Postamputation pain
Sickle cell disease with frequent pain crisis
Chronic illness (e.g., cystic fibrosis)

CRPS I is "a continuous pain in a portion of an extremity after trauma which may include fracture but does not involve major nerve lesions, and is associated with sympathetic hyperactivity" (International Association for Study of Pain). The mechanisms that generate neuropathic pain are varied and complex. The primary loci of increased irritability after injury may be at several levels in the central nervous system, including axonal sprouts or neuromas, the dorsal horn of the spinal cord, and sites more rostral in the central nervous system. Factors contributing to neuropathic pain include disuse of the extremity, fear, anxiety, and repetitive noxious stimuli in a milieu of social pressures and altered family dynamics.

Incidence of Reflex Sympathetic Dystrophy in Children

The incidence is greater in teenage girls than in teenage boys. Pain is seen more frequently in the lower extremity in children; adult RSD patients often have pain in an upper extremity (Table 70-2). Because of underdiagnosis, the incidence of RSD in the pediatric population is less than for adults. Although RSD has been reported in a child as young as 3½ years of age, it is generally seen in children beyond the age of 9 years

TABLE 70–2. DIFFERENCES IN THE PRESENTATION
OF REFLEX SYMPATHETIC DYSTROPHY
IN CHILDREN AND IN ADULTS

Characteristics	Children	Adults
Site	Marked lower extremity predominance (5:1)	Upper extremity commonly involved
Sex ratio	Female preponderance	Mixed occurrence
Treatment strategies	Resolves with TENS, physical therapy, and, rarely, blocks	Early sympathetic blocks
Timing of treatment	Anytime	Early-phase treatment has better results

TENS, transcutaneous electrical nerve stimulation.

299

and is frequently seen in 11- to 13-year-old girls.[1] It is reported in overachievers and competitive athletes.

The clinical triad of CRPS I (RSD) includes the following elements:

1. Sensory
   Allodynia
   Hyperalgesia
   Spontaneous burning pain
   Hyperpathia
2. Autonomic
   Sweating, edema, trophic changes
3. Motor
   Loss of active and passive motion

Evaluation of RSD Patients

A history of the nature of injury, the type and duration of pain, relieving and aggravating factors, and the dependence on medication is important in determining the prognosis and management options.

The following characteristic signs may be identified:

1. Allodynia: Innocuous stimuli (e.g., stroking) elicit excruciating pain. Allodynia in the absence of skin conditions signifies neuropathic pain.
2. Hyperalgesia: The patient has a decreased threshold to pain.
3. Nerve conduction studies: These may give some insight into the location and type of nerve injury. However, invasive monitoring may not be acceptable to the child.
4. Bone scintigraphy: Bone scans in children generally show an increased uptake, but in patients with RSD there is decreased uptake (in contrast to adult patients with RSD).

Noninvasive diagnostic findings include asymmetry of surface temperature by more than 1°C and resting or evoked sudomotor asymmetry. Invasive tests involve the use of systemic α-adrenergic antagonists and sympathetic ganglion blocks.

Treatment

The management of neuropathic pain is frustrating for patients, parents, and caregivers. There is no single proven method to provide these children with adequate and prolonged pain relief. The main goal of therapy is to get the child functional and back in school with his or her peers. Most of the treatment modalities are extrapolated from studies in adults (Table 70–3). Family dynamics and the addition of family therapy are an important aspect of management for pediatric patients with RSD.

Psychological Therapy

Behavioral methods to alleviate pain are used frequently. Biofeedback and visual guided imagery are often used. Structured counseling for coping skills is often used along with distraction techniques.

TABLE 70–3. MANAGEMENT OF NEUROPATHIC PAIN

Nonpharmacological methods
  Hypnosis, biofeedback, visual guided imagery
  TENS and extensive physical therapy
  Family therapy
Pharmacologic methods
  Acetaminophen, nonsteroidal anti-inflammatory drugs
  Tricyclic antidepressants
  Anticonvulsants
  Opioids (reserved for severe debilitating pain)
Regional and sympathetic blockade
  Sympathetic blockade: lumbar sympathetic block, stellate ganglion block
  Epidural and plexus blocks
  Neurolytic blocks for cancer pain

TENS, transcutaneous electrical nerve stimulation.

Physical Therapy

Transcutaneous electrical nerve stimulation (TENS) is widely used and is very effective in children. Rigorous physical therapy is very helpful in these patients and forms the mainstay of management of pediatric RSD.

Medical Therapy

Tricyclic Antidepressants (TCAs). TCAs are very effective for the management of neuropathic pain and are widely used despite the lack of adequate controlled studies in children. Nortriptyline is generally preferred, because it has fewer sedative and cardiovascular side effects. If there are a lot of anticholinergic side effects, trazodone is the preferred drug. A thorough examination of the cardiovascular system is necessary, because TCAs can precipitate sudden death from abnormal cardiac arrhythmias.

Anticonvulsants. Some children benefit from the use of anticonvulsants in the management of neuropathic pain. Carbamazepine, clonazepam, phenytoin, and, more recently, gabapentin have been used to manage pain in patients with RSD.

Opioids. Opioids are helpful in the management of neuropathic pain, especially pain caused by cancer. It is best to titrate the opioids to avoid side effects.

Sympathetic Blockade. Sympathetic blocks are used in pediatric patients who have intractable pain. Lumbar sympathetic blocks, stellate ganglion blocks, continuous epidural infusions, and intravenous regional anesthesia (Bier blocks) have been shown to be effective. Concurrent physical therapy is instituted. An alternative approach to the management of neuropathic pain is to administer adrenergic blocking drugs such as guanethidine or bretylium using intravenous regional techniques. In the event an epidural block is indicated, continuous infusion for a few days is preferable to repeated blocks.

Prognosis

Pediatric RSD can be puzzling and frustrating. A multidisciplinary approach employing physical therapy, psychological interventions, and TCAs can be very useful. The success of management depends on the individual patient and the support from family and the environment.

HEADACHES IN PEDIATRIC PATIENTS

Chronic headaches in pediatric patients have been reported in 75% of all children by their 15th birthday. Headaches are classified into several types (Table 70–4).

It is important for the successful management of headaches to obtain a detailed history. The type of headache, its duration, symptoms, frequency, and quality must be determined. A family history of migraine may be useful in determining a cause.

Precipitating factors for headache may be external (e.g., social stresses, family dysfunction, academic pressures, environmental pressures) or internal (e.g., autonomic hyperactivity, coping deficits, food sensitivities).

Diagnostic Tests

Diagnostic tests include a general physical examination; neurologic examination (cranial circumference, funduscopic examination, cranial nerve examination, mental status, reflexes); laboratory tests; possibly electroencephalography; radiographic examination (magnetic resonance imaging, computed tomography); and psychological tests (Minnesota Multiphasic Personality Inventory, Wechsler's intelligence scale, Woodcock-Johnson achievement battery).

Migraine Headaches

Migraine headaches are very prevalent in teenagers. It is an autosomal dominant disease with a greater penetrance in females. Patients present with paroxysms of vasoconstriction and vasodilatation. Vascular headaches are caused by depolarization of perivascular sensory axons, which leads to pain that is conveyed by axons surrounding cephalic arteries and venous sinuses. This in turn causes local axonal release of vasodilating and permeability-promoting peptides.

Pharmacotherapy of Migraines

Pharmacotherapy of migraines includes the following:

1. Extracranial vasoconstriction: ergotamine, dihydroergotamine
2. Serotonin antagonists: methysergide, cyproheptadine
3. β-Blockers: propranolol, nadolol
4. TCAs: nortriptyline, amitriptyline
5. Nonsteroidal anti-inflammatory drugs (NSAIDs): naproxen, ibuprofen.

TABLE 70–4. CLASSIFICATION OF HEADACHES

Acute	Chronic and nonprogressive
Acute and recurrent	Mixed headache syndrome
Chronic and progressive	

Nonpharmacologic Methods of Headache Management

Several nonpharmacologic methods are available for the management of persistent headache. These include biofeedback, stress management training, psychotherapy, family interventions, and elimination of excess caffeine.

Other Forms of Childhood Headaches

Post-traumatic headache may be sustained during regular childhood activities or at play. These respond very well to the use of nonpharmacologic methods such as biofeedback and family interventions. Anticonvulsants such as carbamazepine and gabapentin have been shown to be very effective.

Children with ventriculoperitoneal shunts may experience recurrent headaches. Patients with hydrocephalus often require revisions of their ventriculoperitoneal shunt. A small segment have repeated headaches despite a functional shunt. This may be caused by a neuropathic component or by causalgia from repeated injury to the nerve during surgical interventions. These patients respond to good physical therapy with neck-strengthening exercises, a small dose of TCAs, and, occasionally, peripheral nerve blockade (greater occipital, supraorbital, and supratrochlear nerve blocks).

Tension-type headaches include episodic and chronic types. These respond very well to nonpharmacologic methods such as biofeedback, family interventions, and mild analgesics including acetaminophen and NSAIDs. Stress reduction is an essential part of management of tension-type headaches.

RECURRENT ABDOMINAL PAIN

Abdominal pain that occurs once a month for three consecutive months and is severe enough to interfere with the child's normal activities is described as recurrent abdominal pain. This occurs in 10% to 17% of school-age children. It exists more commonly in preschool and adolescent children. The pain is usually periumbilical and lasts less than 1 hour, always less than 3 hours. Autonomic symptoms such as perspiration, nausea, vomiting, flushing, and palpitations are seen frequently and can be disconcerting. Pathology must be ruled out, especially if there is weight loss, pain awakening the child at night, fever, dysuria, guaiac-positive stools, anemia, or an elevated erythrocyte sedimentation rate.

Management of Abdominal Pain

Therapeutic steps to treat infectious causes or parasitic infestations are first taken.

School phobia should be treated by a psychologist. Organic disease should be eliminated before a diagnosis of psychogenic pain is entertained. Coping skills are taught, and guided imagery or biofeedback is attempted. A subcategory of children have the equivalent of adult irritable bowel syndrome. Addition of fiber to the diet of such children may reduce the incidence of abdominal pain in this category.

CHEST PAIN

Chest pain is more common in healthy children than in children with congenital heart disease. It leads to physical distress, anxiety, sleep disturbances, school absences, and extensive use of medical resources. After a thorough history has been obtained, a complete examination of the cardiovascular system is performed. Once cardiac pathology has been ruled out, musculoskeletal causes for chest pain should be entertained. Trauma, muscle spasm, costochondritis, and Tietze's syndrome should be ruled out. Fibromyalgia and other myofascial syndromes, although rare, could still occur in children, especially teenagers. Frequent coughing associated with pulmonary pathology is another cause for chest pain.

Conservative management including the use of TENS, biofeedback, heat, massage, and NSAIDs is very effective.

CHILDHOOD CANCER

Pain experienced by patients with cancer can arise from tumor invasion or as a consequence of procedures or therapy.

Cancer-related pain can be recognized from knowledge of the natural history of the tumor. Bone pain usually arises from metastasis of the tumor to the bone. Other less common but important reasons for pain include compression of the spinal cord, tumor involvement of the central or the peripheral nervous system, and obstruction of viscus.

Cancer patients frequently have tests done to check the prognosis or the efficacy of treatment. Bone marrow aspirations, lumbar punctures, and venipunctures are routinely done. These procedures create a lot of anxiety and pain. Biofeedback and distraction techniques have been used. The use of EMLA cream or anxiolytics, or both, can provide a very smooth environment for the child.

Therapy-related pain can be predicted by the type of tumor and the anticancer therapy that is being administered. Peripheral neuropathy, mucositis, surgical incisions, and steroid-induced bone changes and gastritis frequently cause a lot of pain. The analgesic regimen for management of cancer pain depends on the type and rapidity of progression of the lesion (Table 70-5).

PAIN IN TERMINAL ILLNESS

There has recently been a surge in treatment modalities, and children have been part of a cure-oriented, technology-driven health care system. With the help of dedicated organizations like hospice, the care of terminally ill children has developed much the same way as for adults. When children with life-threatening

TABLE 70-5. MANAGEMENT OF CANCER PAIN

Pharmacologic methods
    Opioids (oral, intravenous, patient-controlled)
    Nonsteroidal anti-inflammatory drugs
    Acetaminophen
    Tricyclic antidepressants and anticonvulsants
Regional anesthetics
    Epidural analgesia
    Intrathecal analgesia
Surgical methods
    Tumor debulking
    Neuroablative procedures
Physical therapy
    Acupuncture
    Transcutaneous electrical nerve stimulation
    Ultrasound, whirlpool therapy
Psychological methods
    Guided imagery
    Distraction
    Hypnosis

illnesses have significant setbacks in their lives, there usually are no firm criteria to stop treatment and direct palliative care. Children subjected to chemotherapy or other related aggressive procedures tend to experience significant pain. One of the main tenets of hospice care is to allow patients to live a life that is full and of the best quality possible for what time they have remaining. A variety of acceptable methods are available for the management of cancer pain (see Table 70-5).

Patient-controlled analgesia has been used in a home setting in patients with terminal illness. Indwelling catheters in the epidural or the intrathecal space can be left for palliative care in terminal patients with bony metastasis or in those with extensive involvement of the spinal cord. Anticonvulsants, especially carbamazepine or gabapentin, are very useful for neuropathic cancer pain. Tricyclic antidepressants such as amitriptyline, nortriptyline, and trazodone are useful for decreasing neuropathic pain. Hypnosis, biofeedback, and visual guided imagery are often used in the management of childhood cancers.

Pain in terminal illness must be assessed thoroughly. Other coincident problems such as pressure sores, oral thrush, and constipation must be dealt with along with pain management. Analgesics still form the mainstay of treatment of cancer pain. A gradual progression from mild analgesics to stronger ones, in a stepladder fashion, is recommended by the World Health Organization. Rarely is an as-needed (prn) order sufficient for management of cancer pain. It is important for caregivers to reassess the situation and alter the management as needed.

Strong opioids are usually needed for cancer pain; morphine preparations are widely used. There is no clear role for the use of opioid agonists-antagonists in children. It is important to allay fears of addiction and respiratory depression associated with the use of opioids in a sick and dying child. This also represents acknowledgment by the parents of the terminal nature of their child's illness. Various preparations of morphine are available, including instant-releasing and slow-releasing forms. The type of morphine that is used is based on the degree of pain and the tolerance of the patient. Occasionally, the child is given a small dose of amphetamine to counteract the sedative effect of narcotics. If pain is intolerable, especially that associated with nerve entrapment, a regional anesthetic technique is used. Epidural catheters and intrathecal catheters are placed in the operating room under sterile conditions and tunneled under the skin. This technique can provide long-lasting analgesia, especially with a combination of narcotics and local anesthetics.

Physical reasons are not the only cause for pain in cancer. A strong psychological component of pain is very significant. The progression of the disease and its terminal nature should be discussed with the parents and with the child if possible. Visual guided imagery, hypnosis, and distraction techniques are used frequently for procedural pain in these children.

Parents usually do not want their child to suffer from pain, especially if they have a terminal illness. Excellent pain relief can be achieved regardless of whether the patient is at home or at the hospital.

CONCLUSION

Pediatric patients experience several chronic pain syndromes. The early diagnosis and judicious management of these patients in a multidisciplinary pain clinic allows them to function as normal children and teenagers among their peers. Chronic pain is a disease that needs to be addressed like any infectious process in the child. The availability of pain clinics catering to pediatric patients has made it easier for both patients and parents to understand the need for addressing and managing pain problems in children.

REFERENCES

1. Wilder RT, Berde CB, Wolohan M, et al: Reflex sympathetic dystrophy in children: Clinical characteristics and follow-up of seventy patients. J Bone Joint Surg Am 74:910–919, 1992.
2. Schecter N, Berde CB, Yaster M: Pain in infants, children and adolescents. Baltimore, Williams & Wilkins, 1993.

Cancer Pain

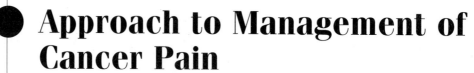

Chapter 71

Approach to Management of Cancer Pain

Charles F. von Gunten, M.D., Ph.D., and Frank D. Ferris, M.D.

EPIDEMIOLOGY OF CANCER PAIN

More than 1 million people in the United States receive a diagnosis of cancer each year. Despite the fact that roughly half of all cancers are cured, there are more than 500,000 deaths from cancer each year, with another 2.5 million Americans living with a diagnosis of cancer.

Pain is highly prevalent in patients with cancer. At the time of diagnosis and early in treatment, 30% to 45% of cancer patients have pain. This increases to 75% of those patients with advanced cancer. Of cancer patients with pain, 40% to 50% describe the pain as moderate to severe and 25% to 30% describe it as very severe or excruciating.

Pain in patients with cancer can be categorized as related to the cancer itself in 70% of patients, related to cancer treatment in 25% of patients, and unrelated to cancer in the remainder. It is important for clinicians to recognize pain syndromes that are common in patients with cancer.

- *Bone metastases.* They are often multiple and are frequently found in vertebrae, pelvis, proximal long bones, and skull. They are uncommonly found in distal extremities. Pain is often described as dull and aching and exacerbated with movement.
- *Epidural metastases and spinal cord compression.* This is a grave consequence of vertebral metastases (except in lymphoma) and is heralded by new or worsened localized back pain, sometimes with radicular components if nerve roots are involved. Diagnosis and definitive treatment before neurological deficits occur is critical to overall preservation of function.
- *Plexopathies.* Cervical, brachial, and lumbosacral plexus may be infiltrated by tumor or damaged by radiation or surgery. Pain may be described with both local and radiating components.
- *Peripheral neuropathies.* Tumor, fibrosis, surgery, chemotherapy, or viral infection may damage peripheral nerves. Pain is often described as dysesthetic and burning in character.

- *Abdominal (visceral) pain.* Pain may be constant or colicky, difficult for the patient to localize, worse after eating, associated with nausea, and referred widely to distant cutaneous sites.
- *Mucositis.* Chemotherapy and/or radiation may cause inflammation and pain in the epithelium of the gastrointestinal tract from mouth to anus. Pain is often intense and interferes with oral intake. Concurrent infection should be sought and treated.

Cancer pain is undertreated in 50% to 80% of patients. The problem persists despite reports of adequate control in more than 90% of patients when simple pharmacologic measures are routinely and systematically employed.

PATHOPHYSIOLOGY OF CANCER PAIN

Cancer pain can be conceptualized in two categories: nociceptive and neuropathic. Nociceptive pain is caused by stimulation of an intact, normally functioning nervous system. Because of the difference in the patterns of innervation, nociceptive pain may be classified as somatic (highly innervated superficial areas with precise localization of pain) or visceral (diffusely innervated organs with poor localization of pain). In contrast, neuropathic pain is caused by a nervous system with disrupted function. In patients with cancer, common causes of neuropathic pain include direct pressure on nerves or nerve invasion by progressive tumor growth, chemotherapy, viral infection, and surgery. Neuropathic pain may persist despite absence of persistent injury.

Because pain is fundamentally an experience of a person rather than merely a nociceptive or neuropathic impulse, the pain clinician must have an appreciation of the "total pain" experienced by patients with cancer, which has four domains: physical, psychological, social, and spiritual (existential). Failure to appreciate these aspects hampers satisfactory pain relief.

MANAGEMENT STRATEGIES

Assessment and reassessment of cancer pain are critical to adequate analgesia. The self-report by the patient is the only reliable indicator of pain. The clinician must believe the patient and presume that nociceptive and/or neuropathic pain mechanisms are responsible even if they cannot be demonstrated or confirmed by objective methods. In addition to an adequate pain history, physical examination, and appropriate diagnostic studies, a pain rating scale should routinely be used to assess pain and its relief.

Pharmacologic methods are the mainstay of cancer pain management. They should be as simple as possible; appropriate to the patient, family, and setting; and be delivered in a timely, logical, and coordinated fashion. Patients should be empowered to control their course to the greatest extent possible. Such empowerment correlates with improved pain management.

Physical modalities such as cutaneous stimulation, heat, cold, massage, pressure, or vibration may be appropriately added to pharmacologic modalities, especially where muscle tension or spasm are present. Physical therapy and occupational therapy may promote and maintain function and improve pain control.

Neurolytic approaches, either chemical or physical, peripheral or central, may help highly selected patients with localized or regional pain syndromes. They are rarely sufficient in isolation from systemic pharmacologic measures.

Cognitive-behavioral approaches such as counseling, guided imagery, relaxation, and biofeedback may play an adjunctive or complementary role in selected patients but should not be substituted for use of systemic analgesics.

Intraspinal delivery of analgesics and coanalgesics, either epidurally or intrathecally, may be required in the minority of patients who do not achieve adequate analgesia with oral or conventional parenteral modalities.

BARRIERS TO APPROPRIATE CANCER PAIN MANAGEMENT

Inadequate cancer pain management results from multiple barriers to achievable pain relief that lie with health care professionals, patients, and the health care system. These barriers chiefly impede the appropriate prescription of opioid analgesics for cancer pain relief. They can be summarized as follows:

- Inordinate and unsupported fear of addiction
- Confusion between psychological and physical dependence
- Inappropriate concern about pharmacologic tolerance
- Exaggerated expectations of side effects and adverse reactions
- Failure to prevent and treat constipation
- Unwarranted concerns about respiratory depression
- Apprehensiveness about regulatory agencies
- Persuasiveness of conventional prescribing practices
- Omission of routine and systematic cancer pain assessment

BIBLIOGRAPHY

Bonica JJ: Cancer pain. *In* Bonica JJ: The Management of Pain. Philadelphia, Lea & Febiger, 1990, pp 400–460.

Doyle D, Hancks G, MacDonald N: Oxford Textbook of Palliative Medicine. New York, Oxford University Press, 1997.

Jacox A, Carr DB, Payne R, et al.: Management of Cancer Pain: Clinical Practice Guideline No. 9. AHCPR Publication No. 94-0592. Rockville, Md: Agency for Health Care Policy and Research, US Department of Health and Human Services, Public Health Service, March 1994.

Levy MH: Pharmacologic treatment of cancer pain. N Engl J Med 35:1124-1132, 1996.

Patt RB: Cancer Pain. Philadelphia, JB Lippincott, 1993.

Chapter 72

Pharmacologic Management of Cancer Pain

Charles F. von Gunten, M.D., Ph.D.,
and Frank D. Ferris, M.D.

Systemic analgesics are the mainstay of pain management. Although many of these approaches have been developed for the management of cancer pain, they may be adapted to other chronic pain states.

Pain is a personal experience rather than a precise neurophysiologic phenomenon. It is influenced by the patient's expectations, fears, hopes, coping styles, witnesses, and attributed meanings. This combination of physiology, sociology, psychology, and spirituality has complicated the study of pain and has led to the concept of "total pain."

In order to simplify the subject there has been an attempt to separate organic pain from psychological/social/spiritual pain. Although this division may be useful for heuristic and conceptual purposes, it has led to the unfortunate labeling of the former as "real" pain and the latter as "not real" pain. This represents both the inappropriate extrapolation of research on acute pain (particularly in laboratory animals) to the management of chronic pain and the general avoidance of emotional, psychological, social, and spiritual issues by physicians trained in the scientific method. Although this chapter reviews pharmacologic management of organic pain, the reader should not suppose that this is the only important component of comprehensive pain management.

ACUTE VS. CHRONIC PAIN

Appropriate pharmacologic management of pain requires the clinician to differentiate acute from chronic pain. Acute pain has been defined as pain lasting less than 6 weeks that is related to a discernible incident such as surgery or trauma. The natural history of acute pain, even in the absence of analgesia, is to resolve. Chronic pain has been defined as pain lasting longer than 6 weeks that is related to an ongoing pathophysiology. Intractable pain is that chronic pain whose cause, if known, is not expected to ameliorate. This may be related to ongoing pathophysiology within the nervous system itself, as in neuropathic pain syndromes.

Recent data suggest that appropriate pharmacologic management may influence the overall severity and duration of pain. Further, documentation is accumulating that preemptive analgesia (analgesics administered before the inciting cause of pain, such as an amputation) and early adequate treatment of acute pain diminish the duration and severity of the acute pain and prevent the development of chronic intractable pain. The concepts of sensitization, windup, and hyperalgesia that underlie these observations and the demonstration that appropriate pharmacologic management mitigates these adverse effects of pain are discussed in Chapters 30 and 31.

THREE-STEP LADDER FOR PAIN MANAGEMENT

In 1988, as part of its efforts to improve public health worldwide, the World Health Organization (WHO) declared cancer pain management a worldwide emergency and adopted the Canadian three-step ladder of analgesic agents for control of nociceptive pain. In addition to influencing government policies about pain control, this ladder provides a useful tool for illustrating and summarizing generally accepted approaches to conventional systemic analgesics. It is not a rigid clinical path that must be traversed in the care of every patient. The clinical judgment of a knowledgeable, experienced clinician is the most important determinant of appropriate pain therapy for any person with pain. The ladder, modified by the authors, is shown in Figure 72-1.

When initiating analgesia, it is important that the patient start at the appropriate step along the ladder—for mild pain start at step 1; for moderate pain, step 2; for severe pain, step 3. As the severity of pain increases, maximize the dosing at the current step and then, if this is insufficient, move up the ladder.

Step One

Acetaminophen and the nonsteroidal anti-inflammatory drugs (NSAIDs) including acetylsalicylic acid (ASA)

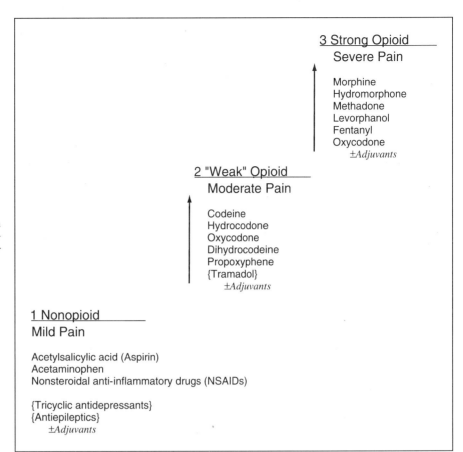

FIGURE 72–1. World Health Organization 3-step ladder for pain management. (Modified from World Health Organization: Cancer Pain Relief. Geneva, WHO, 1986.)

are the mainstay of step 1 of the WHO analgesic ladder for the management of mild pain. They obey first-order kinetics and may be dosed up to recommended maxima (Table 72-1). Many are available without prescription. Sustained-release preparations or drugs with longer half-lives may encourage adherence.

TABLE 72–1. SELECTED STEP-ONE ANALGESICS

Drug	Suggested Maximum Dose
Acetaminophen (APAP, Tylenol)	650 mg po q4h
Acetylsalicylic acid (ASA, Aspirin)	650 mg po q4h
Ibuprofen (Motrin)	800 mg po qid
Choline magnesium trisalicylate (Trilisate)	1500 mg po tid
Diclofenac (Cataflam)	50 mg po qid
Diclofenac-extended release (Voltaren)	75 mg po tid
Diflunisal (Dolobid)	500 mg po tid
Etodolac (Lodine)	400 mg po tid
Indomethacin (Indocin)	50 mg po qid
Ketoprofen (Orudis)	75 mg po qid
Nabumetone (Relafen)	1 g po bid
Naproxen (Naprosyn)	500 mg po tid
Oxaprozin (Daypro)	1800 mg po qd
Sulindac (Clinoril)	200 mg po bid
Salsalate (Disalcid)	1500 mg po tid
Ketorolac (Toradol)	60 mg IM/IV then 30 mg IV/IM q 6h 10 mg po qid not to exceed 5 d

Step Two

Several opioid analgesics are conventionally available in combination with either acetaminophen or ASA and are commonly used to manage moderate pain. They are listed in Figure 72-1 under step 2 of the WHO analgesic ladder. Milligram for milligram, the opioids in this class are close in potency to morphine, with the exceptions of propoxyphene (which truly has weak analgesic activity), tramadol (which has a unique combination of very weak opioid activity with other analgesic properties), and codeine (which has one tenth to one twelfth the potency of morphine). However, they have been termed "weak" opioids because, in combination, they have a ceiling to their analgesic potential due to the maximum amounts of acetaminophen or ASA that can be administered per 24 hours (i.e., 4 g of acetaminophen per 24 hours).

The combination medications of step 2 all obey first-order kinetics and may be dosed up to recommended maxima (Table 72-2). The potential side effects are those of the component drugs.

Frequently, patients are given prescriptions for several step 2 drugs even though pain is poorly controlled. This usually occurs when physicians are reluctant to prescribe a step 3 opioid. Aside from propoxyphene, there is no evidence that maximal dosing of any one medication in this group is better than that of another, and trials of several step 2 medications are likely to prolong the patient's pain. In addition, when a step 2

TABLE 72–2. SELECTED STEP-TWO ANALGESICS

Drug	Suggested Maximum Dose
Codeine 30 mg/325 mg APAP (Tylenol #3)	2 po q4h
Codeine 30 mg/325 mg ASA (Empirin #3)	2 po q4h
Hydrocodone 5 mg/500 mg APAP (Vicodin)	2 po q6h
Hydrocodone 10 mg/650 mg APAP (Lortab)	1 po q 6h
Oxycodone 5 mg/325 mg APAP (Percocet)	2 po q4h
Oxycodone 5 mg/325 mg ASA (Percodan)	2 po q4h
Tramadol (Ultram) 50 mg	2 po q6h

APAP, acetaminophen; ASA, acetylsalicylic acid.

drug inadequately relieves pain, patients may combine two or more medications or take more than the prescribed amount in an attempt to obtain pain relief. In doing so, they may unknowingly put themselves at increased risk for significant toxicity from either the acetaminophen or the ASA component of the medication.

If pain persists or increases despite maximum dosage of a step 2 drug, a step 3 drug should be prescribed instead.

Step Three

Step 3 of the WHO analgesic ladder comprises the pure agonist opioid analgesics. Morphine is the prototypical drug because of its ease of administration and wide availability. Other widely prescribed opioids are listed in Figure 72–1. Many patients with chronic pain are best managed with an appropriately titrated strong opioid that is combined with one or more coanalgesics. In contrast with the step 1 and step 2 analgesics, there is no ceiling effect or upper limit to the dose of opioids when titrating to relieve pain.

"Step Four"

Several studies have demonstrated that application of the WHO three-step ladder results in adequate control of cancer pain in up to 90% of patients. Several authors have informally invoked a "step 4" to indicate approaches that should be reserved for patients whose pain is not controlled by competent use of the analgesic approaches outlined in the first three steps. In general, "step 4" involves invasive approaches for pain relief and can be summarized as follows.

Subcutaneous or intravenous administration of opioid analgesics and coanalgesics may be required for patients for whom oral, buccal mucosal, rectal, or transcutaneous approaches are not possible or practical or if doses of oral opioids lead to undesirable side effects. Side effects may be minimized by the uniform delivery of the drug parenterally, the change in route of administration, or the reduction in first-pass metabolite production. Subcutaneous administration may be preferable to intravenous approaches because it results in equivalent serum levels and analgesia without the risks of thrombosis and infection and is much easier and cheaper to deliver.

Intraspinal administration of opioid analgesics, either epidurally or intrathecally, may be required in selected patients.

Intraventricular application of opioid analgesics and other drugs has been investigated for selected central pain syndromes.

Neuroablative techniques such as peripheral neurolytic blockade, ganglionic blockade, cordotomy, and cingulotomy may be appropriate in highly selected patients.

COMMON ANALGESIC AGENTS

Acetaminophen

Despite its widespread use, the precise mechanism of action of acetaminophen remains unclear. Although it is analgesic and antipyretic, it is not anti-inflammatory, at least systemically. Its analgesic activity is at least additive with that of other analgesic agents, including the NSAIDs and opioids. Acetaminophen is associated with significant liver toxicity. It is generally recommended that the total dose not exceed 4 g per 24 hours.

NSAIDs Including Acetylsalicylic Acid

NSAIDs are anti-inflammatory through their ability to inhibit the enzyme cyclooxygenase, which catalyzes the conversion of arachidonic acid to prostaglandins and leukotrienes. Their effect is to decrease the levels of these inflammatory mediators that sensitize nerve endings to painful stimuli. Because analgesia from NSAIDs is achieved through a different mechanism than analgesia from opioids or other adjuvant analgesics, they may be combined with these drugs to achieve better pain relief than with a single drug alone. Primary analgesia may be achieved at lower doses than those required for anti-inflammatory action. Therefore, when used as an adjuvant for their anti-inflammatory effects, NSAIDs should be given at maximum doses.

The side effects of the NSAIDs are related to their mechanism of action. Inhibition of cyclooxygenase leads to inhibition of platelet aggregation, decreased cytoprotection in the gastric mucosa, and decreased renal perfusion. Consequently, bleeding and renal failure are important side effects. The dyspepsia and abdominal pain that limit use of NSAIDs in some patients do not correlate with significant gastric erosions or gastrointestinal bleeding. Similarly, the use of an H_2-blocking antacid (e.g., cimetidine, ranitidine) to treat NSAID-associated dyspepsia and abdominal pain does not prevent gastric erosions and gastrointestinal bleeding. Only misoprostol, which reverses the effect of NSAIDs on the microarteriolar circulation of the stomach, has been shown to heal gastric erosions and to reduce the risk of significant gastric bleeding.

The nonacetylated salicylates (choline magnesium trisalicylate and salsalate) and nabumetone do not significantly affect platelet aggregation. They may be useful in patients who are thrombocytopenic and for whom other NSAIDs are contraindicated. Sulindac is thought to be least likely to induce renal failure because of its minimal effect on prostaglandin synthesis at the level of the proximal renal tubule. Newer drugs, with specificity for cyclo-oxygenase subtypes and diminished side effect profiles, are in development.

In contrast with the opioids, the NSAIDs and acetaminophen have a ceiling effect to their analgesic potential, do not produce pharmacologic tolerance, and are not associated with physical or psychological dependence.

Opioids

Opioid analgesics act by binding to opioid receptors of three subtypes (μ, κ, and δ). Traditionally, analgesia is thought to be modulated principally by opioid action at central μ-receptors. Recent work suggests that opioids may have other important sites of action. The opioid analgesics in common use may be divided into those that are full μ-receptor agonists, partial agonists, and mixed agonist-antagonists. The pure agonist drugs are the most useful in the treatment of chronic intractable pain.

Opioids to Avoid

The mixed agonist-antagonist opioids (e.g., pentazocine, butorphanol, nalbuphine) and the partial agonist opioids (e.g., buprenorphine) are poor choices for patients with severe pain. They have no advantages over the pure agonist opioids. Besides having a ceiling effect to the analgesia they produce, they have the significant disadvantage that, if combined with a pure opioid agonist, they may precipitate acute pain and opioid withdrawal symptoms.

Meperidine (Demerol) is a synthetic pure agonist opioid that is widely used in the postoperative management of acute pain. However, its continued use has been questioned for three reasons. First, because of its short duration of action in comparison with morphine or other pure agonist opioids, it must be dosed too frequently to provide convenient, adequate analgesia. Second, because its oral absorption is unpredictable, a reliable oral dose cannot be prescribed which corresponds to parenteral doses. Third and most significant, the major liver metabolite normeperidine, which has a longer half-life than meperidine (approximately 6 vs. 3 hours), accumulates with repeat dosing for analgesia and frequently causes significant subclinical or clinical toxicity, including impaired concentration, restlessness, agitation, excessive dreams, hallucinations, myoclonic jerks, and even seizures. This accumulation is particularly accentuated in patients with compromised renal function. The assertions that meperidine is associated with less constipation or spasm of the sphincter of Oddi are not well supported. Its use is best limited to small doses (25 to 50 mg) parenterally to treat rigors associated with fever, drugs, or blood product transfusions.

ANALGESIC PHARMACOLOGY

Appreciation of general pharmacologic principles is essential if systemic analgesics are to be used appropriately to achieve pain relief.

Routes of Administration

The preferred route of analgesic administration for the management of cancer pain is oral. This route provides the simplest, least expensive way to manage up to 90% of all cancer pain. When the oral route is not available, analgesics can be administered buccally, transdermally, or rectally without resorting to more expensive and invasive routes of delivery. In a small number of patients, subcutaneous, intravenous, or intraspinal administration may be required.

Routine Dosing for Constant Pain

When managing pain, it is important to distinguish between constant and intermittent pain. For pain that is constant, such as chronic cancer pain, analgesics should be prescribed on a regular schedule at doses sufficient to keep the pain controlled. Dosing solely on an as-needed (prn) basis is inappropriate because it subjects the patient to unnecessary pain and may increase both the patient's anxiety and the total dose required to control the pain.

Most of the short-acting drugs used for analgesia, particularly acetaminophen, the NSAIDs including ASA, and the opioids, follow first-order kinetics. When prescribed on a routine schedule, they should be administered once every half-life to achieve steady state and maintain constant serum levels (e.g., every 4 hours for oral morphine, hydromorphone, oxycodone; see Tables 72-1 and 72-2 for others). Methadone, with its longer half-life, is administered every 8 to 12 hours.

Titration

When titration is initiated or analgesic therapy is changed, drugs that follow first-order kinetics take five half-lives to reach a pharmacologic steady state. Changes in dosage should be made only after the serum level has reached steady state, such as once every 20 to 24 hours when morphine is given orally or even subcutaneously. Waiting longer does not improve pain control. Increasing the dosage before steady state is reached may lead to unnecessarily high serum levels and undesired side effects.

Sustained-Release Products

Sustained-release medications should not be used to adjust or titrate a patient's uncontrolled pain. Using them for titration unduly prolongs the process of bringing the pain under control. However, once the pain is controlled, changing to a sustained-release product may enhance the patient's quality of life and improve compliance and adherence (due to the decreased frequency of dosing).

Sustained-release preparations of codeine, hydromorphone, morphine, and oxycodone are or soon will be available for oral administration, as will morphine for rectal administration, and should be administered in accordance with the instructions of the manufacturer.

Fentanyl is available as a transdermal preparation that can usually be administered every 72 hours.

Breakthrough or Rescue Dosing for Intermittent Pain

Intermittent pain may occur because of activity (incident pain) or because of a change in the severity of the pain. If the duration and severity of the intermittent pain are sufficient, breakthrough or rescue doses (extra short-acting doses) of the same or a similar medication may be appropriate on an as-needed basis. If a patient requires more than two to four breakthrough doses on a regular basis, then the routine dose should be adjusted upward. For intermittent pain of short duration (seconds to a few minutes), breakthrough dosing, particularly of the opioids, may lead to undesired side effects without increased analgesia.

For most analgesics, the time to reach maximum serum concentration (C_{max}) after a given dose of analgesic correlates closely with the maximum pharmacologic effect. Breakthrough doses of an analgesic can be given safely with a frequency equivalent to the time required to reach C_{max}. For example, a bolus of intravenous morphine achieves C_{max} in 5 to 10 minutes, whereas oral morphine achieves its maximum in 45 to 65 minutes. Therefore, breakthrough doses can be given every 5 to 10 minutes intravenously, every 30 minutes subcutaneously, or every 60 minutes orally. Making the patient wait any longer when the pain is not controlled simply prolongs the time required to establish optimal pain control.

The size of the breakthrough dose should be related to the routine dose. For the strong opioids such as morphine, hydromorphone, and oxycodone, a simple rule of thumb is to administer 10% of the total 24-hour dose per breakthrough. The dose is then adjusted as the routine dose changes or as the intensity of the intermittent pain requires.

Equivalent Doses

The relative abilities of opioid analgesics to relieve pain have been correlated (Table 72-3). These relationships are not scientifically precise, because there is significant interpatient variability. Further, the data from which these equivalencies are derived are often not directly applicable to chronic cancer pain. Nevertheless, the equal analgesia tables are useful to approximate the dose of a new analgesic when a change is contemplated. The dose should then be adjusted based on patient response.

When changing between opioids, the physician must be aware that there is incomplete cross-tolerance between opioids. Some advocate a 25% to 50% reduction in the new drug after the equal analgesic dose is calculated to account for this.

Attempts have been made to correlate the relative analgesia provided by acetaminophen, the NSAIDs, and the opioids. Ketorolac, 10 mg orally, seems to be roughly equivalent to 60 mg codeine/650 mg acetaminophen in cancer pain.

When routes of administration are changed, differences in opioid metabolism (e.g., less first-pass metabolism with intravenous, intramuscular, or subcutaneous administration compared with oral dosing) necessitate adjustments to the opioid dose as indicated in Table 72-3. For example, an equivalent dose of intravenous, intramuscular, or subcutaneous morphine is one half to one third of the amount given orally.

Clearance/Buildup

Acetaminophen is metabolized in the liver and becomes toxic if metabolic pathways become saturated (usually at doses greater than 4 g per 24 hours). Therefore, its use in liver failure or in the setting of significant liver injury is contraindicated. ASA and many of the commonly used NSAIDs (e.g., naproxen, ibuprofen) are also primarily metabolized and/or eliminated by the liver (exceptions include piroxicam).

The opioids are conjugated in the liver, and more than 90% is excreted renally. Although most of the opioid metabolites are inactive, some (e.g., morphine 6-glucuronide) have analgesic activity and several may be responsible for some observed side effects. Mild elevation in transaminases should not significantly impact opioid dosing. Patients with severe liver failure should have their opioid doses decreased and dosing intervals increased.

Impaired renal excretion reduces opioid clearance and may lead to buildup of metabolites. Analgesia is sustained, and the risk of side effects is increased. To reduce the risk of buildup, patients receiving opioids should be well hydrated, and adequate urine output should be maintained. If renal function is impaired, opioid doses should be decreased and dosing intervals increased. The patient with anuria may require very little extra opioid to maintain analgesia. Routine dosing should be discontinued. Maintain analgesia with as-needed (prn) dosing.

Opioid Side Effects

The common and uncommon side effects of the opioid analgesics are listed in Table 72-4.

Common side effects of the opioid analgesics are easily managed. In most patients, pharmacologic tolerance develops to all of the common side effects except

TABLE 72-3. EQUAL ANALGESIA

Oral Dose (mg)	Analgesic	Parenteral Dose (mg)*
150	Meperidine	50
100	Codeine	60
15	Hydrocodone	—
15	Morphine	5
10	Methadone	5
10	Oxycodone	—
4	Hydromorphone	1.5
2	Levorphanol	1
—	Fentanyl	0.050

*Intravenous, subcutaneous, or intramuscular administration.

TABLE 72–4. SIDE EFFECTS OF OPIOID ANALGESICS

Common	Uncommon
Constipation	Dysphoria/delirium
Nausea/vomiting	Bad dreams/hallucinations
Drowsiness	Pruritus/urticaria
Dry mouth	Urinary retention
Sweats	Myoclonic jerks/seizures
	Respiratory depression

constipation within 1 to 2 weeks. Consequently, nausea and vomiting may be treated expectantly with antiemetics for the short period that these symptoms are problematic. If nausea and/or vomiting persists, simply changing the opioid or the route of administration may resolve the problem.

Similarly, patients should be counseled that the drowsiness they experience when initiating an opioid will usually dissipate after the first week or so. Patients can often tolerate a little drowsiness if they are assured that it will not persist for the entire time they are taking opioid analgesics. Once a stable dose of an opioid has been reached, drowsiness will probably settle completely, function will normalize, and most patients on a stable dose of opioid may safely drive a car. Persistent somnolence may be managed by ensuring adequate hydration and renal clearance, changing to a sustained release product to minimize peak effects, changing the opioid, changing the route of administration, or adding a psychostimulant (e.g., methylphenidate, pemoline).

Because patients given opioid analgesics do not develop tolerance to constipation, they should be treated with cathartic laxatives (e.g., Senna, Bisacodyl), osmotic laxatives (e.g., magnesium salts, lactulose), or prokinetic agents (e.g., metoclopramide, cisapride) on a routine basis. Simple stool softeners (e.g., sodium docusate) usually are ineffective.

Persistent side effects of the opioids seem to be somewhat idiosyncratic to the drug and the individual patient. Simply changing to an alternative opioid at an equal analgesic dose often clears the problem.

The uncommon side effects of the opioids are also manageable. The dysphoria and confusion that occasionally occur may be managed by ensuring adequate hydration and renal clearance (thereby minimizing metabolite buildup), lowering the opioid dose, changing to another opioid analgesic, or adding low doses of a neuroleptic drug (e.g., haloperidol, chlorpromazine, risperidone).

The pruritus and urticaria that occur with opioids are not immune mediated but represent a nonspecific release of histamine from mast cells in the skin. This may be managed with long-acting antihistamines or by changing to an alternative opioid analgesic. True allergy presenting as bronchospasm leading to anaphylaxis is extremely rare. Most patients who report allergy have had poorly managed side effects (usually nausea and vomiting and/or constipation) or too much medication given too fast (leading to drowsiness and/or confusion).

The risk of respiratory depression from opioid analgesics in patients with pain is frequently misunderstood.

Pain is a potent stimulus to breathe and a significant stressor. Although the effects of the first dose in an opioid-naive patient are not certain, patients develop pharmacologic tolerance to the respiratory depressant effects of opioids over the same time course as other side effects. Consequently, in the patient with chronic pain taking opioid analgesics for any significant length of time, it is difficult to demonstrate significant respiratory depression even with large doses of opioids.

Too frequently opioids have been withheld or underdosed because of unsubstantiated fear of respiratory depression or the mismanagement of side effects. In the patient with uncontrolled pain, narcotic analgesics can be judiciously but expeditiously and safely titrated until adequate relief is obtained or intolerable side effects are encountered.

Opioid Excess and Overdose

In the setting of pain management, increasing opioid excess manifests first as mild drowsiness and proceeds to persistent somnolence, then to a poorly arousable state, and finally to respiratory depression. These changes may be associated with increasing restlessness, agitation, confusion, dreams, hallucinations, myoclonic jerks, or even sudden onset of seizures.

When assessing a patient for respiratory depression, it is important to remember that a respiratory rate of 8 to 12 is frequently normal, particularly at nighttime and is not associated with any change in blood gases or clinical compromise.

If early or even moderate excess is present without major compromise, the opioid can be withheld and normal metabolism will clear the excess opioid, particularly if the poorly hydrated patient is adequately rehydrated. Naloxone reversal usually is not necessary.

If the patient is not arousable, the respiratory rate is less than 6 to 8 per minute, or there is significant hypoxemia or hypotension, opioid reversal with naloxone may be warranted. Dilute a 0.4 or 1.0 mg ampule of naloxone with 10 mL of saline and administer intravenous boluses of 0.1 to 0.2 mg every 1 to 2 minutes. Subcutaneous or oral administration is not appropriate. Because naloxone has a high affinity for opioid receptors, faster titration, or with larger boluses, may precipitate acute opioid withdrawal that manifests as an acute pain crisis, psychosis, or severe abdominal pain leading to pulmonary edema or even myocardial infarction. Only if several 0.1 to 0.2 mg boluses are ineffective should the bolus size be increased.

Naloxone has a high affinity for lipids and redistributes itself into adipose tissue within 10 to 15 minutes of administration. Often, any improvement seems to disappear within this time frame and signs of toxicity return. Repeated naloxone dosing may be necessary to sustain the reversal until the patient has cleared sufficient opioid to be out of danger. If the overdose is severe and considerable naloxone is needed, a continuous infusion of naloxone may be required until the crisis is over.

If a patient who has been well managed on a stable dose of opioid for some time suddenly develops signs of overdose, the opioid should be stopped and sepsis or other causes should be ruled out. It is unlikely that the opioid alone would be the cause of this "effective overdose."

Addiction vs. Tolerance

Addiction, the psychological dependence on a drug, is also a vastly overrated and misunderstood consequence of the use of opioid analgesics. In patients with chronic pain, the incidence of addiction is less than 1 in 1000 and is usually related to preexisting psychological dependency. Because of its rarity, it is not listed in Table 72-1 with the other side effects of the opioids.

Physical dependence, the development of a withdrawal syndrome on abrupt discontinuation of a drug, is not evidence of addiction. Physical dependence occurs over the same time course in which tolerance develops to the side effects of the opioid analgesics and is the result of changes in the numbers and function of opioid neuroreceptors in the presence of exogenous opioid.

If opioid analgesics are tapered instead of abruptly withdrawn, withdrawal symptoms do not occur. Usually the opioid dose can be reduced by 50% to 75% every 2 to 3 days without ill effect. Occasionally, a small dose of a benzodiazepine (e.g., 0.5 to 1.0 mg of lorazepam) or of methadone (with its longer half-life) may be necessary to settle the feeling of slight uneasiness or restlessness that accompanies the tapering process. If restlessness or agitation is anything more than very mild, the rate of tapering should be slowed.

ADJUVANT PAIN MEDICINES

Adjuvant analgesics are drugs used to enhance the analgesic efficacy of opioids, treat concurrent symptoms that exacerbate pain, and/or provide independent analgesia for specific types of pain. They may be used in all stages of the analgesic ladder. Some of the adjuvants, such as acetaminophen, the NSAIDs, the tricyclic antidepressants, and perhaps the antiepileptics, have primary analgesic activity themselves and may be used alone or as coanalgesics.

Two cancer pain syndromes bear particular mention in this regard. Bone pain from bone metastases is thought to be, in part, mediated by prostaglandins. Consequently, the NSAIDs and/or steroids may be particularly helpful in combination with opioids. Cord compression should always be considered if back pain is severe, increases quickly, or is associated with motor, bowel, or bladder dysfunction.

Neuropathic pain is rarely controlled with opioids alone. Tricyclic antidepressants, antiepileptics, and steroids are often required in combination with the opioids to achieve adequate relief. Commonly used agents are listed here with a few comments about their use.

NSAIDs or acetaminophen, or both, may be added to the opioids for adjuvant analgesia, particularly if inflammatory or peripheral mechanisms are thought to be responsible for the painful stimulus.

Corticosteroids provide a range of effects including anti-inflammatory activity, mood elevation, antiemetic activity, and appetite stimulation. They reduce pain both by their anti-inflammatory effect of reducing arachidonic acid release to form prostaglandins and by decreasing swelling and pressure on nerve endings. Undesirable effects such as hyperglycemia, weight gain, myopathy, and dysphoria or psychosis may complicate prolonged therapy.

Anticonvulsants (e.g., carbamazepine, valproate, clonazepam, phenytoin, gabapentin) are used either alone or in addition to opioids or other coanalgesics to manage neuropathic pain. They have been advocated particularly for neuropathic pain with a shooting or lancinating quality, such as trigeminal neuralgia or nerve root compression.

Tricyclic antidepressants (e.g., amitriptyline, desipramine, imipramine, nortriptyline) are useful in pain management in general, and for neuropathic pain in particular. They have innate analgesic properties and are effective through mechanisms that include enhanced inhibitory modulation of nociceptive impulses at the level of the dorsal horn. If the anticholinergic side effects of tertiary amine tricyclics (amitriptyline, imipramine) are undesirable or troublesome, the secondary amine tricyclics (nortriptyline, desipramine) may be effective analgesics and produce fewer side effects. The selective serotonin reuptake inhibitor class of antidepressants has not been shown to be useful in the same way as the tricyclic antidepressants.

Bisphosphonates (e.g., pamidronate) and *calcitonin* have been used as adjuvant analgesics in the management of bone pain from bone metastases. In cancer, bone pain results in large part from osteoclast-induced bone resorption rather than from the direct effects of the tumor on periosteal or medullary nerve endings. Both the bisphosphonates and calcitonin inhibit osteoclast activity on bone and have been reported to reduce pain significantly in at least some patients.

Neuroleptic medications (e.g., haloperidol, chlorpromazine, risperidone) and anxiolytics (e.g., lorazepam) are used for the management of specific psychiatric disorders that complicate pain management, such as delirium, psychosis, or anxiety disorders. With the exception of methotrimeprazine and clonazepam, none has been shown to have intrinsic analgesic activity.

SUMMARY

Appropriate pharmacologic intervention can effectively manage most pain. Medications should be chosen appropriately, they should be administered with the guidance of pharmacologic principles, and patients monitored closely for undesired side effects. Some frequently associated side effects may also require preventative intervention.

BIBLIOGRAPHY

Bonica JJ: Cancer pain. *In* Bonica JJ (ed): The Management of Pain. Philadelphia, Lea & Febiger, 1990, pp 400-460.

Doyle D, Hancks G, MacDonald N: Oxford Textbook of Palliative Medicine. New York, Oxford University Press, 1997.

Jacox A, Carr DB, Payne R, et al: Management of Cancer Pain: Clinical Practice Guideline No. 9. AHCPR publication No. 94-0592. Rockville, Md, Agency for Health Care Policy and Research, US Department of Health and Human Services, Public Health Service, March 1994.

Levy MH: Pharmacologic treatment of cancer pain. N Engl J Med 35:1124–1132, 1996.

Librach SL, Squires BP: The Pain Manual: Principles and Issues in Cancer Pain Management. Toronto, Pegasus Healthcare International, 1997.

Patt RB: Cancer Pain. Philadelphia, JB Lippincott, 1993.

Chapter 73

Intrathecal and Epidural Neurolysis

Robert E. Molloy, M.D.

Neuraxial neurolytic blockade can be a valuable tool in the management of intractable pain due to advanced malignancy. The goal of these blocks is interruption of nociceptive input from injured tissues at the spinal or epidural level. The desired result is selective destruction of dorsal roots and rootlets between the spinal cord and the dorsal root ganglion. The combined selection of patient position, level of injection, and baricity of the neurolytic agent is designed to produce predictable, segmental sensory loss. The resultant analgesia should be prolonged but not permanent; axonal regeneration does occur over a period of weeks to months. Only a small minority of cancer patients are candidates for neurolytic blockade.[1]

INDICATIONS

Neurolytic subarachnoid blockade should be reserved for intractable cancer pain, particularly when it is well localized in a patient with a short life expectancy.[2] Appropriate anticancer therapy measures should be employed, along with basic analgesic drug therapy. The World Health Organization analgesic ladder should be employed with appropriate adjuvant drug therapy. Neurolytic spinal blockade is ideal for patients with advanced or terminal malignancy; for patients with pain resistant to usual analgesic measures or intolerable side effects of analgesic therapy; and for patients with unilateral pain localized to a few adjacent dermatomes, ideally situated in the trunk, away from the innervation of the extremities and sphincters[2] (Table 73-1). Additional favorable factors are a primary somatic pain mechanism; absence of midline, axial pain; and demonstrated relief with prognostic local anesthetic blocks. The presence of intraspinal tumor is associated with failure of neurolytic spinal blockade. Informed consent from patient and relatives is essential. Patients must be aware of the expected benefits and potential risks of intrathecal neurolysis. Reasonable expectations of localized analgesia, decreased analgesic requirements, and diminished side effects should be tempered by understanding that the

malignancy may continue to progress and produce pain at other sites and that the block will gradually lose effectiveness over time and may have to be repeated. Potential problems include inadequate initial pain relief, inadequate duration of relief, and weakness of the limb muscles or the rectal and bladder sphincters. Any available alternative analgesic strategies should also be discussed with the patient in a similar fashion.[1]

TECHNIQUES

An accurate pain diagnosis after comprehensive evaluation of the patient is necessary to select a technique of neurolytic spinal blockade. Documentation of preblock neurological function is essential along with the location of all malignant lesions. Prognostic spinal anesthetic blockade with a small amount of local anesthetic should be performed in a fashion that mimics the planned neurolytic block as much as possible.[3] Anesthetic baricity and volume, injection site, and patient position should be considered to achieve this goal. In general, neurolytic blockade produces less dramatic effects than the initial prognostic local anesthetic injection. The

TABLE 73-1. INTRATHECAL NEUROLYSIS

Indications for Neurolytic Spinal Block
Intractable cancer pain
Failure of analgesic therapy
Intolerable side effects of analgesic therapy
Advanced or terminal malignancy
Unilateral pain
Pain limited to a few dermatomes
Pain located in the trunk, thorax, abdomen
Primary somatic pain mechanism
Absence of intraspinal tumor spread
Effective analgesia with prognostic block
Fully informed consent of patient
Realistic expectations of patient and family

Derived from Bonica JJ, Buckley FP, Moricca G, et al.: Neurolytic blockade and hypophysectomy. *In* Bonica JJ (ed): The Management of Pain, ed 2. Philadelphia, Lea & Febiger, 1990, p 1980.

TABLE 73-2. AGENTS FOR NEUROLYTIC SPINAL BLOCKADE

Agent	Alcohol	Phenol
Concentration	100%	4-7%
Diluent	None	Glycerin
Patient position	Lateral	Lateral
Added tilt	Semiprone	Semisupine
Painful side	Uppermost	Most dependent
Injection sensations	Immediate burning pain	Painless, warm feeling
Onset of neurolysis	Immediate	Delayed 15 minutes
Cerebrospinal fluid uptake ends	30 minutes	15 minutes
Full effect	3 to 5 days	1 day

choice of hypobaric alcohol or hyperbaric phenol is based on the location of pain and practical patient positioning considerations. There is no clear difference in efficacy (Table 73-2).

INTRATHECAL ALCOHOL

The specific gravity of absolute alcohol is less than 0.8, and that of spinal fluid is almost 1.007. Therefore, alcohol is hypobaric to and tends to move upward in cerebrospinal fluid, in a direction opposite to that of gravity. Dermatome and sclerotome charts (for bone metastases) aid in selection of nerve roots to be blocked.[4] Neurolytic spinal blockade is carried out at the level where the target dorsal root leaves the spinal cord, not where the spinal nerve passes through the intervertebral foramen (Table 73-3). This distinction is important only for lower thoracic and lumbosacral nerve root destruction. The patient must be positioned

TABLE 73-3. RELATIONSHIPS OF SPINAL VERTEBRAE TO SPINAL CORD LEVELS

Interspace Used for Injection	Nerve Rootlets Arising from Cord
C5-6	C6, C7
C6-7	C8
C7-T1	T1, T2
T1-2	T2, T3
T2-3	T3, T4
T3-4	T5
T4-5	T6
T5-6	T7
T6-7	T8, T9
T7-8	T9, T10
T8-9	T10, T11
T9-10	T11, T12
T10-11	T12 to L2
T11-12	L2 to L5
T12-L1	L5 to S5

Derived from Bonica JJ, Buckley FP, Moricca G, et al.: Neurolytic blockade and hypophysectomy. *In* Bonica JJ (ed): The Management of Pain, ed 2. Philadelphia, Lea & Febiger, 1990, p 1980; Cousins MJ, Dwyer B, Bigg D: Chronic pain and neurolytic blockade. *In* Cousins MJ, Bridenbaugh PO (eds): Neural Blockade in Clinical Anesthesia and Management of Pain, ed 2. Philadelphia, JB Lippincott, 1988, p 1043; Winnie AP: Subarachnoid neurolytic blocks. *In* Waldman SD, Winnie AP (eds): Interventional Pain Management. Philadelphia, WB Saunders, 1996, p 401.

to place the target rootlets uppermost in the subarachnoid space. The patient is placed in the lateral position with the side to be blocked uppermost. A combination of pillows, kidney rests, and table extension is used below the injection site to elevate it above adjacent spinal levels. The patient is also turned 45 degrees toward the prone position to raise the dorsal nerve rootlets into a horizontal position, superior to their adjacent ventral rootlets. This position is maintained by restraining the patient with adequate tape to prevent movement at an inopportune time.

Once the patient is in position, a short-bevel 22-gauge needle is inserted at the selected interspace. The epidural space is identified, and then cautious entry into the subarachnoid space is detected by continuous aspiration of the syringe's plunger. The needle is adjusted to ensure the bevel's location just anterior to the arachnoid membrane. Alcohol is then injected in 0.1-mL aliquots using a tuberculin syringe and at least 60 to 90 seconds between injections. Alcohol elicits temporary dermatomal burning, which can be used to confirm needle placement at the painful area. If burning is reported at a level distant from the patient's complaint, a new needle may be placed at involved sites, and 0.1-mL aliquots of alcohol may be injected through each properly placed needle. The total dose of alcohol injected for pain localized to one or two dermatomes should not exceed 0.5 to 0.7 mL. The patient remains immobilized for 30 minutes after injection to allow complete fixation of alcohol to the selected nerve roots, preventing subsequent spread to other levels. The efficacy of alcohol spinal blockade should be assessed after 3 to 5 days. Repeat injection may be necessary in some patients after this time interval.

INTRATHECAL PHENOL

Phenol in glycerin is hyperbaric relative to cerebrospinal fluid, and its spread after injection is determined by gravity. The patient must be positioned with the painful side dependent and the affected rootlets most dependent. Invariably the head of the table is elevated, and often the table is flexed under the injection site. The patient is also turned 45 degrees toward the supine position to place the target dorsal rootlets in the most dependent position. Hyperbaric phenol seems well suited to treat pelvic and perineal pain with unilateral blocks on each side or, alternatively, with a saddle block performed in one sitting.[5] The solution is extremely viscous and difficult to inject, even when a 20-gauge, short-bevel needle is used. Phenol is injected in 0.1-mL increments up to a total dose similar to that used with alcohol.[5] With both agents, the needle should be cleared with 0.2 mL of air before it is withdrawn. Phenol fixes within 15 minutes, but the patient should remain in position for 30 minutes after injection. Phenol produces an initial local anesthetic effect, but no injection pain occurs. The resultant analgesia can be assessed after 1 day, allowing for earlier decisions about repeat injection than after alcohol spinal blockade.

RESULTS

Neurolytic spinal blockade can produce profound unilateral segmental analgesia. Frequently incomplete analgesia occurs, but this may be remedied by repeating the injection. The most likely causes of treatment failure are unreasonable expectations and poor patient selection. The results of published series are difficult to interpret because of differences in tumor type and site; neurolytic agent, dose, and site of injection; and definitions of pain relief. Specific data on drug intake, pain scores, nausea and sleep scales, activity levels, and severity and duration of side effects are not uniformly reported. Bonica and colleagues[1] attempted to compare the best studies reporting the results of subarachnoid alcohol and phenol in three broad categories: good, fair, and poor pain relief. Their conclusions are summarized in Table 73-4.

The superiority of one neurolytic agent over the other has not been established. Many authors believe that pain relief may be better and last longer with alcohol than with phenol.

COMPLICATIONS

Side effects of neurolytic spinal blockade include post–dural puncture headache, rare meningitis, loss of touch and position sense, persistent numbness and paresthesias, and loss of motor function due to unintended neurolysis of ventral rootlets. The most serious complications are muscle weakness of the extremities and paresis of the urinary and rectal sphincters. These latter complications occur relatively frequently. Fortunately, they are usually transient occurrences, resolving within 1 week in many patients. Gerbershagen[6] reviewed reports that provided data on the duration of 303 complications after intrathecal neurolysis and observed when they disappeared: 28% did so within 3 days, 23% within 1 week, 21% within 1 month, 9% within 4 months, and 18% after more than 4 months. Bonica and associates summarized the incidence of serious neurological complications based on 11 studies[1]; these data are adapted and summarized in Table 73-5. The overall incidence of each condition is recorded along with the figure for prolonged or permanent conditions when available.

Acute paraplegia may occur immediately after intrathecal neurolysis when undiagnosed metastatic spinal tumor is present before blockade.[7, 8] The acute neurological deterioration may be related to traumatic needling

TABLE 73-4. SUBARACHNOID BLOCKS
FOR CANCER PAIN RELIEF

Agent	No. of Studies	No. of Patients	Good Results	Fair Results	Poor Results
Alcohol	13	1634	61%	24%	15%
Phenol	12	1982	58%	16%	28%

Data extracted and modified from Bonica JJ, Buckley FP, Moricca G, et al.: Neurolytic blockade and hypophysectomy. *In* Bonica JJ (ed): The Management of Pain, ed 2. Philadelphia, Lea & Febiger, 1990, Table 96-3, p 2007 and Table 96-4, p 2008.

TABLE 73-5. SUBARACHNOID BLOCKADE
FOR CANCER PAIN RELIEF*

Agent	No. of Studies	No. of Patients	Bladder Paresis	Bowel Paresis	Motor Weakness
Alcohol	7	3123	5.7%/0.7%	1.1%/0.3%	4.9%/0.8%
Phenol	4	874	9.7%/0.8%	1.6%/0.3%	4.7%/1.5%

*Complications are given as total %/prolonged %.
Data extracted and modified from Bonica JJ, Buckley FP, Moricca G, et al.: Neurolytic blockade and hypophysectomy. *In* Bonica JJ (ed): The Management of Pain, ed 2. Philadelphia, Lea & Febiger, 1990, Table 96-25, p 2009.

of tumor but also may occur even when spinal injection is performed many segments away from the spinal metastatic disease.

EPIDURAL NEUROLYTIC BLOCK

Epidural neurolysis has been used as an alternative approach to subarachnoid blockade. It provides relief of pain that is bilateral, but analgesia may be less profound than after intrathecal neurolysis. Some of the proposed advantages of this technique are better efficacy for cervical and cervicothoracic junction pain, increased safety, and ease of repeated injections. Some of these advantages remain theoretical. Placement of a thoracic epidural catheter may be less demanding to some practitioners than positioning of multiple needles just barely into the subarachnoid space but not within the substance of the spinal cord.

Technique

Injection may be made through an epidural needle or catheter. The needle should be placed near the vertebral levels corresponding to the dermatomal levels that supply the patient's painful lesion. A large needle is required to inject phenol in glycerin, but a smaller needle or catheter is adequate for aqueous phenol or phenol in saline. Confirmation of correct needle placement can be made with contrast-enhanced radiologic imaging and a test dose of local anesthetic. Use of an epidural catheter allows careful confirmation of epidural position and of pain relief with a small volume (3 to 4 mL) of local anesthetic. Epidural neurolysis can then be performed through the same catheter at a later time. Racz and colleagues[9] developed a soft, nonkinking, wire-embedded epidural catheter for this purpose; it is designed to help prevent false-negative aspiration tests before injection. Aspiration without repeat local anesthetic test dosing can then be used before each injection of 5.5% phenol in saline. The volume injected should correspond to the effective dose of local anesthetic used previously. From 2 to 5 mL may be adequate depending on the injection level.[10] Racz and colleagues recommended daily repeat injection until increasingly positive responses cease to occur or the patient is free of pain after 24 hours. Korevaar[11] used a similar technique but injected ethyl alcohol on a daily basis for 3 days through a thoracic epidural catheter. Local anesthetic test doses were used before each daily dose of 3 to 5 mL of alcohol given over 25 to 30 minutes in 0.2-mL increments.[11]

Results

In four studies, the results of thoracic epidural phenol or alcohol neurolysis were positive for management of cancer pain. Initial pain relief was obtained in about 80% of patients (range, 65% to 100%).[1] The duration of benefit varied with severity of patient disease and in many cases lasted until the time of death. Among survivors, the average duration of analgesia varied from less than 1 month to longer than 3 months in different patient groups. Although some authors noted no serious complications, a greater margin of safety for epidural versus intrathecal neurolysis has not been established. Katz and associates[12] questioned the safety of epidural phenol in a study of the effects of lumbar epidural phenol on primate spinal cord 2 weeks after injection. They demonstrated lower extremity motor weakness clinically. Predominant posterior nerve root damage was observed, but anterior root and spinal cord damage also was seen. Adequate information to support the superiority of epidural versus intrathecal neurolysis is lacking.

PATIENT CARE AFTER INTRASPINAL NEUROLYTIC BLOCK

The patient may experience profound pain relief after the neurolytic block procedure. Failure to decrease long-acting analgesic therapy may result in relative overdose and predictable side effects. However, sudden cessation of all narcotic drugs is likely to lead to a withdrawal syndrome. Careful attention to gradual drug withdrawal and individual titration of opioids to manage any residual pain at the target area or at distant sites is required. Assessment of the procedure's success should include the extent of change in the patient's verbal pain score, 24-hour opioid consumption, side effect profile, sleep, activity tolerance, and the objective assessment of relatives and caregivers. Careful neurological examination to document the extent and duration of any sensory or motor deficits is also required. Should such complications occur, the neurological deficits can be expected to resolve over time. Many do so quickly, and most will resolve after nerve regeneration has occurred. Patient reassurance, analgesia, and protective physical therapy should be provided in such cases. If analgesia is incomplete after appropriate evaluation, repeat injection may be offered.

Because of the anatomic separation of sensory and motor roots in the subarachnoid space, particularly at thoracic levels, intrathecal neurolytic blocks offer the unique potential to provide relatively selective unilateral sensory blockade without concomitant motor blockade. Epidural neurolytic blocks allow for repeat injections near the cervicothoracic junction and for treatment of bilateral pain. Both procedures have potential neurological complications. It is essential that these be discussed with the patient and family before the procedure, and informed consent should be documented. There has been a trend to avoid these procedures and to maximize the use of opioids by the oral, subcutaneous, intravenous, transdermal, and intraspinal routes of administration. There are some selected patients who remain good candidates for neurolytic blockade after aggressive trials of the World Health Organization cancer pain treatment guidelines.[13]

REFERENCES

1. Bonica JJ, Buckley FP, Moricca G, et al: Neurolytic blockade and hypophysectomy. *In* Bonica JJ (ed): The Management of Pain, ed 2. Philadelphia, Lea & Febiger, 1990, p 1980.
2. Cousins MJ, Dwyer B, Bigg D: Chronic pain and neurolytic blockade. *In* Cousins MJ, Bridenbaugh PO (eds): Neural Blockade in Clinical Anesthesia and Management of Pain, ed 2. Philadelphia, JB Lippincott, 1988, p 1043.
3. Swerdlow M: Complications of neurolytic neural blockade. *In* Cousins MJ, Bridenbaugh PO (eds): Neural Blockade in Clinical Anesthesia and Management of Pain, ed 2. Philadelphia, JB Lippincott, 1988, p 719.
4. Winnie AP: Subarachnoid neurolytic blocks. *In* Waldman SD, Winnie AP (eds): Interventional Pain Management. Philadelphia, WB Saunders, 1996, p 401.
5. Swerdlow M: Intrathecal and extradural block and pain relief. *In* Swerdlow M (ed): Relief of Intractable Pain. Amsterdam, Elsevier, 1983, p 175.
6. Gerbershagen HY: Neurolysis: Subarachnoid neurolytic blockade. Acta Anesthesiol Belg 1:45, 1981.
7. Hay RC: Subarachnoid alcohol block in the control of intractable pain: Report of results in 252 patients. Anesth Analg 41:12, 1962.
8. Kuzucu EY, Derrik WS, Wilber SA: Control of intractable pain with subarachnoid alcohol block. JAMA 195:541, 1966.
9. Racz GB, Sabonghy M, Gintautas J, Kline WM: Intractable pain therapy using a new epidural catheter. JAMA 248:579, 1982.
10. Racz GB, Heavner J, Haynsworth R: Repeat epidural phenol injections in chronic pain and spasticity. *In* Lipton S (ed): Persistent Pain: Modern Methods of Treatment, vol 5. New York, Grune & Stratton, 1985, p 157.
11. Korevaar WC: Transcatheter thoracic epidural neurolysis using ethyl alcohol. Anesthesiology 69:989, 1988.
12. Katz JA, Sehlhorst S, Blisard KS: Histopathologic changes in primate spinal cord after single and repeated epidural phenol administration. Reg Anesth 20:283, 1995.
13. Ventafridda V, Tamburini M, Caraceni A, et al: A validation study of the WHO method for cancer pain relief. Cancer 59:850, 1987.

Chapter 74

Celiac Plexus Block

Honorio T. Benzon, M.D.,
and Robert E. Molloy, M.D.

ANATOMY

The celiac plexus is the largest of the prevertebral plexuses in the body. It is subdivided into right and left celiac ganglia, which are located in the epigastrium, on either side of the midline, anterior to the crura of the diaphragm. The plexus extends in front of the lower half of the body of the 12th thoracic vertebra and the entire first lumbar vertebra. Occasionally, it extends to the upper portion of the second lumbar vertebra.

Each celiac ganglion receives the terminal portion of the greater, the lesser, and the least splanchnic nerves. Preganglionic sympathetics from T5–9 form the greater splanchnic nerve, T10–11 the lesser, and T12 the least. Afferent fibers from the viscera travel with these sympathetic efferents through the celiac plexus and the splanchnic nerves back to the viscera. The celiac plexus also receives a branch from both vagus nerves. Several plexuses originate from the celiac plexus; these include the phrenic, hepatic, superior and inferior gastric, splenic, renal and suprarenal ganglia and the superior mesenteric ganglion, which gives rise to the pancreatic plexus. It can be seen from this massive network of ganglia that the celiac plexus innervates all of the abdominal viscera except the left side of the colon and the pelvic viscera; these structures are innervated by the superior hypogastric plexus.

The normal anatomic variations of the celiac plexus have been studied by Ward and associates.[1] The celiac ganglia vary in number from one to five and in location from the T12 to the L1 vertebra. The ganglia are usually less than 1.5 cm in front of the anterior vertebral margin. The vertebral level of the left celiac ganglia is lower than that of the right; most are located opposite the lower or middle third of L1 on the left and above the middle third on the right. Celiac plexus block (CPB) is therefore most likely to be successful if the needle on the left side is placed at the level of the junction of the middle and lower third of the first lumbar vertebra and the needle on the right side is placed approximately 1 cm higher.[1]

TECHNIQUE OF CELIAC PLEXUS BLOCK

Diagnostic magnetic resonance imaging or computed tomography (CT) scans should be reviewed to detect any abnormal anatomy caused by extensive retroperitoneal tumor and to rule out the presence of an abdominal aortic aneurysm. If the anatomy appears unfavorable for needle placement with the classic technique, an alternative approach may be considered.

The posterior approach is the most commonly used technique. The patient lies prone, and a pillow is placed under the abdomen between the ribs and the iliac crests. A 5- or 6-in., 20-gauge needle is inserted 6 to 7.5 cm lateral to the spine of L1 at an angle of 45 degrees with the skin of the back. After contact is made with the body of L1, the needle is withdrawn and reinserted with an increased angle between the needle shaft and the skin. This maneuver is repeated until the needle tip slips off the body of the vertebra and the needle advanced 1 to 1.5 cm (Fig. 74–1). The procedure is repeated on the opposite side of L1. Twenty to 25 mL of local anesthetic (e.g., 0.125% bupivacaine) is injected through each needle. Neurolytic celiac plexus block (NCPB) with either 50% alcohol or 6% phenol is performed 24 to 48 hours later when there is significant relief of pain with the diagnostic block. Although the block can be performed blindly, the use of fluoroscopy or CT is advisable, especially when neurolytic agents are injected. Fluoroscopy can be used to verify needle placement anterior to the L1 vertebral body in the lateral view. The proper distribution of the injected contrast material can be confirmed in both anteroposterior and lateral views. The contrast agent should be seen anterior to the L1 body and the psoas fascia and should not appear to be intravascular.

Moore and colleagues[2] studied CPB with the use of x-rays and CT scans in patients and corpses. They showed that maximum spread of the drug is favored by bilateral placement of needles, injection of at least 25 mL through each needle, and placement of the left

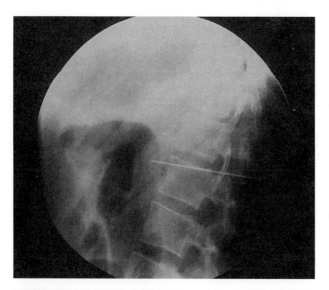

FIGURE 74–1. Lateral radiographic view showing the tip of the needle at 1.0 to 1.5 cm anterior to the body of the L1 vertebra.

needle tip immediately behind the aorta with the right needle adjacent to the lateral wall of the aorta. They recommended that the site of insertion of the needle not exceed 7.5 cm from the spinous process of the lumbar vertebra to avoid puncture of the kidneys.

Singler[3] described the transcrural approach with CT guidance. The celiac artery is located, and the left needle is inserted 4 cm lateral to the midline until its tip is immediately adjacent to the anterolateral wall of the aorta. The right needle is inserted 5 to 10 cm lateral to the midline; both needles pass through the crura of the diaphragm (Fig. 74–2). A smaller volume is required, 10 to 20 mL, compared with the classic technique.

Ischia and co-workers[4] described a transaortic approach designed to provide analgesia with a single needle placement, a low volume of injectate, and avoidance of posterior spread to the sympathetic chain and the lumbar somatic roots. A single left-sided needle is placed slightly closer to the midline and advanced until it passes into and through the aorta, confirmed by saline

loss of resistance to identify the preaortic space. Fluoroscopy confirms needle placement about 4 cm anterior to the L1 vertebral body and appropriate spread of contrast material.

An anterior approach to the celiac plexus can be performed with a single needle placed through the abdominal wall and viscera.[5] It aims to avoid patient discomfort induced by the prone position, to shorten the procedure time, and to decrease the risk of neurological complications. The needle is inserted below the xiphoid process and placed anterior to the aorta before injection of 20 mL of neurolytic agent. CT scanning has been employed to place the needle between the origins of the celiac and superior mesenteric arteries.[5] Ultrasound has also been used to guide needle advancement to the same preaortic location.[6]

The effectiveness of the three posterior percutaneous NCPB techniques—the classic retrocrural approach, the transaortic approach, and the bilateral splanchnicectomy approach—was studied by Ischia and associates.[7] They found no statistical difference in terms of quality or quantity of pain relief, whether immediate (within 5 days) or long-term (up to the time of the patients' death). Morbidity was nil with all three techniques. The incidence of hypotension was less with the transaortic technique, probably because of limited or nonexistent spread of the drug in the psoas compartment, which contains the sympathetic chain.

Some investigators recommend a diagnostic block before the neurolytic block is performed. The advantages of a diagnostic block include evaluation of the effectiveness and physiologic consequences of the block and observation of the patient's response to discontinuation of the opioid. Others recommend against a diagnostic block because several factors limit its prognostic ability, including a placebo effect, differences in local diffusion and mechanism of action between the local anesthetic and the neurolytic agent, and systemic absorption of the local anesthetic resulting in possible analgesia.

Complications of CPB include arterial hypotension from splanchnic vasodilatation, subarachnoid injection, epidural or somatic nerve block, paralysis, kidney punc-

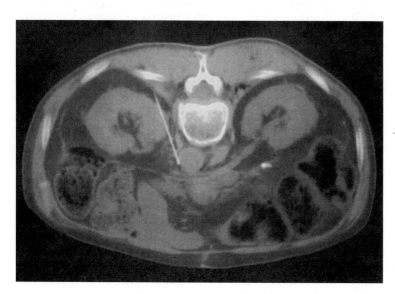

FIGURE 74–2. Computed tomographic (CT) scan showing the needle adjacent to the lateral wall of the aorta, anterior to the crura of the diaphragm.

ture, pneumothorax, back pain, retroperitoneal fibrosis after multiple CPBs, sexual dysfunction, monoparesis with loss of anal and bladder sphincter function, retroperitoneal hematoma, aortic dissection with necrosis of the duodenum and proximal jejenum[8] (evidence of dissection and thrombosis of the superior mesenteric and hepatic arteries), and intravascular injection. Intravascular injection of phenol results in convulsions; phenol increases acetylcholine concentrations, facilitating central synaptic transmission and neuronal hyperexcitability.[9]

Acute paraplegia represents the most serious potential complication. It may occur after unintentional spinal or epidural injection. It has also been attributed to traumatic neurolytic injury to the artery of Adamkiewicz. Exposure to alcohol and phenol induces vasospasm of segmental lumbar arteries in dogs.[10] Low concentrations of ethanol produce significant contractile effects in human aortic smooth muscle cells by increasing the intracellular concentration of ionized calcium.[11]

EFFECTIVENESS OF NEUROLYTIC CELIAC PLEXUS BLOCK

Early clinical studies looked at the effectiveness of NCPB in relieving abdominal pain caused by malignancy.[12, 13] These studies reported success rates of 91% to 94%. Of the 91 patients who responded to NCPB, 48 were pain free until their death, 32 needed mild analgesics, and 11 required morphine during their last few weeks of life. Spread of the cancer to organs beyond the innervation of the celiac plexus was the main reason for opioid intake.

When NCPB was used to relieve the pain of pancreatic cancer, immediate pain relief was reported in 70% to 86% of patients.[7, 14, 15] In the series of Brown and coworkers,[14] 75% of 136 patients had pain relief that lasted until their death. Ischia and colleagues[7] reported that celiac pain was immediately relieved in 70% to 80% of 61 patients; 60% to 75% of the patients had no recurrence of celiac pain before death. In this study celiac pain was only a component of the pancreatic cancer pain. When all types of pain were considered (e.g., hip, shoulder), NCPB was immediately effective in 40% to 52% of the patients, with long-term effectiveness in only 10 to 24%. The authors noted that complete pain relief was significantly greater when the onset of pain occurred less than 2 months before NCPB (72% success rate versus 37%). Later in the patients' clinical course, the malignancy involved extraceliac structures and NCPB alone was ineffective.[7] Combination therapy (i.e., with NSAIDs or opioids) was required and was recommended.

Two reviews on the management of pain secondary to pancreatic cancer concluded that NCPB is a very effective technique when compared with other methods.[16, 17] However, there were numerous methodologic flaws in the published studies. Sharfman and Walsh[17] reviewed 15 papers on NCPB for pancreatic cancer pain and reported satisfactory response in 418 (87%) of 480 patients. Deficiencies in the published studies included

lack of a control group, lack of pre-NCPB analgesic history, and limited postblock data including post-NCPB analgesic dosages. A study that compared NCPB with traditional analgesic management showed a reduction in opioid consumption for about 51 days after NCPB.[18] The administration of analgesics alone resulted in an equal reduction of pain scores (visual analogue scale) until death but with more unpleasant side effects.[18]

Eisenberg and colleagues[19] performed a meta-analysis of the efficacy and safety of NCPB for cancer pain based on 24 papers describing the use of this treatment in 1145 patients (63% of the patients had pancreatic cancer). Good to excellent pain relief was reported in 89% of the patients during the first 2 weeks after NCPB. Partial to complete relief continued in 90% of the patients who were alive at 3 months and in 70% to 90% of the patients until death. Transient side effects included local pain (96%), diarrhea (44%), and hypotension (38%). Neurological complications were reported in 1% of the patients. This analysis failed to demonstrate a higher success rate or a lower incidence of complications when imaging techniques (radiography, fluoroscopy, CT, or ultrasound) were used for guidance.[19]

NCPB is an effective tool for treating the pain of upper abdominal malignancy, especially pancreatic cancer. However, additional anticancer, analgesic, and supportive interventions are required to maximize patient comfort. Future advances to eliminate the risk of neurological injury are desirable.

NEUROLYTIC CELIAC PLEXUS BLOCK AND BENIGN PAIN

An objection to the use of NCPB in patients with chronic benign pain is that it may mask the signs and symptoms of an acute abdomen. Although this has not been observed in patients with cancer pain because the patients die within a few months of their diagnosis, its occurrence is possible in those with chronic benign pain. Hastings and McKay[20] showed that NCPB can be performed safely in such patients and recommended its use when all other treatments fail. They described a woman with severe visceral pain from celiac axis compression syndrome. Bedridden for 4 months, she had four NCPBs which relieved her pain and allowed her to resume her previous lifestyle. The authors pointed out that abdominal pathology, in the presence of a neurolyzed celiac plexus, will ultimately cause pain. Peritoneal irritation causes pain via spinal nerves from the body wall adjacent to the inflamed organ. The large bowel distal to the left colonic flexure and pelvic organs send visceral sympathetic nerves through the hypogastric plexus and retain intact visceral pain sensation. The intraperitoneal organs and the mesentery send afferent nerves directly to the spinal nerves. Finally, bowel obstruction eventually causes vomiting, distention, and cessation of flatus.[20] The fact that patients with bowel ischemia do not always present with pain and that NCPB may mask early signs of bowel obstruction or ischemia calls for vigilance for the signs and symptoms of acute abdomen in the rare patient who has had NCPB for noncancer abdominal pain.

REFERENCES

1. Ward EM, Rorie DK, Nauss LA, et al: The celiac ganglia in man: Normal anatomic variations. Anesth Analg 58:461, 1979.
2. Moore DC, Bush WH, Burnett LL: Celiac plexus block: A roentgenographic, anatomic study of technique and spread of solutions in patients and corpses. Anesth Analg 60:369, 1981.
3. Singler RL: An improved technique for alcohol neurolysis of the celiac plexus. Anesthesiology 56:137, 1982.
4. Ischia S, Luzzani A, Ischia A, et al: A new approach to the neurolytic block of the coeliac plexus: The transaortic technique. Pain 16:333, 1983.
5. Romanelli DF, Beckman CF, Heiss FW: Celiac plexus block: Efficacy and safety of the anterior approach. Am J Roentgenol 160:497, 1993.
6. Gimenez A, Martinez-Noguera A, Donoso L, et al: Percutaneous neurolysis of the celiac plexus via the anterior approach with sonographic guidance. Am J Roentgenol 161:1061, 1993.
7. Ischia S, Ischia A, Polati E, et al: Three posterior percutaneous celiac plexus block techniques. Anesthesiology 76:534, 1992.
8. Kaplan R, Schiff-Keren B, Alt E: Aortic dissection as a complication of celiac plexus block. Anesthesiology 83:632, 1995.
9. Benzon HT: Convulsions secondary to phenol: A hazard of celiac plexus block. Anesth Analg 58:150, 1979.
10. Brown DL, Rorie DK: Altered reactivity of isolated segmental lumbar arteries of dogs following exposure to ethanol and phenol. Pain 56:139, 1994.
11. Johnson ME, Sill JC, Brown DL, et al: The effect of the neurolytic agent ethanol on cytoplasmic calcium in arterial smooth muscle and endothelium. Reg Anesth 21:6, 1996.
12. Thompson GE, Moore DL, Bridenbaugh LD, et al: Abdominal pain and alcohol celiac plexus block. Anesth Analg 56:1, 1977.
13. Jones J, Grough D: Coeliac plexus block with alcohol for relief of upper abdominal pain due to cancer. Ann R Coll Surg Engl 59:46, 1977.
14. Brown DI, Bulley CK, Quiel EL: Neurolytic celiac plexus block for pancreatic cancer pain. Anesth Analg 66:869, 1987.
15. Hegedus V: Relief of pancreatic pain by radiograph guided block. Am J Roentgenol 133:1101, 1979.
16. Lebovits AH, Lefkowitz M: Pain management of pancreatic carcinoma: A review. Pain 36:1, 1989.
17. Sharfman WH, Walsh TD: Has the analgesic efficacy of neurolytic celiac plexus block been demonstrated in pancreatic cancer pain? Pain 41:267, 1990.
18. Mercadante S: Celiac plexus block versus analgesics in pancreatic cancer pain. Pain 52:187, 1993.
19. Eisenberg E, Carr DB, Chalmers TC: Neurolytic celiac plexus block for treatment of cancer pain: A meta-analysis. Anesth Analg 80:290, 1995.
20. Hastings RH, McKay WR: Treatment of chronic benign abdominal pain with neurolytic celiac plexus block. Anesthesiology 75:156, 1991.

Superior Hypogastric Plexus Block Neurolysis for Cancer Pain

Oscar A. de Leon-Casasola, M.D.

Pain associated with cancer may be somatic, visceral, and neuropathic in origin. Visceral pain is typically present in the early stages of cancer when the tumor is localized within a viscus. When visceral structures are stretched, compressed, invaded, or distended, a poorly localized noxious pain is reported. Patients often describe the pain as vague, deep, squeezing, crampy, or colic in nature, and the pain frequently radiates to other parts of the body.

Neurolysis of the sympathetic axis is an important adjunct to pharmacologic therapy for the relief of severe visceral pain experienced by cancer patients. Rarely can these blocks eliminate pain in cancer patients, because somatic and neuropathic pain may also be present. Therefore, other analgesic agents and adjuvant therapy are needed. The goals of neurolytic superior hypogastric plexus blocks are (1) to maximize the analgesic effect of opioid and nonopioid analgesics and (2) to reduce the dosage of these agents so as to alleviate untoward side effects.

SUPERIOR HYPOGASTRIC PLEXUS BLOCK

Pelvic pain associated with either cancer[1, 2] or chronic benign conditions[3, 4] may be alleviated by blockade of the superior hypogastric plexus. Analgesia to the organs in the pelvis is possible because the afferent fibers innervating these structures travel in the sympathetic nerves, trunks, ganglia, and rami. A sympathectomy for visceral pain therefore has the same effect as a peripheral neurectomy or dorsal rhizotomy for somatic pain.[5] Moreover, since visceral pain may be an important component of pelvic pain associated with cancer,[1, 2, 6] significant pain control may be achieved with percutaneous neurolytic blocks of the superior hypogastric plexus.

The superior hypogastric plexus is in the retroperitoneum, bilaterally extending from the lower third of the fifth lumbar vertebral body to the upper third of the first sacral vertebral body (Fig. 75-1).

Efficacy

The efficacy of neurolytic superior hypogastric plexus blocks has been demonstrated in patients with cancer-related pelvic pain who either failed to derive further benefits from oral opioid therapy or experienced excessive side effects from this mode of therapy.[1, 2, 7] The effectiveness of this technique was originally demonstrated by documentation of a significant decrease in pain scores on a visual analogue scale (VAS). In that

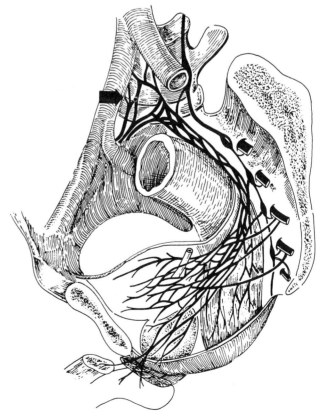

FIGURE 75–1. Simplified anatomy of the pelvis. *Bold arrow* points to the superior hypogastric plexus.

study, Plancarte and colleagues[1] showed that the block was effective in reducing VAS scores in 70% of the patients with pelvic pain associated with cancer.[1] In a subsequent study, our own group reported similar results[2]: 69% of the patients experienced both a decrease in VAS scores and a reduction in mean daily opioid morphine use of 67% in the success group (from 736 ± 633 to 251 ± 191 mg/day) and 45% in the failure group (from 1443 ± 703 to 800 ± 345 mg/day). In a more recent multicenter study,[7] 159 patients with pelvic pain associated with cancer were evaluated. Overall, 115 patients (72%) had satisfactory pain relief after one or two neurolytic procedures. Mean opioid use decreased by 40% (from 58 ± 43 to 35 ± 18 equianalgesic milligrams per day of morphine) at 3 weeks after treatment in all the studied patients. This decrease in opioid consumption was significant for both the success group (56 ± 32 to 32 ± 16 mg/day) and the failure group (65 ± 28 to 48 ± 21 mg/day).

Three important conclusions may be drawn from the results of these three studies. First, reductions in pain scores and in opioid consumption are significant even in advanced stages of cancer disease, suggesting that visceral pain may be an important component of cancer pain even in the late stages of the disease. The visceral component of pelvic cancer pain has been considered important only in the early stages of disease.[8] In our experience, differentiation of somatic pain from visceral pain in advanced stages of pelvic cancer is very difficult. Not only do all components exist, but a continuous acute pain probably occurs as well, in response to an expanding tumor mass.[9]

Second, neurolysis is not as effective in the presence of significant retroperitoneal lymph node involvement (20% vs. 70% response rate). The lack of success may have also been influenced by the involvement of nervous structures (neuropathic pain) or by tumor spread to other somatic structures (somatic pain) within the pelvis. However, patients with extensive retroperitoneal pelvic involvement who showed a confluence of contrast material in the midline (posteroanterior fluoroscopy projections) experienced good results in one of the studies.[2]

Third, considering the cost of pharmacologic therapy, use of this blockade early in the management of pelvic pain associated with cancer may be economically sound. This is based on the opioid reduction experienced by patients in both the failure and the success groups.[2, 7]

Technique

The technique for the performance of the block is straightforward. Patients are admitted to the ambulatory surgery center and then taken to the operating room, where routine monitors are connected. Patients are placed in the prone position with a pillow under the pelvis to flatten the lumbar lordosis. The L4–5 intervertebral space is then found and marked. Antisepsis with an iodine solution and placement of sterile sheets in the lumbosacral area are done. Sedation is provided with combinations of opioids and benzodiazepines. Skin

wheals are raised 5 to 7 cm bilaterally to the midline (depending on the patient's height and girth) at the level of the L4–5 interspace with 1% lidocaine. Two 15-cm, 22-gauge Chiba needles (Cook; Bloomington, Indiana) are then inserted through the skin wheals with the bevels directed medially. Both needles are inserted 45 degrees mesiad (off the coronal plane) and 30 degrees caudad (off the medial sagittal plane) so that the needle tips lie anterolateral to the L5–S1 intervertebral space (Fig. 75–2). Although the transverse process of L5 is frequently encountered, a slight change in the angle of insertion or use of insertion points 1 cm more lateral or more medial to the original point of entry allows needle advancement. When the vertebral body of L5 is encountered, retrieval of the needle to superficial planes and reinsertion with slight concavity of the shaft helps correct placement.

Careful aspiration to determine intravascular placement should always be done. If blood is obtained during aspiration, the needle is advanced while aspiration is continued until no more blood can be obtained. Biplanar fluoroscopy and 2 to 3 mL of water-soluble contrast medium are used to verify accurate placement of the needles and to rule out intravascular injection (Figs. 75–3 and 75–4). Accurate placement of the needles is determined by the collection of contrast medium just anterior to the L5–S1 intervertebral space. A diagnostic block with 8 mL of 0.25% bupivacaine injected through each needle may be performed. If the patient reports a 50% reduction in the pain intensity, a neurolytic block should then be done. Some patients, despite apparent success with the diagnostic block, fail to experience an analgesic response from neurolytic blockade. Variations in the intensity of pain during the day, placebo effect, or differences in needle placement between the diagnostic and the neurolytic block may explain such discrepancies. Moreover, we found extensive retroperitoneal disease in all patients who experienced a favorable response to a diagnostic block but failed to derive any benefits from the neurolytic blocks.[2]

Our practice is to perform a neurolytic block without a diagnostic block. This rationale is based on the low incidence of side effects associated with this block and the savings in hospitalization and patient inconvenience.

For neurolysis, 8 mL of 10% phenol (dissolved in sterile water just before injection) is used on each side.

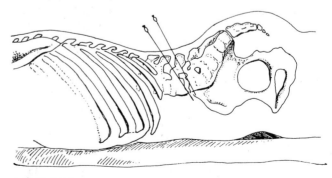

FIGURE 75–2. Cross-lateral view of patient lying in prone position, illustrating the position of the tip of the Chiba needles for performing the superior hypogastric plexus block.

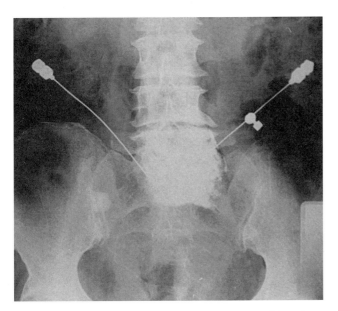

FIGURE 75–3. Posteroanterior radiograph demonstrating bilateral correct needle placement and adequate spread of the contrast medium.

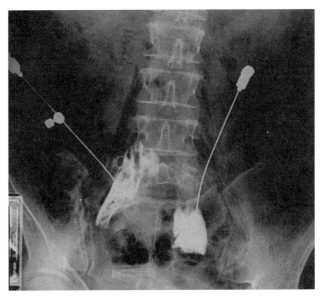

FIGURE 75–5. Anteroposterior radiograph showing correct needle placement but inadequate spread of the contrast medium due to tumor spread.

A suspension may be formed when the phenol is mixed with the sterile water; however, if it is prepared immediately before needle placement has been confirmed, it will be clinically effective.[1, 2, 7]

Some authors have suggested that neurolysis of the superior hypogastric plexus block may be done with a single needle and computed tomographic guidance.[10] This is an appropriate approach provided that there is no evidence of retroperitoneal tumor activity, which would affect the spread of the neurolytic agent[6] (Fig. 75-5).

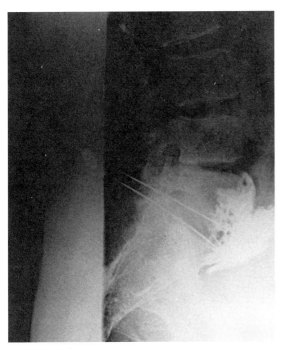

FIGURE 75–4. Cross-lateral radiograph demonstrating correct needle placement and adequate spread of the contrast medium.

Patient Care

After the block, patients are taken to the Post Anesthesia Care Unit (PACU), where VAS scores are evaluated on arrival, 30 minutes later, and 60 minutes later. Patients are then discharged home and re-evaluated by telephone after 24 and 48 hours. If adequate pain control is reported, they are re-evaluated every 2 weeks in the Pain Clinic to assess the quality of pain control and the incidence of side effects. Criteria for success of neurolytic blockade vary. Our group has used the following criteria: (1) a decrease in VAS of at least 60% or a pain intensity level lower than 3 (scale of 0 to 10) during the first 3 weeks after neurolytic blockade, and (2) a decrease in oral opioid requirements of at least 30% at 3 weeks after neurolytic blockade.

Patients with failed blocks after two consecutive attempts should have their pharmacologic therapy optimized and may be candidates for intraspinal opioid analgesia.

On the day of the neurolytic block, patients are asked to reduce their daily opioid dosage by 50%, and morphine sulfate elixir every 3 to 4 hours is prescribed for breakthrough pain. Patients keep a record of their daily oral therapy during the first week of treatment to ease rapid adjustment and optimization of therapy.

Patients who have undergone neurolysis via a transarterial approach are observed in the Ambulatory Center for 4 hours to rule out both "trash foot" and retroperitoneal hematoma. A "trash foot" occurs with the dislodgment of an atherosclerotic plaque from the iliac vessels. Patients experiencing these complications need hospitalization for heparinization. A vascular surgery consultation should always be obtained.

Complications

The three studies[1, 2, 7] available for scrutiny have not reported any major complications associated with this procedure.

REFERENCES

1. Plancarte R, Amescua C, Patt RB, et al: Superior hypogastric plexus block for pelvic cancer pain. Anesthesiology 73:236-239, 1990.
2. de Leon-Casasola OA, Kent E, Lema MJ: Neurolytic superior hypogastric plexus block for chronic pelvic pain associated with cancer. Pain 54:145-151, 1993.
3. Freier A: Pelvic neurectomy in gynecology. Obstet Gynecol 25:48-55, 1965.
4. Lee RB, Stone K, Magelsen D, et al: Presacral neurectomy for chronic pelvic pain. Obstet Gynecol 68:517-521, 1986.
5. Loeser JD, Sweet WH, Tew JM, et al: Neurosurgical operations involving peripheral nerves. In Bonica JJ, Loeser JD, Chapman CR, et al (eds): The Management of Pain. Philadelphia, Lea & Febiger, 1990, pp 2044-2066.
6. Wang JK: Intrathecal morphine for intractable pain secondary to cancer of pelvic organs. Pain 21:99-102, 1985.
7. de Leon-Casasola OA, Plancarte R, Allende S, et al: Neurolytic superior hypogastric plexus block for cancer pain: A multicenter experience with 159 patients. Anesthesiology 83:A843, 1995.
8. Orlandini G: Selection of patients undergoing neurolytic superior hypogastric plexus block [letter]. Pain 56:121, 1994.
9. de Leon-Casasola OA, Lema MJ: Reply. Pain 56:122, 1994.
10. Waldman SD, Wilson WL, Kreps RD: Superior hypogastric plexus block using a single needle and computed tomography guidance: Description of a modified technique. Reg Anesth 16:286-287, 1991.

Chapter 76

Ganglion Impar Block

Bing Xue, M.S., Mark J. Lema, M.D., Ph.D.,
and Oscar A. de Leon-Casasola, M.D.*

The sympathetic nervous system has been associated with various types of cancer pain. Sympathetically mediated pain may be of either visceral or neuropathic origin. Traditionally, blockade of sympathetic pathways has been widely utilized to relieve oncologic pain. In addition to the classic targets of sympatholysis, such as stellate (cervicothoracic) ganglion, celiac plexus, and lumbar ganglia, a new approach to anesthetize or neurolyse the ganglion impar to relieve perineal pain has been undertaken (Fig. 76-1).

NEUROANATOMY

The peripheral part of the sympathetic nervous system consists of (1) two ganglionated paravertebral chains that extend from the base of the skull to the coccyx, (2) several major prevertebral plexuses that surround the abdominal aorta and its large visceral branches (cardiac, celiac, and hypogastric), and (3) numerous small intermediate and terminal ganglia. The paravertebral ganglia are connected with each other by longitudinal fibers and are arranged in a segmental fashion along the anterolateral surface of the vertebral column. They lie anterior to the transverse processes in the cervical region, anterior to the heads of the ribs in the thoracic region, along the sides of the vertebral bodies in the abdomen, and in front of the sacrum in the pelvis. Owing to fusion of adjacent components and anatomic variability among individuals, the number of ganglia varies: 2 or 3 pairs of cervical ganglia, 11 or 12 pairs of thoracic ganglia, 3 or 4 pairs of lumbar ganglia, and 4 or 5 pairs of sacral ganglia are found. In the sacral region, the two sympathetic chains gradually merge together and fuse anterior to the sacrococcygeal junction to form the ganglion impar (also known as Walther's ganglion, the sacrococcygeal ganglion, or the coccygeal ganglion). It is a solitary retroperitoneal structure and

the only unpaired autonomic ganglion in the body (Fig. 76-2).

NEUROPHYSIOLOGY

Intractable pain arising from disorders of the viscera and somatic structures within the pelvis and perineum often poses difficult problems for the pain practitioner. The reason for this difficulty is that the region contains diverse anatomic structures with mixed somatic, visceral, and autonomic innervation affecting bladder and bowel control and sexual function. Clinically, sympathetic pain in the perineum has a distinctly vague, burning, and poorly localized quality and is frequently associated with the sensation of urgency. Although various approaches have been proposed for the management of intractable perineal pain, their efficacy and applications are limited. Historically, neurolytic blockade in this region has been focused mainly on somatic rather than sympathetic components.

Ganglion impar has gray rami communicantes passing to sacral and coccygeal nerves but lacks white rami communicantes. It has been associated with the innervation of perineum, distal rectum, anus, distal urethra, vulva, and distal third of vagina. A study of ganglion impar blockade done by Plancarte and colleagues[1] in 1990 demonstrated its effectiveness in treating perineal pain without significant somatovisceral dysfunctions for patients with advanced cancer. In their report, 16 patients were studied, including 13 women and 3 men, ranging in age from 24 to 87 years (median, 48 years). All patients had advanced cancer (cervix, 9; colon, 2; bladder, 2; rectum, 1; endometrium, 2), and pain had persisted in all cases despite surgery and/or chemotherapy and radiation, analgesics, and psychological support. Localized perineal pain was present in all cases and was characterized as burning and urgent in 8 patients and of a mixed character in 8 patients. Pain was referred to the rectum (7 patients), perineum (6 patients), or vagina (3 patients). After preliminary local anesthetic blockade and subsequent neurolytic block, 8

*Mr. Xue was a summer fellow at Roswell Park Cancer Institute as part of the 1997 National Institutes of Health–National Cancer Institute Clinical Cancer Education Grant.

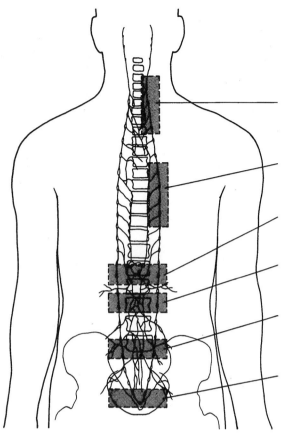

CERVICOTHORACIC GANGLIA
Brain, meninges, eye, ear,
tongue, pharynx, larynx,
glands and skin of head,
neck and upper extremity

THORACIC GANGLIA
Mediastinal contents, esophagus,
trachea, bronchi, pericardium,
heart, thoracic aorta, pleura, lung

CELIAC PLEXUS
GI tract (distal esophagus to
mid-transverse colon), liver,
adrenals, ureters, abdominal vessels

LUMBAR GANGLIA
Skin and vessels of lower extremity,
kidney, ureters, transverse colon,
testes

HYPOGASTRIC PLEXUS
Descending and sigmoid colon, rectum,
vaginal fundus, bladder, prostate,
prostatic urethra, testes,
seminal vesicles, uterus and ovaries

GANGLION IMPAR
Perineum, distal rectum and anus,
distal urethra, vulva and distal
third of vagina

FIGURE 76–1. Schematic drawing of major ganglia and plexuses of sympathetic nervous system and their innervated structures.

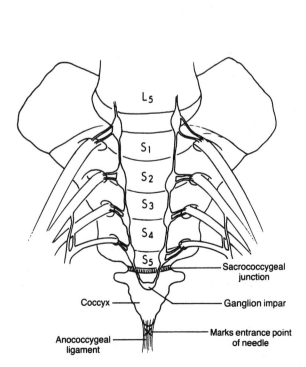
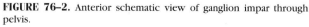

FIGURE 76–2. Anterior schematic view of ganglion impar through pelvis.

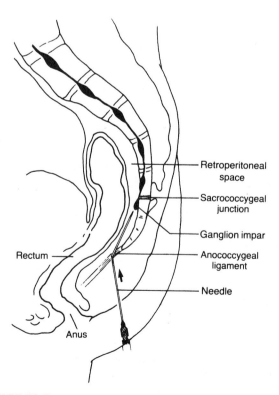

FIGURE 76–3. Lateral schematic view of correct needle placement for blockade of ganglion impar.

patients experienced complete (100%) pain relief, and the remainder experienced significant reduction in pain (60% to 90%) as determined by the visual analogue pain scale. The blocks were repeated in 2 patients, with further improvement.

TECHNIQUE

The patient is positioned in the lateral decubitus position with hips flexed toward the abdomen. The right lateral decubitus position is used if the operator is right-handed. A standard 22-gauge, 3.5-in. spinal needle is manually bent about 1 in. from its hub to form a 25- to 30-degree angle. In some cases, an additional bend of the needle is required to access an abnormal sacrococcygeal vertebral column. This maneuver facilitates positioning of the needle tip anterior to the concavity of the sacrum and coccyx. Then the needle is introduced under local anesthesia through the anococcygeal ligament with its concavity oriented posteriorly and, under fluoroscopic guidance, is directed along the midline to contact bone at or near the sacrococcygeal junction (Fig. 76–3). Retroperitoneal location is verified by observation of the spread of 2 mL of water-soluble contrast medium. Dye spread on the lateral view is shaped like a comma, and in the posteroanterior view it vaguely resembles a fleur-de-lis. Alternatively, patients may be placed in the lithotomy position using stirrups. This position straightens the path from the anococcygeal ligament to the ganglion impar and eliminates the need to bend the needle.

Two alternative approaches have been described for this block. In the transsacrococcygeal approach, a 22-gauge, 3.5-in. needle is directly placed in the retroperitoneal space, in the middle at the level of the sacrococcygeal junction. This approach has the advantage of increasing the patient's tolerance by avoiding the insertion of a finger in the rectum, which may be extremely painful for some patients. This is particularly important in patients with postradiation proctitis. However, fluoroscopic guidance is still needed. The second alternative approach is sometimes used by our group. It requires placing the patient in the lithotomy position. In this position, the curvature of the coccyx is decreased, allowing access to the ganglion impar with a straight 22-gauge spinal needle, and thus facilitating the needle positioning. However, placement of the finger in the rectum and fluoroscopic guidance are still needed. In our experience, the advantages of this approach include easy needle placement and a less cumbersome fluoroscopic evaluation of the needle's tip.

For diagnostic blocks, 4 to 8 mL of 1% lidocaine or 0.25% bupivacaine is used, and for neurolytic blocks 4 to 8 mL of 10% phenol is used. Although the technique is relatively straightforward, care is needed to prevent perforation of the rectum and injection into the periosteum.

SUMMARY

Ganglion impar blockade is an important adjunct to pharmacologic therapy for the relief of intractable perineal pain experienced by advanced cancer patients. It may also be beneficial for patients suffering from malignancies of the pelvis (endometrial, ovarian, rectal, or sarcomatous cancers). Treatment of coccydynia by this technique has not been studied, but it may provide some relief. To date no complications or side effects have been reported with this block. Rarely can this block entirely eliminate pain. It should be considered as part of a multimodal approach to pain management and not as a definitive "cure." The goals of the block are (1) to maximize the analgesic effect of opioid and nonopioid analgesics and (2) to reduce the required dosage of the agents so as to alleviate untoward side effects.

REFERENCE

1. Plancarte R, Amescua C, Patt RB: Presacral blockade of the ganglion impar (ganglion of Walther). Anesthesiology 73:A751, 1990.

FURTHER READING

Carpenter MB: Human Neuroanatomy. Philadelphia, Williams & Wilkins, 1976, pp 191–197.

de Leon-Casasola OA: Superior hypogastric plexus block and ganglion impar neurolysis for pain associated with cancer. Techniques in Reg Anesth Pain Manage 1:31, 1997.

Patt RB: Cancer Pain: Neurolytic Blocks of the Sympathetic Axis. Philadelphia, JB Lippincott, 1993, pp 377–420.

Wemm K, Saberski L: Modified approach to block the ganglion impar (ganglion of Walther) [letter]. Reg Anesth 20:544, 1995.

Chapter 77

Agents Used for Neurolytic Block

Robert E. Molloy, M.D.

Neurolytic blockade is a valuable tool, useful in managing intractable cancer pain. Its use presupposes a thorough assessment of the patient's overall medical condition and application of a multimodal approach to address the patient's many needs. The use of appropriate anticancer therapy, opioid analgesics, and adjuvant drugs is all presumed, as is consideration of other potential invasive therapies and the potential benefits and risks of each intervention. This must be followed by a thorough discussion of reasonable expectations for a neurolytic block; the limitations to any expected pain relief; the probable need for use of analgesic and other drugs in reduced doses; and an honest description of potential complications. Diagnostic or prognostic local anesthetic blocks are also desirable before neurolytic blockade. These procedures should be performed by well-trained, experienced physicians. The patient's response should be monitored by assessing pain levels, pain relief, activity levels, appetite, sleep, mood, and drug intake before and after blockade. The potential for respiratory depression and narcotic withdrawal syndrome after sudden cessation of pain requires carefully titrated opioid withdrawal.[1] The agents available for neurolytic block[2, 3] are described in this chapter.

ALCOHOL

Alcohol is the classic neurolytic agent, reported by Dogliotti for subarachnoid injection in 1931. It produces destruction of nerve fibers and subsequent wallerian degeneration of axonal fibers. A series of events occurs, including neural swelling and dissolution of cellular elements, followed by collapse and digestion of the myelin sheath. However, the basal lamina of the Schwann cell sheath remains intact, allowing for new Schwann cell proliferation and providing a framework for subsequent nerve fiber growth. Therefore, regeneration of axons can occur unless the cell bodies of these nerves have been completely destroyed.[1] Schlosser[4] studied alcohol block of the trigeminal nerve and reported in 1907 that the entire nerve, except for the neurolemma, degenerates and is absorbed. More dilute solutions produce less complete neural destruction of somatic neurons. The concentration of alcohol needed to provide adequate relief of pain with somatic nerve block seems to be 50% to 70%, although Labat and Greene[5] found a 33% concentration to be effective on peripheral nerves without producing significant muscle paralysis. Attempts to find a relatively low concentration of alcohol capable of producing complete sensory loss without any motor deficits have not been ultimately successful.

Alcohol extracts neural cholesterol, phospholipid, and cerebrosides, and it causes precipitation of lipoproteins and neuropeptides.[6] Merrick[7] described the effects of alcohol injection on sympathetic nerves. Injection of the sympathetic ganglion cells produced permanent nerve destruction, whereas injection of preganglionic and postganglionic fibers produced axonal degeneration with limited destruction of ganglion cell bodies and recovery of many neurons. Sympathetic neurons regenerate over the course of 3 to 5 months or longer. Intrathecal alcohol injection results in rapid uptake of alcohol, resultant destruction of the dorsal roots, and variable injury to the surface of the spinal cord and the posterior columns.[8] Alcohol is rapidly absorbed from cerebrospinal fluid (CSF): 10% of the injected dose remains in CSF after 10 minutes, and only 4% after 30 minutes.[9] Alcohol is hypobaric to CSF and quickly floats to the top when injected in CSF. The effective concentration is almost 100% for intrathecal use and 50% for celiac plexus block. Clinically, alcohol neurolysis is employed most often for lumbar sympathetic and celiac plexus blocks, although epidural and cranial nerve blocks have also been reported to be useful. Alcohol produces significant pain on injection, and it may be followed by burning or shooting neuropathic pain which can last for weeks to months. This may occur after peripheral nerve block or with spread to somatic nerve roots after lumbar sympathetic block. Unintended spread of alcohol to adjacent tissues can produce cellular injury or necrosis.

PHENOL

Mandl reported the use of phenol for sympathetic ganglion neurolysis in animals in 1947, and Maher described the results of intrathecal phenol in humans in 1955.[10] Mandl observed complete necrosis within 24 hours, progressive degeneration over 45 days, and regeneration in less than 3 months.[11] This suggests that recovery from sympathetic block with phenol occurs more rapidly than with alcohol. It was also supposed that phenol selectively blocked small nerve fibers while sparing large fibers. Subsequent reports documented transient local anesthetic blockade by dilute intrathecal phenol but widespread neural damage with clinically relevant concentrations. In essence, phenol appears to be just as neurotoxic as alcohol, producing nonselective damage to neural tissues. Phenol coagulates proteins as its primary mechanism of injury. In studies of intrathecal injection in both cats and humans, Smith[12] demonstrated that hyperbaric phenol primarily destroys axons in posterior sensory rootlets, in the posterior columns of the cord, and to a lesser extent in the anterior root axons. It produces nonselective destruction by denaturing proteins of axons and adjacent blood vessels. Degeneration occurred over 2 weeks, and regeneration progressed over 14 weeks. Injected phenol in glycerin appears to fix rapidly within the subarachnoid space. Ichiyanagi and colleagues[13] found that the phenol concentration decreased to 30% of the initial concentration within 1 minute and to 0.1% by 15 minutes. Phenol injection near peripheral nerves produces protein coagulation, axonal degeneration, and subsequent wallerian degeneration. Axonal regeneration occurs more rapidly than after alcohol. Gregg and coworkers[14, 15] performed in vivo electrophysiologic studies of the effects of alcohol and phenol peripheral nerve injections in cats. Alcohol produced significant depression of compound action potentials at 2 months.[14] The effects of phenol seen at 2 weeks had returned to normal by 8 weeks.[15] The maximum aqueous concentration of phenol is just over 6.7%. Mixture with glycerin to a 4% to 10% concentration results in a solution that is hyperbaric to cerebrospinal fluid. The initial injection of phenol is painless. It produces a local anesthetic effect that diminishes over 24 hours, leaving a less intense neurolytic effect. Phenol is used clinically for lumbar sympathetic, celiac plexus, hypogastric plexus, and somatic nerve blocks.

VASCULAR EFFECTS

An added risk of neurolytic block is incurred when alcohol or phenol is injected adjacent to a vascular prosthetic graft. Dacron woven grafts exhibited diminished tensile strength after 72-hour exposure to 50% ethyl alcohol or 6% phenol, whereas Gore-Tex grafts were unchanged. Electron microscopy has demonstrated significant fiber degeneration of Dacron and much less degradation of Gore-Tex by higher concentrations of these agents.[16] Occasional paraplegia after neurolytic celiac plexus block has been postulated to occur because of spinal cord ischemia. Vasospasm of segmental lumbar arteries has been induced in dogs after exposure to ethanol and phenol.[17] This appears to be unrelated to synaptic neurotransmitters or to sodium channels. Johnson and colleagues[18] demonstrated that low concentrations of ethanol induce significant contractile effects in human aortic smooth muscle cells along with increased intracellular concentration of cytoplasmic ionized calcium.

REFERENCES

1. Bonica JJ, Buckley FP, Moricca G, et al: Neurolytic blockade and hypophysectomy. In Bonica JJ, Loeser JD, Chapman CR, et al (eds): The Management of Pain. Philadelphia, Lea & Febiger, 1990, p 1980.
2. Jain S, Gupta R: Neurolytic agents in clinical practice. In Waldman SD, Winnie AP (eds): Interventional Pain Management. Philadelphia, WB Saunders, 1996, p 167.
3. Myers RR, Katz J: Neuropathology of neurolytic and semidestructive agents. In Cousins MJ, Bridenbaugh PO (eds): Neural Blockade in Clinical Anesthesia and Management of Pain. Philadelphia, JB Lippincott, 1988, p 1031.
4. Schlosser H: Erfahrungen in der neuralgiebehandlung mit alkoholeinspritzungen. Verh Cong Innere Med 24:49, 1907.
5. Labat G, Greene MB: Contribution to modern method of diagnosis and treatment of so-called sciatic neuralgias. Am J Surg 11:435, 1931.
6. Rumsby MG Finean JB: The action of organic solvents on the myelin sheaths of peripheral nerve tissue: II. Short-chain aliphatic alcohols. J Neurochem 13:1509, 1966.
7. Merrick RL: Degeneration and recovery of autonomic neurones following alcoholic block. Ann Surg 113:298, 1941.
8. Gallagher HS, Yonezawa T, Hay RC, et al: Subarachnoid alcohol block: II. Histologic changes in the central nervous system. Am J Pathol 35:679, 1961.
9. Matsuki M, Kato Y, Ichiyanagi K: Progressive changes in the concentration of ethyl alcohol in the human and canine subarachnoid spaces. Anesthesiology 36:617, 1972.
10. Maher RM: Relief of pain in incurable cancer. Lancet 1:18, 1955.
11. Mandl F: Aqueous solution of phenol as a substitute for alcohol in sympathetic block. J Int Coll Surg 13:566, 1950.
12. Smith MC: Histological findings following intrathecal injections of phenol solutions for the relief of pain. Anaesthesia 36:387, 1964.
13. Ichiyanagi K, Matsuki M, Kinefuchi J, et al: Progressive changes in the concentration of phenol and glycerin in the human subarachnoid space. Anesthesiology 42:622, 1975.
14. Gregg RV, Constantini CH, Ford DJ, et al.: Electrophysiologic investigation of alcohol as a neurolytic agent. Anesthesiology 63:A250, 1985.
15. Gregg RV, Constantini CH, Ford DJ, et al: Electrophysiologic and histopathologic investigation of phenol in renografin as a neurolytic agent. Anesthesiology 63:A239, 1985.
16. Gale DW, Valley MA, Rogers JN, et al: Effects of neurolytic concentrations of alcohol and phenol on Dacron and Gore-Tex vascular prosthetic grafts. Reg Anesth 19:395, 1994.
17. Brown DL, Rorie DK: Altered reactivity of isolated segmental lumbar arteries of dogs following exposure to ethanol and phenol. Pain 56:139, 1994.
18. Johnson ME, Sill JC, Brown DL, et al: The effect of the neurolytic agent ethanol on cytoplasmic calcium in arterial smooth muscle and endothelium. Reg Anesth 21:6, 1996.

Local Anesthetics and Nerve Blockade

Chapter 78

Physiology of the Nerve Impulse

Gary Strichartz, Ph.D.

The transmission of electrical information in the peripheral and central nervous systems (CNS) occurs through nerve impulses. Sensory coding by energy-selective transducing mechanisms at the distal ends of afferent peripheral nerve fibers located in skin, joints and muscles, and viscera converts stimuli of touch, heat, cold, and pain into trains of nerve impulses which are received and synaptically integrated by the CNS. Similarly, trains of impulses in efferent motor axons are integrated through peripheral junctions to drive contractions of skeletal and smooth muscles, glandular secretions, and the host of homeostatic responses orchestrated by the autonomic nervous system. It is on these impulses that local anesthetics act during peripheral nerve blockade, and an understanding of impulse physiology is essential for any appreciation of the mechanisms of neural blockade.

THE ELECTRICAL POTENTIAL DEPENDS ON ION CHANNELS

Three elements are essential for nerve impulses: an electrically insulating membrane, energy-driven *pumps* to establish and maintain ion (Na+, K+) gradients, and ionic selective pores or *channels*, at least some of which are *voltage gated* (i.e., they can be activated by changes in the membrane potential). Through hydrolysis of adenosine triphosphate, the Na+-K+ pump of the neuronal membrane transfers three Na+ ions from the intracellular to the extracellular compartment while transferring two K+ ions in the opposite direction. Consequently, cells reach a relatively steady-state condition wherein extracellular concentrations of Na+ at about 150 mmol/L and K+ at 3 to 4 mmol/L are juxtaposed across the membrane from intracellular concentrations of Na+ at 5 to 10 and K+ at 120 to 135 mmol/L. These ion concentration gradients provide diffusive forces that result in net fluxes of ions through the ion channels. At the resting condition, the membrane's "resting" K+ channels are often open, allowing a small efflux of K+ ions to the outside and leaving a miniscule excess of

negative over positive ionic charges within the cell. To a large degree, but not exclusively, this charge imbalance accounts for the electrical *membrane potential* at rest. Some Na+ (and occasionally Ca2+) ions enter the cell, through channels or by other exchange systems (e.g., coupled to the active uptake of certain neurotransmitters), and these are removed by a gently stimulated Na+-K+ pump. The overall resting potential results from the summed actions of this Na+ "leak" current (directed inward) and the K+ and pump-associated currents (directed outward). The membrane at rest is thus in a steady state, but is never at equilibrium.

OPEN SODIUM CHANNELS DRIVE THE NERVE IMPULSE

Nerve impulses represent a strong contrast to the resting state. Sodium channels open rapidly in response to small membrane depolarizations and conduct an in-

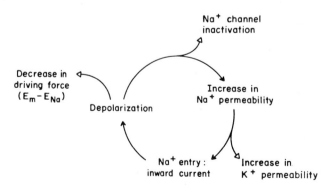

FIGURE 78–1. Ionic contributions to the positive feedback cycle that underlies regenerative action potentials. Each of the three components with *filled arrowhead* in the cycle is increased by the preceding one and, in turn, increases the subsequent one. Each of the diverging components with *open arrowheads* reduces membrane excitability and tends to terminate the action potential. The cycle is usually initiated by a source of inward current "external" to the membrane area being studied, for example, an adjacent excited region, a sensory ending depolarized by a physiologic stimulus, or postsynaptic currents.

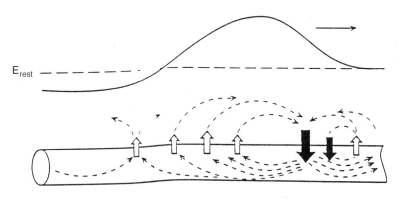

FIGURE 78-2. The spatial distribution of membrane potential and corresponding membrane currents during propagation of action potential in a nonmyelinated axon. *Filled arrows* show net inward current, which depolarizes membrane from the resting potential (E_{rest}). *Open arrows* show net outward current, which repolarizes it. In nonmyelinated fiber, outward current after impulse is large enough to hyperpolarize membrane. *Dashed lines* indicate the direction of longitudinal current carried by ions inside and outside axon.

ward current that drives further depolarization. Small local depolarizations, initiated by sensory stimuli or activated synapses, can induce enough Na^+ channels to open so that the Na^+ current exceeds the responding outward current through the K^+ channels; the resulting *net inward current* further depolarizes the membrane, thereby opening more channels, and catalyzing a large Na^+ current, and so on. This positive feedback cycle (Fig. 78-1) accounts for the depolarizing phase of the nerve impulse. If the instigating stimulus is too small, however, so few Na^+ channels are opened that the responding net current is outward and the membrane repolarizes. The condition whereupon this responding net current turns from outward to inward is called *threshold*.

Figure 78-1 also shows the three factors that repolarize the membrane after the peak of the nerve impulse. Critical among these are the dynamic behavior of the Na^+ and K^+ channels. The former close after some period of openness and cannot again become opened by depolarization until some period of intervening membrane polarization (e.g., to the resting potential); this state of closure is termed *inactivation*. In addition, certain types of K^+ channels are also opened by depolarization and, supporting a further outward current, return the membrane potential back to rest or beyond, whereupon they slowly close. Because each impulse results in some inactivation of Na^+ channels along with activation of K^+ channels, the ability to stimulate a net inward current is at first absent and then for a while compromised after the impulse. The membrane is *refractory* to excitation during this period; the threshold is elevated but gradually subsides to the initial condition.

IMPULSE PROPAGATION IS LOCAL EXCITATION COUPLED TO STIMULATION

Because the inward current entering the membrane undergoing impulse depolarization must flow back to its source (a law of physics), it is distributed along an intracellular pathway (the axoplasm is a conducting, ionic medium) before returning to the extracellular source (Fig. 78-2). Such a *local circuit current* is in essence a local stimulus; each impulse generates inward current that, if sufficient, raises the next region of the membrane beyond threshold. The impulse is a self-propagating wave of depolarization that can travel unattenuated from the site of initiation to the axons's far terminus, invading all the branches that contain enough Na^+ channels.

Impulse failure occurs when Na^+ channels are too few; when at high frequencies of firing the time between impulses is shorter than the refractory period; or when an injured or metabolically compromised nerve becomes "leaky," depolarizes, and is made permanently refractory. Failure also occurs when Na^+ channels are initiated by local anesthetics, as described in detail in the next two chapters.

BIBLIOGRAPHY

Hille B: Ionic Channels in Excitable Membranes, ed 2. Sunderland, Mass., Sinauer Press, 1991.
Kandel EC, Schwartz JH, Jessell TM (eds): Principles of Neural Science, ed 3. Norwalk, Conn, Appleton & Lange, 1991, pp 34-104.

Chapter 79

Mechanisms of Local Anesthetic Action

Gary Strichartz, Ph.D.

Local anesthetics are administered by a variety of routes to prevent or to abolish pain. Among these routes are topical application or subcutaneous infiltration of the skin, percutaneous injection around peripheral nerves, epidural or intrathecal delivery at the spinal cord, and intravenous infusion for the relief of chronic, neuropathic pain. The mechanism of action for peripheral nerve block is relatively certain, and it is often assumed that the same action occurs at all the other locations, but local anesthetics are not very selective drugs and they may alter diverse physiologic processes by actions at a number of molecular targets. Nevertheless, a major use is for peripheral nerve blockade, and that mechanism is the one addressed in this chapter.

LOCAL ANESTHETICS INHIBIT SODIUM ION CHANNELS

Sodium Channels Are the Primary Targets

Chapter 78 described the quintessential role of Na^+ channels for the generation and propagation of nerve impulses. Local anesthetics block nerve impulses by inhibiting these channels. The Na^+ channel is a protein that spans the plasma membrane of the nerve, and the local anesthetic binds to a specific site on the channel. Although there are differently structured and somewhat differently functioning Na^+ channels within individual sensory axons and among nervous tissue and skeletal and cardiac muscle, the general actions of local anesthetics on these channels are the same. The drugs bind to their target sites on the channels in bare nerve membranes rapidly, in 1 to 10 seconds at the 50% inhibitory drug concentration (IC_{50}), and dissociate about as fast. These IC_{50} concentrations are much lower than the clinically injected concentrations; for example, the IC_{50} for channel inhibition by lidocaine is 0.2 mmol/L, but a successful block requires injection of about 1%, almost 40 mmol/L. The reasons for this large difference are primarily pharmacokinetic, as described in Chapter 80.

The Binding Site Is Reached From Either the Cytoplasm or the Membrane

Local anesthetics reach their primary, high-affinity binding site on the Na^+ channel either by passing through the channel's opening *(pore)* from a cytoplasmic compartment or by entering "sideways," from the membrane surrounding the channel (Fig. 79–1). Entry through and exit from the pore pathway requires an open channel; the *channel gate* seems to control access to the binding site from the cytoplasm. Entry from the membrane occurs without requiring an open channel and is probably the major pathway to the binding site during dense, clinical blockade.

Binding Depends on the Configuration of the Sodium Ion Channel

Local anesthetics bind with different affinities to the different states of the Na^+ channel. The weakest binding is to the *resting*, closed state; rapid binding occurs to

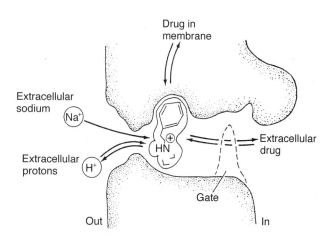

FIGURE 79–1. Na^+ channel block by local anesthetics. Two pathways exist for drug to reach its receptor in the pore. The hydrophilic pathway is unavailable when the gate is closed. Extracellular Na^+ and H^+ ions can reach bound drug molecules through the outer opening of the channel, respectively hastening or retarding their dissociation.

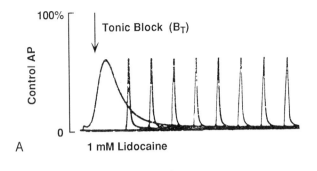

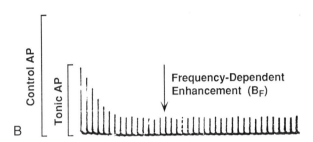

FIGURE 79–2. Inhibition of the nerve impulse at rest (B_T, tonic block) and during repetitive stimulation at 40 sec^{-1} (B_F, frequency-dependent enhancement or use-dependent block). These tracings are from compound action potentials of myelinated axons in isolated sciatic nerve in vitro. Lidocaine (1 mM) was applied for 10 minutes before these records were taken.

the *open* state, and somewhat slower binding to the *inactivated* state. During an impulse, therefore, additional drug binding occurs. Local dissociation of anesthetic from the channel is generally slower than the normal process of recovery from inactivation, so that in the presence of these drugs the apparent refractory period is functionally extended by the process of departure of drug from the channel. Increased binding therefore produces a use-dependent action of local anesthetics that appears as a potentiation of blockade during repetitive stimulation (Fig. 79–2).

Protonated Drugs Dissociate Slowly From the Channel

Being tertiary amine compounds, local anesthetics exist in rapid equilibrium between neutral and protonated, charged forms. The membrane pathway to the site is favored by the neutral species, the pore pathway by the charged species. Once at the binding site, the drug is ionized by protons from the *extracellular compartment*, since the amine nitrogen cannot then be reached from the axoplasm (Fig. 79–1). The protonated drug can unbind from the closed channel about 10 times more slowly than the neutral one can; therefore, the use-dependent actions are much more pronounced and overall binding is enhanced under mildly acidic extracellular conditions, such as in a region of inflammation. On the other hand, extracellular acidification also reduces the fraction of drug molecules in the membrane-permeant neutral form, thereby limiting penetration of extracellular local anesthetics to their sites of action. The overall balance between tighter binding, which produces slower drug dissociation, and reduced concentration, which produces slower association, varies with the individual drug's dissociation constant (pK_a) and hydrophobicity, but in general there is less resting channel block at neutral or slightly acid pH, and more at moderately alkaline pH.

Sodium Ion Channel Activation Is Inhibited by Local Anesthetics

In theory, Na$^+$ channel actions can be inhibited in two ways: Activation gating can be suppressed (*conformational* mechanism), or the pore can be blocked (*occlusion* mechanism). Neutral local anesthetics act primarily by the first mechanism, charged anesthetics by the second. Because the clinically used tertiary amine local anesthetics are in dynamic equilibrium between charged and neutral forms, they inhibit Na$^+$ channels through both mechanisms. Whether they do this by the same molecular action at exactly the same site on the Na$^+$ channel is a question that remains to be answered.

BIBLIOGRAPHY

Butterworth JF, Strichartz GR: Molecular mechanisms of local anesthesia: A review. Anesthesiology 72:711–734, 1990.

Chernoff DM: Kinetic analysis of phasic inhibition of neuronal sodium currents by lidocaine and bupivacaine. Biophys J 58:53–68, 1990.

Hille B: Local anesthetics hydrophilic and hydrophobic pathways for the drug-receptor reaction. J Gen Physiol 69:497–515, 1977.

Ragsdale DS, McPhee JC, Scheuer T, et al.: Molecular determinants of state-dependent block of Na$^+$ channels by local anesthetics. Science 265:1724–1730, 1994.

C h a p t e r   8 0

Local Anesthetic Pharmacology

Gary Strichartz, Ph.D.

In Chapters 78 and 79, the ionic basis of the nerve impulse and the mechanism of local anesthetic action were presented to provide a molecular basis for impulse blockade. This chapter addresses the in vivo situation for a consideration of the clinical pharmacology of local anesthetic blockade.

IMPORTANCE OF DRUG IONIZATION AND HYDROPHOBICITY FOR NERVE BLOCK

During regional nerve blockade, a solution of local anesthetic is injected so close to a peripheral nerve that enough drug enters the nerve to prevent impulse propagation (i.e., to bind a sufficient number of the Na^+ channels on individual axons). Drug penetration through the surrounding perineurial "sheath" depends on drug ionization and hydrophobicity.

The protonated species of drug, although more potent than the neutral species at its site of action on the Na^+ channel (see Chapter 79), passes through the nerve sheath considerably more slowly. As weak bases (Fig. 80–1), local anesthetics equilibrate between protonated and neutral species depending on their dissociation constant (pK_a) and the local pH. The pK_a is the pH at which the drug spends half of the time protonated and half the time in the neutral, uncharged form. Ionization-deionization is very rapid, occurring hundreds of times each second. Local anesthetics have a different pK_a

when they are adsorbed to serum proteins, to membranes, and even to Na^+ channels than when they are free in solution. The pK_a is also dependent on temperature, being as a rule lower at physiologic temperature (37°C) than at room temperature (20 to 22°C). Drugs with a higher pK_a are more likely to be protonated at physiologic pH than drugs with a lower pK_a; therefore, they are more intrinsically potent at the neuronal site of action but less likely to reach that site before being resorbed by the vasculature. Therefore, drugs with a moderately alkaline pK_a (8 to 9.5) are the most effective clinical local anesthetics.

Hydrophobicity is also of mixed value for clinical actions. Moderate hydrophobicity is essential for passage through the ensheathing tissue, and binding at the Na^+ channel site is enhanced by increased hydrophobicity. However, extremely hydrophobic local anesthetics (e.g., etidocaine) have practical limitations, including their limited aqueous solubility, tendency to be strongly adsorbed by local fat and muscle, and very slow penetration through ensheathing tissue.

The most effective local anesthetics are moderately ionized and moderately hydrophobic and can establish a functional block in 5 minutes that lasts from 30 to 500 minutes. The longest duration of blockade occurs with use of relatively hydrophobic drugs that are probably absorbed by extraneural fat as well as by intraneural (e.g., myelin) regions and are slowly released to the sites from whence channel binding and blocking occurs.

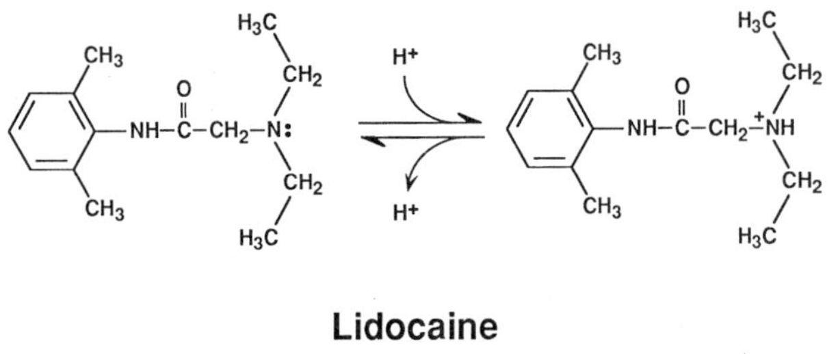

DRUG DELIVERY TO NERVE IS AN INEFFICIENT PROCESS

Little of the local anesthetic injected for clinical blockade actually enters the peripheral nerve. Less than 1 molecule in 20 of the injected dose of a 1% lidocaine solution is found within the nerve during blockade (Fig. 80–2). Similarly, in order to fully block impulses in isolated nerves in vitro, lidocaine concentrations of 0.5 to 1 mmol/L (0.0125% to 0.025%) are required, in com-

Lidocaine

FIGURE 80–1. Structure and rapid ionization of lidocaine.

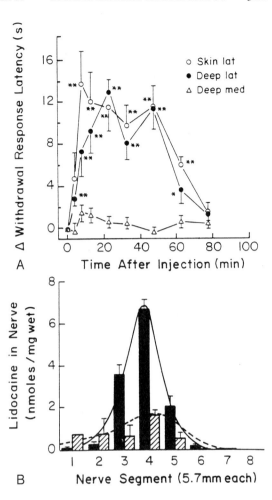

FIGURE 80–2. The time course of analgesia after lidocaine block of rat sciatic nerve (*A*) and the corresponding intraneural lidocaine distribution (*B*). *A,* Time course of changes in withdrawal response latency (WRL) to pinch of a skinfold on the lateral foot ("Skin lat"), and deep pinch at the first ("Deep med") and fifth toe ("Deep lat") during nerve block. Plotted values represent mean values ± SE; *P < 0.05, **P < 0.01, relative to baseline (predrug) values (n = 12). *B,* Distribution of lidocaine along the sciatic nerves removed from rats at two different behavioral end points. *Solid bars* indicate values during profound block (at 15 to 20 minutes postinjection); *striped bars,* return (at 45 to 55 minutes) of withdrawal response to deep pain (toe pinch). At full block, the total of all lidocaine in the nerve, exclusive of the sheath, is less than 5% of the injected dose.

parison to the 40 to 80 mmol/L (1% to 2%) that must be injected for complete functional blockade in vivo. Two major reasons account for this inefficient delivery: (1) The protonated drug is highly predominant (>99%) in most clinical formulations, having a pH of 5 to 6 at most, so that perineurial penetration is poor, and (2) the extraneural and intraneural vasculature rapidly removes lidocaine from the area around the nerve.

Two obvious ways to improve the efficiency of drug delivery, therefore, are to neutralize the injectate, thereby substantially increasing the fraction of uncharged drug molecules, and to co-inject with vasoconstrictors to depress vascular removal. Neutralization should be moderate (e.g., not more than pH 7), because the base is less soluble in aqueous solutions than the

cation and precipitation of drug must be avoided. Vasoconstrictors are only effective in prolonging blockade by those drugs for which vascular removal limits duration; intrinsically vasoconstrictive anesthetics (e.g., bupivacaine) and those that are hydrolyzed by local esterases (e.g., 2-chloroprocaine) are less potentiated than lidocaine by added vasoconstrictors.

BIBLIOGRAPHY

deJong RH: Local Anesthetics. St. Louis, Mosby, 1994.

Greene NM, Brull SJ: Physiology of Spinal Anesthesia. Baltimore, Williams & Wilkins, 1993.

Strichartz GR, Berde CB: Local anesthetics. *In* Miller RD (ed): Anesthesia, ed 4. New York, Churchill Livingstone, 1994, pp 489–521.

Chapter 81

● Local Anesthetics: Clinical Aspects

Spencer S. Liu, M.D.

Local anesthetics are commonly used in the clinical practice of pain medicine. This chapter discusses clinical pharmacology, pharmacokinetics, and toxicity of local anesthetics.

PHARMACOLOGY

Clinical Potencies of Local Anesthetics

Clinical effects of local anesthetics depend on numerous factors other than in vitro potency.[1] Local factors affecting diffusion and spread of local anesthetic have great impact on clinical potencies of local anesthetics[2] and vary with different applications (e.g., peripheral nerve block vs. spinal injection). Furthermore, clinical use may not require absolute suppression of the compound action potential but, rather, a disruption of information coding in the pattern of discharges.[3] Thus, clinical potencies may not exactly concur with potencies determined in experimental models[1] but will more accurately reflect clinical effects (Table 81-1).

Tachyphylaxis

Tachyphylaxis to local anesthetics is a clinical phenomenon, whereby repeated injection of the same dose of local anesthetic leads to decreasing efficacy. Tachyphylaxis has been described after central neuraxial blocks, peripheral nerve blocks, and for many different local anesthetic agents (amides, esters, short acting, long acting). An interesting clinical feature of tachyphylaxis to local anesthetics is its dependence on dosing interval. If dosing intervals are short enough that pain does not occur, then tachyphylaxis does not develop. Conversely, longer periods of patient discomfort before redosing hasten development of tachyphylaxis. Previous studies investigating the etiology of tachyphylaxis have found few pharmacokinetic or dynamic changes from repeated doses of local anesthetics. For example, with the development of clinical tachyphylaxis, there is no difference in local anesthetic spread within or clearance from the epidural space. Changes in pH of the sur-

rounding tissues do not affect the development of tachyphylaxis. Prolonged exposure of peripheral nerve and neural cells to local anesthetic does not affect either flux through sodium channels or propagation of the action potential over time. The clinical observation of the importance of pain for the development of tachyphylaxis suggests a central mechanism of tachyphylaxis via spinal cord sensitization (wind-up), and recent studies lend support to this theory.[4] Further work is needed to fully elucidate spinal mechanisms of tachyphylaxis to local anesthetics.

Additives to Increase Local Anesthetic Activity

Epinephrine

Addition of epinephrine to local anesthetics can prolong duration of local anesthetic block, increase intensity of block, and decrease systemic absorption of local anesthetic.[5] The mechanism whereby epinephrine exerts its effects on local anesthetics remains uncertain. Vasoconstrictive effects of epinephrine probably play an important role, as most local anesthetics (except ropivacaine) produce local vasodilation. Local vasoconstriction would theoretically inhibit systemic absorption of local anesthetic, thus allowing a greater amount available for blocking activity. Further analgesic effects from epinephrine may also occur via interaction with α_2-adrenergic receptors in the brain and spinal cord, especially because local anesthetics increase the vascular uptake of epinephrine.[6] Although most reports support the practice of adding epinephrine, reported effectiveness depends on amount of epinephrine added, local anesthetic used, and type of regional block (Table 81-2).

Alkalinization

The initial rationale for alkalinization was to increase the percent of local anesthetic existing as the lipid soluble, neutral form able to access neural sodium channels. The pH of commercial preparations of local anes-

TABLE 81–1. RELATIVE POTENCY OF LOCAL ANESTHETICS FOR DIFFERENT CLINICAL APPLICATIONS

	Short Duration	Medium Duration		Long Duration		
	2-Chloroprocaine	Lidocaine	Mepivacaine	Bupivacaine	Ropivacaine	Tetracaine
Peripheral nerve	N/A	1.0	2.6	3.6	3.6	N/A
Spinal	N/A	1.0	1.0	9.6	N/A	6.3
Epidural	2.0	1.0	1.0	4.0	4.0	N/A

Data from Hassan HG: Acta Anaesth Scand 38:505, 1994; Langerman L: Br J Anaesth 72:456, 1994; Langerman L: Anesth Analg 79:490, 1994; Smith C: Br J Hosp Med 52:455, 1994; Morrison LM: Br J Anaesth 72:164, 1994; Wahedi W: Reg Anesth 15:66, 1990; Nolte H: Reg Anesth 15:118, 1990; Pateromichelakis S, Porkopion AA: Acta Anaesthesiol Scand 32:672, 1988; and Vainionpaa VA: Anesth Analg 81:534, 1995.

N/A, not available.

thetics ranges from 3.9 to 6.47 and is especially acidic if prepackaged with epinephrine.[7] As the pKa of commonly used local anesthetics ranges from 7.6 to 8.9, less than 3% of the commercially prepared local anesthetic exists as the lipid soluble, neutral form. However, local anesthetics cannot be alkalinized beyond a pH of 6.05 to 8.0 before precipitation occurs,[7] and such pHs will only modestly increase the neutral form to approximately 10%.

Other effects of alkalinization can also increase the clinical effects of local anesthetics. In general, clinical studies demonstrate increased activity of alkalinized local anesthetic only when epinephrine is present, either prepackaged or freshly added. Although prepackaged epinephrine-containing solutions are quite acidic, fresh addition of epinephrine does not alter the pH of the more alkaline plain local anesthetic solutions.[7] Thus, the association between increased local anesthetic activity with alkalinization and epinephrine does not appear to be solely caused by increased acidity with epinephrine-containing solutions. On the other hand, the vasoconstrictive effects of epinephrine are also pH dependent. At a pH of less than 5.6, little vasoconstriction is seen,

and maximal vasoconstriction occurs at a pH of approximately 7.8. Therefore, alkalinization may affect activity of local anesthetic by activation of vasoconstrictive effects of epinephrine.

A series of studies examining desheathed nerve fibers also suggest multiple mechanisms of interaction between bicarbonate and local anesthetic independent of neural penetration.[8] Alkalinization of the local environment by itself inhibited neural impulse conduction. Furthermore, addition of bicarbonate potentiated local anesthetic block of impulse conduction. This finding suggests a specific interaction at the local anesthetic receptor within the sodium channel. Thus, it is likely that alkalinization of local anesthetics works through multiple mechanisms to affect local anesthetic activity.

Opioids

Addition of opioids to local anesthetics has gained recent popularity. Opioids have multiple central neuraxial and peripheral mechanisms of analgesic action. Supraspinal administration of opioids results in analgesia via opiate receptors in multiple sites, via activation of

TABLE 81–2. EFFECTS OF ADDITION OF EPINEPHRINE TO LOCAL ANESTHETICS

	Increase in Duration	Decrease in Blood Levels (%)	Dose or Concentration of Epinephrine
Peripheral Nerve Block			
Bupivacaine	+/−	10–20	1:200,000
Lidocaine	+ +	20–30	1:200,000
Mepivacaine	+ +	20–30	1:200,000
Ropivacaine	− −	0	1:200,000
Epidural			
Bupivacaine	+/−	10–20	1:300,000–1:200,000
Chloroprocaine	+ +		1:200,000
Lidocaine	+ +	20–30	1,600,000–1:200,000
Mepivacaine	+ +	20–30	1:200,000
Ropivacaine	− −	0	1:200,000
Spinal			
Bupivacaine	+/−		0.2 mg
Lidocaine	+ +		0.2 mg
Tetracaine	+ +		0.2 mg

Data from McLintic AJ: Br J Anaesth 67:683, 1991; Noble DW: Br J Anaesth 66:645, 1991; Takasaki M: Can J Anaesth 37:166, 1990; Brose WG: Anesthesiology 69:936, 1988; Ohno H: Anesthesiology 68:625, 1988; Laishley RS: Br J Anaesth 60:180, 1988; Wilson CM: Anaesthesia 43:12, 1988; Eisenach JC: Anesth Analg 66:447, 1987; Abboud TK: Anesth Analg 66:71, 1987; Burm AG: Anesth Analg 65:1281, 1986; Abboud TK: Anesth Analg 64:585, 1985; Takasaki M: Anesth Analg 66:337, 1987; Johnson MD: J Cardiothorac Anesth 4:200, 1990; Gaumann D: Anesth Analg 75:69, 1992; Eledjam JJ: Can J Anaesth 38:870, 1991; Abouleish E: Anesth Analg 77:457, 1993; Hurley RJ: Reg Anesth 16:303, 1991; Cederholm I: Reg Anesth 19:18, 1994; Cederholm I: Acta Anaesthesiol Scand 38:322, 1994; Renck H: Acta Anaesthesiol Scand 36:387, 1992; Hickey R: Can J Anaesth 37:732, 1990; Quist Christensen L: Acta Anaesthesiol Scand 38:15, 1994.

+ +, Overall supported; − −, overall not supported; +/−, unclear.

descending spinal pathways, and via activation of non-opioid analgesic pathways. Spinal administration of opioids provides analgesia primarily by attenuating C-fiber nociception and is independent of supraspinal mechanisms.[9] Coadministration of opioids with local anesthetics epidurally and intrathecally results in synergistic analgesia.[10]

The recent discovery of peripheral opioid receptors offers yet another avenue where the coadministration of local anesthetics and opioids may be useful.[11] The most promising clinical results have been from intra-articular administration of local anesthetic with opioid for postoperative analgesia, whereas combining local anesthetics and opioids for nerve blocks appears to be ineffective.[11] There are several reasons for a predicted lack of effect of coadministration of local anesthetic and opioid for peripheral nerve blocks. Anatomically, peripheral opioid receptors are found primarily at the end terminals of afferent fibers.[12] However, peripheral nerves are commonly blocked by deposition of anesthetic proximal to the end terminals of nerve fibers. In addition, common sites for peripheral nerve blocks are encased in multiple layers of connective tissue, which the anesthetics must traverse before accessing peripheral opioid receptors. Finally, previous studies have demonstrated the importance of concomitant local tissue inflammation for analgesic effectiveness of peripheral opioid receptors.[11] Mechanism for the underlying dependence on local inflammation is speculative and may involve upregulation or activation of peripheral opioid receptors or "loosening" of intercellular junctions to allow passage of opioids to receptors. Nonetheless, lack of inflammation at the site of a peripheral nerve block may also reduce the effects of coadministration of local anesthetic and opioid. All of these factors combine to decrease the theoretical effectiveness of combinations of local anesthetics and opioids for peripheral nerve blocks.

α_2-Agonists

α_2-Agonists may also be a useful adjuvant to local anesthetics. α_2-Agonists, such as clonidine, produce analgesia via supraspinal and spinal adrenergic receptors.[13] Clonidine also has direct inhibitory effects on peripheral nerve conduction (A and C nerve fibers). Thus, addition of clonidine may have multiple routes of action, depending on type of application. Preliminary evidence suggests that coadministration of α_2-agonist and local anesthetic results in central neuraxial and peripheral nerve analgesic synergy, whereas systemic (supraspinal) effects are additive.[14] Central neuraxial synergy may be partially due to reductions in spinal cord metabolism and vasoconstriction of spinal cord blood flow by clonidine. Overall, clinical trials indicate that addition of clonidine to intrathecal, epidural, and peripheral applications of local anesthetics enhances local anesthetic activity.

Systemic Analgesia From Local Anesthetics

Intravenous administration of lidocaine (1 to 5 mg/kg) has been used to treat postoperative, cancer, and chronic neuropathic pain. The mechanism of analgesia remains unclear but does not involve blockade of impulse conduction in peripheral nerves.[15] In fact, multiple mechanisms of systemic analgesia have been proposed. A peripheral mechanism has been demonstrated, as systemic local anesthetics at sub-blocking concentrations (1 to 20 µg/mL) reversibly depress generation of spontaneous electrical activity in injured C and Aδ nerve fibers and dorsal root ganglia. The ability of sub-blocking concentrations of local anesthetic to inhibit electrical coding of sensory information represents another peripheral mechanism for systemic analgesia.[3] Central mechanisms have also been demonstrated by inhibition of tonic electrical activity of hippocampal pyramidal cells and inhibition of nociceptive reflexes and central sensitization in the spinal cord.[16] In addition, orally administered tocainide and mexiletine (class I antiarrhythmic agents that are structurally and electrophysiologically similar to lidocaine) have been successfully used to treat chronic pain conditions.

CLINICAL PHARMACOKINETICS

Systemic absorption of local anesthetics after clinical use can produce blood levels resulting in central nervous system and cardiovascular toxicity. In general, local anesthetics with decreased systemic absorption have a greater margin of safety. Rate and extent of absorption depend on numerous factors, the most important of which are site of injection, dose of local anesthetic, physicochemical properties of local anesthetic, and addition of epinephrine.

The relative amounts of fat and vascularity surrounding the site of injection interact with the physicochemical properties of the local anesthetic to affect rate of systemic uptake. In general, areas with greater vascularity have more rapid and complete uptake, as compared with those with more fat, regardless of type of local anesthetic. Thus, rates of absorption generally decrease in the following order: intercostal, caudal, epidural, brachial plexus, sciatic or femoral (Table 81–3).

The greater the total dose of local anesthetic injected, the greater the systemic absorption and peak blood levels (C_{max}). This relationship is nearly linear and is relatively unaffected by anesthetic concentration and speed of injection.

Physicochemical properties of local anesthetics affect systemic absorption. In general, the more potent agents with greater lipid solubility and protein binding result in lower systemic absorption and C_{max}. Increased binding to neural and non-neural tissue probably explains this observation.

Epinephrine can counteract the inherent vasodilating characteristics of most local anesthetics. The reduction in C_{max} with epinephrine is most effective for the less potent, shorter-acting agents (see Table 81–2), as increased tissue binding rather than local blood flow may be a greater determinant of absorption for the long-acting agents.

TABLE 81–3. TYPICAL PEAK BLOOD LEVELS AFTER CLINICAL USE OF LOCAL ANESTHETICS

Local Anesthetic	Technique	Dose (mg)	C_{max} ($\mu g/mL$)	T_{max} (min)	Toxic Plasma Concentration ($\mu g/mL$)
Bupivacaine	Brachial plexus	150.0	1.0	20	3
	Celiac plexus	100.0	1.50	17	
	Epidural	150.0	1.26	20	
	Intercostal	140.0	0.90	30	
	Lumbar sympathetic	52.5	0.49	24	
	Sciatic/Femoral	400.0	1.89	15	
Lidocaine	Brachial plexus	400.0	4.0	25	5
	Epidural	400.0	4.27	20	
	Intercostal	400.0	6.8	15	
Mepivacaine	Brachial plexus	500.0	3.68	24	5
	Epidural	500.0	4.95	16	
	Intercostal	500.0	8.06	9	
	Sciatic/Femoral	500.0	3.59	31	
Ropivacaine	Brachial plexus	190.0	1.3	53	3
	Epidural	150.0	1.07	40	
	Intercostal	140.0	1.10	21	

Data from Kopacz DJ: Anesthesiology 81:1139, 1994; Katz JA: Anesth Analg 70:16, 1990; Tucker GT: Properties, absorption, and disposition of local anesthetic agents. *In* Cousins MJ, Bridenbaugh PO (eds): Neural Blockade in Clinical Anesthesia and Management of Pain. Philadelphia, JB Lippincott, 1988, p 47.

C_{max}, Peak plasma levels; T_{max}, time until C_{max}.

TOXICITY OF LOCAL ANESTHETICS

Central Nervous System Toxicity of Local Anesthetics

Systemic Central Nervous System Toxicity

Systemic central nervous system (CNS) toxicity due to local anesthetics is dose dependent (Table 81–4). Local anesthetic potency for systemic CNS toxicity approximately parallels action potential–blocking potency (Table 81–5). External factors can increase potency for CNS toxicity, such as acidosis and increased PCO_2, perhaps via increased cerebral perfusion or decreased protein binding of local anesthetic. There are also external factors that can decrease local anesthetic potency for generalized CNS toxicity. For example, seizure thresholds of local anesthetics are increased by administration of barbiturates and benzodiazepines.[17]

Local Central Nervous System Toxicity

Recent interest has focused on potential local CNS toxicity from administration of local anesthetics. Previous studies have demonstrated that local anesthetics in clinically used concentrations are safe for peripheral

nerves. However, all clinically used local anesthetics can cause concentration dependent nerve fiber damage in peripheral nerves when used in high enough concentrations.[18] Mechanisms for local anesthetic neurotoxicity remain speculative, but previous studies have demonstrated local anesthetic–induced injury to Schwann cells, inhibition of fast axonal transport, and disruption of the blood-nerve barrier.[18] Local anesthetics may also indirectly damage nerves by decreasing neural blood flow and thus causing ischemia, possibly through effects on prostaglandin metabolism.[18]

Intrathecal use of lidocaine (5% in 7.5% dextrose) has received special interest because of reports of persistent sensory deficits after administration via small-bore intrathecal catheter and single injection.[19] Multiple factors, such as rate of injection, size of injection device, and pooling of lidocaine in the sacral area, may be involved.[19] Nonetheless, lidocaine does appear to possess an inherently higher potential for intrathecal neurotoxicity than other clinically used local anesthetics. As multiple clinical factors are involved in the potential neurotoxicity of intrathecal 5% hyperbaric lidocaine,

TABLE 81–4. SYSTEMIC EFFECTS OF LIDOCAINE

Plasma Concentration ($\mu g/mL$)	Effect
1–5	Analgesia
5–10	Lightheadedness
	Tinnitus
	Numbness of tongue
10–15	Seizures
	Unconsciousness
15–25	Coma
	Respiratory arrest
>25	Cardiovascular depression

TABLE 81–5. THRESHOLD DOSE FOR PRODUCTION OF GENERALIZED CENTRAL NERVOUS SYSTEM TOXICITY BY LOCAL ANESTHETICS IN HUMANS AND CARDIOVASCULAR SYSTEM-TO-CENTRAL NERVOUS SYSTEM TOXICITY IN ANIMALS

Agent	Dose (mg/kg)	CVS:CNS Toxic Dose Ratio
Bupivacaine	1.6	2.0
Chloroprocaine	22.8	3.7
Etidocaine	3.4	4.4
Lidocaine	6.4	7.1
Mepivacaine	9.8	7.1
Ropivacaine	2.4	2.2

Data from Rosenberg PH: Acta Anaesthesiol Scand 37:751, 1993; Covino BG: Acta Anaesthesiol Belg 39:159, 1988; Santos AC: Anesthesiology 82:734, 1995; Reiz S: Acta Anaesthesiol Scand 33:93, 1989; Scott B: Anesth Analg 69:563, 1989.

further studies are needed before conclusions can be drawn.

Cardiovascular System Toxicity of Local Anesthetics

In general, much greater doses of local anesthetics are required to produce cardiovascular system (CVS) toxicity then CNS toxicity. Similar to CNS toxicity, potency for CVS toxicity reflects the anesthetic potency of the agent (Table 81-5). The more potent, more lipid-soluble agents (bupivacaine, etidocaine, ropivacaine) appear to have a different sequence of CVS toxicity than less-potent agents. For example, increasing doses of lidocaine lead to hypotension, bradycardia, and hypoxia, whereas bupivacaine often results in sudden cardiovascular collapse due to ventricular dysrhythmias that are resistant to resuscitation.[20] There are several possible systemic and local mechanisms for increased cardiotoxicity from potent local anesthetics.

Systemic Cardiovascular System Toxicity

Recent studies have demonstrated that the central and peripheral nervous systems may be involved in the increased cardiotoxicity with bupivacaine. The nucleus tractus solitarii in the medulla is an important region for autonomic control of the cardiovascular system. Neural activity in the nucleus tractus solitarii of rats is markedly diminished by intravenous doses of bupivacaine immediately prior to development of hypotension. Furthermore, direct intracerebral injection of bupivacaine can elicit sudden dysthymias and cardiovascular collapse.[17]

Peripheral effects of bupivacaine on the autonomic and vasomotor systems may also augment its CVS toxicity. Bupivacaine possesses potent peripheral inhibitory effects on sympathetic reflexes that have been observed even at blood concentrations similar to those measured after uncomplicated regional anesthesia.[21] Finally, bupivacaine also has potent direct vasodilating properties, which may exacerbate cardiovascular collapse.

Local Cardiovascular System Toxicity

The more potent local anesthetics appear to possess greater potential for electrophysiologic toxicity. A previous study examining lidocaine, bupivacaine, and ropivacaine in rats has demonstrated equivalent peak effects on myocardial contractility but much greater effects on electrophysiology (prolongation of QRS) from bupivacaine and ropivacaine than lidocaine.[22] Although all local anesthetics block the cardiac conduction system via a dose-dependent block of sodium channels, two features of the sodium-channel–blocking abilities of bupivacaine may enhance its cardiotoxicity. First, bupivacaine exhibits a much stronger binding affinity to resting and inactivated sodium channels than lidocaine.[23] Second, bupivacaine dissociates slowly from sodium channels during cardiac diastole, and bupivacaine conduction block accumulates at physiologic heart rates (60 to 180 bpm). In contrast, lidocaine fully dissociates from sodium channels during diastole, and little accumulation of conduction block occurs at physiologic heart rates.[23]

Increased potency for direct myocardial depression from the more-potent local anesthetics is another contributing factor to increased cardiotoxicity. Bupivacaine is the most completely studied potent local anesthetic, and it possesses a high affinity for sodium and potassium channels in the cardiac myocyte.[24] Furthermore, bupivacaine inhibits calcium channels, release of calcium from sarcoplasmic reticulum, and mitochondrial energy metabolism.[25] Thus, multiple direct effects of bupivacaine on activity of the cardiac myocyte may enhance the cardiotoxicity of bupivacaine.

REFERENCES

1. Pateromichelakis S, Porkopiou AA: Local anaesthesia efficacy: Discrepancies between in vitro and in vivo studies. Acta Anaesthesiol Scand 32:672, 1988.
2. Popitz-Bergez FA, Leeson S, Thalhammer JG, Strichartz GR: Relation between functional deficit and intraneural local anesthetic during peripheral nerve block. Anesthesiology 83:583, 1995.
3. Raymond SA: Subblocking concentrations of local anesthetics: Effects on impulse generation and conduction in single myelinated sciatic nerve axons in frog. Anesth Analg 75:906, 1992.
4. Lee K-C, Wilder RT, Smith RL, Berde CB: Thermal hyperalgesia accelerates and MK-801 prevents the development of tachyphylaxis to rat sciatic nerve blockade. Anesthesiology 81:1284, 1994.
5. Tucker GT: Safety in numbers. The role of pharmacokinetics in local anesthetic toxicity: The 1993 ASRA lecture. Reg Anesth 19:155, 1994.
6. Ueda W, Hirakawa M, Mori K: Acceleration of epinephrine absorption by lidocaine. Anesthesiology 63:717, 1985.
7. Ikuta PT, Raza SM, Durrani Z, et al.: pH adjustment schedule for the amide local anesthetics. Reg Anesth 14:229, 1989.
8. Wang GK, Strichartz GR, Raymond SA: On the mechanisms of potentiation of local anesthetics by bicarbonate buffer: Drug structure-activity studies on isolated peripheral nerve. Anesth Analg 76:131, 1993.
9. Niv D, Nemirovsky A, Rudick V, et al.: Antinociception induced by simultaneous intrathecal and intraperitoneal administration of low doses of morphine. Anesth Analg 80:886, 1995.
10. Kaneko M, Saito Y, Kirihara Y, et al.: Synergistic antinociception after epidural coadministration of morphine and lidocaine in rats. Anesthesiology 80:137, 1994.
11. Stein C: Peripheral mechanisms of opioid analgesia. Anesth Analg 76:182, 1993.
12. Fields HL, Emson PC, Leigh BK, et al.: Multiple opiate receptor sites on primary afferent fibres. Nature 284:351, 1980.
13. Eisenach JC, De Kock M, Klimscha W: Alpha2-adrenergic agonists for regional anesthesia. A clinical review of clonidine (1984–1995). Anesthesiology 85:655, 1996.
14. Pertovaara A, Hamalainen MM: Spinal potentiation and supraspinal additivity in the antinociceptive interaction between systemically administered α_2-adrenoreceptor agonist and cocaine in the rat. Anesth Analg 79:261, 1994.
15. Chaplan SR, Bach FW, Shafer SL, Yaksh TL: Prolonged alleviation of tactile allodynia by intravenous lidocaine in neuropathic rats. Anesthesiology 83:775, 1995.
16. Abram SE, Yaksh TL: Systemic lidocaine block nerve injury-induced hyperalgesia and nociceptor driven spinal sensitization in rats. Anesthesiology 80:383, 1994.
17. Bernards CM, Artru AA: Hexamethonium and midazolam terminate dysrhythmias and hypertension caused by intracerebroventricular bupivacaine in rabbits. Anesthesiology 74:89, 1991.
18. Kalichman MW: Physiologic mechanisms by which local anesthetics may cause injury to nerve and spinal cord. Reg Anesth 18:448, 1993.
19. Beardsley D, Holman S, Gantt R, et al.: Transient neurologic deficit after spinal anesthesia: Local anesthetic maldistribution with pencil point needles? Anesth Analg 81:314, 1995.

20. Nancarrow C, Rutten AJ, Runciman WB, Mather LE: Myocardial and cerebral drug concentrations and the mechanisms of death after fatal intravenous doses of lidocaine, bupivacaine, and ropivacaine in sheep. Anesth Analg 69:276, 1989.

21. Chang KSK, Yang M, Andresen MC: Clinically relevant concentrations of bupivacaine inhibit rat aortic baroreceptors. Anesth Analg 78:501, 1994.

22. Reiz S: Cardiotoxicity of ropivacaine—a new amide local anaesthetic agent. Acta Anaesthesiol Scand 33:93, 1989.

23. Guo XT, Castle NA, Chernoff DM, Strichartz GR: Comparative inhibition of voltage-gated cation channels by local anesthetics. Ann N Y Acad Sci 625:181, 1991.

24. Berman MF, Lipka LJ: Relative sodium current block by bupivacaine and lidocaine in neonatal rat myocytes. Anesth Analg 79:350, 1994.

25. Sztark F, Tueux O, Emy P, et al.: Effects of bupivacaine on cellular oxygen consumption and adenine nucleotide metabolism. Anesth Analg 78:335, 1994.

Chapter 82

Complications

Gary Strichartz, Ph.D.

In the course of clinical use, local anesthetics occasionally result in undesirable effects. Some of these are minor, such as local allergic responses; some are more severe but temporary, such as so-called "transient radicular irritation"; and some are genuinely life threatening, such as cardiac dysrhythmias following accidental intravenous injection. In this chapter, the complications of local anesthetics documented during clinical anesthesia are reviewed.

Categorically separated, there are local and systemic complications from local anesthetics (LAs). Local inflammation or irritation from LAs is apparent after skin infiltration and has been used historically as a convenient assay for drug potency. True allergic reactions to local (or systemic) drug applications are very rare, occur most often with ester-linked drugs, and have sometimes been attributed to preservatives (e.g., methylparaben) rather than the LA per se.

Pain from injection of local anesthetics is acute and frequent but arises largely from the acidic pH of pharmaceutical drug formulations and is ameliorated if drug solutions are neutralized before injection (e.g., by addition of bicarbonate).

Local anesthetics, at certain concentrations, often are vasoconstrictive. (At other doses, the same drug may be vasodilatory.) Tissue damage arising from this vasoconstriction, either from the LA itself or from co-injected vasoconstrictors (e.g., epinephrine), is not clinically apparent, even though direct application of LA drugs to nerves in vivo has been shown to strongly reduce local blood flow and leads to marked neuropathologic changes days later.

The direct neurotoxic actions of local anesthetics are irrefutable. Isolated nerves without their perineural covering totally lose impulse conducting capacity after only 5 to 15 minutes of incubation in 5% lidocaine. Even 2% lidocaine produces partial conduction deficits, which persist for the several days that the nerves can be studied in vitro. Rats receiving these lidocaine concentrations through intrathecal catheters develop irreversible neurologic deficits, and frequent reports of

cauda equina syndrome in humans from concentrated LAs given spinally testify to the potential clinical neurotoxicity of these drugs. Because lower concentrations of LA given in sufficient volume are equally effective, it seems prudent and rational to avoid the use of lidocaine above 2%.

The major systemic complications of local anesthetics are on the central nervous system (CNS) and the cardiovascular system. Although LAs are usually inhibitory in their cellular actions, the early CNS signs from systemic administration are excitatory. Facial paresthesias, tinnitus, anxiety, dizziness, nausea, and, ultimately, convulsions all may occur when LAs enter the brain. The mechanistic basis for these effects is unknown. Some have suggested as a cause the early inhibition of tonic inhibitory circuits, leading to unbalanced excitation in the brain, but it is also known that local anesthetics can directly increase intracellular Ca^{2+} and might elevate background as well as stimulated release of neurotransmitters by this action and thus enhance general excitation of the CNS.

Convulsions from systemic local anesthetics are treated successfully by intravenous barbiturates or benzodiazepines. The CNS symptoms usually develop over a time course of minutes (rather than seconds) that permits pharmacologic intervention before frank seizures begin. Luckily, CNS symptoms develop before cardiovascular ones and so can forewarn the anesthesiologist of potential pending problems.

Cardiovascular complications of local anesthesia are both immediately life threatening and difficult to treat. Although some bradycardia may occur, the crisis result is usually ventricular tachycardia leading to ventricular fibrillation and death. Curiously, atrioventricular conduction slowing and block often accompanies this circumstance, suggesting that part of the action involves slow Ca^{2+}-dependent conduction in addition to the recognized effects on Na^+ channels. LAs applied to strips of myocardial tissue or perfused through isolated hearts are only inhibitory, with clear negative inotropic and chronotropic actions. Interestingly, local anesthetics injected into the cerebral ventricles of the brain rapidly result in cardiac arrhythmias, suggesting that at least part of systemic cardiac dysfunction originates in the CNS.

Treatment of cardiovascular toxicity is controversial. Electrical cardioversion may be more difficult in cases of LA-induced toxicity, possibly because of the CNS contribution. Traditional antiarrhythmics such as bretylium or amrinone have some reported success in animals, but epinephrine seems of limited utility in resuscitation protocols. Part of the limitations of pharmacologic interventions for CVS toxicity may be explained by the inhibitory actions of the instigating LA on the receptor pathway sought for therapeutic activation. Nevertheless, and regardless of the particular strategy, intervention should be quick and aggressive and, obviously, every effort should be made to maintain oxygen supply to the brain.

BIBLIOGRAPHY

Covino BG: Toxicity and systemic effect of local anesthetic agents. In Strichartz GR (ed): Local Anesthetics. Berlin, Heidelberg, Springer-Verlag, 1987, pp 187–212.

de Jong RH, Bonin JD: Toxicity of local anesthetic mixtures. Toxicol Appl Pharmacol 54:501–507, 1980.

Feldman HS: Toxicity of local anesthetic agents. In Rice SA, Fish KJ, (eds): Anesthetic Toxicity. New York, Raven Press, 1994, pp 107–133.

Scott DB: Toxic effects of local anaesthetic agents on the central nervous system. Br J Anaesth 58:732–735, 1986.

Strichartz GR, Berde CB: Local anesthetics. In Miller RD (ed): Anesthesia. New York, Churchill Livingstone, 1994, pp 489–521.

Wagman IH, DeJong RH, Prince DA: Effects of lidocaine on the central nervous system. Anesthesiology 28:155–172, 1967.

Chapter 83

Spinal Anesthesia

Radha Sukhani, M.D.,
and Rom A. Stevens, M.D.

Spinal, also called subarachnoid, anesthesia is the fastest, most predictable and reliable form of central neuraxis regional anesthesia. Professor August Bier administered the first true spinal anesthetic in August 1898 in Germany. Two San Francisco surgeons, F. Dudley Tait and Guido E. Caglier, are credited with administering the first spinal anesthetic in the United States a year later.[1] Spinal anesthesia is unique, in that a very small amount of local anesthetic solution, too small to result in systemic toxicity even if injected intravenously, can result in profound and long-lasting sensory and motor block. By altering the baricity or adding small amounts of adjuncts, such as epinephrine or morphine, the duration of anesthesia and analgesia can be significantly prolonged. As a sole anesthetic technique, spinal anesthesia is ideally suited for lower abdominal, pelvic, perineal, and lower-extremity surgery. The ability to provide a block potentially limited to sacral nerve roots makes it superior to epidural anesthesia for ankle, pelvic, and perineal surgery.

Spinally administered local anesthetics and opioids have been used for surgical anesthesia and for long-term management of cancer pain. This chapter covers only the surgical applications of spinal anesthesia.

ANATOMY

The spinal cord begins at the level of foramen magnum and terminates as the conus medullaris at the level of the first lumbar interspace in an adult. The newborn spinal cord extends more distally to the level of L3. To avoid injury to the spinal cord, the spinal needle is inserted at the second through the fifth lumbar interspaces in adults and fourth or fifth lumbar interspaces in infants. The subarachnoid space surrounding the spinal cord is filled with cerebrospinal fluid (CSF) and extends to the second sacral vertebra, where the dural sac terminates. The spinal subarachnoid space is in free communication with the cranial subarachnoid space and subarachnoid space surrounding the nerve roots. There are four curves on the spine that can influence the distribution of local anesthetic solutions in the subarachnoid space: sacral kyphosis, lumbar lordosis, thoracic kyphosis, and cervical lordosis.

CEREBROSPINAL FLUID VOLUME, SPECIFIC GRAVITY, AND BARICITY

Cerebrospinal fluid dilutes local anesthetic drugs injected into the spinal subarachnoid space. The distribution and degree of dilution of local anesthetics within the CSF determine the extent of nerve blockade during spinal anesthesia. Recent work by Hogan and co-workers[2] using magnetic resonance imaging on live human subjects has demonstrated that CSF volume is widely variable among individuals. From the T11 to T12 disc to the sacral terminus of the dural sac, the mean CSF volume was 49 ± 20 mL (range, 28 to 80 mL). Subjects with high body mass index had lower average CSF volumes and static abdominal compression decreased CSF volume by 3.6 ± 3.2 mL.[2] This may contribute to relatively greater spread of local anesthetics and higher block in obese and in gravid patients.

At 37°C, the specific gravity of CSF ranges from 1.003 to 1.009, with a mean of 1.006. Local anesthetic solutions used for spinal anesthesia are classified as hypobaric, isobaric, or hyperbaric, depending on their specific gravity relative to CSF. Local anesthetic solutions with baricity less than 0.9998 at 37°C are hypobaric, and those with baricity greater than 1.009 are hyperbaric. Hyperbaric solutions are prepared by adding dextrose to increase the specific gravity of local anesthetic solution to greater than 1.009. Hypobaric solutions are prepared by diluting local anesthetic solutions with distilled water. Solutions of 0.1% to 0.33% tetracaine in distilled water are hypobaric. Because of its high anesthetic potency, tetracaine in these low concentrations produces reliable sensory and motor block. Isobaric solutions of tetracaine are prepared by diluting tetracaine niphanoid crystals with CSF. Commercial preparations of 0.5% bupivacaine and lidocaine 2% without dextrose are isobaric or slightly hypobaric.

GUIDELINES FOR USE OF HYPERBARIC, ISOBARIC, AND HYPOBARIC SOLUTIONS

In principle, the isobaric solutions remain in the vicinity of the injection site; hypobaric solutions float upward to nondependent regions, and hyperbaric solutions gravitate to dependent areas in the spinal subarachnoid space.

Hyperbaric Solutions

Hyperbaric solutions of local anesthetics are most popular. Distribution of hyperbaric local anesthetic solutions is determined by the position of the patient during the first 20 to 30 minutes following injection. The head-down position enhances the thoracic spread, and the seated position limits spread to the lumbar and sacral dermatomes. The curvature of spine also influences the spread of local anesthetic. In the supine recumbent position, the highest point of the spinal curvature is L3 (apex of lumbar lordosis), and the lowest point is at thoracic kyphosis at T6. Injection below the apex of the lumbar lordosis may result in preferential flow of hyperbaric solution toward the sacral kyphosis, resulting in inadequate anesthesia of thoracic dermatomes. To ensure cephalad spread with low lumbar injections (L4 to 5 interspace and below), the patient should be placed in the head-down position to ensure that hyperbaric solution surmounts the lumbar lordosis to reach thoracic kyphosis.[3] Maldistribution resulting in accumulation of large doses of hyperbaric local anesthetic solution in the sacral area below the summit of lumbar convexity has been implicated in the etiology of neurologic deficits following continuous spinal anesthesia.[4]

Isobaric Solutions

Isobaric local anesthetic solutions offer a major clinical advantage, in that patient position after local anesthetic injection should not affect the distribution of local anesthetic and therefore the final level of spinal anesthesia. Because the isobaric solutions tend to remain at the level of injection and diffuse away from this point by mass diffusion, surgical procedures most suitable for isobaric spinal anesthesia are those below L1 dermatome; e.g., lower-limb procedures.

Hypobaric Solutions

Hypobaric solutions are most suitable for surgical procedures done with patients in the head-down or lateral position; e.g., total hip arthroplasty. The patient is placed in position appropriate for the surgery, with the surgical site uppermost before the local anesthetic injection. The hypobaric solution floats upward to block the nerves that innervate the nondependent surgical site.

FACTORS INFLUENCING THE SPREAD OF LOCAL ANESTHETIC WITHIN THE SUBARACHNOID SPACE

Twenty-five factors have been cited as having potential influence on the spread of local anesthetic solution within CSF.[5] Factors that have been shown to have no demonstrable effect on spread include weight (except for morbid obesity), height, gender, rate of injection and/or barbotage, concentration of local anesthetic injected, addition of vasoconstrictors to the local anesthetic solution, and direction of needle bevel.[5] Factors that influence the spread of local anesthetic solution in CSF and therefore the level of block after subarachnoid injection are (1) patient age, (2) site of injection, (3) anatomic configuration of spine, (4) volume of spinal CSF, (5) baricity of local anesthetic solution, (6) local anesthetic dose (dose = volume × concentration), and (7) position of the patient with hypobaric or hyperbaric solutions.[5] Hogan and colleagues[2] suggested that decreased CSF volume that results from increased abdominal pressure, as seen in morbid obesity or pregnancy, may produce more extensive neuraxial blockade through increased spread of local anesthetic. With pencil-point needles, such as Whitacre and Sprotte, orientation of the needle aperture also has been demonstrated to have a minor effect on spread with isobaric local anesthetic solutions.[6]

TECHNICAL ASPECTS OF SUBARACHNOID BLOCK

To minimize the potential risk of injuring the spinal cord, lumbar puncture for subarachnoid injection of local anesthetics is performed at vertebral interspaces below L2 vertebra. Patient position for lumbar puncture can be lateral decubitus, sitting, or prone. In obese patients and in patients with scoliosis, a sitting position facilitates the location of midline. In patients undergoing rectal and perineal procedures, a prone position may be more time efficient, as it allows the patient to be placed in the actual surgical position prior to administration of hypobaric spinal anesthesia.

There are three principal approaches for entering subarachnoid space: midline, paramedian, and lumbosacral (Taylor) (Fig. 83–1). The midline approach is technically the easiest to learn, because the anesthesiologist directs the needle in only one plane; i.e., perpendicular to the skin and parallel to the spinous processes. A paramedian approach is most suitable in clinical situations where there is a narrowing of the "target interspinous area." Examples of such situations include calcified interspinous spaces (e.g., in elderly patients) and inability to overcome lumbar lordosis and achieve ideal patient position due to obesity or pain (e.g., in fracture of hip and lower-extremity bones). For the paramedian approach, one should identify the tip of the spinous process caudad to the selected intervertebral space and insert the spinal needle 1 cm lateral to it. The direction

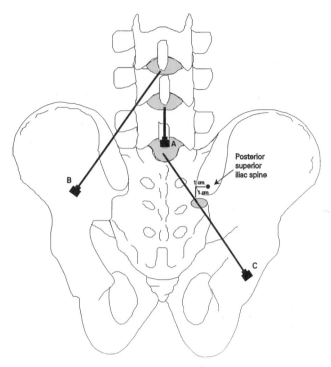

FIGURE 83–1. Midline *(A)*, paramedian *(B)*, and Taylor *(C)* approaches for entering subarachnoid space (see text for details).

of the needle is 15 degrees to 20 degrees toward midline.

The largest interlaminar space in the body is the L5/S1 interspace. The paramedian approach through this interspace is called the "Taylor approach." The spinal needle is inserted at a point, 1 cm medial and 1 cm caudad to the posterior superior iliac spine. The needle is directed on an angle of 45 degrees cephalad and medially toward the L5/S1 interspace. If periosteum over the sacrum is encountered, the needle is withdrawn and redirected cephalad until it reaches the L5/S1 interspace.

CONTINUOUS SPINAL ANESTHESIA (SUBARACHNOID CATHETER)

Continuous spinal anesthesia (CSA) via a subarachnoid catheter has potential advantages over "the single-shot" spinal anesthesia, in that the duration of block can be prolonged by repeated doses of local anesthetic. It also has an advantage over epidural anesthesia because a small dose of local anesthetic, too small to result in systemic toxicity, can produce profound and long-lasting sensory and motor block. CSA has been considered as an effective option for urgent cesarian delivery in a parturient with difficult airway.[7] Continuous spinal anesthesia is a relatively old technique with a reasonable safety margin, provided appropriate catheter placement and local anesthetic dose guidelines are followed. Sacral maldistribution associated with sacrally directed microcatheters and administration of high doses of hyperbaric local anesthetics can cause neurotoxicity.[4] If maldistri-

bution occurs, neurotoxicity may occur even with therapeutic doses of local anesthetics. Rigler and associates[4] propose the following recommendations to reduce potential neurotoxicity with continuous spinal anesthesia: (1) the catheter should be inserted no more than 2 to 3 cm into the subarachnoid space; (2) the lowest effective concentration of local anesthetic should be injected; (3) after a test dose, extent of block should be assessed, and if level is inadequate for that dose, maldistribution should be suspected; (4) the maneuvers to overcome maldistribution, such as changing patient position, altering lumbosacral curvature, changing baricity of local anesthetic, and manipulation of catheter, should be carried out; and (5) if these maneuvers fail to correct inadequate block, the technique should be abandoned. Because of the risk of neurotoxicity, use of microcatheters and lidocaine for CSA has been discouraged. For CSA, one can safely use a commercially available 20-gauge spinal needle with a 22- or 24-gauge catheter or an 18-gauge Tuohy needle with a 20- to 22-gauge catheter (commercial epidural needles and catheters). A standard midline or paramedian approach should be used, with the bevel of the needle directed cephalad. When a free flow of CSF is obtained, the needle should be advanced 1 to 2 mm to ensure that the entire bevel of the needle is within the subarachnoid space. The catheter should be threaded no more than 2 to 3 cm into the subarachnoid space. Once clear CSF flow is identified through catheter, local anesthetic solution is injected in increments to achieve appropriate sensory level.

LOCAL ANESTHETIC DOSE FOR CSA

A major advantage of CSA over single-dose spinal anesthesia is the ability to control level and duration of block. Furthermore, because the duration can be extended by injecting supplemental doses of local anesthetic through the catheter, use of adjuncts such as epinephrine to prolong duration of block is unnecessary.

For CSA, the block can be initiated with 6 to 10 mg of bupivacaine or tetracaine. Increments of 2 mg can be injected until the desired level is obtained. After a two-segment regression of the block, a subsequent dose of local anesthetic through the catheter should be 30% to 50% of the initial dose. With bupivacaine and tetracaine, two-segment regression of anesthesia should be expected to occur in 70 to 100 minutes.

CHOICE OF LOCAL ANESTHETIC DRUG, DOSE, ADJUNCTS, AND DURATION OF SPINAL ANESTHESIA

Local anesthetic drugs most commonly used for spinal anesthesia are lidocaine, bupivacaine, and tetracaine. Dibucaine is no longer available in the United States but is still available in Europe. Procaine is available but not widely used. Ropivacaine produces spinal anesthesia similar in intensity and duration to that produced by bupivacaine.

TABLE 83–1. LOCAL ANESTHETIC DRUG, DOSE, AND DURATION OF SURGICAL ANESTHESIA (HYPERBARIC SOLUTIONS)*

	Dermatome Level/Dose (mg)			Duration of Surgical Anesthesia	
	L1	*T10*	*T4*	*No Epinephrine*	*Epinephrine, 0.2 mg*
Procaine	50–75	100	150	30–45	60–75
Lidocaine	50	75	100	45–60	60–90
Bupivacaine	6–8	10–12	15–20	90–120	90–120
Tetracaine	6	8–10	12–14	90–120	120–180

*Duration of surgical anesthesia is dependent on several factors besides dose of local anesthetic and use of vasoconstrictor adjuncts (see text).

Duration of spinal anesthesia depends on age, choice of local anesthetic drug, concentration of local anesthetic in CSF (dose), baricity of local anesthetic drug, and additives to local anesthetic solutions such as epinephrine, phenylephrine, and clonidine.[8] In geriatric patients, duration of spinal anesthesia is longer than in younger patients. This has been attributed to decreased vascular uptake of local anesthetics from relatively diminished vascularity of spinal cord and meninges in the elderly. Lower doses of local anesthetics provide less-intense neural blockade of shorter duration because less drug spreads over a larger number of spinal segments.[9]

Vasoconstrictors (epinephrine and phenylephrine) have been used since the beginning of this century to prolong the duration of spinal anesthesia. Despite diminished vascularity of the spinal cord, use of vasoconstrictors in elderly patients is not associated with neurologic complications.[8] The dose of epinephrine used for prolonging spinal anesthesia is 0.2 to 0.3 mg, and that for phenylephrine is 2 to 5 mg. When used in these equipotent doses, both epinephrine and phenylephrine produce comparable prolongation in duration of tetracaine spinal anesthesia.[10] Studies that measured two-segment regression of analgesia have failed to demonstrate prolongation of lidocaine and bupivacaine spinal anesthesia with epinephrine.[11, 12] However, studies that considered recovery of anesthesia from lumbosacral dermatomes have demonstrated significant prolongation of lidocaine spinal anesthesia with supplemental epinephrine.[13] Local anesthetic drugs commonly used for spinal anesthesia, their doses, and corresponding duration of surgical anesthesia are depicted in Table 83-1.

Success with spinal anesthesia, as with epidural anesthesia, is related in large part to experience with technique (i.e., ability to perform alternative approaches such as paramedian and Taylor's approach when the standard midline approach has failed). Perhaps equally important in achieving high success with spinal anesthesia is clinical experience with the technique (i.e., judgment with respect to pharmacologic factors, such as choice of drug, dose, baricity, and proper positioning of the patient) (Table 83-2).[14]

PHYSIOLOGIC SIDE EFFECTS AND COMPLICATIONS

Hypotension, bradycardia, and nausea and vomiting are well-known side effects of spinal anesthesia. Hypotension and bradycardia are related to partial interruption of sympathetic fibers resulting in vasodilation, peripheral venous pooling, and decreased cardiac filling. Nausea and vomiting have been attributed to hypotension, cerebral hypoxia, and/or unopposed vagal activity in the presence of sympathetic block. Incidence of these side effects and associated risk factors were addressed in a recent study by Carpenter and associates.[15] Risk factors for bradycardia are (1) patient factors, such as older age, low baseline heart rate, low baseline blood pressure, and preoperative use of β-adrenergic block drugs; and (2) anesthetic factors, including high peak block height (>T5 dermatome), addition of vasoconstrictors, higher lumbar puncture site, and use of supplemental general anesthesia.

Hypotension during spinal anesthesia is treated by intravenous fluids to augment venous return and ephedrine and/or atropine to increase cardiac output. Bradycardia is usually treated with atropine and/or ephedrine. Severe bradycardia (heart rate < 40 beats per minute) is best treated with immediate intravenous epinephrine, 10 to 20 μg. Chest compressions may be necessary to circulate the epinephrine in cases of severe bradycardia. Nausea and vomiting are treated by correcting hypotension and administrating vagolytic agents such as atropine and glycopyrrolate. Administration of supplemental oxygen is recommended when patients are sedated to avoid hypoxemia.

SEVERE BRADYCARDIA AND ASYSTOLE DURING SPINAL ANESTHESIA

The phenomenon of abrupt, severe bradycardia and asystole with spinal anesthesia has received significant

TABLE 83–2. FACTORS AFFECTING SUCCESS OR FAILURE OF SPINAL ANESTHESIA

Technical Factors

1. Identification of subarachnoid space; ability to utilize different approaches
2. Documentation of free cerebrospinal fluid flow before and after injection

Pharmacologic Factors (Clinical Judgment)

1. Selection of appropriate local anesthetic drug; addition of vasoconstrictor, depending on duration of surgery
2. Selection of appropriate dose and baricity, depending on extent of block
3. Appropriate patient position and choice of interspace, depending on site of surgery

attention recently.[16, 17] A reflex mechanism (Bezold-Jarisch reflex) in response to decreased ventricular filling volume has been cited as the possible mechanism.[17] Strategies to minimize this catastrophic complication include vigilant monitoring and prompt pharmacologic intervention when bradyarrhythmias occur during spinal anesthesia and avoidance of hypovolemia during and after surgery through adequate volume replacement.[16, 17]

POST–DURAL PUNCTURE HEADACHE

Post–dural puncture headache (PDPH) is the most frequent complication of spinal anesthesia. PDPH has been attributed to low CSF pressure caused by a leak of CSF from the dural hole created by spinal needle. Although the exact mechanism of PDPH has not yet been elucidated, it is thought that low CSF pressure causes sagging of the brain and pain-sensitive meninges when the patient assumes an upright position. PDPH may be of variable intensity, and associated symptoms may include nausea, vomiting, dizziness, photophobia, diplopia from abducens palsy, and auditory disturbances.

Incidence of PDPH is increased primarily by factors such as younger age, female gender, larger needle diameter (gauge), needle tip configuration (cutting vs. atraumatic pencil point), and, finally, use of the paramedian approach to lumbar puncture. Of all these factors, the two most important are perhaps spinal needle diameter and tip configuration. A recent meta-analysis that examined correlation of PDPH and spinal needle design demonstrated a significant reduction in incidence of PDPH with pencil-point Whitacre and Sprotte spinal needles compared with cutting Quincke needles.[18]

Reducing the needle gauge minimizes risk of PDPH; however, it has practical limits, because use of needles smaller than 27 gauge reduces technical success of spinal anesthesia. Failed spinal anesthesia with small-gauge needles may be the result of technical difficulty with needle insertion (stiffness factor), difficulty in ascertaining subarachnoid placement because of poor back flow of CSF, and slow drug injection leading to poor local anesthetic spread. The best compromise between high technical success and low incidence of PDPH is the use of a 25-gauge atraumatic Whitacre needle, which offers a technical success of 98% and PDPH in the range of 1% to 2%.[19] Use of atraumatic spinal needles not only reduces incidence of PDPH but also may reduce the requirement for epidural patch; PDPH, when it occurs, is usually mild and responds to conservative therapy.

Treatment of Post–Dural Puncture Headache

Mild forms of PDPH are usually transient and respond to bed rest and analgesics. Intravenous hydration is not necessary unless the patient has protracted vomiting. If PDPH limits physical activity beyond 24 hours, especially in patients in whom surgery has not produced restriction of activity, an epidural blood patch should be offered. Other causes of headache, such as migraine headache, meningitis, sagittal sinus thrombosis, and pre-existing headaches, however, should be considered in the differential diagnosis. Complications associated with epidural blood patch are infrequent in the absence of bacteremia and anticoagulation. Low backache and nuchal rigidity reported with epidural blood patch resolve over 24 to 48 hours. Crawford reported a 70% success rate with epidural blood patch, using 6 to 15 mL of autologous blood; this increased to 98% when the volume of injected blood was increased to 20 mL.[20] If PDPH does not resolve with one epidural blood patch, a second blood patch can be used after 24 hours.

BACKACHE AND TRANSIENT RADICULAR IRRITATION

Backache is a common postoperative complaint, occurring in approximately 25% to 30% of patients during the postoperative period.[21] Recently, the phenomenon of transient radicular irritation (TRI), characterized by pain and/or dysesthesias in buttocks, thighs, and lower extremities, has been described in association with lidocaine spinal anesthesia.[22, 23] Reported incidence of TRI in patients receiving lidocaine spinal anesthesia is in the range of 16% to 30%. Reduction of lidocaine concentration from 5% to 2% and changing its baricity does not reduce the risk.[22, 23] Objective evidence of neurotoxicity has not been reported in patients with TRI symptoms, but severe bilateral sciatic pain may persist up to 24 hours. Based on its long-term safety record, it has been proposed that the use of lidocaine for spinal anesthesia should continue until another local anesthetic with a better clinical profile is identified.[24] However, the clinical entity of TRI should be taken into consideration when choosing a local anesthetic for spinal anesthesia, especially in an ambulatory patient.

NEUROLOGIC COMPLICATIONS

Serious neurologic complications are rare after spinal anesthesia. Trauma during needle placement (paresthesia) and local anesthetic neurotoxicity from prolonged exposure to high concentrations of local anesthetics are the two major factors that have been correlated with neurologic deficits following spinal anesthesia.[4, 25] Although preexisting conditions such as spinal stenosis, lumbar radiculopathy, and peripheral neuropathy had previously been considered relative contraindications, a recent review of 4767 consecutive spinal anesthetics failed to demonstrate any adverse effect of spinal anesthesia in patients with such preexisting neurologic deficits.[25]

SPINAL ANESTHESIA FOR AMBULATORY SURGERY

When used judiciously, spinal anesthesia can serve as an optimal and cost-effective anesthetic technique for ambulatory surgery. Patients recovering from spinal anesthesia utilize minimal nursing resources because they are pain free, have minimal or no nausea and vomiting, are alert, and have no airway problems. However, there are three potential disadvantages of spinal anesthesia in an ambulatory patient: prolonged time to ambulation, PDPH, and prolonged time to urination. These disadvantages can be negated by judicious selection of local anesthetic drug and dose, use of smaller-gauge atraumatic spinal needles, and appropriate clinical management. Small doses of short-acting local anesthetics such as lidocaine (40 to 75 mg) and procaine (50 to 75 mg) are desirable for ambulatory spinal anesthesia. Times to ambulation and voiding (home discharge) are related to drug, dose, and addition of adjuncts. Motor recovery and times to micturition are prolonged when epinephrine is used as an adjunct to lidocaine for ambulatory spinal anesthesia.[26] On the other hand, addition of 20 μg fentanyl prolongs duration of surgical anesthesia without prolonging times to motor recovery and micturition.[27]

Concentration and baricity of local anesthetic solution also have importance for motor recovery and time until recovery of micturition. Use of 1.5% hyperbaric lidocaine provides a significantly shorter recovery time when compared with 5% hyperbaric lidocaine.[28] Besides use of appropriate local anesthetic drug, dose, and baricity, delays in voiding following ambulatory anesthesia can be minimized by restriction of intravenous fluids during and after surgery to less than 10 mL/kg, early mobilization, and psychologic encouragement.

COMBINED SPINAL-EPIDURAL ANESTHESIA

Combined spinal-epidural anesthesia (CSE) overcomes the limitations of spinal, as well as epidural, anesthesia. It offers several advantages: rapid onset of profound anesthesia, reduced requirement of local anesthetics compared with epidural block and therefore reduced risk of systemic toxicity, flexibility in extent and duration of anesthesia, rapid recovery, and ability to provide prolonged postoperative analgesia. Because of these advantages, CSE is specifically suited for obstetric patients, ambulatory patients, and patients requiring surgical anesthesia of lumbosacral dermatomes.[29]

LOCAL ANESTHETIC DOSING FOR COMBINED SPINAL-EPIDURAL ANESTHESIA

Subarachnoid Dose

Because of the ability to "top-off" the block via the indwelling epidural catheter, smaller than usual doses of local anesthetics suffice to initiate the block; e.g., 40 to 60 mg lidocaine or 6 to 8 mg bupivacaine. In an ambulatory patient, use of this dose of lidocaine for intrathecal component of CSE facilitates rapid recovery and discharge.[30]

Epidural Dose

The amount of epidural local anesthetic dose for supplementing the initial spinal block during CSE may require more volume of local anesthetic per segment than supplementing routine continuous lumbar epidural anesthesia. An explanation for this phenomenon may be that epidural local anesthetic in CSE is being used to initiate an epidural nerve block and not for reinforcing an already existing epidural block, as is the case with routine epidural anesthesia. The dose range is between 1.5 and 3 mL per segment of routinely used epidural local anesthetics, such as 1.5% lidocaine or 0.5% bupivacaine.[30]

Technique of Combined Spinal-Epidural Anesthesia

Combined spinal-epidural anesthesia can be performed through a single spinal segment technique (SST) using a long (25- to 28-gauge) spinal needle through a 16- to 17-gauge epidural needle as an introducer. CSE can also be performed using a double spinal segment technique (DST), in which the spinal needle is introduced through one intervertebral space and the epidural needle, through the adjacent next intervertebral space. Use of SST is more prevalent because it is more convenient and causes less pain than the two-segment technique. DST carries a theoretical risk of damage to the epidural catheter, because lumbar puncture for the spinal anesthesia component is done after epidural catheter placement. One of the limitations of SST is that spinal local anesthetic is injected before epidural catheter placement. Therefore, if one uses hyperbaric local anesthetic with the patient in the lateral decubitus position, a unilateral block may occur, especially if placement of the epidural catheter is delayed because of technical difficulties. Use of isobaric solutions for the spinal anesthesia component can overcome this limitation.

Packaged sets are now available for doing CSE by SST. One can choose between two kinds of epidural needles: a single-lumen epidural needle for the needle-through-needle approach for dural puncture, and the double-lumen epidural needle approach, in which the spinal needle is guided through a parallel tube incorporated within the epidural needle.

LIMITATIONS OF COMBINED SPINAL-EPIDURAL ANESTHESIA

Two limitations of CSE are the occasional inability to puncture the dura with the needle-through-needle technique and difficulty with test dosing of the epidural catheter and confirming appropriate catheter location in the presence of preexisting spinal block. Technical failure related to dural puncture can be minimized by adhering to the midline approach, minimizing cephalad angulation of the epidural needle and adequate length of the spinal needle with the spinal needle tip extending 12 to 15 mm beyond the epidural needle bevel.

CONTROVERSIES IN SPINAL ANESTHESIA

Spinal Anesthesia in Patients With Previous Laminectomies

Lumbar puncture can be technically difficult in patients who have had prior laminectomies because of loss of normal anatomic landmarks. Spread of local anesthetic solution and extent of spinal anesthesia, however, are not altered. Use of alternate approaches, such as choosing an interspace above the scar, and the Taylor approach, may increase the success rate of spinal anesthesia in these patients.

Spinal Anesthesia in Febrile Patients and Patients With Human Immunodeficiency Virus Infection

The anesthesiologist may have concerns performing spinal anesthesia in a febrile bacteremic patient because of an assumed risk of subsequent meningitis. Available epidemiologic data and a recent animal study, however, have failed to bear out the validity of that assumption.[31] Recommended guidelines for administration of spinal anesthesia in these patients dictate the initiation of appropriate antibiotic therapy prior to dural puncture. The natural history of type 1 human immunodeficiency virus includes central nervous system infection early in the clinical course. Although some reports have cautioned against the use of central neuraxial blocks in these patients, recent experience suggests that central neuraxial blocks are without increased incidence of adverse sequelae.[32] No neurologic sequelae have been reported in follow-up of human immunodeficiency virus–positive patients after autologous blood patch.

Spinal Anesthesia in Patients Receiving Anticoagulants and Antiplatelet Drugs

Central neuraxial blockade in patients with hemostatic abnormalities carries the potential risk of spinal hematoma, with potentially devastating neurologic consequences. Following common-sense guidelines may minimize the risk of spinal hematoma in patients who are receiving anticoagulants in the perioperative period.[33]

Thrombolytic Therapy (Streptokinase, Urokinase)

The risk of hemorrhage following thrombolytic therapy is very high for several hours after initiation of therapy. These agents dissolve the clots that are already formed. Although safe guidelines have not been established, in the opinion of the authors, spinal anesthesia should not be attempted in patients who have received thrombolytic therapy in the preceding 36 to 48 hours. Coagulation profile should be assessed prior to needle placement. Thrombolytic therapy similarly should not be initiated 36 to 48 hours after the block placement. Neurologic status of these patients should be closely monitored.

Systemic Heparinization

Initiation of systemic heparinization more than 1 hour after performing spinal anesthesia is probably safe. Activated partial thromboplastin time (aPTT) should be monitored in these patients and should not be allowed to exceed 1.5 to 2 times the control. For patients who are on heparin preoperatively, heparin should be discontinued for 6 hours, and normal aPTT or activated clotting time (ACT) should be confirmed prior to instituting spinal anesthesia.

Subcutaneous Heparin

Small doses of heparin (5000 units every 8 to 12 hours) are used commonly for prophylaxis against deep venous thrombosis. Anticoagulant effect of a single dose occurs in 40 to 50 minutes and lasts 4 to 6 hours. Because potential of anticoagulation is minimal after this time, spinal anesthesia can be safely performed. Patients who have received multiple doses of subcutaneous heparin, however, may develop thrombocytopenia. A normal platelet count and a normal aPPT or ACT under 180 seconds should be confirmed prior to planning spinal anesthesia in these patients.

Low–Molecular-Weight Heparin

This preparation of heparin has higher bioavailability and longer half-life (10 to 12 hours) than regular subcutaneous heparin. Very little data are available at present concerning the duration of hemostatic abnormality after low–molecular-weight heparin (LMWH) administration. This is clearly an area where more research is needed. Spinal anesthesia should be delayed for 12 hours after subcutaneous LMWH. Ideally, preoperative administration of LMWH should be avoided until after the spinal anesthetic has been performed. LMWH can be administered safely 1 to 2 hours after administration of spinal anesthesia.

Low-Dose Oral Anticoagulants

The anticoagulant effect of warfarin begins in 48 to 72 hours after the initial dose. Spinal anesthesia is safe in patients who have received one or two doses of oral warfarin for deep vein thrombosis prophylaxis. A prothrombin time of 14 seconds or less or internal reference range of less than 1.4, however, should be confirmed prior to procedure because anticoagulant effect can be variable among individual patients.

Antiplatelet Drugs

Spinal anesthesia can be safely performed in patients receiving antiplatelet drugs such as aspirin and nonsteroidal anti-inflammatory agents.

SUMMARY

Spinal anesthesia is the fastest and most predictable form of regional anesthesia; it has been in use for almost 100 years. Over the past decade, considerable investigational work has been done. It has provided insights into CSF volume characteristics, risk factors for side effects, and neurologic complications of spinal anesthesia. Introduction of atraumatic spinal needles has reduced the incidence of PDPH and re-energized the use of spinal anesthesia in obstetric and ambulatory patients. Application of spinal anesthesia is expected to expand further as we resort to more cost-effective anesthetic techniques and to newer central neuraxial block techniques such as combined spinal-epidural anesthesia.

REFERENCES

1. Larson MD: Tait and Caglieri: The first spinal anesthetic in America. Anesthesiology 85:913-919, 1996.
2. Hogan QH, Prost R, Kulier A, et al: Magnetic resonance imaging of cerebrospinal fluid volume and the influence of body habitus and abdominal pressure. Anesthesiology 84:1341-1349, 1996.
3. Lee JA, Atkinson RS, Watt MJ: Intradural analgesia (subarachnoid block). In Lee JA (ed): Sir Robert Macintosh's Lumbar Puncture and Spinal Analgesia, ed 5. New York, Churchill Livingstone, 1985, pp 188-207.
4. Rigler ML, Drasner K, Krejcie TC, et al: Cauda equina syndrome after continuous spinal anesthesia. Anesth Analg 72:275-281, 1991.
5. Greene NM: Distribution of local anesthetic solutions within the subarachnoid space. Anesth Analg 64:715-730, 1985.
6. Urmey WF, Stanton J, Bassin P, et al: The direction of the Whitacre needle aperture affects the extent and duration of isobaric spinal anesthesia. Anesth Analg 84:337-341, 1997.
7. Malon TP, Johnson MD: The difficult airway in obstetric anesthesia: Technique for airway management and the role of regional anesthesia. J Clin Anesth 1:473-480, 1988.
8. Greene NM: Uptake and elimination of local anesthetics during spinal anesthesia. Anesth Analg 62:1013-1024, 1983.
9. Lambert DH: Factors influencing spinal anesthesia. Int Anesthesiol Clin 27:13-19, 1989.
10. Concepcion M, Maddi R, Francis D, et al: Vasoconstrictors in spinal anesthesia with tetracaine—A comparison of epinephrine and phenylephrine. Anesth Analg 63:134-138, 1984.
11. Chambers WA, Littlewood DG, Scott DB: Spinal anesthesia with bupivacaine: Effect of added vasoconstrictors. Anesth Analg 61:49-52, 1982.
12. Chambers WA, Littlewood DG, Logan MR, et al: Effect of added epinephrine on spinal anesthesia with lidocaine. Anesth Analg 60:417-420, 1981.
13. Chiu AA, Liu S, Carpenter RL, et al: The effects of epinephrine on lidocaine spinal anesthesia: A cross-over study. Anesth Analg 80:735-739, 1995.
14. Munhall RJ, Sukhani R, Winnie AP: Incidence and etiology of failed spinal anesthetics in a university hospital: A prospective study. Anesth Analg 67:843-848, 1988.
15. Carpenter RL, Caplan RA, Brown DL, et al: Incidence and risk factors for side effects of spinal anesthesia. Anesthesiology 76:906-916, 1992.
16. Caplan RA, Ward RJ, Posner K, et al: Unexpected cardiac arrest during spinal anesthesia: A closed claims analysis of predisposing factors. Anesthesiology 68:5-11, 1988.
17. Mackey DC, Carpenter RL, Thompson GE, et al: Bradycardia and asystole during spinal anesthesia: A report of three cases without morbidity. Anesthesiology 70:866-868, 1989.
18. Halpern S, Preston R: Postdural puncture headache and spinal needle design. Anesthesiology 81:1376-1383, 1994.
19. Lynch J, Krings-Emst I, Strick K, et al: Use of a 25-gauge Whitacre needle to reduce the incidence of postdural puncture headache. Br J Anaesth 67:690-693, 1991.
20. Crawford JS: Experience with epidural blood patch. Anaesthesia 513-515, 1980.
21. Middleton MJ, Bell CR: Postoperative backache: Attempts to reduce incidence. Anesth Analg 44:446-448, 1965.
22. Pollack JE, Neal JM, Stephenson CA, et al: Prospective study of the incidence of transient radicular irritation in patients undergoing spinal anesthesia. Anesthesiology 84:1361-1367, 1996.
23. Hampl KF, Schneider MC, Pargger H, et al: A similar incidence of transient neurologic symptoms after spinal anesthesia with 2% and 5% lidocaine. Anesth Analg 83:1051-1054, 1996.
24. Carpenter RL: Hyperbaric lidocaine spinal anesthesia: Do we need an alternative? Anesth Analg 81:1125-1128, 1995.
25. Horlocker TT, McGregor DG, Matsushige DK, et al: A retrospective review of 4767 consecutive spinal anesthetics: Central nervous system complications. Anesth Analg 84:578-584, 1997.
26. Chiu AA, Liu S, Carpenter RL, et al: The effects of epinephrine on lidocaine spinal anesthesia: A cross-over study. Anesth Analg 80:735-739, 1995.
27. Liu S, Chiu AA, Carpenter RL, et al: Fentanyl prolongs lidocaine spinal anesthesia without prolonging recovery. Anesth Analg 80:730-734, 1995.
28. Liu S, Pollock JE, Mulroy MF, et al: Comparison of 5% with dextrose, 1.5% with dextrose, and 1.5% dextrose-free lidocaine solution for spinal anesthesia in human volunteers. Anesth Analg 81:697-702, 1995.
29. Felsby S, Juelsgaard P: Combined spinal and epidural anesthesia. Anesth Analg 80:821-826, 1995.
30. Urmey WF, Stanton J, Peterson M, et al: Combined spinal-epidural anesthesia for outpatient surgery. Anesthesiology 83:528-534, 1995.
31. Chestnut DH: Spinal anesthesia in the febrile patient. Anesthesiology 76:667-669, 1992.
32. Hughes SC, Dailey PA, Landers D, et al: Parturients injected with human immunodeficiency virus and regional anesthesia. Anesthesiology 82:32-37, 1995.
33. Vandermeulen EP, Van Aken H, Vermylen J: Anticoagulants and spinal-epidural anesthesia. Anesth Analg 79:1165-1177, 1994.

Chapter 84

● Epidural Anesthesia

Rom A. Stevens, M.D.,
and Nigel E. Sharrock, M.B., B.Ch.

Epidural anesthesia has been used in one form or another since shortly after the start of the 20th century.[1] The advent of the Tuohy needle and the indwelling catheter in the 1940s led to an interest in caudal and lumbar epidural anesthesia for the provision of labor analgesia. During the past 20 years a great deal of new information about the physiology and anatomy relevant to the practice of epidural anesthesia has led to greater clinical success with this technique. Currently, in North America and Europe, epidural anesthesia with or without light general anesthesia is a very popular technique for operative anesthesia with the ability to extend epidural analgesia into the postoperative period for several days or weeks.

ANATOMY

The epidural space is a potential space which exists within the bony confines of the spinal canal outside the dura mater. For this reason, the term *extradural anesthesia* is used in the United Kingdom and Ireland, and *peridural anesthesia* is used in the German- and Spanish-speaking countries. The epidural space extends from the sacrococcygeal ligament to the foramen magnum. This space contains fat and blood vessels at some levels but is only a potential space at other levels. Hogan[2] demonstrated the discontinuous nature of the epidural space. Hogan showed that the epidural space contains fat and blood vessels, but only near the spinal interspaces (Fig. 84–1). Between these areas there are no contents in the space, and the dura is in contact with the bony walls of the spinal canal. This apparently discontinuous space can be made continuous by injection of local anesthetic (or contrast dye), and small-gauge catheters can be passed for some distance cephalad to the insertion point, provided radiologic guidance is used to ascertain that the catheter does not coil near the level of insertion.

Starting from the plane of the back, there are three ligaments through which an epidural needle must pass to reach the epidural space: (1) the supraspinous liga-

ment, a thin ligament of little consequence which joins the tips of the spinous processes; (2) the interspinous ligament, which connects adjacent spinous processes and can degenerate to form cavities, sometimes resulting in a false-positive loss of resistance test (described later); and (3) the ligamentum flavum, which is an embryologically bilateral structure fused in the midline, sometimes incompletely.[2] As the epidural needle is advanced from the interspinous ligament into the more dense ligamentum flavum, an increase in the resistance to injection is felt, and sometimes a "gritty" sensation is noted. Loss of resistance should occur within approximately 5 mm of needle entry into the ligamentum flavum.

The depth from the skin to the epidural space in adults is dependent on the amount of adipose tissue present. Gutierrez measured the distance from skin to loss of resistance in adults[3] (Fig. 84–2). The most frequently encountered distance was 5 cm, but the range

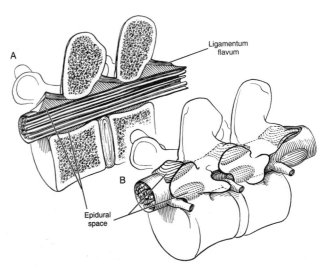

FIGURE 84–1. A three-dimensional view of the epidural space, showing the discontinuous nature of the epidural space contents. (From Brown DL (ed): Regional Anesthesia and Analgesia. Philadelphia, WB Saunders, 1996.)

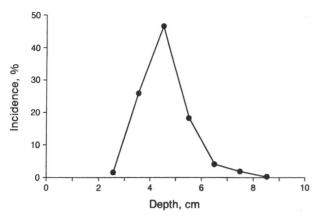

FIGURE 84–2. Distance from skin to epidural space. (From Brown DL (ed): Regional Anesthesia and Analgesia. Philadelphia, WB Saunders, 1996.)

was 2.5 to 9 cm. With some experience it is possible to accurately predict the needle depth at which loss of resistance should be encountered. If a loss of resistance is encountered more superficially than expected, particularly if needle entry into the ligamentum flavum is not felt, then one should be suspicious of a false loss of resistance.

The problem of a false-positive loss of resistance can be largely avoided by use of the paramedian approach. With this technique, the lamina is first located just lateral to the spinous process and the Tuohy needle is advanced cephalad and medially into the ligamentum flavum. At this point, resistance should be encountered. The subsequent loss of resistance heralds epidural entry.

SELECTION OF INTERSPACE AND APPROACH

The epidural space can in theory be entered at any vertebral interspace between C2 and the sacral hiatus. In usual clinical practice, the most cephalad interspace used is C7–T1 and the most caudad is the sacral hiatus. The guiding principle behind the choice of interspace is to place the epidural catheter as closely as possible to the dermatome in the middle of the surgical incision (Fig. 84–3). For example, if the patient is to undergo a gastrectomy (incision at T6–11), the epidural catheter should ideally be placed between T8 and T10. If the patient is to undergo a total knee replacement (incision at L3 dermatome), the epidural puncture should be made between L2 and L4. Following this principle results in delivery of the maximum concentration of local anesthetic or opioid at the dermatomes where anesthesia, analgesia, and/or motor block are required.

There are two standard approaches to the epidural space: midline and paramedian. They differ in the angle of the needle with respect to the plane of the back and in the exact location of needle puncture of the skin. The actual point of needle entry into the epidural space does not differ substantially between these two approaches. For the beginner, the midline approach is the easiest to learn, because the needle is inserted perpen-

dicular to the skin and parallel to the spinous processes at that spinal level. For epidural punctures in the midthoracic region (T5–9), the angulating and in some cases overlapping spinous processes require a very acute angle of insertion when the midline approach is attempted; a paramedian approach is easier in this region. In the elderly population, degeneration of the interspinous ligaments may result in cavitation and a false loss of resistance to injection.[4] Additionally, osteophytic growth of the laminae may result in narrowing of the target area available with the midline approach. The paramedian approach provides a larger target area. Therefore, there are several situations in which the paramedian approach has advantages over the midline approach.

The largest interspace in the body is the L5–S1 interspace. The paramedian approach to this interspace is called the *Taylor approach*. The needle is inserted at a point 1 cm medial and 1 cm caudal to the posterior superior iliac spine, and is advanced at a 45-degree angle cephalad and medially toward the interspace. In patients with advanced stages of calcification of the spine, the Taylor approach may provide the best opportunity to gain access to the lumbar epidural space.

IDENTIFICATION OF THE EPIDURAL SPACE

A variety of different techniques for identifying needle entry into the epidural space have been described.[5]

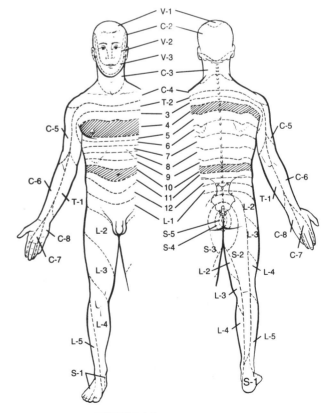

FIGURE 84–3. Dermatome chart.

Most commonly used are the *hanging drop technique* of Gutierrez[6] and the *loss of resistance technique*. Studies have shown that the thoracic epidural space has a subatmospheric pressure, probably related to the negative intrapleural pressure, and will suck up a drop of fluid placed at the hub of the Tuohy needle as the needle is advanced from the ligamentum flavum into the epidural space. Presence of a negative pressure in the lumbar epidural space is not as reliable; therefore Bromage does not recommend the use of the hanging drop technique in the lumbar region, particularly in laboring women, in whom the epidural space pressure may be increased during contractions of the uterus.[6]

Loss of resistance to air or saline is probably the most widely used technique to identify needle entry into the epidural space. The sensation felt on the syringe is quite different with air and with saline. Air is compressible, and the feeling is "bouncy" as the epidural needle is advanced through the interspinous and yellow ligaments. Saline is not compressible, and there is a rapid change from resistance to little resistance to injection when the needle enters the epidural space. Use of air has the advantage that no fluid is injected into the epidural space; therefore, if fluid is aspirated from the Tuohy needle, it clearly is cerebrospinal fluid. In addition, any saline that is injected into the epidural space dilutes the local anesthetic that is subsequently injected. Disadvantages of using air include rare cases of venous air embolus, pneumocephalus, nerve root compression, persistence of epidural air bubbles for longer than 24 hours, expansion of these air bubbles if nitrous oxide is inhaled, and possibly resultant inadequate anesthesia.[7] The authors believe that in the hands of an expert there is no clear advantage of one technique over the other, so long as large volumes of air (more than 3 mL) are not injected. Whether air or saline is used should be left up to the preference of the anesthesiologist.

FACTORS AFFECTING SPREAD OF LOCAL ANESTHETICS WITHIN THE EPIDURAL SPACE

Major factors that have generally been accepted to have a clinically significant effect on the spread of blockade after epidural injection of local anesthetic are dose of local anesthetic (volume and concentration), age of patient, and site of injection (thoracic vs. lumbar).[8] Minor factors are morbid obesity and pregnancy. Factors that have been shown to have little or no effect on spread are (1) gender, (2) height, (3) weight (except for morbid obesity), (4) direction of Tuohy needle orientation, (5) speed of injection, (6) arteriosclerosis, (7) mode of injection (fractionated vs. bolus injection), and (8) position of patient. Doses of local anesthetics should be reduced with thoracic as compared with lumbar injection, in patients older than 70 years of age, and to a lesser extent in patients who are morbidly obese and/or pregnant.

For example, a 40-year-old patient undergoing a thoracotomy has an epidural catheter placed at T3-4. After injection of 15 mL (75 mg) of bupivacaine 0.5%, analgesia develops over the T2 through L2 dermatomes (12 dermatomes). In a 70-year-old patient, the same spread of analgesia could be obtained after injection of 10 mL (50 mg). Similarly, if the 15-mL injection were given to the 40-year-old patient at the L2-3 level, a block from T10 through L5 might be obtained (8 dermatomes), whereas in an 80-year-old patient the same injection would be expected to produce analgesia from T4 to S5 (19 dermatomes). It is difficult to quantitate this age-related decrease in local anesthetic requirements, because the relationship is nonlinear.[9] To roughly calculate anesthetic spread after lumbar injection of 2% lidocaine in a young person, the figures of 1.25 mL per segment for lumbar injection and 0.75 mL per segment for thoracic injection can be used for a 40-year-old patient.[10]

CHOICE OF DRUG, DOSE, AND DURATION OF ACTION

For epidural anesthesia, the choice of drug is essentially a question of the desired duration of anesthesia. Generally, for outpatient surgery, 2-chloroprocaine 3% and lidocaine 2%, with or without epinephrine, are the drugs of choice, because patients usually meet discharge criteria within 3 to 4 hours after a 20-mL dose.[11] Mepivacaine 2% produces a longer duration of sensory anesthesia than does lidocaine 2%, as well as a significantly longer time to discharge from the ambulatory surgery center.

Bupivacaine 0.5% to 0.75% and ropivacaine 0.75% to 1.0% are the drugs of choice for inpatient surgery because of their longer duration of action. The 1% solution of ropivacaine and the 0.75% solution of bupivacaine are roughly equivalent in terms of duration and quality of sensory and motor blockade.[12] The time required to obtain surgical anesthesia and motor block is somewhat longer with the less concentrated solutions. The concentrated solutions produce more complete motor block and more complete block of the S1 nerve root, which sometimes remains unblocked after lumbar epidural anesthesia.[13] Anesthesia of this dermatome is important for ankle surgery and must be confirmed by sensory testing before the patient is draped for surgery. A more intense blockade of the S1 nerve root can be achieved by alkalinizing the local anesthetic.[14]

Epinephrine (1:200,000) usually is added to epidural solutions because it serves as a marker for intravascular injection should either the epidural needle or the catheter be placed into a blood vessel at any time. By monitoring the heart rate during and for 2 minutes after epidural local anesthetic injection, and by injecting no more than a 5-mL aliquot at once, an intravascular injection of local anesthetic can be detected and catastrophic local anesthetic toxicity can be avoided.

One way to compare duration of action among different local anesthetics is the *time to two-segment regression* (Fig. 84-4). Table 84-1 lists the times to two-segment regression for commonly used local anesthetics.[15] However, in current clinical practice, the times to full recovery of motor function of the lower extremities,

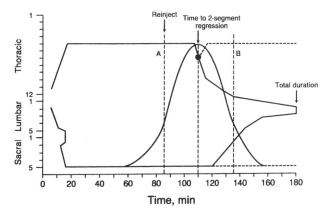

FIGURE 84-4. Onset and regression of epidural analgesia. (From Brown DL (ed): Regional Anesthesia and Analgesia. Philadelphia, WB Saunders, 1996.)

to ambulation, and to voiding seem more relevant to discharge criteria from ambulatory surgery centers.

QUALITY OF EPIDURAL BLOCKADE

A common criticism of epidural anesthesia by surgeons unfamiliar with this technique is that the blocks are not effective for surgical anesthesia. In the authors' experience, this result is caused by two factors: inaccurate needle placement or lack of understanding of factors influencing the quality of epidural blockade. Surgical anesthesia requires both sensory and complete motor blockade at the surgical site. To achieve this, epidural injection should be made at the appropriate interspace and a sufficient dose of local anesthetic should be given. To further intensify the block, epinephrine, clonidine, or opioids can be added. Topping up through the catheter provides more intense, longer-acting blockade; this is described by Bromage as "repainting the fence."

If larger doses of local anesthetic are used, more intense blockade will be achieved but circulatory instability may result. This problem can be managed with intravenous epinephrine or ephedrine. Use of larger doses provides for an intense anesthesia (much like a spinal anesthesia), requiring a lesser degree of sedation. If lower doses of local anesthetic are used, additional

sedation or general anesthesia may be required for surgical procedures.

COMPLICATIONS

Failed Block

Among beginners, the most common complication of epidural anesthesia is a failed block. In experienced hands, the failure rate of epidural anesthesia should be less than 1%. The most common explanation for failure, in the opinion of the authors, is encounter of a false loss of resistance, with subsequent insertion of the epidural catheter and injection of local anesthetic into a space other than the epidural space. A false loss of resistance can be encountered with the Tuohy needle tip in a variety of places, including a cavitated interspinous ligament,[4] the paravertebral space, and the prevertebral space. To avoid a failed epidural block in the practice of surgical anesthesia, the following procedures are recommended:

1. A thorough knowledge of spinal anatomy is necessary.

2. The level of needle puncture should be guided by the dermatomal site of surgery (see previous discussion).

3. An adequate dose of concentrated local anesthetic (0.75% bupivacaine, 0.75% ropivacaine, 3% 2-chloroprocaine, or 2% lidocaine) should be injected via the needle to set up the block with minimal delay and to facilitate passage of the epidural catheter.

4. The epidural catheter must then, after verification of negative aspiration, be tested for intravascular and intrathecal placement by injection of 3 mL of a local anesthetic solution containing epinephrine 15 µg and concurrent monitoring of the heart rate.

Uncertain Block

If it is unclear whether the block is working, the following procedures are recommended:

1. If it is certain that the needle tip is in the epidural space (i.e., good loss of resistance and the catheter passed well), add more local anesthetic via the catheter in 5-mL aliquots, because the problem may be insufficient local anesthetic.

TABLE 84-1. TIME TO TWO-SEGMENT REGRESSION FOR VARIOUS LOCAL ANESTHETICS*

Local Anesthetic	Initial Latency	Time to Maximum Spread	Time to Two-Segment Regression (Plain)	Two-Segment Regression With Epinephrine (1:200,000)
3% 2-Chloroprocaine	4.9	12.3	45	57±7
2% Lidocaine	5.0±1.1	16.2±2.6	46±5	97.5±19
2% Mepivacaine	6.2	17.5	—	117
0.5% Bupivacaine	5.8	18.2	165	196±31
0.75% Bupivacaine	5.0	16.8	164±46	201±40
1% Ropivacaine (plain)	6.0	24.5	177.5	—
1% Etidocaine	3.6	10.9	128±43	170±57

*Time in minutes (mean ± SD). All solutions with epinephrine 1:200,000, unless noted.
Data from Bromage PR: Epidural Analgesia. Philadelphia, WB Saunders, 1978.

2. If the placement of the epidural block is uncertain, do not top up the catheter, because this only limits one's options. After 10 minutes, either repeat the epidural block or, if the dose already given is large, change to a spinal or general anesthetic. The choice of alternatives depends on the indications for the type of anesthetic used. Within 10 minutes, some evidence of epidural anesthesia should be evident—either proximal muscle weakness, abolition of pain, or a decline in blood pressure.

Dural Puncture

Dural puncture should occur with a frequency of less than 1% in experienced hands. In training programs, the incidence of unintentional dural puncture may be as high as 3%. In patients younger than 40 years of age, the rate of headache after puncture of the dura with a 17-gauge epidural needle may be as high as 75%.[16] If a dural puncture occurs, an epidural catheter can be inserted one interspace higher and carefully tested to rule out intrathecal placement. If properly placed, this new epidural catheter can be used to provide surgical or obstetric anesthesia/analgesia. Alternatively, a spinal or general anesthetic can be used. At the end of surgery or labor, a prophylactic autologous blood patch, using 10 to 15 mL sterile autologous blood, can be injected via the epidural catheter. This approach prevents post–dural puncture headache in more than 50% of cases.[17] The epidural catheter is then removed. If a positional headache recurs, a conventional epidural blood patch is made, injecting 10 to 15 mL sterile autologous blood via a Tuohy needle, preferably inserted at the interspace at which the dural puncture occurred. The success rate of a conventional blood patch in treating post–dural puncture headache is greater than 95%.[18] The authors believe that early treatment of a post–dural puncture headache is important because it decreases time to discharge from hospital and may prevent the headache from becoming a chronic problem.[19]

Other Complications

Hypotension

Hypotension is almost an inevitable consequence of conduction blockade due to venous and arterial dilatation and subsequent venous blood pooling in the legs and in the splanchnic bed. Severe hypotension is apt to occur with volume depletion or extensive blockade. Treatment with appropriate volume and support of the circulation with α- and β-adrenergic agonists is effective treatment. Bradycardia and/or asystole can occur with a reduction of preload, especially in patients with extensive blockade. All patients receiving conduction anesthesia require close observation of their circulatory status.[20]

Core hypothermia can occur in patients with epidural or spinal anesthesia due to vasodilatation of blood vessels to the skin of the lower extremities and abdomen, redistribution of heat from the core to the legs, and increased heat loss.[21] In addition, patients with extensive central neuraxis blockade have a lowered shivering threshold. During epidural or spinal anesthesia, patients are at a risk for hypothermia similar to the risk with general anesthesia.[22] Therefore, monitoring of body temperature and proactive warming of intravenous fluids and of the patient (warming blanket) are important with prolonged epidural or spinal anesthesia.

Hypotension can be a serious problem if the patient is or becomes hypovolemic during the course of epidural anesthesia. Hypotension during epidural or spinal anesthesia usually is treated with intravenous ephedrine in boluses of 5 to 10 mg and volume replacement by a balanced salt solution. Blood volume should be monitored by assessment of urine output via a Foley catheter or by measurement of central venous pressures if large blood losses are expected or if bleeding or third-space losses are expected to continue into the postoperative period. Sudden bradycardia can occur during epidural or spinal anesthesia in the presence of hypovolemia (Bezold-Jarisch reflex).[23] To prevent bradycardia, which can lead to cardiac arrest, avoidance of hypovolemia and prophylactic treatment with an intravenous infusion of epinephrine (1 to 4 μg/minute) or other vasopressors can be helpful.[24]

Epidural Hematoma

Epidural hematoma is a serious but very rare complication of epidural or spinal anesthesia. In almost all of the reported cases of this complication, patients with central neuraxis anesthesia had received heparin, warfarin (Coumadin), or an antiplatelet drug before initiation of the anesthetic. Studies performed at the Mayo Clinic convincingly suggest that preoperative use of nonsteroidal anti-inflammatory medications does not place patients at risk for this complication,[25] nor does use of aspirin.[26] Intraoperative anticoagulation with heparin is probably safe as long as the epidural catheter is neither inserted nor removed while the patient has an abnormal coagulation profile.[27]

Definitive diagnosis of epidural hematoma is made by computed tomography or magnetic resonance scanning. Clinical signs are (1) new development of a motor and/or sensory block of the lower extremities, or persistence of a motor or sensory block after the anesthesia should have dissipated; (2) loss of deep tendon reflexes in the lower extremities; and (3) possibly severe back pain localized to the level of the hematoma. Should this complication be suspected, emergency scanning should be done immediately. If the diagnosis is confirmed, a neurosurgeon or orthopedic surgeon should be consulted to immediately decompress the spinal canal. There are cases of full neurologic recovery if decompression is carried out within 4 to 6 hours after the onset of symptoms.[28] Late decompression usually does not result in functional recovery, and poor neurologic outcome is a poor prognostic indicator for longevity.

In the authors' practices, specific recommendations for minimal coagulation parameters before placement of an epidural or spinal needle are as follows: (1) platelet count >80,000/mm³, (2) prothrombin time ≤2 seconds longer than control, (3) partial thromboplastin time <45 seconds, (4) activated clotting time <180 seconds, (5) bleeding time not grossly abnormal (<15 minutes). Attention to these parameters are particularly important in patients who have received anticoagulants in the preoperative period or who are at risk for development of a coagulopathy owing to comorbidities.

Infection

Catheter site infection and epidural abscess are also very rare complications of epidural or spinal anesthesia. DuPen and colleagues[29] studied the incidence and etiologic organisms of epidural catheter tract infections in cancer patients with indwelling epidural catheters. They found that the responsible organism is almost always a skin contaminant. The risk of catheter tract infection increases the longer an epidural catheter is in place. Therefore, in the authors' practices, epidural catheters left in place for postoperative pain control are inspected daily by the Acute Pain Management Service. If signs of infection are detected, the catheter is discontinued, the catheter insertion site is cleaned with antiseptic solution, and consideration is given to treatment of the patient with a first-generation cephalosporin. In general, unless it is tunneled, the authors do not recommend leaving an epidural catheter in place for postoperative analgesia longer than 4 days.

Very rarely, an epidural catheter tract infection may progress to epidural abscess. The definitive diagnosis is again made by computed tomography or magnetic resonance imaging. Clinical signs and symptoms are (1) severe pain at the vertebral level of the abscess, (2) fever and leukocytosis, and (3) new onset of sensory and/or motor block of the lower extremities. Treatment of an epidural abscess is usually by decompression and intravenous antibiotics. However, DuPen's group[29] reported several cases in which cancer patients were treated successfully with antibiotics via the indwelling epidural catheter.

PREPARATION AND POSITIONING OF THE PATIENT

It is very helpful to explain to the patient what to expect during placement of an epidural or spinal block. A judicious amount of intravenous midazolam (2 to 4 mg) is titrated to produce a drowsy and amnestic patient. This point is particularly important when a physician is learning to perform regional anesthesia, because more than one attempt may be required. The patient is preferably positioned in the lateral decubitus position, which is more comfortable and safer for the sedated patient than the sitting position. If the patient is so obese that the spinous processes cannot be palpated, then the patient is placed in the sitting position, preferably with the arms on a Mayo stand. During placement of the epidural or spinal block, the patient is monitored with a pulse oximeter and a blood pressure cuff. After sterile preparation of the skin and sterile draping, a generous amount of local anesthetic (3 to 5 mL) is injected into the skin and interspinous ligament using a 3-cm 25- or 27-gauge needle.

INTRAOPERATIVE MANAGEMENT

If the surgery continues beyond the expected time to two-segment regression for the local anesthetic being used, a re-dose (top-up) dose is necessary. Bromage recommends that the top-up dose be given before the actual time to two-segment regression to avoid intraoperative dissipation of the block. Therefore, for 3% 2-chloroprocaine with epinephrine the recommended time to re-injection is 45 minutes; for 2% lidocaine with epinephrine it is 60 minutes; and for 0.5% bupivacaine it is 120 minutes.

One half to two thirds of the initial volume is given as a top-up dose. For surgical procedures lasting longer than 3 hours, a continuous infusion of 0.5% bupivacaine or 0.75% ropivacaine can be given at a rate of 3 to 5 mL/hour depending on the extent of block desired, the location of the epidural catheter, and the dermatome location of surgery. Use of a continuous infusion vs. top-up dosing has the advantage in that it avoids the hypotension that is not infrequently observed 10 to 15 minutes after a top-up dose is given.

SEDATION AND COMBINED EPIDURAL AND GENERAL ANESTHESIA

For surgical procedures lasting less than 2 hours, it is reasonable to provide intravenous sedation to maintain patient comfort and amnesia during surgery. This can be accomplished with an initial intravenous bolus of midazolam (2 to 4 mg), followed by a continuous intravenous infusion of propofol (25 to 75 μg/kg/minute). When surgical procedures are performed with the patient under regional anesthesia plus intravenous sedation, it is important first to make the patient comfortable on the operating table by placing padding underneath all pressure points. Particularly important during hip replacement surgery with the patient in the lateral decubitus position is that the dependent shoulder must be well padded. A comfortably positioned patient has less need for heavy intravenous sedation.

For surgical procedures lasting 2.5 hours or longer, addition of light general anesthesia to the epidural or spinal anesthetic is often indicated and is preferable to intravenous sedation. For surgical procedures of the thorax and upper abdomen, endotracheal intubation and mechanical ventilation is indicated. For procedures involving the lower abdomen and lower extremities, a laryngeal mask airway and spontaneous ventilation is often adequate. Whichever option of airway management is elected, it is important to realize that epidural local anesthetics provide anesthesia and motor block while the general anesthetic agent provides amnesia and ability to tolerate the artificial airway. Therefore only low concentrations of anesthetic gases are needed to maintain general anesthesia (i.e., less than one half of the minimal alveolar concentration of the inhalation agent). Neuromuscular blocking agents are used only for insertion of the endotracheal tube; they then are allowed to dissipate. In this way, should the patient have too little general anesthetic to prevent recall, movement of the head, neck, or upper extremities will alert the anesthesiologist that a higher inspired concentration of anesthetic is necessary.

ADVANTAGES OF EPIDURAL ANESTHESIA

The advantages of epidural anesthesia include avoidance of airway problems, minimization of the risk of gastric aspiration, reduction of intraoperative blood loss, facilitation of postoperative pain management with epidural analgesia, augmentation of postoperative rehabilitation,[30] and enhanced recovery of colonic function after bowel surgery.[31] In addition, epidural anesthesia is associated with less risk of thromboembolic complications, both deep vein thrombosis in orthopedic surgery[32] and arterial thrombosis after peripheral vascular surgery.[33] For these reasons, epidural anesthesia is now the preferred anesthetic technique, in both obstetrics and many other surgical procedures, either alone or in combination with light general anesthesia.

SUMMARY

Epidural anesthesia is both a science and an art; when mastered, it is a useful addition to the anesthesiologist's armamentarium. Recent advances in the understanding of epidural anesthesia have contributed to the popularity and safety of this technique.

REFERENCES

1. Bromage PR: Epidural Analgesia. Philadelphia, WB Saunders, 1978, pp 1-4.
2. Hogan Q: Epidural anatomy examined by cryomicrotome section: Influence of age, vertebral level, and disease. Reg Anesth 21:395-406, 1996.
3. Gutierrez A: Anesthesia extradural. Rev Cir Buenos Aires 18:52, 1939.
4. Sharrock NE: Recording of, and an anatomical explanation for false positive loss of resistance during lumbar extradural anesthesia. Br J Anaesth 51:253-258, 1979.
5. Bromage PR: Identification of the epidural space. *In* Bromage PR (ed): Epidural Analgesia. Philadelphia, WB Saunders, 1978, pp 176-214.
6. Gutierrez A: Valor de la aspiracion liquida en el espacio peridural en la anestesia peridural. Rev Cir Buenos Aires 12:225, 1933.
7. Saberski LR, Kondamuri S, Osinubi OYO: Identification of the epidural space: Is loss of resistance to air a safe technique? A review of the complications related to use of air. Reg Anesth 22:3-15, 1997.
8. Park WY: Factors influencing distribution of local anesthetics in the epidural space. Reg Anesth 13:49-57, 1988.
9. Sharrock NE: Epidural anesthetic dose responses in patients 20 to 80 years old. Anesthesiology 49:425-428, 1978.
10. Bromage PR: Mechanism of action. *In* Bromage PR (ed): Epidural Analgesia. Philadelphia, WB Saunders, 1978, pp 131-135.
11. Kopacz DJ, Mulroy MF: Chloroprocaine and lidocaine decrease hospital stay and admission rate after outpatient epidural anesthesia. Reg Anesth 15:19-25, 1990.
12. Wood MB, Rubin AP: A comparison of epidural 1% ropivacaine and 0.75% bupivacaine for lower abdominal gynecologic surgery. Anesth Analg 76: 1274-1278, 1993.
13. Galindo A, Benavides O, Ortega de Munoz S, et al.: Comparison of anesthetic solutions used in lumbar and caudal peridural anesthesia. Anesth Analg 57:175-179, 1978.
14. Benzon HT, Toleikis JR, Dixit P, et al.: Onset, intensity of blockade and somatosensory evoked potential changes of the lumbosacral dermatomes after epidural anesthesia with alkalinized lidocaine. Anesth Analg 76:328-332, 1993.
15. Stevens RA: Neuraxial blocks. *In* Brown DL (ed): Regional Anesthesia and Analgesia. Philadelphia, WB Saunders, 1996, p 342.
16. Lambert DH, Hurley RJ, Hertwig L, et al.: Role of needle gauge and tip configuration in the production of lumbar puncture headache. Reg Anesth 22:66-72, 1997.
17. Cheek T, Banner R, Sauter J, et al.: Prophylactic extradural blood patch is effective: A preliminary communication. Br J Anaesth 61:340-342, 1988.
18. Ostheimer GW, Palahnuik RJ, Snider SM: Epidural blood patch for post lumbar puncture headache. Anesthesiology 41:307, 1974.
19. Stevens RA, Jorgensen N: Successful treatment of dural puncture headache with epidural saline infusion after failure of epidural blood patch. Acta Anaesthesiol Scand 32:429-431, 1988.
20. Liguri GA, Sharrock NE: Asystole and severe bradycardia during epidural anesthesia in orthopedic patients. Anesthesiology 86:250-257, 1997.
21. Glosten B, Sessler DI, Faure EAM, et al.: Central temperature changes are not perceived during epidural anesthesia. Anesthesiology 77:10-16, 1992.
22. Frank SM, Beattie C, Christopherson R, et al.: Epidural versus general anesthesia, ambient operating room temperature, and patient age as predictors of inadvertent hypothermia. Anesthesiology 77:252-257, 1992.
23. Mark AL: The Bezold-Jarisch reflex revisited: Clinical implications of inhibitory reflexes originating in the heart. J Am Coll Cardiol 1:90-102, 1983.
24. Sharrock NE, Mineo R, Urquhart B: Hemodynamic response to low-dose epinephrine infusion during hypotensive epidural anesthesia for total hip replacement. Reg Anesth 15:295-299, 1990.
25. Horlocker TT, Wedel DJ, Offord KP: Does perioperative antiplatelet therapy increase the risk of hemorrhagic complications associated with regional anesthesia? Anesth Analg 70:631-634, 1990.
26. Benzon HT, Brunner EA, Valisrub N: Bleeding time and nerve blocks in patients who had aspirin. Reg Anesth 9:86-89, 1984.
27. Rao TKL, El-Etr AA: Anticoagulation following placement of epidural and subarachnoid catheters: An evaluation of neurologic sequelae. Anesthesiology 55:618-620, 1981.
28. Bromage PR: Complications and contraindications. *In* Bromage PR (ed): Epidural Analgesia. Philadelphia, WB Saunders, 1978, pp 668-672.
29. DuPen SL, Peterson DG, Williams A, et al.: Infection during chronic epidural catheterization: Diagnosis and treatment. Anesthesiology 70:905-909, 1990.
30. Williams-Russo P, Sharrock NE, Haas S, et al.: Randomized trial of epidural versus general anesthesia: Outcomes after primary total knee replacement. Clin Orthop 331:199-208, 1966.
31. Liu SS, Carpenter R, Mackey D, et al.: Effects of perioperative analgesic technique on rate of recovery after colon surgery. Anesthesiology 83:757-765, 1995.
32. Sharrock NE, Ranawat CS, Urquhart B, et al.: Factors influencing deep vein thrombosis following total hip arthroplasty. Anesth Analg 76:765-771, 1993.
33. Christopherson R, Beattie C, Frank SM, et al.: The perioperative ischemia randomized anesthesia trial study group: Perioperative morbidity in patients randomized to epidural or general anesthesia for lower extremity vascular surgery. Anesthesiology 79:422-434, 1993.

Chapter 85

Combined Spinal-Epidural Technique

William F. Urmey, M.D.

Combined spinal-epidural anesthesia (CSE) is a regional anesthetic technique which combines an initial single subarachnoid injection with continuous epidural anesthesia and/or analgesia. This technique, first described for obstetric anesthesia by Brownridge,[1] initially involved a separate subarachnoid injection of local anesthetic at one spinal interspace followed by epidural catheter placement at a second interspace. Subsequently, a needle-through-needle technique utilizing a single interspace was reported by Coates,[2] who used it for orthopedic surgical anesthesia.

CSE offers advantages for surgical anesthesia and postoperative acute pain management. Whereas identification of the epidural space is sometimes associated with a vague or uncertain end point, the CSE technique allows more certain confirmation of proper needle position by the appearance of cerebrospinal fluid (CSF) in the spinal needle hub. Therefore, the certainty and quick onset of spinal anesthesia is combined with the flexibility and safe track record of continuous lumbar epidural anesthesia.

The CSE technique has been used safely for 15 years. No reports of unique or major complications specific to the technique have been reported.[3,4]

CSE is also beneficial for outpatient surgery because of more optimal control of duration of spinal anesthesia by facilitating use of minimal drug doses. Smaller intrathecal local anesthetic doses have been reported to result in shorter anesthetic duration. CSE allows one to decrease the initial dose of subarachnoid local anesthetic with the "safety net" of an epidural catheter. If the surgery is longer than anticipated, the short-acting spinal can be easily converted to an epidural.[5] Decreased spinal anesthetic dose may diminish the incidence of side effects, including nausea, vomiting, bradycardia, and hypotension, which have been associated with higher thoracic levels of spinal anesthesia.

Rawal and coworkers[6] found that CSE offered advantages for cesarean section. These same investigators also demonstrated advantages for major orthopedic surgery, specifically hip and knee arthroplasty.[3] The results of a prospective, randomized study of 75 patients showed that CSE had shorter anesthesia onset, better quality block, and a better success rate than epidural anesthesia.

In a study of 90 outpatients having arthroscopic surgery on the knee, Urmey and Stanton[7] found that all 90 had excellent surgical anesthesia. Reduction of the initial subarachnoid dose of lidocaine from 80 or 60 mg to 40 mg allowed these authors to discharge patients considerably earlier.

CSE with the needle-through-needle technique takes less time to place than routine epidural anesthesia and has a faster onset time.[7]

TECHNIQUE

The needle-through-needle technique for CSE has largely supplanted the original technique described by Brownridge in 1981,[1] which utilized separate needle placement for spinal and epidural anesthesia at two interspaces. The needle-through-needle technique with properly matched needles has a high success rate and eliminates the need for a second needle stick in approximately 90% of cases.[4]

Smaller-gauge, pencil-point spinal needles have made CSE acceptable for younger patients, obstetric patients, and outpatients. Use of a 27-gauge Whitacre spinal needle through an epidural needle is associated with a minimal risk of post–dural puncture headache but affords reliable CSF flow. However, smaller-gauge needles (e.g., 29- or 30-gauge) may be associated with lower success rates due to inability to ascertain spontaneous flow of CSF.[8, 9] Assurance of adequate spinal needle protrusion length allows for a success rate with maximal stability of the needle combination, ideally with the needles partially or fully adjoined.

MANAGEMENT

Contraindications and possible complications of CSE are the same as for spinal or epidural anesthesia alone.

TABLE 85–1. INITIAL INTRATHECAL DOSE WITH THE NEEDLE-THROUGH-NEEDLE TECHNIQUE

Type of Surgery	Type of Local Anesthetic	Dose	Sensory Level	Duration (min)
Cephalad to L1 dermatome level (e.g., hernia repair, gynecologic procedures, retrograde pyelography, laparoscopy)	Hyperbaric lidocaine 2%	50–75 mg (2.5–3.75 mL)	T5*	60
Cephalad to L1 dermatome level	Hyperbaric bupivacaine 0.75%	7–15 mg (1–2 mL)	T5*	90–120
Caudad to L1 dermatome level (e.g., knee arthroscopy, anterior cruciate ligament reconstruction, cystoscopy, transurethal prostate resection, Bartholin's cyst drainage, ankle arthroscopy)	Isobaric lidocaine 2%*	40–80 mg (2–4 mL)	T6†	60–90†
Caudad to L1 dermatome level	Isobaric mepivacaine 1.5%–2%	40–80 mg (2–5 mL)	T6†	90–150†

*Level of anesthesia with hyperbaric local anesthetics depends on positioning and spinal curvature. Isobaric local anesthetics are not approved by the U.S. Food and Drug Administration but are commonly used, and their use is described throughout the literature. There is evidence that isobaric preparations may offer advantages from isolated nerve data. It is not necessary to use α-adrenergic agents such as epinephrine or phenylephrine to prolong spinal anesthesia with this technique. α-Adrenergic agents increase variability of duration and may prolong discharge. I recommend the use of plain local anesthetics when using the CSE technique.

†Dose dependent; this represents approximate sensory level to pin-prick. Actual surgical anesthetic level with isobaric spinal is reliably L1.

In contrast to epidural anesthesia, CSE placement, like spinal anesthesia, should be limited to the L2-S1 interspaces, caudal to the termination of the spinal cord.

Short-acting local anesthetics that are preservative free are recommended for the outpatient. Shorter discharge times and decreased incidences of complications, including urinary retention, can be achieved with small doses of shorter-acting local anesthetics. The recommended initial subarachnoid local anesthetics and reinforcement epidural doses and timing are outlined in Tables 85–1 and 85–2.

It is important to consider the distribution of subarachnoid local anesthetic solutions when planning CSE. Plain local anesthetics listed in Tables 85–1 and 85–2 have been shown to be relatively isobaric with regard to CSF. The distribution of the bulk of such solutions therefore is limited to the injection area (i.e., the lumbar subarachnoid space), with minimal amounts of diffusion (Fig. 85–1). These solutions are not greatly affected by patient anatomy or position. Use of isobaric solutions is ideal for lower-extremity surgery, such as orthopedic or vascular procedures, that are performed below the L1 dermatome level.

By contrast, hyperbaric solutions typically are distributed above L1 and pool in the thoracic kyphotic region of the subarachnoid space (see Fig. 85–1). This results in characteristic midthoracic levels of anesthesia that are required for abdominal surgical procedures, including cesarean section. With either hyperbaric or isobaric solutions, direction of the aperture of the pencil-point spinal needle can further alter the distribution of local anesthetic and the resulting characteristics of spinal anesthesia.[5]

SPECIFIC APPLICATIONS

Patients With History of Spine Surgery

CSE can overcome some of the problems associated with epidural anesthesia in patients who have previously undergone spine surgery. Scarring, resulting in complete or partial obliteration of the epidural potential space, may occur in such patients.[10] Partial or failed epidural block may result. CSE overcomes problems in the majority of such patients, and postoperative epidural analgesia can still be effective.

TABLE 85–2. REINFORCEMENT BY EPIDURAL CATHETER AFTER THE INITIAL NEEDLE-THROUGH-NEEDLE DOSE

Type of Surgery	Type of Local Anesthetic	Time to Epidural Reinforcement (min)	Reinforcement Anesthetic	Reinforcement Dose	Epidural Reinforcement Duration (min)
Cephalad to L1 dermatome level	Hyperbaric lidocaine, 2%	45	Lidocaine, 2%, plain	10–15 mL*	45–60
Caudad to L1 dermatome level	Isobaric lidocaine, 2%	60–75	Lidocaine, 2%, plain	10–15 mL*	45–60
Caudad to L1 dermatome level	Isobaric mepivacaine, 1.5%–2%	90	Lidocaine, 2%, plain	10–15 mL*	45–60

*Reinforcement of the initial spinal anesthetic by the epidural route may require more volume than reinforcement of routine continuous lumbar epidural anesthesia. Ten to 15 mL is the total reinforcement dose; it should be given in smaller increments with divided doses after aspiration. This is because the CSE technique requires the anesthetic to be converted to epidural rather than merely to reinforce an established epidural anesthetic. As with epidural anesthesia, safety dictates that small aliquots (3–5 mL) be titrated to accomplish adequate reinforcement. Careful aspiration should be done to rule out intrathecal or intravascular catheter position before each incremental anesthetic dose is given.

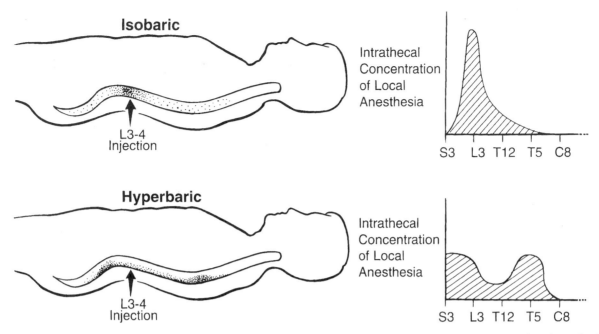

FIGURE 85–1. Distribution of isobaric and hyperbaric local anesthetic in the subdural space. (From Urmey WF: Combined spinal-epidural anesthesia for orthopedic surgery. Tech Reg Anesth Pain 1:123, 1997.)

Sacral Anesthesia

Perineal or ankle surgery presents an obstacle for patients having continuous lumbar epidural anesthesia. Large local anesthetic doses injected in the lumbar epidural space may still prove inadequate for surgical sacral anesthesia. CSE can easily overcome the problem of insufficient sacral anesthesia.

Postoperative Analgesia

As with spinal anesthesia, single-dose intrathecal analgesics can be used and are very effective for labor or cesarean section. Postoperative epidural analgesia by infusion can also be used, however, providing added flexibility. Postoperative epidural analgesics have been found to be more effective for pain control in patients undergoing major orthopedic surgery.[11-14]

Preservative-free epidural opioids (e.g., fentanyl, 50 to 100 μg as a single dose) or opioid/local anesthetic combinations (e.g., bupivacaine or ropivacaine, 0.06% to 0.1%,[15] with fentanyl, 3 to 5 μg/mL, given as a continuous infusion) may be used with the CSE technique.

THEORETICAL DIFFICULTIES

Subarachnoid Migration of the Epidural Catheter

Epidural anesthesia or CSE may be associated with rare inadvertent migration of the epidural catheter into the subarachnoid space. With properly matched needle sets using a 27-gauge spinal needle and a 20-gauge epidural catheter, this is no more likely to occur with CSE than with continuous epidural anesthesia. Holmström and associates[16] were unable to deliberately pass a 20-

gauge catheter through a 25-gauge dural hole in a study using fresh cadavers and periduroscopic visualization.[16] In addition, the epidural catheter advances at a different angle than the stiffer spinal needle does (Fig. 85–2).

Inability to Puncture the Dura When Using the Needle-Through-Needle Technique

An adequate protrusion length of spinal needle projecting beyond the epidural needle is necessary for suc-

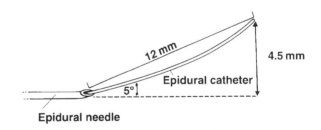

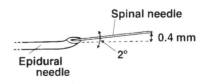

FIGURE 85–2. Schematic illustration showing the different routes (and points of dural contact) for spinal needle and epidural catheter inserted through 18 gauge Weiss needle. (Measurements made from Becton-Dickinson Durasafe matched needle set with Burron epidural catheter.) (From Urmey WF: Combined spinal-epidural anesthesia for orthopedic surgery. Tech Reg Anesth Pain 1:123, 1997.)

cessful needle-through-needle CSE. Twelve to 15 mm should be adequate for an almost 100% rate of success. Further increase in spinal needle lengths is unwieldy and results in instability of the needle combination. In approximately 10% of cases, the spinal needle encounters bone, indicating that it is off midline. When this occurs, the needle-through-needle technique can be abandoned in deference to a separate spinal and epidural, double-injection technique, as originally performed by Brownridge, in the same or separate interspaces.

SUMMARY

CSE is a developing technique that offers many advantages over spinal or epidural anesthesia while keeping complications at an acceptably minimal level.

REFERENCES

1. Brownridge P: Epidural and subarachnoid analgesia for elective caesarean section [letter]. Anaesthesia 36:70, 1981.
2. Coates MB: Combined subarachnoid and epidural anesthesia [letter]. Anaesthesia 37:89, 1982.
3. Holmström B, Laugaland K, Rawal N, et al: Combined spinal epidural block versus spinal and epidural block for orthopaedic surgery. Can J Anaesth 40:601, 1993.
4. Urmey WF, Stanton J, Peterson M, et al: Combined spinal-epidural anesthesia for outpatient surgery: Dose-response characteristics of intrathecal isobaric lidocaine using a 27-gauge Whitacre spinal needle. Anesthesiology 83:528, 1995.
5. Urmey WF, Stanton JS, Bassin P, et al: Direction of Whitacre needle aperture affects extent and duration of isobaric spinal anesthesia. Anesth Analg 84:337–341, 1996.
6. Rawal N, Schollin J, Wesström G: Epidural versus combined spinal epidural block for cesarean section. Acta Anaesthesiol Scand 32:61, 1988.
7. Urmey WF, Stanton J: Combined spinal epidural vs epidural anesthesia for outpatient knee arthroscopy [abstract]. Reg Anesth 22:6, 1997.
8. Lesser P, Bembridge M, Lyons G, et al: An evaluation of a 30-gauge needle for spinal anaesthesia for caesarean section. Anaesthesia 45:767, 1990.
9. Lyons G, Macdonald R, Mikl B: Combined epidural/spinal anaesthesia for caesarean section: Through the needle or in separate spaces? Anaesthesia 47:199, 1992.
10. Sharrock NE, Urquhart B, Mineo R: Extradural anaesthesia in patients with previous lumbar spine surgery. Br J Anaesth 65:237, 1990.
11. Ilahi OA, Davidson JP, Tullos HS: Continuous epidural analgesia using fentanyl and bupivacaine after total knee arthroplasty. Clin Orthop 299:44, 1994.
12. Mahoney OM, Noble PC, Davidson J, et al: The effect of continuous epidural analgesia on postoperative pain, rehabilitation, and duration of hospitalization in total knee arthroplasty. Clin Orthop 260:30, 1990.
13. Moiniche S, Hjorsto NC, Hansen BL, et al: The effect of balanced analgesia on early convalescence after major orthopaedic surgery. Acta Anaesthesiol Scand 38:328, 1994.
14. Pettine KA, Wedel DJ, Cabanela ME, et al: The use of epidural bupivacaine following total knee arthroplasty. Orthop Rev 18:894, 1989.
15. Badner NH, Reid D, Sullivan P, et al: Continuous epidural ropivacaine infusion for prevention of postoperative pain after major orthopedic surgery: A dose finding study. Can J Anaesth 43:17, 1996.
16. Holmström B, Rawal N, Axelsson K, et al: Risk of catheter migration during combined spinal epidural block: Percutaneous epiduroscopy study. Anesth Analg 80:747, 1995.
17. Urmey WF: Combined spinal-epidural anesthesia for orthopedic surgery. Tech Reg Anesth Pain 1:123, 1997.

Chapter 86

Caudal Anesthesia

Charles E. Laurito, M.D.

The caudal canal is, in essence, the lowermost aspect of the epidural space. A defect in the posterior bony covering of the lower aspects of the sacrum is termed the sacral hiatus. This defect has several normal anatomic variants and, in approximately 5% of adults, is completely ossified, such that needle entry is impossible. In most patients, however, the space is present and allows for the easy passage of a needle into the caudal epidural space. The gap in bone (sacral hiatus) is bounded by the sacral cornua laterally and covered with a tough sacrococcygeal ligament (Fig. 86–1). The ligament is analogous to both the supraspinous and intraspinous ligaments, which are present in more discrete forms at higher levels of the spinal canal. These fused ligaments are also adherent to the ligamentum flavum at this level, making the sacrococcygeal ligament a very dense tissue to traverse with a needle. Immediately ventral to this ligament is the sacral canal itself. This canal contains the dural sac and the anterior and posterior divisions of the sacral nerves with their dorsal root ganglia. It is also filled with epidural fat, areolar connective tissue, and epidural veins. Immediately anterior to the canal is the solid body of the sacrum, which consists of dense bone.

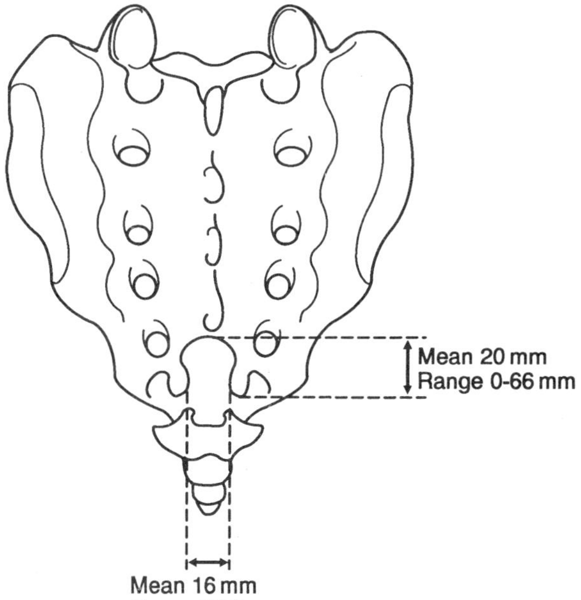

PERFORMANCE OF THE BLOCKADE

The block is usually performed with the patient prone, with a rolled blanket placed under the pelvis to elevate the lower sacrum. It is often beneficial to have the patient position the feet so that the toes are pointed inward and the heels outward. This makes gluteal muscle contraction more difficult and allows for easier palpation of the sacral cornua. A gauze sponge is placed into the gluteal fold to prevent the prep solution from dripping to the perineum, and the area is prepped and draped. The sacral hiatus is identified by palpation. With a little practice, the area can be easily felt as a softer gap between the hard, bony cornua. The lowermost aspect of the hiatus is usually 2 cm superior to the tip of the coccyx. The center of the hiatus is also one of the three points of an equilateral triangle. The other two points are each of the posterior superior iliac spines. Once the structure is identified, a skin wheal of local anesthetic is raised and time is allotted for the agent to work. The area is particularly sensitive. Typically, a 22-gauge 5-cm needle is advanced perpendicular to the skin and through the ligament until dense bone is encountered. At this point, the needle is withdrawn 1 mm and the hub is lowered from a 90-degree angle down to approximately a 30- to 45-degree angle to the surface of the skin (Fig. 86–2). The needle tip is advanced 1 cm, which is usually enough to ensure entry into the epidural space while avoiding penetration of the dural sac, which commonly ends at the S2 level.

A test dose of 2 to 4 mL of normal saline is injected

Mean 20 mm
Range 0–66 mm

Mean 16 mm
Range 7–28 mm

FIGURE 86–1. Dorsal surface of the sacrum. (From Martin LVH: Sacral epidural (caudal) block. *In* Wildsmith JAW, Armitage EN (eds): Principles and Practice of Regional Anesthesia. New York, Churchill-Livingstone, 1987, pp 127–134.)

rapidly through the needle to be sure the needle tip is indeed within the canal and not placed more posteriorly. During the injection, the palm of the nondominant hand is firmly placed at a site on the sacrum that corresponds to the needle tip. If the needle has been inadvertently placed posterior to the canal, the injection will be felt. The practitioner will know to repeat the sequence to place the needle more anteriorly so that it will be appropriately placed within the caudal canal. A test dose of an epinephrine containing solution is used to indicate that no vein has been entered, and the local anesthetic is injected in fractionated doses. In a 70-kg adult, approximately 15 mL are needed to fill the caudal canal. An additional 1 to 2 mL are needed to anesthetize each additional spinal segment. Commonly, 30 mL of local anesthetic are used to provide surgical anesthesia to approximately the T10 level.

In pediatric patients, the performance of the block is similar to that in the adult. Most agree that the technique is easier in children because the sacral hiatus is more easily identified and the ligament is softer and less calcified than it is in the adult. With children, particular care must be made to avoid dural penetration with the needle tip. The child has a much smaller sacral canal, and the most inferior aspect of the dura is closer to the sacral hiatus. Special caution must be used to prevent an accidental intrathecal injection of a dose of anesthetic intended for the epidural space. With either the child or adult, a Touhy needle can be placed through the sacrococcygeal ligament and an epidural catheter threaded into the caudal canal. This catheter can then be used for a continuous infusion of agent to provide surgical anesthesia for prolonged cases or for the infusion of more dilute agents to provide postoperative analgesia. The catheter can be kept in place with a benzoin preparation to make the skin stickier and a clear plastic bandage (Tagaderm) to provide an occlusive, waterproof barrier.

Because the caudal canal is continuous with the epidural space, the use of a larger dose will result in a higher level of epidural blockade. One can induce a midthoracic or even a high thoracic block with the use of a large dose of local anesthetic. This can be a dangerous technique, however, because caudal blockade, in particular, results in elevated blood levels of the anesthetic agent used. When thoracic blockade is required, it is preferable to enter the epidural space at the thoracic level of the spinal canal. Over the past few years, the use of lumbar and thoracic approaches to the epidural space has become more popular. The level of blockade is more appropriate to these surgical sites, and data have shown the techniques to be both well accepted and safe. During this same time period, the use of caudal blockade has waned.

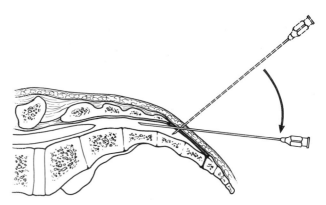

FIGURE 86–2. Technique of caudal blockade (see text). (From Martin LVH: Sacral epidural (caudal) block. *In* Wildsmith JAW, Armitage EN (eds): Principles and Practice of Regional Anesthesia. New York, Churchill-Livingstone, 1987, pp 127–134.)

INDICATIONS AND CONTRAINDICATIONS

The block is very useful for surgical and obstetric procedures on the perineum and lower abdomen. The technique is especially well suited for anal surgery because the operations are performed in the same position that is used for placement of the block. Dense surgical anesthesia can be provided with little spread to more superior levels. The technique is also useful because a catheter can be inserted and medications infused or reinjected for prolonged postoperative pain relief.

Contraindications to the use of the technique are similar to the contraindications to the use of any central blockade. The patient must give full, informed consent to the procedure, have no bleeding diathesis, not be taking anticoagulants, and have no skin infection in the area. Sacral decubiti can occur at sites near the cornua, and, if present, mandate the use of another anesthetic technique.

BIBLIOGRAPHY

Brown DL: Atlas of Regional Anesthesia. Philadelphia, WB Saunders, 1992, pp 293–301.

Brown DL: Spinal, epidural, and caudal anesthesia. *In* Miller RD (ed): Anesthesia, ed 4. New York, Churchill Livingstone, 1994, pp 1522–1530.

Lofstrom B: Caudal anaesthesia. *In* Eriksson E (ed): Illustrated Handbook in Local Anaesthesia, ed 2. Philadelphia, WB Saunders, 1980, pp 133–138.

Raj P, Pai U: Techniques of nerve blocking. *In* Raj PP (ed): Handbook of Regional Anesthesia. New York, Churchill Livingstone, 1985, pp 237–243.

Moore DC: Regional Block, ed 4. Springfield, Ill, Charles C Thomas Publisher, 1965, pp 439–451.

Chapter 87

Cervical Plexus Block

Robert E. Molloy, M.D.

ANATOMY

The original cervical plexus block technique was reported by Kappis in 1912, using a posterior approach. Heidenbeim described a lateral technique for this block in 1914, and this general approach has gained widespread acceptance.[1] The cervical plexus is formed from the upper four cervical nerves. Their dorsal and ventral roots join to form a spinal nerve as they exit through an intervertebral foramen. The cervical spinal nerves then split into anterior and posterior divisions. The C1 spinal nerve is formed almost entirely from a ventral root, and it is primarily a motor nerve. It actually emerges between the occiput and the arch of the atlas as the suboccipital nerve, and it is not directly blocked during cervical plexus block. The anterior primary rami of C2–4 travel laterally along the sulcus in their respective transverse processes, passing posterior to the vertebral artery. Lateral to the transverse process, these cervical nerves are enclosed in a fascial space derived from the fascia of the muscles attached to the tubercles of the transverse processes. This space is continuous with the interscalene fascial plane inferior to it, allowing for single-injection techniques of cervical plexus block.

The anterior primary rami of C2–4 form three loops, which are referred to as the cervical plexus. This plexus lies behind the sternomastoid muscle, giving off both superficial and deep branches[1] (Fig. 87–1). The superficial branches pierce the deep cervical fascia posterior to the sternomastoid muscle and supply skin and superficial tissues in the head, neck, and shoulder. The four distinct branches of the superficial cervical plexus are the lesser occipital, the great auricular, the transverse cervical, and the supraclavicular nerves.[2] The first two branches pass superiorly to the area of the ear, the mastoid, and the angle of the mandible. The transverse cervical nerve passes anteriorly to supply most of the anterolateral neck between the chin and the sternal notch and clavicles. The supraclavicular nerves descend to supply the anterolateral shoulder and the upper pectoral region. The deep branches of the cervical plexus innervate the deeper structures, including the muscles of the anterior and lateral neck as well as the diaphragm via the phrenic nerve.[2]

INDICATIONS

Cervical plexus blockade is indicated for many surgical procedures of the anterior and lateral neck and the supraclavicular fossa (Table 87–1). Unilateral block is adequate for procedures that do not extend to the midline.[1] For surgery of the thyroid gland,[3] larynx, and trachea, bilateral block and intravenous sedation are required. Bilateral deep cervical plexus block is usually avoided because of the added risks involved, particularly respiratory compromise. Superficial cervical plexus block facilitates awake placement of pulmonary artery catheters[5] and central venous catheters.[6] Combined with midazolam, superficial cervical plexus block has been found to be a safe, reliable, and well-tolerated alternative to general anesthesia in pediatric patients with mediastinal masses.[4]

Various types of carotid artery surgery have been performed under combined superficial and deep cervical plexus block.[7-12] The major advantages of performing carotid endarterectomy with this approach include the ability to assess neurologic function (and therefore the need for vascular shunting) in the awake patient.[8-10] Davies and colleagues[10] reported high patient acceptance of this technique, a low incidence of neurologic complications, and an acceptable rate of cardiovascular complications. Corson and colleagues[11] observed an apparent decrease in the incidence of neurologic complications after carotid endarterectomy performed with cervical plexus block when compared with general anesthesia. Benjamin and associates[8] reported that awake neurologic monitoring during carotid endarterectomy allowed for prompt, accurate identification of patients with cerebral ischemia who would clearly benefit from intraoperative shunting. Preoperative clinical status and vascular anatomy were not reliable predictors of the need for shunting. Adequate anesthesia for transvenous pacemaker insertion has been observed after cervical

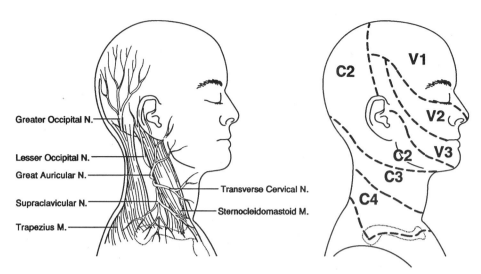

FIGURE 87–1. Peripheral cutaneous *(left)* and dermatomal *(right)* innervation of the head and neck, including the branches of the superficial cervical plexus and the greater occipital nerve.

plexus block combined with block of the second through the fourth intercostal nerves.[14] Complete anesthesia of the dermatomes from C3–T4 was obtained, without anesthesia of the brachial plexus.

TECHNIQUE

Superficial Cervical Plexus Block

For superficial cervical plexus block,[15, 16] the patient is placed in the supine position with the arms resting at the sides and the head turned slightly away from the side to be blocked. The head is lifted off the table to bring the sternomastoid muscle and its posterior border into prominence. The midpoint of the muscle's posterior border is identified, and a 22-gauge, 4- to 5-cm needle is inserted subcutaneously, posterior and immediately deep to the sternomastoid muscle, injecting 5 mL of local anesthetic. Two additional 5-mL injections are made along the posterior border of the muscle as the needle is redirected both superiorly and inferiorly. A lower concentration of local anesthetic is effective, such as 0.5% to 0.75% lidocaine with epinephrine, 5 μg/mL.[1]

TABLE 87–1. POTENTIAL INDICATIONS FOR CERVICAL PLEXUS BLOCK

Superficial neck procedures
Neck dissection procedures
Thyroglossal and branchial cysts
Thyroidectomy[3]
Lymph node excision
Cervical node biopsy in a child with a mediastinal mass[4]
Insertion of a pulmonary artery catheter[5]
Internal jugular and subclavian venous cannulation[6]
Percutaneous carotid balloon angioplasty[7]
Carotid endarterectomy with awake neurological monitoring[8–12]
Relief of metastatic pharyngeal cancer pain[1]
Relief of occipital and other neuralgias[1]
Relief of postoperative pain after neurosurgical operations[13]
Transvenous cardiac pacemaker insertion[14]

Deep Cervical Plexus Block

The patient is positioned just as for superficial cervical plexus block. This procedure is essentially a cervical paravertebral somatic block of the C2, C3, and C4 spinal nerves at the lateral edge of their transverse processes[1, 2, 15, 16] (Fig. 87–2). A lateral approach has been proven to be simple and more reliable than the posterior approach for deep cervical plexus block. Traditionally three needles are inserted at the C2–4 levels.[15] The insertion sites are located along a reference line drawn on the patient's neck. This line connects the tip of the mastoid process to the anterior tubercle of the C6 transverse process, which is easily palpated at the level of the cricoid cartilage. Some authors recommend drawing a second reference line parallel to and 1 cm posterior to the original line to better approximate the location of the underlying transverse processes, which are then located by palpation.[2] The C2 transverse process is located 1 to 2 cm below the mastoid along the reference line, while C3 and C4 are sought 1.5 cm and 3 cm inferior to C2.[1] The C3 transverse process is located at the level of the hyoid bone. The C4 transverse process may be found at the level of the upper border of the thyroid cartilage or, alternatively, at the lower level of the mandibular ramus.[15]

The deep cervical plexus block is performed with a 22-gauge needle directed medially and caudally to avoid an excessive depth of insertion and unintentional spinal, epidural, or subdural blockade or vertebral artery injection. The first end point for needle placement is contact with the bony transverse processes at a depth of 1.5 to 3 cm; the more inferior processes tend to become more superficial. The second end point is production of a paresthesia, which may require redirecting the needle in anterior and posterior directions along the tip of the transverse process. At each level, 3 to 5 mL of local anesthetic is injected, using a relatively higher concentration such as 1.5% lidocaine with epinephrine, 5 μg/mL.

Deep cervical plexus block can also be produced with a single injection at one level using a larger volume of local anesthetic. A single-needle interscalene cervical

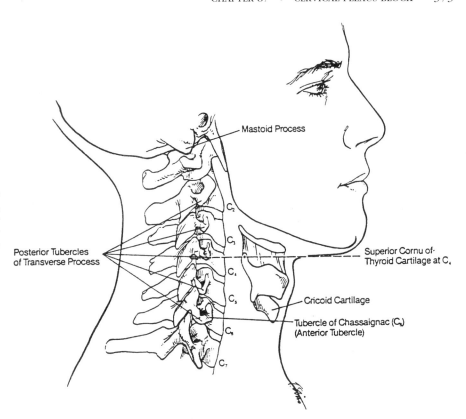

FIGURE 87–2. Bony landmarks for deep cervical plexus block. (From Raj PP, Pai U, Rawal N: Techniques of regional anesthesia in adults. *In* Raj PP (ed): Clinical Practice of Regional Anesthesia. New York, Churchill Livingstone, 1991, p 271.)

plexus block has been described with injection at the C4 level.[17] The interscalene cervical plexus block is performed in a fashion similar to that for brachial plexus block but at a more cephalad level. If a nerve stimulator is used, a deltoid muscle motor response is sought, and 10 to 15 mL of local anesthetic is injected. Incomplete analgesia may occur during procedures such as carotid endarterectomy. This is occasionally noted at the upper extent of a cervical incision, where glossopharyngeal nerve innervation is encountered.[1] Incision of the carotid sheath may also produce pain during an otherwise satisfactory block. This sheath is traversed by branches of the upper and lower roots of the ansa cervicalis.[18] Local infiltration by the surgeon is often effective in these situations.

Local Anesthetics

Shorter-duration block may be produced with lidocaine or mepivacaine, longer block with bupivacaine or ropivacaine. More dilute solutions can be used for superficial cervical plexus block. Several studies have measured blood levels of local anesthetic after cervical plexus block without detecting clinical or laboratory evidence of toxicity.[19-22] Dawson and colleagues[19] observed mean peak lidocaine blood levels of about 5 μg/mL after injection of 6 mg/kg of 1.5% lidocaine with epinephrine, 5 μg/mL. These levels are similar to those found after multiple, bilateral intercostal nerve blockade, the regional anesthetic technique widely considered to produce the highest systemic levels of local anesthetic.[19] Molnar and colleagues[20] demonstrated the effect of epinephrine 5 μg/mL on lidocaine blood lev-

els.[20] After 7 mg/kg of 1.5% lidocaine, mean peak blood levels were about 7.5 μg/mL with clonidine added and 4.5 μg/mL with epinephrine.

COMPLICATIONS

Because of the proximity of the vertebral artery, accidental intra-arterial injection may result in almost instantaneous CNS toxicity consisting of convulsions, loss of consciousness, and blindness.[15, 23] Intraneural or transforaminal needle placement may result in unintentional spinal anesthesia.[15] Local anesthetic may spread to the epidural or subdural space, resulting in bilateral cervicothoracic anesthesia.[24, 25] Phrenic nerve block can be anticipated, with a resultant decrement in inspiratory capacity.[26] Bilateral cervical plexus block is generally avoided to prevent serious respiratory compromise, particularly in the presence of pulmonary disease. Bradycardia from bilateral sympathetic block and airway obstruction may also occur.[27] Local anesthetic deposition or spread superficial to the deep cervical fascia can block the sympathetic chain and the recurrent laryngeal nerve, resulting in Horner's syndrome and hoarseness.[15] Systemic toxicity may occur after accidental injection of the vertebral, external jugular, or internal jugular veins with either deep and superficial cervical plexus blocks. Careful aspiration tests and the initial injection of 1 mL of anesthetic with deep cervical plexus block are used to detect intrathecal, intravascular, or vertebral artery injection. Limiting needle insertion to the depth of the lateral edge of the transverse process may also decrease complications.

REFERENCES

1. Pappas JL, Kahn CH, Warfield CA: Cervical plexus blockade. *In* Waldman SD, Winnie AP (eds): Interventional Pain Management. Philadelphia, WB Saunders, 1996, p 247.
2. Tucker JH, Flynn JF: Head and neck regional blocks. *In* Brown DL (ed): Regional Anesthesia and Analgesia. Philadelphia, WB Saunders, 1996, p 240.
3. LoGerfo P, Ditkoff BA, Chabot J, et al: Thyroid surgery using monitored care: An alternative to general anesthesia. Thyroid 4:437, 1994.
4. Brownlow RC, Berman J, Brown RE: Superficial cervical plexus block for cervical node biopsy in a child with a large mediastinal mass. J Ark Med Soc 90:378, 1994.
5. Brull SJ: Superficial cervical plexus block for pulmonary artery catheter insertion. Crit Care Med 20:1362, 1992.
6. Chauhan S, Baronia AK, Maheshwari A, et al: Superficial cervical plexus block for internal jugular and subclavian venous cannulation in awake patients. Reg Anesth 20:459, 1995.
7. Alessandri C, Bergeron P: Local anesthesia in carotid angioplasty. J Endovasc Surg 3:31, 1996.
8. Benjamin ME, Silva MB, Watt C, et al: Awake patient monitoring to determine the need for shunting during carotid endarterectomy. Surgery 114:673, 1993.
9. Davies MJ, Mooney PH, Scott DA, et al: Neurologic changes during carotid endarterectomy under cervical plexus block predict a high risk of postoperative stroke. Anesthesiology 78:829, 1993.
10. Davies MJ, Murrell GC, Cronin KD, et al: Carotid endarterectomy under cervical plexus block: A prospective clinical audit. Anaesth Intensive Care 18:219, 1990.
11. Corson JD, Chang BB, Karmody AM: The influence of anesthetic choice on carotid endarterectomy outcome. Arch Surg 122:807, 1987.
12. Castresana MR, Balser JS, Newman WH, et al: Cervical block for carotid endarterectomy followed immediately by general anesthesia for coronary artery bypass and aortic valve replacement. Anesth Analg 77:186, 1993.
13. Niijima K, Malis LI: Preventive superficial cervical plexus block for postoperative cervicocephalic pain in neurosurgery. Neurol Med Chir (Tokyo) 33:365, 1993.
14. Raza SM, Vasireddy AR, Candido KD, et al: A complete regional anesthesia technique for cardiac pacemaker insertion. J Cardiothorac Vasc Anesth 5:54, 1991.
15. Murphy TM: Somatic blockade of head and neck. *In* Cousins MJ, Bridenbaugh PO (eds): Neural Blockade in Clinical Anesthesia and Management of Pain, ed 2. Philadelphia, JB Lippincott, 1988, p 533.
16. Raj PP, Pai U, Rawal N: Techniques of regional anesthesia in adults. *In* Raj PP (ed): Clinical Practice of Regional Anesthesia. New York, Churchill Livingstone, 1991, 271.
17. Winnie AP, Ramamurthy S, Durrani Z, et al: Interscalene cervical plexus block: A single injection technique. Anesth Analg 54:370, 1975.
18. Einav S, Landesberg G, Prus D, et al: A case of nerves. Reg Anesth 21:168, 1996.
19. Dawson AR, Dysart RH, Amerena JV, et al: Arterial lignocaine concentrations following cervical plexus blockade for carotid endarterectomy. Anaesth Intensive Care 19:197, 1991.
20. Molnar RR, Davies MJ, Scott DA, et al: Comparison of clonidine and epinephrine in lidocaine for cervical plexus block. Reg Anesth 22:137, 1997.
21. Tissot S, Frering B, Gagnieu MC, et al: Plasma concentrations of lidocaine and bupivacaine after cervical plexus block for carotid surgery. Anesth Analg 84:1377, 1997.
22. Neill RS, Watson R: Plasma bupivacaine concentration during combined regional and general anesthesia for resection and reconstruction of head and neck carcinomata. Br J Anaesth 56:485, 1984.
23. Szeinfeld M, Laurencio M, Pallares VS: Total reversible blindness following stellate ganglion block. Anesth Analg 60:689, 1981.
24. Kumar A, Battit GE, Froese AB, et al: Bilateral cervical and thoracic epidural blockade complicating interscalene brachial plexus block: Report of two cases. Anesthesiology 35:650, 1971.
25. Huang KC, Fitzgerald MR, Tsueda K: Bilateral block of cervical and brachial plexuses following interscalene block. Anaesth Intensive Care 14:87, 1986.
26. Castresana MR, Masters RD, Castresana EJ, et al: Incidence and clinical significance of hemidiaphragmatic paresis in patients undergoing carotid endarterectomy during cervical plexus block anesthesia. J Neurosurg Anesthesiol 6:21, 1994.
27. Levelle JP, Martinez OA: Airway obstruction after bilateral carotid endarterectomy. Anesthesiology 63:220, 1985.

Chapter 88

Occipital Nerve Block

Robert E. Molloy, M.D

Blockade of the greater occipital nerve provides anesthesia of the medial part of the posterior scalp. It is most often employed in the diagnosis and therapy of chronic pain conditions.[1] Most headaches are either muscular or vascular in nature. Occipital pain may rarely occur with cranial malignancy, infection, or congenital abnormalities, and a careful history and physical examination are always indicated to rule out serious underlying causes of headache.[2] Myofascial trigger points in the posterior cervical muscles (e.g., the upper semispinalis cervicis) produce dull, aching occipital pain, whereas trigger points in the splenius capitis produce referred headache near the vertex. They may be managed with better posture, massage, stretching exercises, and trigger point injections. Arthritis of the cervical spine may also be associated with occipital headaches. Exaggerated muscle tension or contraction of the semispinalis capitis muscle may be theorized to produce occipital neuralgia by direct compression of the greater occipital nerve. However, the role of greater occipital nerve compression may be relatively minor.[3] Occipital neuralgia produces continuous throbbing pain in the suboccipital area, perhaps aggravated by pressure over the greater occipital nerve.[4] By definition, occipital neuralgia is relieved by diagnostic blockade of the greater occipital nerve.[5] This may include referred pain to the head and neck outside the typical distribution of the greater occipital nerve. A series of occipital nerve blocks with local anesthetic and depot steroid may be therapeutic for occipital neuralgia.[6]

Bovim and Sand[7] evaluated the response to diagnostic greater occipital nerve block in patients with cervicogenic headache, migraine without aura, and tension-type headache. They defined cervicogenic headache according the criteria proposed by Sjaastad and associates,[4] the most important of which are as follows:

1. Unilateral headache; always on the same side
2. Symptoms and signs of neck involvement
   Pain due to neck pressure or head position
   Ipsilateral neck, shoulder, or arm pain
   Reduced cervical flexibility

3. Pain characteristics
   Episodic or continuous pain
   Moderate, nonthrobbing neck pain with
      radiation
   History of neck trauma
   Female sex

Occipital nerve block reduced pain in 19 of 22 patients with cervicogenic headache. At least 40% pain relief (visual analogue scale) was noted in 80% of cervicogenic headache patients, but in none of those with migraine or tension-type headache. Forehead pain was also relieved in 17 of 22 patients with cervicogenic headache, suggesting the presence of referred pain to the trigeminal nerve distribution. Pain relief outside the area blocked was rare with the other two headache types.[7]

ANATOMY

The sensory innervation of the posterior head and neck arises from the second and third cervical nerves.[1] The lateral section of the posterior scalp is supplied by the lesser occipital and great auricular nerves, branches of the cervical plexus (see Fig. 87—1 in Chapter 87). They are accessible for blockade laterally near the superior nuchal line or, alternatively, at the posterior edge of the sternomastoid muscle, in its middle one third. The medial section of the posterior scalp is supplied by the greater occipital nerve, the termination of the medial branch of the dorsal ramus of C2.[2] This nerve arises between the atlas and axis laterally and travels posteriorly and medially before turning cephalad, deep to the semispinalis capitis muscle.[8] Near the base of the skull, the greater occipital nerve passes posteriorly through the semispinalis capitis muscle and then continues under the trapezius muscle to travel cephalad and laterally, passing between the insertions of the trapezius and sternomastoid muscles to reach a subcutaneous position.[2] In its subcutaneous course over the posterior scalp, the nerve lies adjacent and medial to the occipital

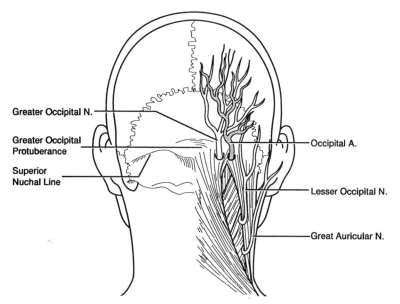

FIGURE 88–1. Technique of greater occipital nerve block, demonstrating the position of the greater occipital nerve and the occipital artery above the superior nuchal line. (Modified from Tucker JH, Flynn JF: Head and neck regional anesthesia. *In* Brown DL (ed): Regional Anesthesia and Analgesia. Philadelphia, WB Saunders, 1996, p 240.)

artery, which serves as the prime landmark for blockade of the greater occipital nerve[1] (Fig. 88–1).

TECHNIQUE

The greater occipital nerve is blocked with the seated patient's head and neck flexed forward, chin to chest.[2] Three landmarks are identified: the mastoid process, the greater occipital protuberance, and the superior nuchal line. The occipital arterial pulse is identified along this line, approximately one third of the distance from the greater occipital protuberance toward the mastoid.[1] Injection of 3 to 5 mL of local anesthetic just medial to the artery, with or without prior elicitation of paresthesia, produces occipital anesthesia. An initial diagnostic block is best performed with only 1 to 2 mL of drug after a paresthesia has been obtained. When the arterial pulse is not palpable, a wider area of subcutaneous infiltration may be required. Anesthesia of the scalp should develop in 5 to 10 minutes.[2]

There are no common complications to this block that do not apply to any superficial, perivascular injections. This presumes that the skull is intact and that an accidental suboccipital injection is avoided.[2]

REFERENCES

1. Tucker JH, Flynn JF: Head and neck regional blocks. *In* Brown DL (ed): Regional Anesthesia and Analgesia. Philadelphia, WB Saunders, 1996, p 240.
2. Brown DL, Wong GY: Occipital nerve block. *In* Waldman SD, Winnie AP: Interventional Pain Management. Philadelphia, WB Saunders, 1996, p 226.
3. Bovim G, Bonamico L, Fredriksen TA, et al: Topographic variations in the peripheral course of the greater occipital nerve. Spine 16:475, 1991.
4. Sjaastad O, Fredriksen TA, Pfaffenrath V: Cervicogenic headache: Diagnostic criteria. Headache 30:725, 1990.
5. Headache Classification Committee of the International Headache Society: Classification and diagnostic criteria for headache disorders, cranial neuralgias, and facial pain. Cephalalgia 8(suppl 7):1, 1988.
6. Anthony M: Headache and the greater occipital nerve. Clin Neurol Neurosurg 94:297, 1992.
7. Bovim TG, Sand T: Cervicogenic headache, migraine without aura and tension-type headache: Diagnostic blockade of greater occipital and supra-orbital nerves. Pain 51:43, 1992.
8. Vital JM, Grenier F, Dantheribes M, et al: An anatomic and dynamic study of the greater occipital nerve (n. of Arnold): Applications to the treatment of Arnold's neuralgia. Surg Radiol Anat 11:205, 1989.
9. Neill RS: Head, neck and airway. *In* Wildsmith JAW, Armitage EN (eds): Principles and Practice of Regional Anaesthesia, ed 2. Edinburgh, Churchill Livingstone, 1993, p 203.

Chapter 89

Maxillary, Mandibular, and Glossopharyngeal Nerve Blocks

Umeshraya T. Pai, M.D., and Rajeshri Nayak, M.D.

TRIGEMINAL NERVE

The trigeminal nerve is the fifth cranial nerve and has three divisions: ophthalmic, maxillary, and mandibular. It is predominantly a sensory nerve, with a small motor component that is contained in the mandibular division. Proximally, the sensory component of the trigeminal nerve is connected to the ventral aspect of the pons. Distally, the sensory component leaves from the medial concave border of the trigeminal (semilunar) ganglion. The trigeminal ganglion is located at the apex of the petrous temporal bone in the posterior medial part of the middle cranial fossa. The ganglion is also related to the inferior lateral aspect of the cavernous sinus. The minor motor component of the trigeminal nerve is at the medial side of the nerve at the attachment to the pons and runs inferior to the ganglion to exit through the foramen ovale, with the mandibular division as its motor branches.

MAXILLARY NERVE BLOCK

Anatomy

The maxillary nerve is the second division of the trigeminal nerve and is also known as the V2 division. This nerve is the middle division of the trigeminal nerve and is attached to the distal convex border of the trigeminal ganglion. The maxillary nerve exits from the cranial cavity through the foramen rotundum. From this point, the nerve traverses the superior part of the pterygopalatine fossa and swings laterally to traverse the inferior orbital fissure toward the maxillary sinus. As the nerve runs along the roof of the maxillary sinus, it supplies the maxillary sinus itself and the anterior teeth of the upper jaw via the anterior and middle superior alveolar nerves. The nerve then exits through the infraorbital foramen to innervate the skin of the face and the underlying mucosa extending from the lower eyelid to the upper lip. While the nerve is at the pterygopalatine fossa, it is connected to the pterygopalatine ganglion, through which it gives off branches to the nasal cavity,

pharynx, and palate. In addition, the nerve gives off the zygomatic nerve and the posterior superior alveolar nerve. The zygomatic nerve supplies the lateral portion of the face and the posterior superior alveolar nerve, which supplies the upper molar region.

Indications for Maxillary Nerve Blocks

1. Maxillofacial procedures
2. Surgical procedures on the teeth of the upper jaw
3. Chronic pain conditions involving tumors of the maxillary sinus
4. Assessment and diagnosis of pain syndromes in the distribution of the nerve

Contraindications

1. Infection at the site of entry
2. Coagulopathy
3. Preexisting neurologic deficits

Landmarks

1. Midpoint of the zygomatic arch of the temporal bone
2. Condyle of the mandibular head
3. Coronoid process of the mandible
4. Mandibular notch between the condyle and the coronoid process

Technique

There are two approaches in performing a maxillary nerve block, both of which are discussed here (Fig. 89-1).

Lateral Approach

The patient is supine with the head turned away from the side of the intended block. The side of the face is prepared and draped in a sterile manner. The landmarks are palpated, and the midpoint of the zygomatic arch is

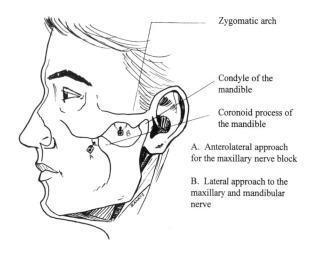

Entry point of the needle for the
    A. Anterolateral approach for the maxillary nerve block
    B. Lateral approach for the maxillary and mandibular nerve block

FIGURE 89–1. Two approaches to performing a maxillary nerve block.

marked. The skin is infiltrated with local anesthetic in the area of the mandibular notch between the condyle and the coronoid process of the mandible below the midpoint of the zygomatic arch.

After infiltration, a 22-gauge, 3-in. needle is introduced perpendicular below the midpoint of the zygomatic arch and walked onto the lateral pterygoid plate. A depth marker can be placed on the needle to the anticipated depth (approximately 0.5 to 1 cm from the initial depth to the lateral pterygoid plate). The needle is then withdrawn and redirected and advanced anteromedially into the pterygopalatine fossa (Fig. 89–2). A nerve stimulator may be helpful if available, because paresthesias may or may not be elicited. After aspiration to rule out intravascular placement of the needle, 2 to 3 mL of local anesthetic is deposited for the desired effect.

Anterolateral Approach

The patient is positioned and prepared in the manner described previously. The angle between the inferior border of the zygomatic bone and the coronoid process of the mandible is located and marked. After a skin wheal is raised at this angle, a 3-in., 22-gauge needle is directed medially, superiorly, and posteriorly to lay along the posterior surface of the maxilla and further advanced approximately 4 to 5 cm, depending on the extent of subcutaneous tissue. Once the needle tip walks off the maxilla, a paresthesia may be elicited when the needle tip reaches the pterygopalatine fossa. As before, a nerve stimulator may be helpful to verify the position of the needle. Once the position is determined, local anesthetic is deposited after negative aspiration.

Complications

1. If the needle is placed too deep and anterior, direct injection into the optic nerve is possible, resulting in transient blindness with local anesthetic use or permanent blindness with the use of neurolytic agent.

2. Because of vascularity of the region secondary to the rich venous plexus and the third part of the maxillary artery and its five to six branches, intravascular injection is a possibility.

3. Hematoma can develop, the extent of which depends on the size of the needle.

MANDIBULAR NERVE BLOCK

Anatomy

The mandibular nerve is the third division of the trigeminal nerve and is also referred to as the V3 division. It arises from the lower part of the distal convexity of the trigeminal ganglion and then joins the motor component. From this point, the nerve exits through the foramen ovale to enter the infratemporal fossa. It then divides into a smaller anterior division and a larger posterior division. The anterior division is predominantly motor, except for the buccal branch, which provides sensation to the cheek. The motor branches innervate the muscles of mastication. The posterior division is predominantly sensory, except for the myelohyoid branch, which provides motor innervation to the myelohyoid muscle and the anterior belly of the digastric muscle. The sensory portion of the mandibular nerve innervates the meninges (via the recurrent meningeal branch), the temporomandibular joint, the ear, and the outer surface of the tympanic membrane, anterior two thirds of the mouth, and adjoining part of the floor of the mouth, and the mandible with its associated teeth. The sensory portion terminates as the mental nerve, which supplies the chin. All of these areas are innervated through the following branches: auriculotemporal, lingual, and inferior alveolar.

Indications

1. Surgical procedures in the cutaneous distribution of the nerve

2. Surgery of the mandible (i.e., open reduction and internal fixation of the mandible), associated teeth and gums, and anterior two thirds of the tongue

3. Postoperative pain control in the area of distribution of the nerve

4. Treatment of chronic pain syndromes; i.e., carcinoma of the tongue, lower jaw, and floor of the mouth

Contraindications

Contraindications are similar to those described for the maxillary nerve block.

Landmarks

Landmarks are similar to those described for the maxillary nerve block.

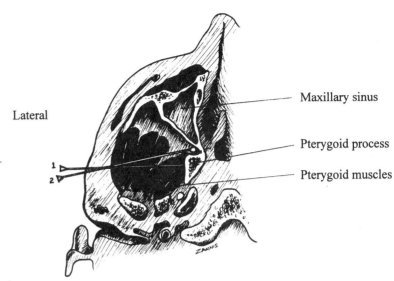

FIGURE 89–2. Maxillary nerve block, transverse section.

1. Pterygoid plate
2. Maxillary nerve

Maxillary Nerve Block

Technique

The patient is positioned and prepared in a manner similar to that described for the maxillary nerve block. The landmarks are palpated, and a point below the midpoint of the zygomatic arch in the mandibular notch is marked. After infiltration of the overlying skin with local anesthetic, a 22-gauge, 3-in. needle is inserted perpendicular to the skin and advanced posteromedially to a depth of approximately 4 to 5 cm, at which point paresthesias in the distribution of the nerve may be elicited. Local anesthetic is deposited after negative aspi- ration to achieve the desired effect. On the other hand, if bone (lateral pterygoid plate) is contacted, the needle is withdrawn and redirected more posteriorly in an attempt to elicit paresthesia (Fig. 89–3). Once again, a nerve stimulator may be useful if there is difficulty in eliciting paresthesias. The landmarks for this block are similar to those for the lateral approach to the maxillary block, the difference between the two being the direc- tion of advancement of the needle: The lateral approach to the maxillary block involves advancing the needle anteromedially, whereas the mandibular block involves advancing the needle posteromedially.

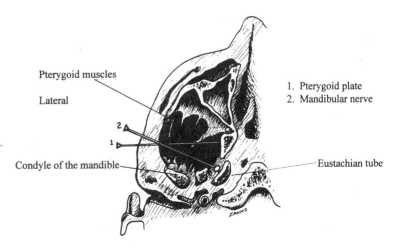

FIGURE 89–3. Mandibular nerve block, transverse section.

1. Pterygoid plate
2. Mandibular nerve

Mandibular Nerve Block

Complications

1. Intravascular injection is a potential complication because of the proximity of the pterygoid plexus of veins, maxillary artery, and its branch, the middle meningeal artery.

2. If the needle is inserted too deep, the superior constrictor muscle can be pierced, resulting in entry into the pharynx.

GLOSSOPHARYNGEAL NERVE BLOCK

Anatomy

The glossopharyngeal nerve is the ninth cranial nerve. It arises from the cranial part of the medulla and exits from the cranial cavity through the intermediate compartment of the jugular foramen. The nerve then runs between the internal carotid artery and internal jugular vein, after which it swings around the stylopharyngeus muscle toward the pharynx and the tongue. During its course, it lies deep to the styloid process. The nerve supplies motor fibers to the pharyngeal muscles and sensory fibers to the middle ear, posterior third of the tongue, and the pharynx. It also innervates the carotid sinus and the carotid body. The nerve is in close proximity to the vagus nerve, accessory nerve, and sympathetic trunk.

Indications

1. Diagnosis and treatment of glossopharyngeal neuralgia
2. Control of pain arising from cancer of the tongue and pharynx
3. Control of pain during awake endoscopy

Contraindications

Contraindications are similar to those mentioned for the earlier-described blocks.

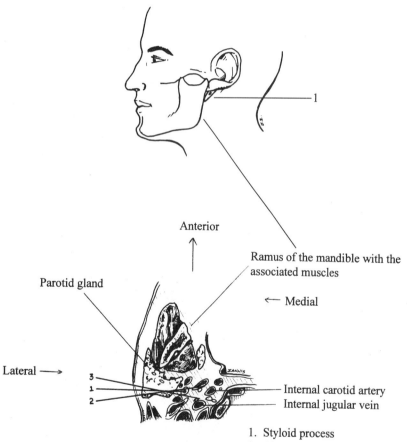

Anterior

Ramus of the mandible with the associated muscles

← Medial

Parotid gland

Lateral →

3
1
2

Internal carotid artery
Internal jugular vein

1. Styloid process
2. Glossopharyngeal nerve with stylopharyngeus muscle
   Hypoglossal nerve
3. Accessory nerve

Transverse Section to Show the Position
of the Needle for the Glossopharyngeal Nerve Block

FIGURE 89–4. Glossopharyngeal nerve block, transverse section.

Landmarks

1. Mastoid process, posteriorly
2. Angle of the mandible, anteriorly
3. Styloid process of the temporal bone, in the middle

Technique

Appropriate monitoring and intravenous access are required before proceeding with the block. The patient is supine, with the head turned to the side opposite of the block. The lateral face and portion of the neck below the ear are prepared in sterile manner.

The angle of the mandible and the mastoid process are marked. The point midway between these two landmarks inferior to the ear corresponds to the position of the styloid process of the temporal bone. The skin overlying the styloid process is infiltrated with local anesthetic. A 22-gauge, 3-in. needle is then inserted perpendicular to the skin and advanced toward the styloid process. Once the styloid process is contacted, a depth marker is placed 0.5 cm from the skin. The needle is then withdrawn and reinserted anterior to the styloid process to the depth marker. This corresponds to the location of the glossopharyngeal nerve as it curves around the stylopharyngeus muscle (Fig. 89–4). Two to 3 mL of local anesthetic is injected after negative aspiration.

Complications

1. Intravascular injection into the internal carotid artery or internal jugular vein is a potential risk. Injection into the carotid artery can result in seizures and possible cardiovascular collapse.
2. Hematoma from trauma to the above-mentioned vessels can occur.
3. Proximity to the vagus and accessory nerves can result in block of these nerves as well.
4. Bilateral block of the glossopharyngeal nerves can result in total pharyngeal paralysis with associated risk of aspiration.

Chapter 90

Orbital Nerve Blocks

Robert C. Hamilton, M.B., B.Ch., F.R.C.P.C.

A necessary prerequisite for performing orbital nerve blocks is a sound knowledge of the anatomy of the orbit and its contents. To embark on orbital regional anesthesia blocks without this knowledge is to subject patients to unacceptable risk of serious sequelae. Cadaver dissection provides a superb grounding in the three-dimensional aspects of the anatomy of this small but vital part of the human body and is highly recommended. An atlas of orbital anatomy[1, 2] and a human skull are worthwhile resources. Observation of, and subsequent initial supervision by, colleagues with wide clinical experience and knowledge is ideal.

ANATOMY AND APPLIED ANATOMY

The paired orbits are mirror-imaged, bilaterally symmetrical, bony cavities located on each side of the midline sagittal plane of the skull. Each is made up from seven bones as illustrated in Fig. 90–1. The facial, or anterior, aspect of the orbit, known as the orbit rim, forms a protecting buttress for the vital structures held within and comprises three robust bones: zygomatic, frontal, and maxillary. The surface anatomy of the orbit rim, as palpated through its superficial periorbital coverings, is the key to successful regional orbital anesthesia. The rim forms the rounded rectangular base of a pear-shaped pyramid which tapers posteriorly to form a tight apex. The greatest diameter of the orbit is that portion immediately inside the rim. The volume of the adult orbit averages 30 mL, and that of the globe is about 6.5 mL. The typical dimensions at the rim are 35 mm vertically and 40 mm horizontally. The depth of the orbit from inferior orbit rim to the optic foramen ranges from 42 to 54 mm.[3] The lateral orbit rim is set back 12 to 18 mm behind the cornea, allowing exposure of the globe to its equator (Fig. 90–2).

The medial wall of each orbit is in the sagittal plane and parallel to the contralateral medial orbit wall. The lateral wall of each orbit forms a 90-degree angle with

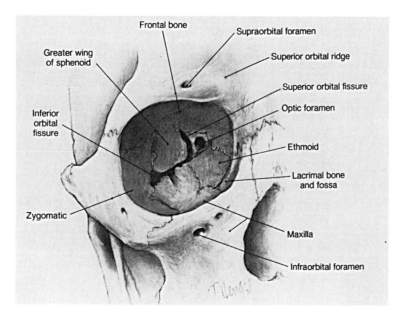

FIGURE 90–1. Frontal view of the orbit. The skull is rotated slightly to the left to visualize more clearly the orbital apex. (From Doxanas MT, Anderson RL: Clinical Orbital Anatomy. Baltimore, Williams & Wilkins, 1984.)

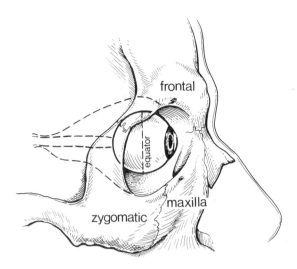

FIGURE 90–2. The lateral orbital rim is set back in line with the globe equator. The orbit, in sagittal section, is C-shaped rather than U-shaped, with a greater overhang superiorly. (From Grizzard WS: Ophthalmic anesthesia. *In* Reinecke RD (ed): Ophthalmology Annual. New York, Raven Press, 1989, pp 265–294.)

the contralateral lateral orbit wall. The medial and lateral walls of each orbit make a 45-degree angle with each other. The orbit apex and optic foramen are in the same sagittal plane as the medial orbit wall. Thus the optic foramen is located both posteriorly and medially in the orbit, and is not directly behind the globe. The globe occupies the front half of each orbit and projects anteriorly beyond it (see Fig. 90–2). The visual axis (eye in primary gaze) is sagittal.

The periosteum of the orbit is known as *periorbita*. It blends with the facial bone periosteum and with the orbital septum circumferentially at the anterior orbital margin (Fig. 90–3). Posteriorly, at the orbital apex, periorbita is continuous through the optic canal with the pericranium and with the dural sheath of the optic nerve. The orbital septum defines the anatomic anterior border of the orbit and on the nasal side has attachments with both the anterior and posterior lacrimal crests. Its central attachments are in the upper and lower eyelids, and it lies deep to the orbicularis oculi muscle.

A diffuse connective tissue matrix which radiates from the fascial sheaths of the extraocular muscles out to the periorbita (see Fig. 90–3) permits the muscles to function and suspends the globe within the orbital cavity. Intermuscular septa span the intervals between the rectus muscles, especially anteriorly, dividing the orbital fat into compartments respectively inside and outside the cone of rectus muscles. In the central or *intracone* compartment, the fat is arranged in large fusiform lobules held in loose alignment with and surrounding the optic nerve, allowing its maximum mobility as the globe rotates, along with the ciliary vessels and nerves which transmit the motor, autonomic, and sensory nerves and blood vessels to the globe. The intraorbital part of the optic nerve is about 4 mm in diameter, averages slightly more than 3 cm in length, and has a winding course across the 2.5-cm gap between the optic foramen and

the hind surface of the globe which it enters 3 mm to the nasal side of its posterior pole; within the orbit, therefore, the nerve has about 7 mm of "excess play." The peripheral or *pericone* fat compartment is composed of less mobile, smaller fat lobules arranged into four lobes.

The globe is in the shape of a sphere about 23.5 mm in diameter on the average (but great variations exist, commonly ranging from 20 to 30 mm or more, and rarely outside these limits), with an anterior bulge, the cornea, having a smaller radius of curvature.

The anatomic relationships of the three branches of the ophthalmic nerve and the three oculomotor nerves to the bony orbit and its contained muscles are illustrated in Fig. 90–4. The ciliary ganglion, a peripheral ganglion of the parasympathetic nervous system, is situated in the posterior intracone space at a distance of 1 cm from the orbital apex and 1.5 cm posterior to the globe. It lies between the optic nerve and the ophthalmic artery (medially) and the lateral rectus muscle (laterally). The nasociliary branch of the ophthalmic nerve, in addition to communications with the ciliary ganglion, provides sensation to the iris, ciliary body, cornea, and perilimbal (central) conjunctiva. It courses through the intracone space, where it is effectively blocked by small-volume intracone local anesthetic injection. Its most anterior division, the infratrochlear nerve (see Fig. 90–4), runs along the superior border of the medial rectus muscle and penetrates the orbital septum to innervate the peripheral conjunctiva on the nasal side, including the caruncle, the lacrimal sac, and adjacent skin of the nose and eyelids (Fig. 90–5). The remaining peripheral conjunctival sensation is mediated via the lacrimal, frontal, and infraorbital nerves (see Fig. 90–5), all lying outside of the cone of rectus muscles (see Fig. 90–4); this explains the incomplete conjunctival anesthesia resulting from small-volume intracone local anesthetic injection.

The orientation of the six extraocular muscles is shown in Figure 90–6; Figures 90–3, 90–4, and 90–6 show the orientation of the levator muscle of the upper eyelid, which is superimposed on the superior rectus muscle. Of the rectus muscles, only the medial is significantly separated from the adjacent bony orbit wall by an adipose tissue compartment. Within this compartment, at the level of the equator of the globe, a consolidation of connective tissue extending nasally to the medial orbit wall produces the medial check ligament (Fig. 90–7). Local anesthetic injected medial to the caruncle and through the medial check ligament spreads anteriorly around the check ligament (both above and below it) and through defects in the orbital septum into the preseptal space of the upper and lower eyelids in a tissue plane on the deep surface of the orbicularis oculi muscle, where the fine terminal motor branches of the seventh nerve are readily blocked. In addition, medial-compartment local anesthetic injection spreads around the remaining pericone fat compartments to block peripheral conjunctival sensation and, by spreading posteriorly, blocks the motor nerve of the superior oblique muscle lying outside the muscle cone (see Fig. 90–4).

The distribution of the orbital arterial system is de-

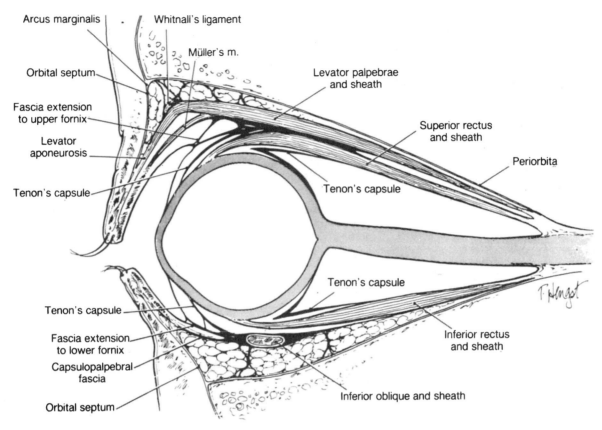

FIGURE 90–3. Connective tissue systems of the orbit. Sagittal section of the orbit demonstrating the diffuse attachments of the extraocular muscles to the periorbita and Tenon's capsule. (From Doxanas MT, Anderson RL: Clinical Orbital Anatomy. Baltimore, Williams & Wilkins, 1984.)

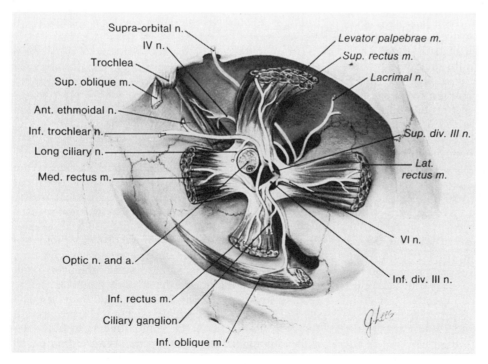

FIGURE 90–4. This illustration includes detail of the motor innervation of the extraocular muscles. The four rectus muscles are innervated from their conal surfaces. Note the long course of the nerve to the inferior oblique (branch of *Inf. div. III n.*). The trochlear *(IV n.)* remains outside the muscle cone and enters the superior oblique at its superolateral edge. (From Miller NR: Walsh and Hoyt's Clinical Neuro-ophthalmology, ed 4. Baltimore, Williams & Wilkins, 1982.)

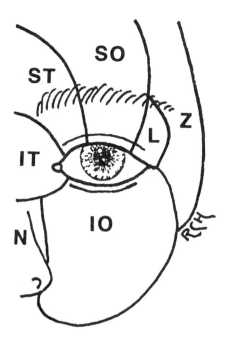

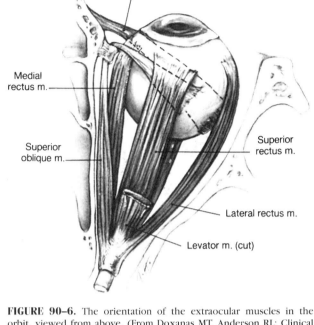

FIGURE 90–5. The cutaneous nerve supply to the periorbital region. IT, infratrochlear nerve; ST, supratrochlear nerve; SO, supraorbital nerve; L, lacrimal nerve; Z, zygomaticotemporal and zygomaticofacial nerves; IO, infraorbital nerve; N, nasal nerve. (From Gimbel Educational Services, Gimbel Eye Centre, Calgary, Alberta, Canada.)

FIGURE 90–6. The orientation of the extraocular muscles in the orbit, viewed from above. (From Doxanas MT, Anderson RL: Clinical Orbital Anatomy. Baltimore, Williams & Wilkins, 1984.)

picted in Figure 90-8. Because large vessels, the potential sources of vision-threatening bleeding, are located in the apex of the orbit along with tightly packed vital structures (optic nerve and extraocular muscle origins) that are subject to serious damage, regional anesthesia needles should not be introduced into the posterior 1.5 cm of the orbit. The superonasal quadrant of the orbit should be avoided as an injection site because it contains the end arteries of the ophthalmic artery and large venous connections between the facial angular vein and the superior orbital vein, as well as the trochlear

mechanism of the superior oblique muscle. There are, however, three adipose tissue compartments in the anterior and middle orbit which are relatively avascular and serve as the preferred sites for local anesthetic injection: the inferotemporal compartment (adjacent to the intermuscular septum between the inferior and lateral rectus muscles); the superotemporal compartment (close to the orbit roof in the plane lying between the lacrimal gland and the levator/superior rectus complex); and the medial compartment (located medially to the medial rectus muscle and between it and the medial orbit wall).

FIGURE 90–7. Transverse section through right orbit, viewed from above. *Dotted line* shows the path and depth of penetration of a 12-mm, 30-gauge disposable needle traversing the medial check ligament and entering the fat compartment on the nasal side of the medial rectus muscle. (From Gills JP, Loyd T, Cherchio M: Anesthesia, preoperative, and postoperative medications. Curr Opin Ophthalmol 6:131, 1995.)

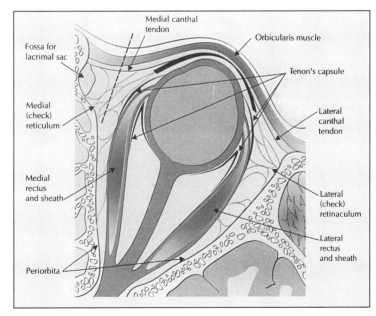

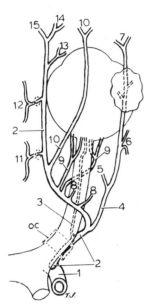

FIGURE 90–8. Arterial supply to the orbit. *1*, internal carotid artery; *2*, ophthalmic artery; *3*, central artery of the retina; *4*, lacrimal artery; *5*, muscular branch of the lacrimal artery; *6*, zygomatic branches of lacrimal artery; *7*, lateral palpebral arteries; *8*, muscular branches of ophthalmic artery; *9*, long and short posterior ciliary arteries; *10*, supraorbital artery; *11*, posterior ethmoidal artery; *12*, anterior ethmoidal artery; *13*, medial palpebral arteries; *14*, supratrochlear artery; *15*, dorsal nasal artery; OC, optic canal. (From McCord CD: Oculoplastic Surgery. New York, Raven Press, 1987, p 47.)

ORBITAL BLOCK TECHNIQUES

When analgesia alone is being sought, lidocaine in a concentration of 0.25% to 1.0%, or the equivalent, is used. If motor blockade is required lidocaine, 2.0% or the equivalent is recommended. Longer surgical procedures call for longer-acting agents, commonly bupivacaine. Epinephrine in 1:200,000 concentration may be added to the injectate to prolong neural contact time and may be used in higher concentration to reduce bleeding in eyelid surgery. The addition of hyaluronidase to the injectate promotes bulk spread of local anesthetics after injection.[4] Mechanical orbital decompression devices are frequently used for efficient production of globe hypotony after intraorbital local anesthetic injection.[5] Orbital nerve blocks are done both transconjunctivally and percutaneously, the advantage of the former being that a preliminary topical local anesthetic agent may be used to abolish the pain of needle insertion. If on digital retraction of the patient's lower eyelid the lid margin is found to be tightly held against the globe, if the globe is deeply recessed within the orbit, if there is a wide lateral canthal fold, or if the patient is blinking uncontrollably, a percutaneous approach is favored. In all cases the axial length measurement of the globe is carefully noted; in the presence of high myopia, the globe is at increased risk of penetration or perforation from regional block techniques.[6]

"Painless Local" Injection

The recommended sequence is as follows: (1) topical drops to the conjunctival sac; (2) "painless local" anes-

thetic injection using a sharp, 12-mm, 30-gauge disposable needle at the site of proposed full-strength injection (Fig. 90–9); (3) full-strength local anesthetic injection. "Painless local" anesthetic mixture[7] is made up by adding 1.5 mL of any full-strength local anesthetic to a 15-mL plastic bottle of sterile balanced salt solution (available in all ophthalmologists' offices). This technique sequence is extremely helpful in patient management in four ways:

- Without producing any stinging stimulus, excellent analgesia is produced in the area injected.
- Having experienced no pain, the patient relaxes and has confidence in the anesthesiologist for the subsequent procedures.
- The anesthesiologist obtains objective evidence of the patient's psychological status by observing his or her reactivity to being approached with a needle and receiving a minor stimulus.
- Frequently it is unnecessary to administer any sedative or systemic analgesic drug for the full-strength local anesthetic injection technique to follow.

Retrobulbar (Intracone) Block

Intracone regional block is still the most popular and dependable regional block for cataract extraction, the most commonly performed of all eye surgeries. Common surgical requirements for intraocular surgery using regional anesthesia are threefold: globe and conjunctival anesthesia; globe, lid, and periorbital akinesia; and intraocular hypotony.

Although there is commonality between the fat compartments within and outside the geometric confines of the cone of rectus muscles, injectate placed in midorbit intraconally, compared with periconally, is more effective in producing globe akinesia. Precision placement is the key to avoidance of complications (Fig. 90–10).

Peribulbar (Pericone) Blocks

In peribulbar (pericone) blocks, local anesthetic agent is injected into one of the lobes of the peripheral orbital fat compartment, no attempt being made to direct the needle within the cone of rectus muscles. Because larger volumes are necessary to achieve effective blocks than with the intracone method, it is recommended that a two-site technique be routinely used. Peribulbar techniques were introduced[8] in the expectation that the incidence of complications would be reduced, but this expectation has not been realized. Knowledge of orbital anatomy is as important as with intracone techniques. There are many variations of the pericone technique, a common one being placement in two locations, one inferotemporal and the other superonasal. A preferable alternative to the latter site of injection is the fat compartment on the nasal side of the medial rectus muscle (see Fig. 90–7).[9] A failure rate of up to 50% for achieving akinesia with periconal blocking has been reported.[10]

The routine combination of inferotemporal intracone injection with complemental pericone injection (medial

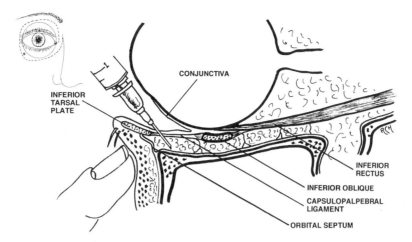

FIGURE 90–9. Injection of "painless local" in inferotemporal quadrant, viewed from lateral side. After gently retracting the lower eyelid with a finger, the tip of a 30-gauge, 12-mm needle enters transconjunctivally and inferotemporally just posterior to the inferior tarsal plate, with the shaft of the needle placed tangential to the globe. Following test aspiration, the initial injection is of 1.0 mL "painless local" to a depth of 1 cm from the conjunctiva. The needle has easily and painlessly (because preliminary topical anesthesia drops were applied) penetrated the conjunctiva, deep to the capsulopalpebral fascia. The needle entry point is at the lower end of the lateral orbit rim (small inset). Landmarks for transcutaneous injection of "painless local" are the same, but without lower eyelid retraction. The needle in this case passes inferior to the inferior tarsal plate, but otherwise follows an identical path, with its shaft tangential to the globe and directed toward the orbit floor. (From Gimbel Educational Services, Gimbel Eye Centre, Calgary, Alberta, Canada.)

compartment block recommended) produces a standard of globe anesthesia/akinesia, intraoperative patient comfort, and eyelid akinesia better than other techniqes.[10, 11]

When regional anesthesia is used for scleral buckling procedures, bupivacaine in 0.75% concentration is an excellent choice for these longer operations. I find that, in addition to inferotemporal intracone and medial pericone injections, a superotemporal pericone block is needed to obtund the surgical stimulation in the upper orbit (Fig. 90–11).

Facial Nerve Blocks

Facial nerve conduction block removes tone in the orbicularis oculi muscle, hence protecting the surgically opened eye from external pressure exerted by eyelid squeezing. Various methods of seventh nerve conduction block were in common use in earlier decades and deposited local anesthetics at some point along the distribution of the nerve from its emergence from the base of the skull at the stylomastoid foramen to its terminal branches on the deep surface of the orbicularis oculi muscle. However, when hyaluronidase is mixed with local anesthetics, injected into the orbit in higher volume, and used in combination with orbital decompression devices, effective spread from the orbit through the orbital septum occurs to achieve eyelid akinesia[12] without resorting to painful percutaneous seventh nerve blocking techniques.

Non-akinetic Block Techniques

With modern small-incision phacoemulsification cataract extraction techniques, it is no longer essential that the operating conditions be maintained as in the former era, with complete anesthesia and akinesia of the globe and adnexae. These procedures fall into three groups: subconjunctival (perilimbal) anesthesia; injection of local anesthetic by needle or cannula within Tenon's capsule; and modified topical corneoconjunctival anesthesia (topical anesthetic drops to the conjunctival sac plus the introduction of preservative-free 1.0% lidocaine into the anterior chamber of the eye during surgery).

Individual Sensory Nerve Blocks

The sensory nerves emerge from the orbit to supply the periorbital skin, as illustrated in Figure 90-5. Each of these nerves may be blocked as clinically required by injecting 0.5 to 1.0 mL of local anesthetic solution through a 30- or 27-gauge sharp disposable needle directed tangential to the globe over the adjacent orbit rim. In the nasal, inferior, and temporal orbit this can usually be achieved transconjunctivally (infratrochlear, infraorbital, and zygomatic nerves), whereas in the superior orbit the percutaneous route is the more usual. In addition to the transconjunctival method, the infraorbital nerve may be blocked percutaneously on the cheek at the infraorbital foramen or by the transoral approach, in which the needle is inserted through the superior buccal sulcus and directed upward to the intraorbital foramen which is being palpated by the other hand.

It is recommended that a "painless local" injection (see Fig. 90–9) be used before any of these blocks. The medial compartment block technique (see Fig. 90–7) effectively anesthetizes the infratrochlear nerve, including the peripheral medial conjunctiva, caruncle, semilunar fold, and lacrimal duct system.[9] The superotemporal block technique (see Fig. 90–11) anesthetizes the frontal (supraorbital and supratrochlear) and lacrimal nerves for surgery to the anterior two thirds of the scalp (unilateral). It is essential after any of these orbit rim blocks

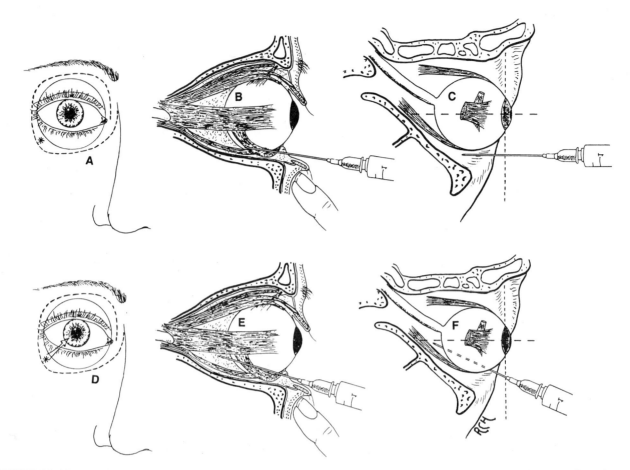

FIGURE 90–10. Inferotemporal intracone block: *A* and *D,* Views from in front. *B* and *E,* Views from lateral side. *C* and *F,* Views from above. A 27-gauge, 31-mm sharp disposable needle is used. The figure illustrates the transconjunctival approach but is equally applicable to transcutaneous injection (if the transcutaneous route were used, the lower lid would not be retracted, and needle tip entry would be inferior to the tarsal plate). The globe is in primary gaze. The needle tip enters at the lower temporal orbit rim, slightly up from the orbit floor *(A)* and very close to the bone. The needle track initially passes backward in the sagittal plane *(C)* and parallel to the orbit floor (i.e., with a 10-degree elevation from the transverse plane) *(B)* until the midshaft of the needle has reached the plane of the iris and the needle tip has passed the globe equator *(B* and *C).* (If the needle were further advanced in the sagittal plane, contact with the lateral wall of the orbit would occur.) Following this, the needle is directed medially and slightly upward *(D),* aiming for an imaginary point behind the globe on the axis formed by the pupil and the macula, so that the needle tip approaches but does not pass the midsagittal plane of the globe *(F).* The needle enters the intracone space by passing through the intermuscular septum just inferior to the lower border of the lateral rectus muscle *(E).* The globe is continuously observed during needle placement to detect globe rotation that would indicate engagement of the sclera by the needle tip. During needle placement, continuing observation of the relationship between the needle-hub junction and the plane of the iris establishes an appropriate depth of orbit insertion *(E* and *F).* In a globe with normal axial length, as illustrated here, when the needle-hub junction has reached the plane of the iris, the tip of the needle lies 5 to 7 mm beyond the hind surface of the globe *(E* and *F).* Following test aspiration, up to 4 mL of anesthetic solution is very slowly injected. (From Gimbel Educational Services, Gimbel Eye Centre, Calgary, Alberta, Canada.)

that the eyelids be taped closed at the completion of the procedure for the duration of the anesthetic action of the chosen injectate, until full corneal sensitivity and eyelid function recover.

Subcutaneous Lid Infiltration Anesthesia

Oculoplastic surgeons frequently use subcutaneous local infiltration anesthesia for upper and lower blepharoplasties. Small volumes only are injected, to avoid distortion of the tissues and, in the case of ptosis surgery, to permit continuing levator muscle function, which is essential in the assessment of eyelid position. Hyaluronidase in the mixture promotes spreading, and

higher concentrations of epinephrine—up to 1:50,000 (acceptable because of the small volumes involved)—may be used to reduce bleeding.

COMPLICATIONS OF ORBITAL NERVE BLOCKS

Techniques requiring multiple needle placements are associated with an increased incidence of complications when compared with a single injection or a reduced number of injections. Techniques in which the patient is momentarily rendered unconscious, using rapid-acting intravenous anesthetics for the duration of the orbital

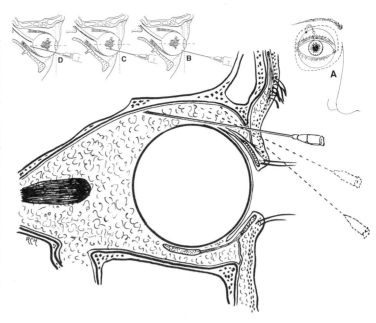

FIGURE 90–11. Superotemporal pericone block: Detail of needle placement depicted in a section of the orbit through the lateral limbus at a 5 degree nasal angle from the true sagittal section of the head. The plane is lateral to the cornea and the inferior rectus, superior rectus, and levator palpebrae muscles, but the front portion of the levator aponeurosis, consisting of anterior (Muller's muscle inserting on the upper edge of the superior tarsal plate) and posterior lamellae, is seen. An oblique slice of the lateral rectus muscle appears posteriorly, and a cross-section of the inferior oblique muscle appears below the globe. The needle tip is inserted through the skin of the lid, 3 mm lateral to the sagittal plane of the lateral limbus at the level of the superior orbit rim, and is aimed up markedly toward the roof of the orbit (A), with a medial angle of about 5 degrees in a plane lateral to the superior rectus–levator complex (B–D). The needle tip "walks" along the periorbita of the orbit roof (full-size illustration) in curvilinear fashion (A) until the needle tip is at a depth of 25 to 30 mm, at which point the injection is made with the usual precautions. (From Gimbel Educational Services, Gimbel Eye Centre, Calgary, Alberta, Canada.)

injection, have the inherent risk of abolishing patient complaint of pain as an indicator of therapeutic mishap.

Hemorrhage

When serious bleeding occurs within the orbit there is not only the problem of general orbital pressure increase, making surgery difficult, but also the potential for obstruction of the blood supply to and from the globe. Because the orbit apex contains large vessels, the depth to which needles are inserted should be limited to 31 mm from the orbit rim.[3] If the three relatively avascular anterior orbital sites described previously are chosen for anesthetic injection, and fine disposable needles are used, significant orbital hemorrhage is avoided.

Brain-Stem Anesthesia

Brain-stem anesthesia is caused by direct spread of local anesthetic to the brain from the orbit along submeningeal pathways after anesthetic invasion of the dural sheath which surrounds the optic nerve (Fig. 90–12).[13] It should be suspected if there is onset of any of the following: mental confusion or loss of contact with the patient, signs of extraocular paresis or amaurosis of the contralateral eye, shivering bordering on convulsant behavior, nausea or vomiting, dysphagia, sudden swings in the cardiovascular vital signs, dyspnea, or respiratory depression. Management of these differing manifestations of central spread includes reassurance, ventilatory support with oxygen, intravenous fluid therapy, and pharmacologic circulatory support with vagolytics, vasopressors, vasodilators, or adrenergic blocking agents as appropriate and as dictated by close vital sign monitoring. This complication is avoided by requesting patients to direct their eyes in primary gaze during intracone needle placement and by limiting the depth of needle penetration to a maximum of 31 mm.[3, 14]

Globe Penetration and Perforation

Factors that contribute to globe penetration (entry only) and globe perforation (both entry and exit) include failure to understand the extra risk inherent when dealing with long ovoid eyes and the presence of a preexisting scleral buckle from earlier retinal detachment surgery. In these cases, it is important that the globe be held in primary gaze during needle placement[6, 14]; pericone techniques may be more prudent than intra-

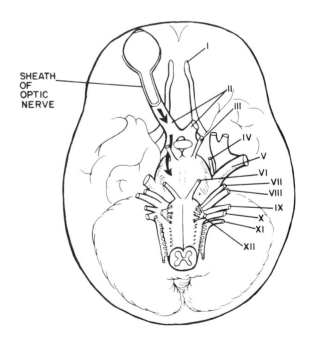

FIGURE 90–12. Illustration of the base of the brain and the pathway for spread of local anesthetic inadvertently injected into the subarachnoid space surrounding the optic nerve. Note that this pathway includes the cranial nerves, pons, and midbrain. (From Javitt JC, Addiego R, Friedberg HL, et al. Brain stem anesthesia after retrobulbar block. Ophthalmology 94:718, 1987.)

cone techniques, and general anesthesia should be considered as an alternative to both. In blocks of the upper orbit, a failure to appreciate the closeness of the globe to the orbit roof and the overhang of the roof itself may contribute to globe injury (see Fig. 90-2). Detailed anatomic knowledge is again stressed. Access to the intracone space is facilitated by moving the entry point for inferotemporal intracone blocking to the temporal side.[15, 16] Grizzard and colleagues[17] stated that tactile discrimination is progressively reduced with increasing needle size; they found that penetration or perforation of the eye from use of larger dull needles caused more serious damage than when fine disposable ones were used, and questioned the arguments advanced in their favor in the earlier literature. The appropriate management of scleral penetration and perforation is complex; once confirmed, it is imperative that a surgical retinal specialist be consulted as soon as possible.[18]

Myotoxicity

A common cause of prolonged extraocular muscle malfunction, presenting as postoperative diplopia, is intramuscular injection. A good three-dimensional knowledge of the anatomy of the orbit and its contents is essential to accurately place injections (see Fig. 90-6). Damage to the inferior rectus muscle is most common and is caused by inadequate elevation of the needle tip from the orbit floor during attempted intracone placement. However, the superior rectus may be damaged,[19] as may also the inferior oblique.[20]

Optic Nerve Damage

Injection at the orbital apex has the potential of frank optic nerve injury.[3] The needle length introduced beyond the orbital rim for both intraconal and periconal injections should not exceed 31 mm to assuredly avoid damage to the optic nerve in all patients.[3]

Oculocardiac Reflex

Use of dull, larger-gauge needles or a rapid injection rate, or both, is most likely the reason that the oculocardiac reflex has been reported as the most common complication of orbital regional anesthesia.[21] Other workers, reporting large regional block series, failed to find the reflex a problem when finer needles and slower injection rates were employed.[11, 22, 23]

Therapeutic Misadventures

Orbital injections of depot steroid medications and antibiotics are frequently employed at the time of ophthalmic surgery for their anti-inflammatory and anti-infective properties. Their inadvertent injection into the vitreous has serious implications.[24, 25]

Seventh Nerve Block Complications

Seventh nerve conduction blockade, produced by deposition of local anesthetics at some point along the distribution of the nerve from its emergence from the base of the skull at the stylomastoid foramen to its terminal branches on the deep surface of the orbicularis oculi muscle, is often used to reduce muscle tone in that muscle. Complications with blocking of the main trunk of the facial nerve at the base of the skull have resulted in swallowing difficulty and respiratory obstruction related to unilateral vagus, glossopharyngeal, and spinal accessory blockade.[26] For facial blockade at this site, it is prudent to inject no deeper than 12 mm and to avoid hyaluronidase in the injectate. When hyaluronidase is mixed with local anesthetics, injected into the orbit in higher volume, and used in combination with orbital decompression devices, effective spread from the orbit through the orbital septum occurs to achieve eyelid akinesia without definitive seventh nerve block (see previous discussion).[12]

REFERENCES

1. Doxanas MT, Anderson RL: Clinical Orbital Anatomy. Baltimore, Williams & Wilkins, 1984.
2. Dutton JJ: Atlas of Clinical and Surgical Orbital Anatomy. Philadelphia, WB Saunders, 1994.
3. Katsev DA, Drews RC, Rose BT: An anatomic study of retrobulbar needle path length. Ophthalmology 96:1221, 1989.
4. Nicoll JMV, Treuren B, Acharya PA, et al: Retrobulbar anesthesia: The role of hyaluronidase. Anesth Analg 65:1324, 1986.
5. Davidson B, Kratz R, Mazzoco T: An evaluation of the Honan intraocular pressure reducer. Am Intra-ocular Implant Soc J 5:237, 1979.
6. Duker JS, Belmont JB, Benson WE, et al: Inadvertent globe perforation during retrobulbar and peribulbar anesthesia. Ophthalmology 98:519, 1991.
7. Farley JS, Hustead RF, Becker KE: Diluting lidocaine and mepivacaine in balanced salt solution reduces the pain of intradermal injection. Reg Anesth 19:48-51, 1994.
8. Davis DB, Mandel MR: Posterior peribulbar anesthesia: An alternative to retrobulbar anesthesia. J Cataract Refract Surg 12:182, 1986.
9. Hustead RF, Hamilton RC, Loken RG: Periocular local anesthesia: Medial orbital as an alternative to superior nasal injection. J Cataract Refract Surg 20:197, 1994.
10. Loots JH, Koorts AS, Venter JA: Peribulbar anesthesia: A prospective statistical analysis of the efficacy and predictability of bupivacaine and a lignocaine/bupivacaine mixture. J Cataract Refract Surg 19:72, 1993.
11. Hamilton RC, Gimbel HV, Strunin L: Regional anaesthesia for 12,000 cataract extraction and intraocular lens implantation procedures. Can J Anaesth 35:615, 1988.
12. Martin SR, Baker SS, Muenzler WS: Retrobulbar anesthesia and orbicularis akinesia. Ophthalmic Surg 17:232, 1986.
13. Hamilton RC: Brain-stem anesthesia as a complication of regional anesthesia for ophthalmic surgery. Can J Ophthalmol 27:323, 1992.
14. Unsld R, Stanley JA, DeGroot J: The CT-topography of retrobulbar anesthesia. Græfes Arch Clin Exp Ophthalmol 217:125, 1981
15. Hamed LM: Strabismus presenting after cataract surgery. Ophthalmology 98:247, 1991.
16. Hamilton RC: Retrobulbar block revisited and revised. J Cataract Refract Surg 22:1147, 1996.
17. Grizzard WS, Kirk NM, Pavan PR, et al: Perforating ocular injuries caused by anesthesia personnel. Ophthalmology 98:1011, 1991.
18. Rinkoff JS, Doft BH, Lobes LA: Management of ocular penetration from injection of local anesthesia preceding cataract surgery. Arch Ophthalmol 109:1421, 1991.
19. Cap H, Roth E, Johnson T, et al: Vertical strabismus after cataract surgery. Ophthalmology 103:918, 1996.
20. Hunter DG, Lam GC, Guyton DL: Inferior oblique muscle injury

from local anesthesia for cataract surgery. Ophthalmology 102:501, 1995.

21. Meyers EF: Anesthesia. *In* Krupin T, Waltman SR (eds): Complications in Ophthalmic Surgery. Philadelphia, JB Lippincott, 1984, p 1.

22. Nicoll JMV, Acharya PA, Ahlen K, et al: Central nervous system complications after 6,000 retrobulbar blocks. Anesth Analg 66:1298, 1987.

23. Wong DHW: Review article: Regional anaesthesia for intraocular surgery. Can J Anaesth 40:635, 1993.

24. Brown GC, Eagle RC, Shakin EP, et al: Retinal toxicity of intravitreal gentamicin. Arch Ophthalmol 108:1740, 1990.

25. Schlaegal TF, Wilson FM: Accidental intraocular injection of depot corticosteroids. Trans Am Acad Ophthalmol Otolaryngol 78:847, 1974.

26. Lindquist TD, Kopietz LA, Spigelman AV, et al: Complications of Nadbath facial nerve block and review of the literature. Ophthalmic Surg 19:271, 1988.

Chapter 91

Brachial Plexus Anatomy

David R. Walega, M.D.

The brachial plexus provides the majority of sensory and motor innervation of the upper extremity.[1] Cutaneous innervation of the shoulder is provided by the supraclavicular nerve, a branch of the cervical plexus, and by the suprascapular nerve, a branch of the upper trunk of the brachial plexus. Sensory innervation of the medial aspect of the upper extremity is provided by three nerves. Innervation of the upper medial arm is derived from the intercostobrachial branch of the second intercostal nerve. Cutaneous innervation of the medial aspect of the distal portion of the upper arm and

forearm is derived from two branches of the medial cord of the brachial plexus: the medial cutaneous nerves of the arm and forearm (Fig. 91–1). A continuous fascial sheath extends from the cervical transverse processes to several centimeters beyond the axilla to enclose the entire brachial plexus from the cervical roots to the terminal nerves of the upper arm.[2]

The *roots* of the brachial plexus are formed by the anterior primary rami of the fifth, sixth, seventh, and eighth cervical nerves and the first thoracic nerve. In two thirds of patients the fourth cervical nerve contrib-

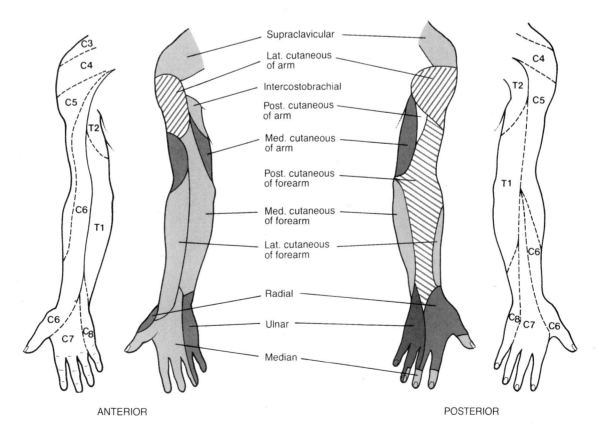

FIGURE 91–1. Cutaneous innervation of the upper extremity. (From Hughes JJ, Desgrand DA: Upper limb blocks. *In* Wildsmith JAW, Armitage EN (eds): Principles and Practice of Regional Anesthesia, ed 2. Edinburgh, Churchill Livingstone, 1993, p 169.)

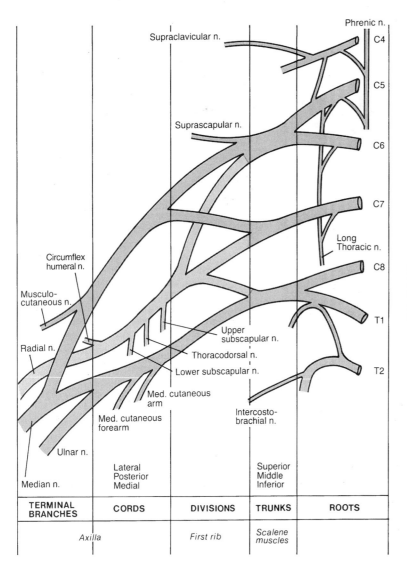

FIGURE 91–2. Anatomy of the brachial plexus. (From Hughes JJ, Desgrand DA: Upper limb blocks. *In* Wildsmith JAW, Armitage EN (eds): Principles and Practice of Regional Anesthesia, ed 2. Edinburgh, Churchill Livingstone, 1993, p 169.)

utes to the brachial plexus, and in one third of patients the second thoracic nerve contributes to the brachial plexus.[3] The nerve roots emerge from the intervertebral foramina and course behind the vertebral artery. They then pass anterolaterally and inferiorly between the anterior and middle scalene muscles, where they form the *superior* (C5, C6), *middle* (C7), and *inferior* (C8, T1) *trunks* of the brachial plexus (Fig. 91-2). Note that the phrenic nerve (C3-5) lies anterior to the anterior scalene muscle and is susceptible to blockade during interscalene brachial plexus block.

The trunks emerge from the interscalene groove, pass cephalad and posterior to the subclavian artery, and at the lateral portion of the first rib divide into *anterior* and *posterior divisions*. These divisions pass below the midportion of the clavicle to enter the axilla through its apex. The fibers of the plexus then recombine to form the three *cords* of the brachial plexus. The cords are named in relation to the axillary artery.[4] The *lateral cord* is formed by the union of the anterior division of the superior and middle trunks. The *medial cord* is a continuation of the anterior division of the inferior trunk. The *posterior cord* is formed by the posterior divisions of all three trunks.

At the lateral border of the pectoralis minor muscle, the three cords divide to form the peripheral nerves of the upper extremity. The lateral and medial cords give off branches to form the lateral and medial heads of the median nerve. The lateral cord continues as the musculocutaneous nerve. The medial cord also gives rise to the ulnar nerve. The posterior cord divides into the axillary nerve and the radial nerve.

REFERENCES

1. Hughes TJ, Desgrand DA: Upper limb blocks. *In* Wildsmith JAW, Armitage EN (eds): Principles and Practice of Regional Anesthesia, ed 2. Edinburgh, Churchill Livingstone, 1993, p 169.
2. Bridenbaugh LD: The upper extremity: Somatic blockade. *In* Cousins MJ, Bridenbaugh PO (eds): Neural Blockade in Clinical Anesthesia and Management of Pain, ed 2. Philadelphia, JB Lippincott, 1988, p 387.
3. Winnie AP: Anatomical considerations. Plexus Anesthesia: Perivascular Techniques of Brachial Plexus Block. Philadelphia, WB Saunders, 1983, p 11.
4. Brown D: Brachial plexus anesthesia: An analysis of options. Yale J Biol Med 66:415, 1993.

Chapter 92

Use of Nerve Stimulators for Peripheral Nerve Blocks

Jeffrey A. Katz, M.D.

OVERVIEW

Although much has been written on the use of nerve stimulators in peripheral nerve blockade, there remains controversy about its role relative to other approaches, such as the elicitation of paresthesia or the use of transarterial methods.[1] Nonetheless, it has particular advantage in those situations where the surrounding anatomy is not consistent relative to the target nerve's location (e.g., obturator or popliteal nerve block) or where patient cooperation may not be present. With the development of equipment specially suited for peripheral nerve stimulation for regional anesthesia and the increasing availability of associated equipment such as insulated needles, it would appear that the use of nerve stimulation in regional anesthesia will likely increase over the next several years.

HISTORY

In 1912, about 1 year after Kulenkampff's description of brachial plexus blockade via the axillary approach, Perthes used electrical stimulation to locate the brachial plexus.[2, 3] However, because his equipment was cumbersome and inconvenient and required the use of needles insulated with lacquer, it was largely disregarded. In 1955, Pearson demonstrated how motor nerve stimulation could be used to locate peripheral nerves, but it was the introduction in 1962 by Greenblatt and Denson of a convenient transistorized unit that the method became practical.[1] They demonstrated how motor nerves could be stimulated using voltages (later demonstrated to be a crude parameter relative to current) without eliciting pain and how the voltage required reflected the distance of the needle from the target nerve.[2]

Later issues addressed the concern that insulated needles of that time (using modified needles or plastic catheters) altered the tactile sensitivity during the procedure, so studies on uninsulated needles were performed. It was found that standard, unsheathed needles could be used successfully for nerve localization for regional anesthesia.[4]

TECHNICAL ISSUES

Excellent reviews have been published on the technical aspects of nerve stimulator design and application.[5] To appreciate the design and application of nerve stimulators for regional anesthesia, it is useful to understand the electrophysiology of stimulation.

The ability to stimulate a nerve depends on both the current applied (pulse amplitude) and the duration of current application (pulse width). Smaller nerve fibers (Aδ or C) require longer current durations than larger fibers (Aα motor) to be stimulated for a given current. Hence, in mixed peripheral nerves, by limiting the duration of the pulse width, it is possible to stimulate only motor fibers without triggering pain. A short pulse width of 50 to 100 μsec is optimal. Furthermore, shorter pulse widths provide better discrimination of the distance of the needle tip from the nerve; i.e., longer pulse widths are more likely to stimulate a nerve when the tip is too far away, whereas with short pulse widths it takes much more current to stimulate distant nerves.[5]

Another important consideration in the design and use of nerve stimulators is in the assignment of the (negative) cathode to the exploring needle and the (positive) anode to the ground lead. Less current is required to stimulate a nerve in this configuration, because when the needle is the cathode, current flows toward it, causing depolarization of nerve tissue near the needle; if the needle is the anode, then hyperpolarization of the nerve occurs.[6, 7] This has been shown to have clinical relevance during brachial plexus blockade, with the current required for stimulation being tripled when the positive lead is connected to the needle.[8]

The basis of nerve stimulation for regional anesthesia is the concept that the current required to stimulate the nerve is directly related to the distance of the needle tip from the nerve. Current density diminishes quickly as one moves further from the stimulating needle tip. For example, if a stimulus of 0.1 mA is needed to depolarize a nerve when the needle is touching the nerve, at 0.5 cm from the nerve 2.5 mA will be needed, and at 1 cm, 10 mA will be needed.[5] Based on these theoretical calculations, it is very unlikely that a nerve will be stimulated until the needle tip is within 1 cm. An early study of obturator nerve blocks demonstrated that 0.5 mA was needed for direct stimulation of the obturator nerve, and when 1 to 3 mA was needed to elicit motor response, the subsequent block was usually unsuccessful.[9] Another study examining interscalene, supraclavicular, and axillary approaches to the brachial plexus found that currents ranging from 0.2 to 1.5 mA were "readily obtainable and sufficient for localization" of the plexus in all locations.[10]

A debated issue relating to accuracy of needle placement concerns the use of insulated vs. uninsulated needles for stimulation. Uninsulated needles are effective despite the fact that current may escape along their entire length, because the greatest current density is at the tip (Fig. 92-1). Some even take the position that the pattern of current spread from uninsulated needles allows more precise positioning of the needle tip next to the nerve than insulated needles.[11] However, uninsulated needles can mislead needle placement by stimulating a nerve even though the tip of the needle has passed the nerve. Furthermore, higher currents are needed to stimulate nerves using uninsulated vs. insulated needles.[12] Using the saphenous nerve of an in vivo cat model, it was found that, on average, a minimally stimulating current of 0.5 mA (range, 0.2 to 0.9 mA) located the tip of an insulated needle an average of 0 cm from the nerve (range, 0 to 0.2 cm past the nerve). This is in comparison to an average minimally stimulating current of 1.2 mA (range, 0.7 to 1.5 mA) and a distance of 0.4 cm past the nerve (0 to 0.8 cm past the nerve) using uninsulated needles.[12] Despite the slight advantages insulated needles may have, it is generally held in most clinical discussions that either needle type can be used with equal likelihood of clinical success.

The stimulator should provide a reliable and constant current in the face of changing resistance as the needle passes through various tissues. This predictability greatly facilitates the use of current strength as an indicator of needle proximity to the nerve. The resistance to current flow may vary during a procedure by a factor of 20. Furthermore, the current should be displayed to confirm the "dose" of electricity being given.[5] Constant current in the face of changing resistance can be provided through the use of current multipliers in the stimulator.[13]

Other considerations in the design of a nerve stimulator are a low battery indicator, a current output range of at least 0.1 to 5.0 mA, and a linear scale current controller (i.e., half of a dial turn provides half the current of a full dial turn).

CLINICAL ISSUES

It should be emphasized that use of a nerve stimulator for regional anesthesia still necessitates knowledge of the anatomy involved and of the pharmacology of the agents being used. Simply demonstrating nerve stimulation at a low current is not enough to ensure that subsequent injection of local anesthetic will provide adequate block.[14]

Axillary approach toward the brachial plexus is perhaps not the optimal regional anesthetic in which to examine nerve stimulation, because other established techniques exist. However, the transarterial approach does present a risk for hematoma, and paresthesias have repeatedly been targeted as a possible cause of persistent dysesthesia following plexus blockade.[15-17] Of note is that not everyone agrees that use of a nerve stimulator reduces the risk of post-block dysesthesia, as cases of paresthesia and nerve injury occurring while using nerve stimulators have been reported.[18]

One study comparing three techniques of axillary block (transarterial, paresthesia, and nerve stimulation) found use of the nerve stimulator to provide no greater success than the other two methods; in fact, it appeared that a trend toward nerve stimulation being least effective existed.[19] Studies conducted even by strong proponents of the technique have found that in axillary block, nerve stimulation does not offer higher success rates than other methods, but it still requires the additional equipment and preparation.[20] Others using nerve stimulation to facilitate interscalene blocks (compared to paresthesia technique) also found it to provide no greater likelihood of success.[14, 21]

Nerve stimulation may have its greatest advantage in situations in which there are no clear anatomic landmarks indicating precise nerve location (e.g., popliteal nerve,[22] lateral femoral cutaneous nerve,[23] sciatic nerve, lumbar plexus) or in situations in which production of paresthesia might be unreliable (e.g., in the recovery room or following opioid administration). One study demonstrated that, despite the design of the stimulator

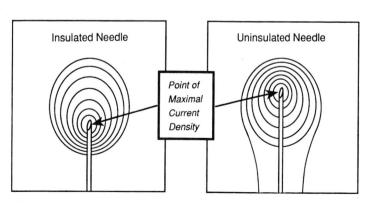

FIGURE 92-1. The differences between the current densities for insulated and uninsulated needles. Lines represent points of equal current density. Note that for the uninsulated needle, the center is proximal to the needle tip, and the pattern extends up the shaft. (From Pither C: Nerve stimulation. *In* Raj P (ed): Clinical Practice of Regional Anesthesia. New York, Churchill Livingstone, 1991, p 164.)

to target primarily motor nerves, purely sensory nerves could be successfully identified and blocked with a stimulator. Although localization of the lateral femoral cutaneous nerve took significantly longer using the nerve stimulator, successful block rates were much higher and onset of block began within 1 minute vs. 7 minutes for infiltration techniques. The end point used was a paresthesia referred to the lateral aspect of the knee at 0.6 mA.[23]

METHOD

Preparation for blockade using a nerve stimulator should be no different than other techniques, except for the stimulator equipment. Following preparation of medications and airway materials, placement of appropriate monitors, and preparation of the injection site, a ground electrode (positive) from the stimulator should be placed on the patient at a site distant from the block site and away from superficial peripheral nerves. The needle can be attached to the negative electrode of the stimulator, either through connections in specially designed needles or using an alligator clip attached to the proximal end of the needle. Although not always documented in the literature, many patients may find the motor twitching of the stimulator unpleasant. Therefore, because total alertness is not a requirement for this technique, sedation should be considered.

Once the needle has entered the skin, the nerve stimulator should be turned on and set to pulse at 1 to 2 Hz, with an initial current of 1 to 2 mA. As the needle is advanced, motor response to the nerve stimulator in the distribution of the target nerve should be monitored. When any motor response occurs, whether to local stimulation from the needle passing through a muscle or from the target muscles, the current output should be decreased immediately to limit the twitching to the minimum amount needed to confirm motor response. Excessive motor twitching can be extremely unpleasant and should be minimized.

As the needle approaches the target nerve, the current output should be able to be decreased. Optimally, currents of 0.5 mA with target motor response are desired, but some report consistent success with currents less than 1 mA. Remember that uninsulated needles require higher currents than insulated needles.

Another marker sometimes used to indicate appropriate needle placement is the sudden reduction in motor response following the injection of only 2 mL of solution.[24] This rapid response is not the result of neural blockade, but rather the result of the nerve being displaced away from the needle tip. This has been confirmed in studies where air produced the same sudden response as local anesthetic.[2] If the needle is past the nerve and the shaft of the needle is causing stimulation, then injection will not change the motor response and the needle should be slightly withdrawn and the test repeated. However, this test is not commonly mentioned in published reports describing nerve stimulation for regional anesthesia and so is likely little used.

CONCLUSIONS

Although nerve stimulation as a method of facilitating regional anesthesia offers several advantages over other methods, including the avoidance of hematoma and possible nerve damage through paresthesia, it also requires costly equipment. These costs are further increased if specially purchased insulated needles are used. It also requires the use of an assistant to manipulate the stimulator (although there are reports of various work-arounds for this obstacle, including foot-pedal controllers and using makeshift sterile attachments to the stimulator control dials) and may require additional time to locate the nerve. However, it offers an additional option toward approaching blocks that might otherwise be difficult due to anatomic or patient considerations and should be available in any institution wanting to offer regional anesthesia.

REFERENCES

1. Winnie A: Plexus Anesthesia. Philadelphia, WB Saunders, 1983, pp 215–217.
2. Raj P: Adjuvant techniques in regional anesthesia. In Raj P (ed): Handbook of Regional Anesthesia. New York, Churchill Livingstone, 1985, pp 250–258.
3. Perthes von G: Uker leitungsanasthesie unter zuhilfenahme elektrischer reizung. Medizinische Monatsschrift 47:2545–2548, 1912.
4. Raj P, Montgomery S, Nettles D, et al: Infraclavicular brachial plexus block: A new approach. Anesth Analg 52:897, 1973.
5. Pither C, Raj P, Ford D: The use of peripheral nerve stimulators for regional anesthesia: A review of experimental characteristics, technique, and clinical applications. Reg Anesth 10:49–58, 1985.
6. Ford D, Pither C, Raj P: Electrical characteristics of peripheral nerve stimulators: Implications for nerve localization. Reg Anesth 9:73–77, 1984.
7. Rosenberg H, Greenhow D: Peripheral nerve stimulator performance: The influence of output polarity and electrode placement. Can Anaesth Soc J 25:424–426, 1978.
8. Tulchinsky A, Weller R, Rosenblum M, et al: Nerve stimulator polarity and brachial plexus block. Anesth Analg 77:100, 1993.
9. Magora E, Rozin R, Ben-Menachem Y, et al: Obturator nerve block: An evaluation of technique. Br J Anaesth 41:695, 1969.
10. Riegler F: Brachial plexus block with the nerve stimulator: Motor response characteristics at three sites. Reg Anesthesia 17:295–299, 1992.
11. Jones R, De Jonge M, Smith B: Voltage fields surrounding needles used in regional anaesthesia. Br J Anaesthesia 68:515–518, 1992.
12. Ford D, Pither C, Raj P: Comparison of insulated and uninsulated needles for locating peripheral nerves with a peripheral nerve stimulator. Anesth Analg 63:925–928, 1984.
13. Technical Data Sheet. Munich, Braun Medical, Inc, 1992.
14. Smith B: Efficacy of a nerve stimulator in regional anaesthesia: Experience in a resident training programme. Anaesthesia 31:778, 1976.
15. Selander D, Edshage S, Wolff T: Paresthesiae or no paresthesiae—nerve lesions after axillary blocks. Acta Anaesth Scand 23:27–33, 1979.
16. Plevak D, Linstromberg J, Danielson D: Paresthesia vs. non-paresthesia, the axillary block [abstract]. Anesthesiology 59:A216, 1983.
17. Selander D: Axillary plexus block: Paresthetic or perivascular. Anesthesiology 66:726–728, 1987.
18. Moore D, Mulroy M, Thompson G: Peripheral nerve damage and regional anaesthesia [editorial]. Br J Anaesth 73:435, 1994.
19. Goldberg M, Gregg C, Larijani G, et al: A comparison of three

methods of axillary approach to brachial plexus blockade for upper extremity surgery. Anesthesiology 66:814–816, 1987.

20. Baranowski A, Pither C: A comparison of three methods of axillary brachial plexus anaesthesia. Anaesthesia 45:362, 1990.

21. McClain D, Finucane B: Interscalene approach to the brachial plexus: Paresthesia vs. nerve stimulator [abstract]. Reg Anesth 8:39, 1983.

22. Singelyn F, Gouverneur J, Gribomont B: Popliteal sciatic nerve block aided by a nerve stimulator. Reg Anesth 16:278–281, 1991.

23. Shannon J, Lang S, Yip R, et al: Lateral femoral cutaneous nerve block revisited. Reg Anesth 20:100–104, 1995.

24. Montgomery S, Raj P, Nettles D, et al: The use of the nerve stimulator with standard unsheathed needles in nerve blockade. Anesth Analg (Cleve) 52:827, 1973.

Chapter 93

Axillary Brachial Plexus Block

Robert E. Molloy, M.D.

Brachial plexus anesthesia has the greatest potential application of all regional anesthetic techniques, with the exception of intraspinal anesthesia. Essentially all upper extremity surgical procedures may be performed with a regional block technique. The choice of a specific approach depends on the surgical site, the experience of the anesthesiologist, and the inherent advantages and disadvantages of each technique. Some unique features of each approach are summarized in Table 93-1.

The popularity of axillary block for brachial plexus anesthesia can be explained by the simplicity of technique, the presence of easily located superficial landmarks, the relative absence of significant complications, and the reliable anesthesia of the hand, forearm, and elbow that is produced.[1] This technique blocks (or fails to block) terminal peripheral nerves. The axillary and musculocutaneous nerves tend to be missed because they depart from the axillary sheath high in the axilla; the radial nerve, which lies deep to the axillary artery, may be missed with approaches that use a superficial injection. Anesthesia of the median and ulnar nerves, which have a more superficial location, occurs most reliably with this approach. Success of the axillary block is evaluated by testing motor and cutaneous sensory function in a peripheral nerve distribution[2, 3] (see Fig. 91-1 in Chapter 91).

ANATOMY

High in the axilla, the three cords of the brachial plexus form the peripheral nerves of the upper extremity: the axillary, radial, musculocutaneous, median, ulnar, medial brachial cutaneous, and medial antebrachial cutaneous nerves. The axillary and musculocutaneous nerves quickly exit from the perivascular sheath. At the level of injection for axillary block, the neurovascular bundle contains the axillary artery and vein; the radial, median, ulnar, and medial antebrachial cutaneous nerves; and the surrounding fascia. The intercostobrachial nerve, often the medial brachial cutaneous nerve, and occasionally the axillary vein are located subcutaneously, outside this fascial layer.[4] The typical arrangement of the nerves around the axillary artery is demonstrated with some common variations in Figure 93-1.

TECHNIQUE

The patient may be sedated for axillary block but should retain the ability to quickly report the onset of paresthesias and the early signs of local anesthetic toxicity. The supine patient's shoulder is abducted and the elbow is flexed to about 90 degrees. Two landmarks are identified: the coracobrachialis muscle and, slightly

TABLE 93-1. TECHNIQUES OF BRACHIAL PLEXUS BLOCKADE

Technique	Area of Anesthesia	Advantages	Disadvantages
Axillary	Hand, forearm, and elbow	Simple; good landmarks and end points; minimal complications	No upper arm; may miss musculocutaneous nerve; positioning in abduction
Interscalene	Shoulder, arm, elbow, lateral forearm and hand	Blocks lower cervical and upper brachial plexus for shoulder surgery	May miss lower dermatomes (C8-T1) of brachial plexus
Subclavian perivascular	Entire arm except for shoulder	Entire brachial plexus blocked	Pneumothorax risk; more difficult
Infraclavicular	Entire arm except for shoulder	Facilitates catheter secured to chest wall	Very difficult; painful (classic technique); requires nerve stimulator

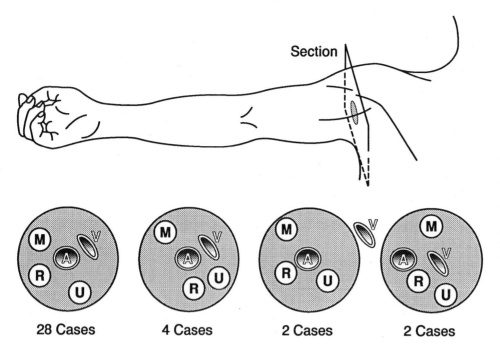

FIGURE 93–1. Variable anatomy of the axillary sheath seen in 36 axillary dissections in cadavers. Cross-sections taken at labeled site in proximal arm demonstrate the relative positions of the axillary artery (A) and vein (V), and the median (M), ulnar (U), and radial (R) nerves. (Modified from Partridge B, Katz J, Benirschke K: Functional anatomy of the brachial plexus: Implications for anesthesia. Anesthesiology 66:743, 1987.)

Section

28 Cases　　4 Cases　　2 Cases　　2 Cases

caudad to it, the axillary artery. The artery is fixed against the humerus, high in the axilla, with the index and long fingers of the nondominant hand. Four end points have been used to identify the brachial plexus: feeling a fascial pop or click, eliciting paresthesias, entering the artery, and electrical stimulation of muscle movement. Single or multiple injections may be selected. To produce the most reliable yet safe anesthesia, relatively large volumes of local anesthetic can be employed. The ideal total volume to be injected is 40 to 50 mL.[2] With all of these techniques, a subcutaneous injection of 3 to 5 mL superficial to the axillary artery blocks the intercostobrachial and medial brachial cutaneous nerves (Fig. 93-2). The various techniques are summarized in Table 93-2.

Paresthesia Techniques

The use of a small (22- to 25-gauge), short-bevel needle to elicit paresthesias is a classic axillary block technique. From one to four paresthesias may be sought, injecting 10 mL or more at each location.[5] Multiple injections with paresthesias may both improve anesthetic effectiveness and increase the risk of intraneural injection and traumatic injury to nerves.[6] An association of this technique with postoperative neurologic deficits has been suggested but never proved.[7] Careful initial drug injection, confirming that the patient does not report painful paresthesias, may help prevent intraneural injection. Many authors prefer to avoid seeking multiple paresthesias, particularly after some local anesthetic has been injected. The goals of greater simplicity and safety have led to the use of other techniques of axillary block.

Perivascular Sheath Techniques

Perivascular sheath techniques emphasize the role of surrounding fascia in containing injected local anes-

thetic to the neurovascular bundle, allowing the injectate under the influence of distal digital pressure to travel proximally and block the musculocutaneous nerve.[8] When a relatively blunt needle, aimed cephalad and at the artery, is passed through this fascial layer, a fascial "pop" is appreciated.[1] This technique is highly dependent on operator skills. The misdirected needle may encounter false fascial clicks that simulate entry into the sheath. The success rate with this technique is quite variable in the literature.

Transarterial Techniques

Transarterial techniques use entry into the artery to confirm needle placement within the neurovascular sheath.[9] Entry into the vein is not reliable, for this structure may reside outside the axillary sheath. A relatively sharp needle is placed into and slowly just through the artery before the local anesthetic is injected. The needle may be withdrawn into the artery and again slowly advanced until blood return ceases during the procedure to reconfirm exact placement of the needle outside the arterial lumen and wall but still within the sheath. Some authors inject up to one half of the volume anterior to the artery, whereas others inject all 40 to 50 mL posterior to the artery.[10] This deeper, posterior injection technique is inherently designed to increase the success rate of radial nerve block. It is essential to use frequent aspiration to avoid intravascular injection, particularly with this technique. Digital pressure over the injection site and careful inspection aim to prevent axillary hematoma formation.

Nerve Stimulator Techniques

Nerve stimulator techniques attempt to use low current near a nerve to stimulate a painless muscle contraction without eliciting paresthesias.[11] Achieving the great-

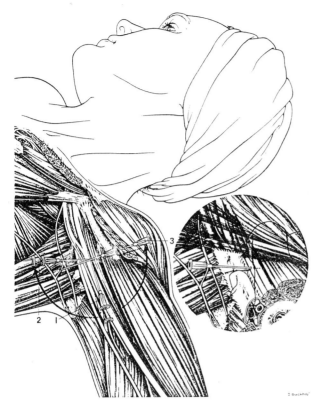

FIGURE 93-2. Axillary block technique. *1,* Perivascular injection adjacent to the median nerve. *2,* Musculocutaneous nerve block with 5 mL injected superiorly into the coracobrachialis muscle (see insert for detail). *3,* Subcutaneous infiltration of intercostobrachial and medial brachial cutaneous nerves superficial to the axillary artery. (From Winnie AP: Plexus Anesthesia: Perivascular Techniques of Brachial Plexus Block. Philadelphia, WB Saunders, 1983.)

est success requires these elements: use of an insulated needle, producing movement at the wrist or hand rather than at the elbow,[12] with the lowest possible current (less than 0.5 to 1.0 mA), and immediate cessation of motor response after injection of 1 mL of local anesthetic.[13] This technique is dependent on additional equipment and the services of an assistant. Its advantage may be more easily demonstrated in locating less superficial neural structures (e.g., the sciatic nerve). The nerve stimulator may best be wedded to single-injection nerve block techniques, so that previously injected drug does not interfere with subsequent identification of additional motor responses. However, overall success rates may increase with the number of nerves stimulated as well as the number of paresthesias elicited.[14] The nerve stimulator technique does not offer success rates superior to those obtained with the transarterial or paresthesia techniques.

Continuous Catheter Techniques

Continuous catheter techniques may be used to provide analgesia of the hand, forearm, and elbow after surgery.[15-17] A nerve stimulator may be used to place an axillary catheter with a large initial bolus of local anesthetic. This is followed by a dilute infusion of a long-acting agent or by intermittent bolus injections before physical therapy, dressing changes, or other painful events. This single injection catheter approach may be more reliable for postoperative analgesia than for initial surgical anesthesia. Catheter dislodgment, infection, and accidental injection of drugs meant for intravenous administration may complicate this technique.

Single-Injection Technique

Many authors who minimize the significance of fascial compartmentalization of the axillary sheath recommend a single-injection technique for its simplicity and purported safety. Numerous studies with single-injection, nonparesthesia techniques of axillary block have reported success rates not much greater than 85%.[17] It is not unusual for a single or even two nerves to be spared with axillary block. The highest success rates, approaching 100% (with high concentrations and large doses of local anesthetic), were reported for single injections posterior to the artery with a transarterial technique.[9] This approach has been recommended for the novice regional anesthetist.[18]

Multiple-Injection Techniques

Authors who emphasize the compartmentalization of the axillary sheath recommend the use of multiple injections and are willing to incorporate various end points so as to minimize the number of needle insertions.[19] This may include splitting the dose posterior and anterior to the artery with a transarterial approach; additional injection into the coracobrachialis muscle to

TABLE 93-2. VARIATIONS IN AXILLARY BRACHIAL PLEXUS BLOCK TECHNIQUE

Techniques	Advantages	Disadvantages
Paresthesia technique	Reliable anesthesia	Multiple punctures; painful; possibly increased nerve trauma
Perivascular sheath technique	Simple; single-injection; nontraumatic	Sparing of single nerves; inherent failure rate
Transarterial technique	Easy end point; high success rate with high dose	Risks of hematoma and systemic toxicity
Nerve stimulator technique	Nontraumatic; good for obese patients or poor anatomic landmarks	Extra equipment and assistant required; no increase in success
Single-injection technique	Simple; nontraumatic	Sparing of single nerves
Multiple-injection technique	Reliable anesthesia	Possibly increased nerve trauma
High-concentration, high-dose technique	Increased success	Risk of systemic toxicity

block the musculocutaneous nerve (see Fig. 93–2); infiltration around the artery in the vicinity of each nerve, whether or not a paresthesia has been elicited; and willingness to switch techniques when a paresthesia or arterial blood is unintentionally detected.

LOCAL ANESTHETICS

Intermediate-acting local anesthetics are selected to provide surgical anesthesia with rapid onset and variable duration from 2 to 5 hours. Lidocaine and mepivacaine, in a 1.0% to 1.5% concentration, with added epinephrine provide excellent anesthesia and low toxicity even when up to 750 mg is used for axillary block (40 to 50 mL). Longer-acting agents provide anesthesia of much greater duration (twice that of mepivacaine), with delayed onset of block. The dose of 0.5% bupivacaine or ropivacaine is limited to 200 mg. A 0.25% concentration is used for infusion at 6 to 10 mL/hour with continuous catheter techniques.[16] Plasma local anesthetic concentrations are relatively lower after brachial plexus block, compared with epidural, intercostal, or infiltration techniques. However, in a French survey,[20] use of large-volume, moderate-concentration techniques for brachial plexus block appeared to increase the incidence of systemic toxicity by seven-fold, compared with epidural anesthesia employing much lower doses of local anesthetic.

Adjuvants

Epinephrine is added to the local anesthetic solution to achieve a concentration of 5 μg/mL. This aims to improve the quality, duration, and safety of blockade. Sodium bicarbonate is added to lidocaine and mepivacaine only, to achieve a maximum concentration of 0.1 mEq/mL. This aims to improve onset and quality of anesthesia. Adjuvants are not added to continuous infusions.

SUPPLEMENTAL DISTAL BLOCKS

Incomplete brachial plexus blockade may be supplemented by reinjection of the plexus, at the same site or at an alternate site. Distal block at the elbow is not routinely useful, with the exception of blockade of the lateral cutaneous nerve of the forearm (musculocutaneous), lateral to the biceps tendon and proximal to the elbow crease in the distal arm.[21] Injection of the ulnar nerve at the elbow may risk added nerve injury, and it fails to block the medial forearm, being limited to anesthesia of the medial hand. Wrist blocks may be used to supplement brachial plexus blockade for hand surgery. Approximately 5 mL of local anesthetic is used for each nerve via a 25- to 27-gauge needle. The median nerve can be blocked medial to the flexor carpi radialis tendon, just deep to the fascia. The ulnar nerve is also blocked deep to the wrist fascia between the ulnar artery and the tendon of flexor carpi ulnaris. The radial nerve is blocked more superficially, infiltrating from lat-

eral to the radial artery around to the dorsal surface of the wrist.

SIDE EFFECTS AND COMPLICATIONS

Local anesthetic toxicity is a potential risk of axillary blockade because of the large volumes of local anesthetic used and accidental or intentional vessel puncture. Dose fractionation, frequent aspiration, and close patient monitoring are essential. Hematoma formation, vascular injury, and local infection are rare complications of axillary blockade. Traumatic nerve injury, persistent paresthesias, and usually transient deficits may occur rarely. Postoperative neural complaints may be reported by 0.3% to 2.8% of patients.[6, 22, 23]

REFERENCES

1. de Jong RH: Axillary block of the brachial plexus. Anesthesiology 22:215, 1961.
2. Vester-Andersen T, Husum B, Lindeberg T, et al: Perivascular axillary block IV: Blockade following 40, 50, or 60 ml of mepivacaine 1% with adrenaline. Acta Anaesthesiol Scand 28:99, 1984.
3. Lanz E, Theiss D, Janovic D: The extent of blockade following various techniques of brachial plexus block. Anesth Analg 62:58, 1983.
4. Partridge B, Katz J, Bernirschke K: Functional anatomy of the brachial plexus: Implications for anesthesia. Anesthesiology 66:743, 1987.
5. Bridenbaugh LD: The upper extremity: Somatic blockade. In Cousins MJ, Bridenbaugh PO (eds): Neural Blockade in Clinical Anesthesia and Management of Pain, ed 2. Philadelphia, JB Lippincott, 1988, p 387.
6. Selander D, Edshage S, Wolff T: Paresthesiae or no paresthesiae? Nerve lesions after axillary block. Acta Anaesthesiol Scand 23:27, 1979.
7. Wedel DJ: Nerve blocks. In Miller RD (ed): Anesthesia, ed 4. New York, Churchill Livingstone, 1994, p 1535.
8. Winnie AP: Perivascular techniques of brachial plexus block. Plexus Anesthesia: Perivascular Techniques of Brachial Plexus Block. Philadelphia, WB Saunders, 1983, p 117.
9. Cockings E, Moore P, Lewis RC: Transarterial brachial plexus blockade using 50 mL of 1.5% mepivacaine. Reg Anesth 12:159, 1987.
10. Hickey R, Hoffman J, Tingle IJ, et al: Comparison of the clinical efficacy of three perivascular techniques for axillary brachial plexus block. Reg Anesth 78:335, 1993.
11. Montgomery SJ, Raj PP, Nettles D, et al: The use of the nerve stimulator with standard unsheathed needles in nerve blockade. Anesth Analg 52:827, 1973.
12. Riegler FX: Brachial plexus block with the nerve stimulator: Motor response characteristics at three sites. Reg Anesth 17:295, 1992.
13. Pither CE, Raj PP, Ford DJ: The use of peripheral nerve stimulation for regional anesthesia: A review of experimental characteristics, techniques, and clinical applications. Reg Anesth 10:49, 1985.
14. Baranowski PA, Pither CE: A comparison of three methods of axillary brachial plexus anesthesia. Anaesthesia 45:362, 1990.
15. Selander D: Catheter technique in axillary plexus block. Acta Anaesthesiol Scand 21:324, 1977.
16. Tuominen M, Rosenberg P, Kalso E: Blood levels of bupivacaine after single dose, supplementary dose, and continuous infusion in axillary plexus block. Acta Anaesthesiol Scand 27:303, 1983.
17. Selander D: Axillary plexus block: Paresthetic or perivascular? Anesthesiology 66:726, 1987.
18. Urmey WF: Upper extremity blocks. In Brown DL (ed): Regional Anesthesia and Analgesia. Philadelphia, WB Saunders, 1996, p 254.

19. Thompson G, Rorie D: Functional anatomy of the brachial plexus sheath. Anesthesiology 59:117, 1983.

20. Auroy Y, Narchi P, Messick A, et al: Enquete prospective sur les complications toxiques systemiques des anesthesies locoregionales en France. Ann Fr Anesth Reanim 14:R218, 1995.

21. de Jong RH: Modified axillary block: With block of the lateral antebrachial cutaneous (terminal musculo-cutaneous) nerve. Anesthesiology 26:615, 1965.

22. Plevak DJ, Linstromberg JW, Danielson DR: Paresthesia vs. non paresthesia: The axillary block. Anesthesiology 59:A216, 1983.

23. Winchell SW, Wolfe R: The incidence of neuropathy following upper extremity nerve blocks. Reg Anesth 10:12, 1985.

Chapter 94

Interscalene Brachial Plexus Block

Dinna Billote, M.D.

One basic regional anesthesia approach to the brachial plexus is the interscalene block. This technique is well suited to clavicular, shoulder, and upper arm surgery, because the interscalene approach preferentially blocks the caudad nerves of the cervical plexus (C3–4) and the cephalad nerves of the brachial plexus (C5–7).[1] If blockade of the inferior trunk of the brachial plexus is required, supplementation of this technique may be necessary, as the ulnar nerve (C8–T1) is often incompletely blocked. Easily palpable landmarks, the lack of significant patient positioning requirements, and the need for minimal patient cooperation make the interscalene approach to the brachial plexus for regional anesthesia popular.

The interscalene block is particularly useful in the ambulatory surgical setting. With proper preparation, the interscalene approach requires less total nonsurgical intraoperative time and decreased postanesthesia recovery unit time. Other benefits include reduced blood loss[2] and fewer unplanned admissions for the treatment of nausea and vomiting, sedation, or severe pain when compared with those for general anesthesia.[3] The overall success rate of interscalene brachial plexus block is 90% to 100%.

TECHNIQUE

The patient lies supine and slightly rotates the neck to expose the side of the brachial plexus intended for blockade. The patient adducts the desired arm and extends the forearm toward the leg. One landmark is the lateral border of the sternocleidomastoid muscle, which may be easily identified by asking the patient to lift the head. Once the lateral edge of the sternocleidomastoid muscle is palpated at the level of the cricoid cartilage (C6), the anesthesiologist rolls his or her fingers into the interscalene groove bordered by the anterior and middle scalene muscles. Deep inspiration by the patient to contract the scalene muscles accentuates this groove and enables the anesthesiologist to differentiate between the interscalene groove and the more medial

space between the sternocleidomastoid and anterior scalene muscle.[4] Within this narrow space at the level of the cricoid cartilage, a 1½-in., short-bevel, 22-gauge needle is inserted perpendicular to the skin in all planes (Fig. 94–1). It is advanced until the patient reports paresthesias below the elbow or until hand muscle contractions are elicited using a nerve stimulator. A "click" may be detected as the needle punctures the prevertebral fascia. This fascial sheath surrounds the cervicobrachial plexus from the cervical spine to the axilla and is the basis for potentially successful block of any part of the plexus by a single local anesthetic injection.[6] Once the plexus is identified, the anesthesiologist aspirates the needle to ensure against intravascular or

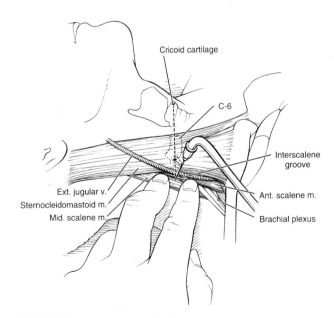

FIGURE 94–1. Interscalene block technique demonstrating these landmarks: cricoid cartilage, transverse process of C6, and sternomastoid, anterior, and middle scalene muscles. Needle insertion is shown between the palpating fingers of the nondominant hand in the interscalene groove. (From Urmey WF: Upper extremity blocks. *In* Brown DL (ed): Regional Anesthesia and Analgesia. Philadelphia, WB Saunders, 1996, p 254.)

intrathecal injection. After negative aspiration, the anesthesiologist usually injects 20 to 40 mL of local anesthetic in 5-mL increments. The amount of local anesthetic utilized depends on the extent of blockade desired. The interscalene approach can miss the inferior trunk of the brachial plexus if insufficient volume of local anesthetic is used. Radiographic studies have demonstrated that 40 mL of solution will cover the entire cervical and brachial plexus.[6]

A nerve stimulator facilitates the identification of the brachial plexus. Eliciting muscle contraction below the elbow with an electrical stimulus of at most .5 to .6 mA demonstrates close proximity to the brachial plexus and predicts with confidence that an adequate block will be achieved. If contraction of the diaphragm is observed, the needle lies on the anterior surface of the anterior scalene muscle and must be repositioned more lateral to lie within the groove. If periosteum is encountered, the needle is probably touching transverse process and should be redirected systematically in a cranial or caudal fashion until the patient reports paresthesia or the desired muscle contractions are observed.

Signs of successful brachial plexus block can be observed within minutes after local anesthetic injection. Motor blockade develops prior to sensory blockade and is attributed to the motor fibers being in the mantle and sensory fibers being in the core of the trunks and cords.[7]

COMPLICATIONS AND SIDE EFFECTS

Spinal Block or Epidural Block

Significant patient compromise requiring intubation, fluids, and vasopressors can rapidly develop if unintentional intrathecal or epidural block occurs. Winnie emphasizes that the direction of needle insertion should be slightly caudal, dorsal, and mesial to avoid direct horizontal insertion of the needle, which can lead to peridural or subarachnoid injection.[6] Unexpected life-threatening complications include apnea, loss of consciousness, seizures, profound hypotension, and bilateral sensory and motor blockade.

Intravascular Injection

This complication arises from vertebral artery injection and can quickly lead to seizures. Aspiration and incremental injection of local anesthetic allow early detection and expedient treatment.

Stellate Ganglion Block

The cervical sympathetic chain can be blocked by the spread of local anesthetic anteriorly through the fascial sheath, causing Horner's syndrome (ptosis, miosis, and enophthalmos). The patient should be warned of this minor, transient complication.

Vagus/Recurrent Laryngeal Nerve Block

The patient may experience hoarseness secondary to unilateral vocal cord paralysis and may only need reassurance until it resolves.

Pneumothorax

This is a rare but possible complication, as the level of needle insertion is above the dome of the lung.

Ipsilateral Phrenic Nerve Block

The interscalene technique commonly blocks the phrenic nerve because of the anterior spread of the local anesthetic over the anterior scalene muscle.[8] A 25% reduction in forced vital capacity (FVC) should be anticipated.[9] This rarely causes significant respiratory compromise, although the patient may require reassurance about the subjective symptom of dyspnea.

Nerve Damage or Neuritis

Intraneural injection or multiple attempts leading to neuronal trauma cause this uncommon complication. Transient paresthesias may be reported as the needle mechanically stimulates a nerve, but the anesthesiologist should not inject local anesthetic if the patient reports continuous pain. Unexpected postoperative neurologic damage may be due to the regional block performed, to patient positioning causing excessive compression or stretching of nerves, or to the surgery itself. When it is important to avoid confusion about this, an interscalene block placed for postoperative pain relief should be conducted in an awake patient after ascertaining that no previous neurologic damage has occurred.

Vasovagal Episodes

Interscalene block for shoulder arthroscopy in the sitting position may cause a neurocardiogenic syncopal episode mediated by the Bezold-Jarisch reflex.[10] This phenomenon is commonly seen by cardiologists and neurologists during tilt-table testing in the evaluation of syncope. Intraoperatively, the patient complains of feeling faint and experiences hypotension and/or profound bradycardia. The proposed mechanism of this vasodepressor episode involves venous blood pooling from the sitting position reducing end-diastolic volume (decreased preload) and increased cardiac contractility reflexively responding to a low preload state by concomitant catecholamine release. This in turn results in increased activity of mechanoreceptors in the left ventricle, which causes parasympathetic mediated vasodilation and/or bradycardia. Epinephrine in doses used for interscalene blocks or found in orthopedic irrigating solutions may yield sufficient catecholamine levels to help trigger the vasodepressor response. This reflex may be prevented by intravenous fluid administration to achieve adequate preload and atropine, 0.4 mg intravenously.

REFERENCES

1. Lanz E, Theiss D, Jankovic D: The extent of blockade following various techniques of brachial plexus block. Anesth Analg 62:55, 1983.
2. Tetzlaff J, Yoon H, Brems J: Interscalene brachial plexus block for shoulder surgery. Reg Anesth 19:339, 1994.
3. D'Alessio JG, Rosenblum M, Shea K, et al: A retrospective comparison of interscalene block and general anesthesia for ambulatory surgery shoulder arthroscopy. Reg Anesth 20:62, 1995.
4. Harrock NE, Bruce G: An improved technique for locating the interscalene groove. Anesthesiology 44:431, 1976.
5. Urmey WF: Upper extremity blocks. In Brown DL (ed): Regional Anesthesia and Analgesia. Philadelphia, WB Saunders, 1996, p 254.
6. Winnie AP: Interscalene brachial plexus block. Anesth Analg 49:455, 1970.
7. Winnie AP, Tay C, Patel KP, et al: Pharmacokinetics of local anesthetics during plexus blocks. Anesth Analg 56:852, 1977.
8. Urmey WF, Talts KH, Sharrock NE: One hundred percent incidence of hemidiaphragmatic paresis associated with interscalene brachial plexus anesthesia as diagnosed by ultrasonography. Anesth Analg 72:498, 1991.
9. Urmey WF, McDonald M: Hemidiaphragmatic paresis during interscalene brachial plexus block: Effects on pulmonary function and chest wall mechanics. Anesth Analg 74:352, 1992.
10. D'Alessio J, Weller R, Rosenblum M: Activation of the Bezold-Jarisch reflex in the sitting position for shoulder arthroscopy using interscalene block. Anesth Analg 80:1158, 1995.

FURTHER READINGS

Blanchard J, Ramamurthy S: Brachial plexus. In Benumof JL (ed): Clinical Procedures in Anesthesia and Intensive Care. Philadelphia, JB Lippincott, 1992, p 760.

Wedel DJ: Nerve blocks. In Miller RD (ed): Anesthesia, ed 4. New York, Churchill Livingstone, 1994, p 1535.

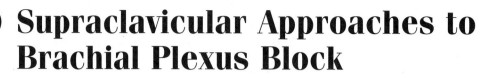

Chapter 95

Supraclavicular Approaches to Brachial Plexus Block

Edward P. Grimes, M.D.

SUPRACLAVICULAR BRACHIAL PLEXUS BLOCK

Anesthesia of the upper extremity can be provided by blocking the brachial plexus using a supraclavicular approach. The plexus is blocked where it is most compactly arranged, at the level of the nerve trunks. As a result, a block with a rapid onset can be achieved. This approach can be performed with the upper extremity in any position and is especially useful in patients who cannot circumduct the humerus for the axillary approach. The supraclavicular approach also offers a high success rate for hand surgery because all the branches of the brachial plexus can be reliably blocked.[1] It avoids the sparing of the ulnar nerve that frequently occurs with an interscalene block and provides good musculocutaneous anesthesia, which is often missed with an axillary block. One should be aware that this approach carries a greater risk of pneumothorax than either the axillary or the interscalene approach.[2] Thus, this approach is best avoided in patients who are uncooperative, have unclear anatomic landmarks, or have significant pulmonary disease.

Anatomy

As the superior, middle, and inferior trunks of the brachial plexus emerge from between the scalene muscles, they form a bundle that lies dorsal and inferior to the midpoint of the clavicle. These three trunks pass inferior to the clavicle and superior to the first rib to enter the axilla. In a frontal plane, the lateral aspect of the first rib lies at approximately the midpoint of the clavicle. Just dorsal to the midpoint of the clavicle, the subclavian artery can usually be palpated in the interscalene groove. At this level, the trunks lie dorsal to the subclavian artery and are enclosed by a sheath derived from prevertebral and scalene fascia.

Technique

With the patient in a supine position with the head turned toward the nonoperative side, the interscalene groove is identified. The medial and lateral borders of the clavicle should be identified and the midpoint of the clavicle should be marked. The first rib lies dorsal to the midpoint of the clavicle in most cases. A 23-gauge, 32-mm short-bevel needle is inserted 1 cm dorsal to the midpoint of the clavicle. The direction of the needle should be directly caudal, with a slight posterior and medial inclination. In some patients, it may be easier to find the nerve trunks by inserting the needle 2 to 3 cm behind the clavicle. If a paresthesia is not obtained using this method, the needle should be advanced down to the first rib. The needle is "walked" along the rib in a dorsal and ventral direction until paresthesia is obtained. Small adjustments in needle trajectory are required so as not to miss the relatively narrow plexus at this level. If the subclavian artery is contacted, the needle must be redirected more posteriorly.

Once a hand or forearm paresthesia is obtained, an attempt is made to aspirate from the needle. If no blood return is evident, a small test injection is made to check for intraneural position of the needle tip. If no persistent paresthesia is obtained on test injection, local anesthetic is injected in 5-mL increments, each preceded by an attempt to aspirate blood. If no blood is obtained, a total of 15 to 35 mL of local anesthetic is injected.

Complications

One potential complication of supraclavicular brachial plexus block is pneumothorax. The frequency of this complication has been estimated to be between 0.5% and 6%.[3] Clinically significant pneumothorax or tension pneumothorax is rare. Dyspnea, cough, or pleuritic chest pain are symptoms that may herald the development of pneumothorax. If it is suspected, a chest x-ray should be obtained. The treatment of pneumothorax depends on its size and the patient's symptoms. For extensive pneumothorax (greater than 50% of normal lung volume), the air should be removed with a chest tube. With lesser percentages of pneumothorax, the air should be removed by needle aspiration only if it is causing symptoms.

Other complications of this technique include spread of local anesthetic to other nerve fibers. Phrenic nerve blockade occurs in 40% to 60% of cases but usually causes no symptoms. Caution must be taken in patients with significant pulmonary disease. When large volumes of local anesthetic (50 mL or more) are used for brachial plexus block, Horner's syndrome from stellate ganglion blockade is common. Nerve damage is uncommon but can occur as a result of intraneural injection or faulty positioning of the anesthetized arm during surgery. Local anesthetic toxicity can also occur either as a result of overdose or, more commonly, from unintentional intravascular injection.

SUBCLAVIAN PERIVASCULAR BLOCK

Modifications of the supraclavicular approach to the brachial plexus have been suggested because of a concern about the potential for pneumothorax. Recognizing that the nerves of the brachial plexus exist in a perivascular sheath, Winnie and Collins[4] recommended use of the "subclavian perivascular technique." Prevertebral fascia envelops the brachial plexus from the cervical vertebrae to the distal axilla. These authors demonstrated that a single injection of local anesthetic into this sheath was sufficient to provide brachial plexus anesthesia. They further demonstrated that the extent of anesthesia depended on the volume of local anesthetic injected into the perivascular sheath.

Prior to the description of the subclavian perivascular technique, the supraclavicular approach to the brachial plexus involved multiple injections and a needle direction pointing mesial, caudal, and dorsal. Considering the anatomy of the brachial plexus sheath, it appeared that a needle insertion site more cephalad in the interscalene groove resulted in a much greater depth to the perivascular sheath, and it allowed much greater movement of the needle without leaving the space (Fig. 95-1). The perivascular technique effectively utilized a single injection, demonstrating that multiple injections were unnecessary.

Technique

With the patient supine and the head turned to the nonoperative side, the interscalene groove is palpated. Palpate inferiorly along the interscalene groove until the subclavian artery pulse is found. The block needle should be inserted cephalad to this point and should point directly caudal, but not mesial or dorsal, as would be used with the classic supraclavicular approach. The level of insertion is high in the triangular perivascular space. A single injection of local anesthetic is made at this point. The direction of needle insertion, the use of a short-bevel needle, and the use of a single injection decrease the risk of pneumothorax. Because it confirms that the tip of the needle is within the perivascular sheath, the ability to elicit paresthesia is essential to obtaining a high degree of success with this block. The volume of local anesthetic recommended is 25 to 35 mL.

Complications

The risk of pneumothorax with this approach should be less than with the classic supraclavicular approach, because no attempt is made to seek contact with the first rib. Once paresthesia is obtained, the local anesthetic should be injected. Other complications are similar to those described for the supraclavicular block and include phrenic nerve blockade, Horner's syndrome, nerve damage, and local anesthetic toxicity.

PLUMB-BOB TECHNIQUE

Additional modifications to the classic supraclavicular block have included various parascalene methods.[5,6] Perhaps the simplest modification is the plumb-bob technique described by Brown and Bridenbaugh[7] and Brown

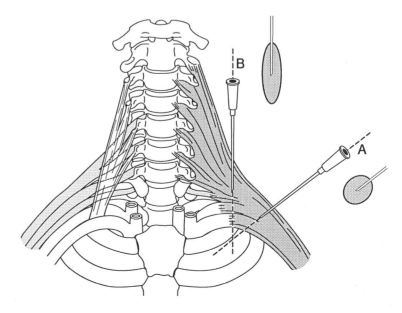

FIGURE 95–1. Anatomy of the subclavian perivascular space, illustrating the fascial sheath after the adjacent muscles and vessels have been removed. *A* shows a cross-section through the space at the level of the classic block technique. *B* demonstrates a section at the level of the subclavian perivascular technique. (Redrawn from Winnie AR, Collins VJ: The subclavian perivascular technique of brachial plexus anesthesia. Anesthesiology 25:353, 1964.)

and colleagues,[8] which was designed to reduce the incidence of pneumothorax and to simplify the technique. It utilizes readily identified skin landmarks and anatomic planes for needle insertion and uses a systemic method for locating the brachial plexus (Fig. 95–2). This simplicity of technique may be associated with greater ease of teaching the method to trainees.[8]

Technique

The patient lies supine with the head turned away from the side to be blocked. The skin entry site is marked at the insertion of the most lateral edge of the sternocleidomastoid muscle on the superior border of the clavicle. Needle insertion is made perpendicular to the plane of the operating room table. A blunt, short-bevel needle is advanced until paresthesia is elicited or the first rib is contacted. If neither occurs, the needle is redirected cephalad in the parasagittal plane in small steps until paresthesia is obtained or a 30-degree angulation of the needle results. If this fails, similar gradual adjustments are made in a caudad direction with a 30-degree angle limit. Cephalad angulation is commonly required in smaller, thin patients, whereas caudad angulation is commonly required for larger or more muscular individuals. The brachial plexus is located immediately cephalad and posterior to the subclavian artery, dictating the direction of needle adjustment necessary should the latter vessel be accidentally entered.

Complications

This modification of supraclavicular block has been shown by careful analysis to be anatomically sound, and it appears to be associated with a low incidence of pneumothorax.

REFERENCES

1. Mulroy MF, Thompson GE: Supraclavicular approach. *In* Hahn MB, McQuillan PM, Sheplock GJ (eds): Regional Anesthesia. St Louis, Mosby–Year Book, 1996, p 101.
2. Tetzlaff JE: Peripheral nerve block. *In* Morgan GE, Mikhail MS

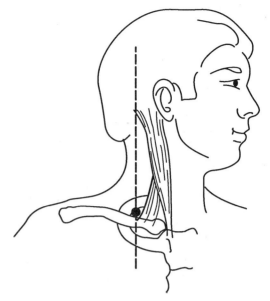

FIGURE 95–2. Modified supraclavicular block using the plumb-bob approach. The needle entry site (marked with a *black dot*) is just lateral to the clavicular head of the sternocleidomastoid muscle and immediately cephalad to the clavicle. The needle is inserted perpendicular to the table and "walked" cephalad, then caudally, along the sagittal plane, which is identified by the *dotted line*. (Redrawn from Brown DL, Cahill DR, Bridenbaugh LD: Supraclavicular nerve block: Anatomic analysis of a method to prevent pneumothorax. Anesth Analg 76:530, 1993.)

   (eds): Clinical Anesthesiology, ed 2. East Norwalk, Conn, Appleton & Lange, 1995, p 249.
3. Bridenbaugh LD: The upper extremity somatic blockade. *In* Cousins MJ, Bridenbaugh PO (eds): Neural Blockade in Clinical Anesthesia and Management of Pain, ed 2. Philadelphia, JB Lippincott, 1988, p 387.
4. Winnie AP, Collins VJ: The subclavian perivascular technique of brachial plexus anesthesia. Anesthesiology 25:353, 1964.
5. Vongvises P, Panijayanond T: A parascalene technique of brachial plexus anesthesia. Anesth Analg 58:267, 1979.
6. Dalens B, Vanneuville G, Tanguy A: A new parascalene approach to the brachial plexus in children: Comparison with the supraclavicular approach. Anesth Analg 66:1264, 1987.
7. Brown DL, Bridenbaugh LD: Physics applied to regional anesthesia results in an improved supraclavicular nerve block: The "plumb-bob" technique. Anesthesiology 3(suppl):A376, 1988.
8. Brown DL, Cahill DR, Bridenbaugh LD: Supraclavicular nerve block: Anatomic analysis of a method to prevent pneumothorax. Anesth Analg 76:530, 1993.

Chapter 96

Infraclavicular Brachial Plexus Block

Honorio T. Benzon, M.D.

ANATOMY

The axilla is located in the infraclavicular space between the medial side of the arm and the upper lateral part of the chest. It has a base, an apex, and four walls.[1] The base is formed by the skin and the axillary fascia. The apex faces the root of the neck and is limited by the superior border of the scapula, the outer border of the first rib, and the posterior surface of the clavicle. The walls consists of the pectoralis major and pectoralis minor muscles anteriorly; the subscapularis, teres major, and latissimus dorsi muscles posteriorly; the first four ribs medially; and medial side of the arm laterally. The axilla contains the brachial plexus, axillary vessels, lymph glands, fat, and loose areolar tissue.

TECHNIQUE

The classic technique was described by Raj and coworkers.[1] The patient is supine with the head turned away from the arm to be blocked. The arm is abducted to 90 degrees. The midpoint of the clavicle, the site at which the subclavian artery usually dips under the clavicle, is marked. The C6 tubercle in the neck and the brachial artery in the arm are marked. A line is drawn from the C6 tubercle to the brachial artery in the arm, passing through the midpoint of the clavicle. The site of insertion of the needle is 1 in. below the inferior border of the midpoint of the clavicle (Fig. 96–1). A skin wheal is made, and an insulated needle is inserted at an angle of 45 degrees. With the nerve stimulator set at 1 to 2 V, the needle is advanced laterally toward the brachial artery. Movements of the wrist or fingers with a voltage of less than 1 mA, preferably 0.3 to 0.7 mA, signify proximity of the needle to the brachial plexus. Injection of 1 to 2 mL of local anesthetic results in prompt disappearance of the previously elicited muscle movement. Twenty-five to 30 mL of local anesthetic is injected.

MODIFIED INFRACLAVICULAR BRACHIAL PLEXUS BLOCK

The classic approach can be painful and difficult to master. Because of this, Sims[2] modified the classic approach, in which the site of needle insertion is closer to the brachial plexus. The index finger is placed in the groove between the coracoid process of the scapula

FIGURE 96–1. Landmarks and technique involved in the classic approach to infraclavicular brachial plexus blockade. The needle is inserted at X. The cross-section at the level of the axilla shows the orientation of the artery (A), vein (V), and medial (M), radial (R), and ulnar (U) nerves within the axillary sheath.

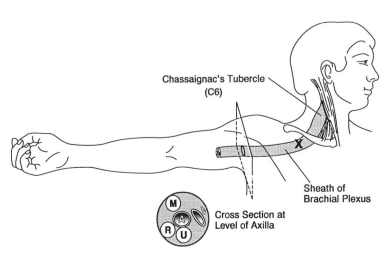

Chassaignac's Tubercle
(C6)

Sheath of
Brachial Plexus

Cross Section at
Level of Axilla

and the inferior border of the clavicle. The fingertip is then advanced inferiorly and medially until it falls into a depression bordered by the superior portion of the pectoralis major inferiorly and medially, the coracoid process of the scapula laterally, and the clavicle superiorly. This area is medial to the pectoralis minor muscle and superficial to the pectoralis major muscle. A skin wheal is made at this point, and the needle is advanced inferiorly, laterally, and posteriorly toward the apex of the axilla (Fig. 96-2). The brachial plexus is usually reached 2 to 3 cm from the skin wheal. The use of an insulated needle and a nerve stimulator is recommended, as above. Thirty-five to 40 mL of local anesthetic is injected.

CORACOID TECHNIQUE OF THE INFRACLAVICULAR BRACHIAL PLEXUS BLOCK

Whiffler[3] described the coracoid modification of the infraclavicular brachial plexus block. In this technique, the arm is abducted 45 degrees from the chest wall, and the ipsilateral shoulder is depressed (this maneuver brings the axillary sheath and its contents closer to the coracoid process of the scapula). The midpoint of the clavicle is identified, and the subclavian artery is palpated. The artery is followed laterally until it disappears under the clavicle; this point is marked X1. The coracoid process is identified and marked, and the axillary artery is palpated as high as possible in the axilla. The site on the anterior surface of the chest wall where the axillary artery is palpated is marked X2. This point (X2) usually lies in the deltopectoral groove, just below the head of the humerus. A line is drawn along points X1 and X2, passing immediately inferior and medial to the coracoid process. The site of needle insertion is inferomedial to the coracoid process and advanced along the line toward the axillary artery. Whiffler used a 21-gauge, 51-mm needle and, in most instances, found it necessary to insert the needle all the way to its hub. Thirty to 35 mL of local anesthetic is injected.

Wilson and colleagues[4] studied the orientation and the depth of insertion of the needle in coracoid block. They found that infraclavicular brachial plexus block can be achieved with the needle inserted directly posterior from a point located 2 cm medial and 2 cm caudal to the coracoid process. The mean distance from the skin to the axillary artery (the brachial plexus surrounds the second portion of the axillary artery) was 4.2 ± 1.5 cm (range, 2.25 to 7.75 cm) in men and 4.0 ± 1.3 cm (range, 2.25 to 6.5 cm) in women.[4]

ADVANTAGES OF THE INFRACLAVICULAR BRACHIAL PLEXUS BLOCK

The block avoids the neurovascular structures of the neck, and it can be performed with the arm adducted.

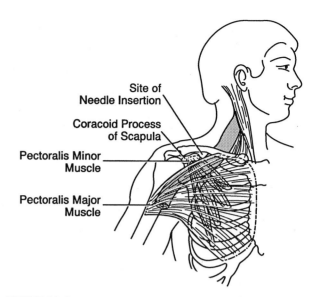

FIGURE 96–2. Landmarks and needle position involved in the modified technique of infraclavicular brachial plexus blockade.

The musculocutaneous nerve is more consistently blocked, which is not the case with block of the brachial plexus at the axilla.[4] Compared to the supraclavicular approach, the risk of pneumothorax is smaller. Finally, if a continuous block with a catheter is desired, the approach allows easy fixation of a catheter with less chance of dislodgment than the axillary, interscalene, or supraclavicular approaches.[1-4]

CHOICE OF TECHNIQUE OF BRACHIAL PLEXUS BLOCKADE AS DICTATED BY THE SITE OF SURGERY

The technique of blockade of the brachial plexus can be tailored to fit the site of surgery.[5] Raj divided the upper extremity into four regions: (1) shoulder, (2) elbow, (3) forearm, and (4) wrist and hand. The *shoulder* is innervated by the C3, C4, C5, and C6 nerve roots, and the interscalene approach to the brachial plexus is the recommended technique. If deeper tissues, or the shoulder joint, are to be operated on, then Raj recommended that the T1 and T2 nerve roots be blocked also. Operations at the *elbow* (e.g., ulnar transposition, skin graft, closed or open reduction of the elbow joint) require blocking the C5, C6, C7, C8, T1, and T2 nerve roots or their branches. Blockade of the C5-8 is critical for operations on the lateral or posterolateral aspect of the elbow, whereas blockade of the C8, T1, and T2 nerve roots are required for operations on the medial aspect of the elbow. The use of a tourniquet requires blocking of the superficial branches of the C5 to T2 nerve roots. The best approach to surgery on the elbow is the infraclavicular approach followed by the supraclavicular approach[5] (the T2 nerve root may be missed with the supraclavicular approach). Surgery of the *forearm region* requires blockade of the musculocutaneous nerve (C5-7) on the lateral aspect, the median nerve

(C6-T1), the ulnar nerve (C8-T1) on the anteromedial aspect, the posterior nerve (C5-8), which is derived from the radial nerve, and the medial cutaneous nerve of the forearm (C8-T1), which is derived from the medial cord of the brachial plexus. All of these are branches of the brachial plexus formed by the C5-T1 nerve roots, and the infraclavicular approach is the technique of choice because it blocks all these nerves at the cord level. The supraclavicular, interscalene, and axillary approaches can be performed but are not as effective as the infraclavicular approach. For surgery of the *wrist and the hand*, the median nerve (which innervates the anterolateral aspect), the radial nerve (which innervates the posterolateral aspect), and the musculocutaneous nerve (which innervates the superolateral aspect) must all be blocked. The interscalene and supraclavicular approaches are the recommended techniques for surgery of the base of the thumb. For median nerve decompression, surgery on the ulnar aspect of the wrist, or surgery of the hand and digits, the axillary approach is ideal.[5]

REFERENCES

1. Raj PP, Montgomery SJ, Nettles D, et al: Infraclavicular brachial plexus block: A new approach. Anesth Analg 52:897, 1973.
2. Sims JK: A modification of the landmarks for infraclavicular approach to brachial plexus block. Anesth Analg 56:554, 1977.
3. Whiffler K: Coracoid block: A safe and easy technique. Br J Anaesth 53:845, 1981.
4. Wilson JL, Brown DL, Wong GY, et al: Infraclavicular nerve block: Needle insertion orientation and depth important for coracoid block. Anesthesiology 87:A769, 1997.
5. Raj PP: Ancillary measures to assure success. Reg Anesth 5:9, 1980.

Chapter 97

Nerve Blocks at Elbow and Wrist

Charles E. Laurito, M.D.

Isolated radial, median, or ulnar nerve blocks usually are performed as supplements to spotty brachial plexus blockades. The site to be blocked corresponds to the exact site of surgery to be performed and the experience of the individual practitioner. Aside from this setting, there is almost no indication for selective radial nerve blockade. In contrast, an isolated median nerve block can be performed at elbow or wrist immediately before a carpal tunnel release. An isolated ulnar nerve block has as an indication a few specific surgical procedures, such as open reduction of a fifth metacarpal fracture. A clear understanding of the anatomic course of each of the three nerves is essential to performance of the nerve blockade. A realization of the risks of intraneural blockade is particularly important in a patient who has already received a partial block proximal to the site of supplementation. The risk of neural damage is always present when a peripheral nerve block is performed in this setting.

BASIC ANATOMIC CONSIDERATIONS

The radial nerve is a branch of the posterior cord of the brachial plexus. It courses through the axilla and lies posterior to the humerus. At this site it innervates the triceps muscle, then enters the spiral grove of the humerus as it travels laterally. As it approaches the lateral epicondyle, it moves anterior to the elbow joint and branches into two distinct rami: superficial and deep. The superficial ramus joins the radial artery in its course and innervates both the radial aspects of the dorsal wrist and the dorsolateral three and one-half fingers. The deep ramus travels close to the periosteum to innervate extensor muscles of the forearm.

The median nerve arises from segments of the medial and lateral cords of the brachial plexus. It enters the arm and travels medial to the brachial artery. At the antecubital space, it is located between the brachial artery and the terminal insertion of the tendon of the biceps muscle. Distal to this site, the nerve gives off several motor branches to superficial and deep flexors of the wrist and fingers. At the level of the most proximal wrist flexion crease, the nerve is located within the carpal tunnel between the palmaris longus and the flexor carpi radialis.

The ulnar nerve is a continuation of the medial cord of the brachial plexus. It travels from the axilla with the axillary artery until it reaches the distal third of the humerus, where it moves medially and passes posterior to the medial epicondyle. The nerve can be palpated at this site in many patients. From here, the nerve continues on its course; it provides motor branches to the muscles of the forearm and then divides at the distal forearm into terminal dorsal and palmar branches. At the level of the wrist, the nerve is found lateral to the tendon of the flexor carpi ulnaris muscle and medial to the ulnar artery.

PERFORMANCE OF INDIVIDUAL BLOCKS

Radial Nerve Block

Radial nerve block at the elbow is performed where the lateral aspect of the biceps tendon is identified at the level of the elbow crease. After a skin wheal is raised at this site, a small-gauge needle is advanced toward the lateral epicondyle of the radial head until a paresthesia is elicited or bone is encountered (Fig. 97-1). If a nerve stimulator is used, evoked wrist extensions can be elicited at low amperages (<1 mA) to guide injection. Usually 5 mL of local anesthetic is adequate to provide dense analgesia. If a paresthesia is elicited, care is taken to withdraw the needle tip a few millimeters before injection.

At the wrist, the landmark for blockade is found at the level of the radial styloid. At this site, the sensory branches of the radial nerve travel to the lateral side of the thumb and lie between the radial artery and the flexor carpi radialis tendon. Adequate anesthesia can be provided by subcutaneous injection of 5 mL of local anesthetic at this site, as illustrated in Figure 97-2.

414

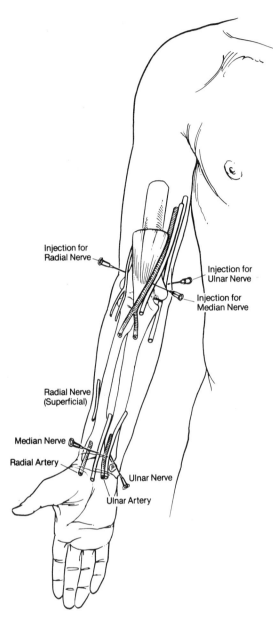

FIGURE 97–1. Blockade of the radial, ulnar, and median nerves at the elbow and wrist. (From Raj PP, Pai U, Rawal N: Techniques of regional anesthesia in adults. *In* Raj PP (ed): Clinical Practice of Regional Anesthesia. New York, Churchill Livingstone, 1991, pp 271–363.)

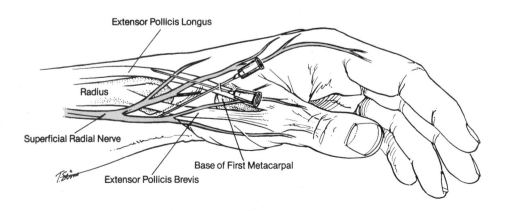

FIGURE 97–2. Blockade of the superficial radial nerve of the wrist. (From Raj PP, Pai U, Rawal N: Techniques of regional anesthesia in adults. *In* Raj PP (ed): Clinical Practice of Regional Anesthesia. New York, Churchill Livingstone, 1991, pp 271–363.)

Median Nerve Block

Median nerve block at the elbow is performed at the level of the antecubital crease. For this block, the medial aspect of the insertion of the biceps tendon is identified. Care is also taken to identify the medial and lateral aspects of the brachial artery. Successful blockade is performed by placing a small-gauge needle just medial to the brachial artery. The needle is advanced through skin that has been anesthetized toward the medial epicondyle until a paresthesia is induced or bone is encountered (Fig. 97-1). If a paresthesia is obtained, the needle tip is withdrawn a few millimeters before injection. If bone is encountered, the needle tip is withdrawn 0.5 to 1 cm before injection. A more reliable method for localizing the nerve is the use of a peripheral nerve stimulator. With this device, the needle is advanced and a characteristic wrist flexion is elicited at a low amperage. When this is documented, the injection of 3 to 5 mL of anesthetic usually provides adequate analgesia corresponding to the distribution of the nerve.

At the wrist, the median nerve is easily identified at the proximal wrist flexion crease (Fig. 97-1). It lies deep to the flexor retinaculum between the palmaris longus and the flexor carpi radialis (Fig. 97-3). Both of these tendons can be identified easily in a cooperative patient. The tendon of the flexor carpi radialis is prominent with wrist flexion against resistance, and the tendon of the palmaris longis muscle is prominent when the thumb and little finger are forcefully opposed with the wrist slightly flexed. The needle is advanced at this site proximal to the flexor retinaculum, and 3 mL of local anesthetic is injected. For this particular block, paresthesias are not deliberately elicited for fear of damage to the nerve.

Ulnar Nerve Block

Ulnar nerve block at the elbow is performed as illustrated in Figure 97-1. The nerve is fixed in its position posterior to the medial epicondyle and can be injured if the needle is directed within this space. Instead, a small-gauge needle is advanced through a skin wheal of local anesthetic that is raised 2 cm proximal to this epicondyle. If a paresthesia is elicited, care is taken to withdraw until the patient notes relief from the sensation. If a nerve stimulator is used, the typical motor response is ulnar deviation of the fingers which corresponds to the rate of electrical stimulation at a low amperage. When this is seen, 3 to 5 mL of local anesthetic is injected.

At the wrist, the ulnar nerve is just medial to the ulnar artery. If the artery is palpable, it is identified at the proximal wrist crease. At this point, the needle is advanced through a skin wheal of local anesthetic just medial to the arterial pulsation (Figs. 97-1 and 97-3). If a paresthesia is elicited, the needle is withdrawn a few millimeters and 3 to 5 mL of anesthetic is injected.

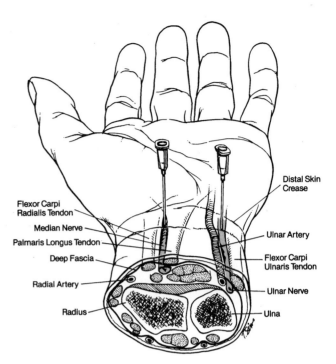

FIGURE 97-3. Wrist block of the median and ulnar nerves. (From Raj PP, Pai U, Rawal N: Techniques of regional anesthesia in adults. *In* Raj PP (ed): Clinical Practice of Regional Anesthesia. New York, Churchill Livingstone, 1991, pp 271-363.)

INDICATIONS AND CONTRAINDICATIONS

Because these blocks performed at the elbow and wrist are often attempts to salvage spotty brachial plexus blockades, the danger of nerve damage must always be considered. The practitioner must weigh the risks of placing a needle near this more distal neural tissue against the benefits of successful blockade. Nerve damage from the physical contact of the needle tip or contact coupled with intraneural injection of the local anesthetic must be considered. In addition, because the nerves travel in close approximation with arteries, the risk of arterial perforation or intra-arterial injection must be considered. This is particularly relevant when arterial structures are used as landmarks and lie immediately adjacent to the nerve tissue.

BIBLIOGRAPHY

Lofstrom B: Nerve block at the elbow and wrist. *In* Eriksson E (ed): Illustrated Handbook in Local Anaesthesia, ed 2. Philadelphia, WB Saunders, 1980, pp 86-92.
Moore DC: Regional Block, ed 4. Springfield, Ill.: CC Thomas, 1965, pp 257-274.
Raj P, Pai U: Techniques of nerve blocking. *In* Raj PP (ed): Handbook of Regional Anesthesia. New York, Churchill Livingstone, 1985, pp 181-186.
Brown DL: Atlas of Regional Anesthesia. Philadelphia, WB Saunders, 1992, pp 47-53.
Wedel DJ: Nerve blocks. *In* Miller RD (ed): Anesthesia, ed 4. New York, Churchill Livingstone, 1994, pp 1543-1545.

Chapter 98

Suprascapular Nerve Block

Honorio T. Benzon, M.D.

ANATOMY

The suprascapular nerve originates from the upper trunk of the brachial plexus (C4-6), crosses the posterior triangle of the neck, and passes deep to the trapezius muscle. The nerve traverses the suprascapular notch and descends deep to the supraspinatus and the infraspinatus muscles,[1] supplying the two muscles and the shoulder joint.[2]

INDICATIONS

Suprascapular nerve block is indicated for relief of pain in the shoulder, which may be due to bursitis, capsular tear, or other causes.[2] The author has found it useful in patients who have had stroke and developed adhesive capsulitis of the shoulder. The block is performed before physical therapy, which is used to increase the range of motion of the involved shoulder.

TECHNIQUE

The patient sits on the table or cart, preferably with the arms folded across the abdomen. A line is drawn along the spine of the scapula from the tip of the acromion to the scapular border. The midpoint of this line is noted, and a vertical line, parallel to the vertebral spines, is drawn through it. The angle of the upper outer quadrant is bisected with a line; the site of insertion of the needle is 1 in. from the apex of the angle. The area is prepared and draped and a skin wheal is made. A 3-in. (7.5-cm), 22-gauge needle is inserted perpendicular to the skin in all planes, (i.e., downward, inward, and forward) (Fig. 98-1). After contacting bone (i.e. the area surrounding the suprascapular notch) at approximately 2 to 2½ in., the needle is slightly withdrawn and redirected medially, laterally, or superiorly until it is felt to slide into the notch. Ten milliliters of local anesthetic is injected. The position of the needle

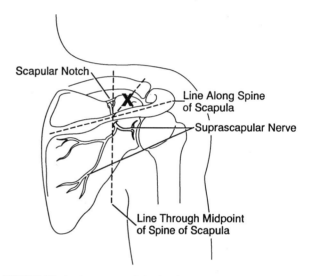

FIGURE 98-1. Anatomy and landmarks involved in suprascapular nerve block. X is the site of needle insertion. (Adapted from Moore DC: Regional Block: A Handbook for Use in the Clinical Practice of Medicine and Surgery, ed 4. Springfield, Ill, Charles C. Thomas, 1979, pp 300-303.)

tip is checked by withdrawing the needle and reinserting it laterally or medially to contact the walls of the suprascapular notch. Pneumothorax, which occurs in fewer than 1% of cases, is caused by deeper-than-recommended advancement of the needle.

A successful block is indicated by the subjective relief of the patient's symptoms and the ability of the patient to tolerate manipulation of the shoulder. No skin analgesia results from the block.

REFERENCES

1. Ellis H, Feldman S: Anatomy for Anaesthetists, ed 3. London, Blackwell Scientific Publications, 1977, p 186.
2. Moore DC: Regional Block: A Handbook for Use in the Clinical Practice of Medicine and Surgery, ed 4. Springfield, Ill, Charles C Thomas, 1979, pp 300-303.

Chapter 99

● Intercostal Nerve Block

Robert E. Molloy, M.D.

Intercostal nerve blocks provide analgesia of the chest or abdominal wall for patients with surgical incisions, rib fractures, chest tubes, thoracic herpes zoster, and rib lesions.[1-4] Intercostal block has been combined with light general anesthesia and celiac plexus block to provide anesthesia for abdominal surgical procedures. Repeated blocks may be required for acute traumatic pain states. The usefulness of this block would be enhanced by the introduction of a safe, ultra–long-acting local anesthetic agent. Intercostal block may be helpful as one diagnostic tool in the evaluation of patients with abdominal or thoracic pain, particularly in detection of somatic rather than visceral mechanisms of pain. Intercostal blocks produce minimal effects on pulmonary function studies.[5] They do reduce the decline in 1-second forced expiratory volume (FEV_1) seen in the initial postoperative period after truncal incisions,[6, 7] and they may decrease the incidence of postoperative pulmonary complications.[8] Bilateral intercostal nerve blocks are infrequently performed because of the possibility of bilateral pneumothorax and local anesthetic toxic effects.

ANATOMY

Thoracic nerve roots emerge from the intervertebral foramina into the paravertebral space. Here they send white rami communicantes to the sympathetic chain, receive gray rami communicantes in return, and send a posterior cutaneous branch to supply the paravertebral skin and muscles and the posterior ligaments and articulations of the vertebral column. As the nerves leave the paravertebral space, they enter the intercostal space below the respective rib of each, lying between the innermost intercostal muscle and the pleura. Lateral to the paravertebral muscles, the prominent angles of the ribs are palpable as the primary landmark for intercostal nerve block. At the angle of the rib, the nerve lies between the innermost intercostal muscle and the inner intercostal muscle. At this distance, the costal groove is at its widest. Here the nerve is positioned below the intercostal vein and artery, under or below the rib (Fig. 99-1). A cadaver study found that the intercostal nerve remained in a classic subcostal position only 17% of the time.[10] It was shown to be in a midcostal location most frequently (73%), and it was supracostal in some cadavers (10%). Just beyond the midaxillary line, the lateral cutaneous branch of the nerve arises, providing sensory innervation anteriorly and posteriorly to much of the thoracic and abdominal wall. The terminal anterior cutaneous branches of the intercostal nerves supply the tissues near the midline of the thorax and abdomen[11] (Fig. 99-2).

The ideal location for intercostal nerve block is at the posterior angle of the rib, just lateral to the paravertebral muscle mass, except for the uppermost nerves, because of the interposition of the scapula. Block may also be performed just posterior to the midaxillary line without missing the lateral cutaneous nerve.[12] However, the intercostal space is narrower here, and the lower edge of the rib becomes sharper and more narrow.[13]

The intercostal nerves are the primary rami of thoracic nerves T1-11. Most of the T1 nerve fibers combine with C8 to form the lower trunk of the brachial plexus. Fibers from T2 and T3 form the intercostobrachial nerve; they also supply the upper chest wall above the nipple line, along with the supraclavicular nerves from the cervical plexus. Intercostal nerves T4-11 supply the thoracoabdominal wall from the nipple line to below the umbilicus. The T12 nerve is actually a subcostal nerve that contributes branches to the iliohypogastric and ilioinguinal nerves.[14]

TECHNIQUE

Patient Position

The ideal patient position is prone, with a pillow under the abdomen and both upper extremities hanging over the sides of the table, which maximizes retraction of the scapulae away from the upper ribs. This allows for bilateral blockade and posterior access to the angles of the ribs to enhance safety and success of the proce-

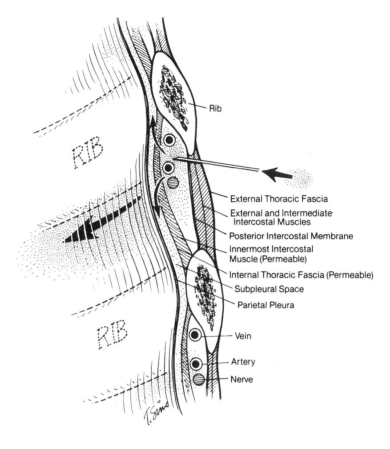

FIGURE 99–1. Anatomy of the intercostal nerve at the angle of the rib, the site of needle placement for classic intercostal nerve block. (From Raj PP, Pai U, Rawal N: Techniques of regional anesthesia in adults. *In* Raj PP (ed): Clinical Practice of Regional Anesthesia. New York, Churchill Livingstone, 1991, p 271.)

Rib

External Thoracic Fascia

External and Intermediate Intercostal Muscles

Posterior Intercostal Membrane

Innermost Intercostal Muscle (Permeable)

Internal Thoracic Fascia (Permeable)

Subpleural Space

Parietal Pleura

Vein

Artery

Nerve

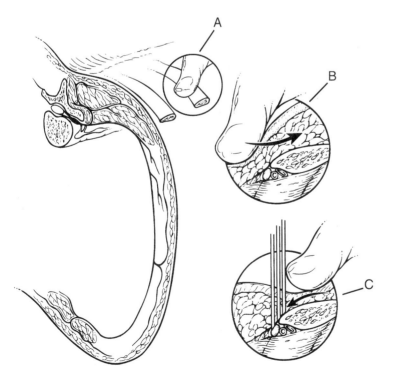

FIGURE 99–2. Anatomy of the intercostal nerve and technique of classic intercostal nerve block near the angle of the rib. (From Thompson GE: Intercostal nerve block. *In* Waldman SD, Winnie AP (eds): Interventional Pain Management. Philadelphia, WB Saunders, 1996, p 311.)

TABLE 99–1. POSITIONING THE PATIENT FOR INTERCOSTAL NERVE BLOCK

Patient Position	Site of Block	Advantages and Disadvantages
Prone	Angle of ribs	Best access for bilateral block; simplest technique
Lateral	Angle of ribs	Ideal for patient comfort and unilateral block; position change for bilateral blocks
Supine	Midaxillary line	Bilateral blocks under general anesthesia, avoids position change, more difficult
Intrathoracic	Intrapleural; direct injection of nerve	Technically difficult to inject, total spinal anesthesia may occur

dure. The lateral decubitus position is also quite satisfactory for unilateral block after rib fractures and lateral thoracotomy and for chest tube placement. The supine position has been utilized for bilateral block under general anesthesia, which avoids the need to turn the patient. The anatomy of the intercostal space is less ideal near the midaxillary line (Table 99–1).

After intravenous access has been established, with the patient positioned and monitored, the landmarks for block are drawn with a marking pen. The midline spinous processes are marked, and bilateral lines are drawn through the angles of the ribs where they are first easily palpated lateral to the paraspinal muscles. This may be 8 cm lateral to the midline inferiorly and less than 6 cm superiorly, to avoid the scapula. An intersecting line is drawn at the inferior border of each rib to be blocked, beginning with the 12th rib. Appropriate intravenous sedation is required, and skin wheals are raised at each intersecting line. A 22- to 25-gauge short-bevel needle attached to a 10-mL control syringe is used, beginning at the most caudal nerve to be blocked. The index finger of the left (nondominant) hand pulls the skin up over the rib, and the right (dominant) hand inserts the needle with syringe, angled slightly cephalad, close to the tip of the index finger and onto the rib. The left hand now grasps the needle hub, anchored to the chest wall, and both controls the needle and "walks" it off the lower rib margin. It is advanced about 3 mm beyond the lower rib margin. The right hand injects 3 to 5 mL of local anesthetic while the left hand either remains motionless or jiggles the needle in and out about 1 mm. The needle is then replaced on the same rib or removed altogether, before the left hand begins to palpate the next rib margin in a cephalad direction (see Fig. 99–2). This process is repeated for each nerve to be blocked. It is important to retain control of the syringe and needle at all times, so that the physician's advancement of the syringe and the patient's unexpected movements will not allow the needle to penetrate the pleura.[11, 13, 14]

SIDE EFFECTS AND COMPLICATIONS

Intercostal block is avoided by many physicians to avoid the risk of pneumothorax, which has been thought to occur relatively frequently, in 1% to 2% of patients. The rate of pneumothorax detected by x-ray has been reported to be 0.42% by Moore and Bridenbaugh,[15] and clinically obvious pneumothorax occurs at a much lower rate. Chest tube insertion is rarely needed, even when a small pneumothorax occurs. Systemic local anesthetic toxic effects are a concern with multiple intercostal nerve blocks because of multiple injections and relatively rapid absorption from this site. The local anesthetic agent selected and the total dose employed are important contributing factors. Epinephrine, 5 μg/mL, decreases absorption of the local anesthetic agent. Drug concentration must be reduced when large volumes are used to avoid exceeding maximum recommended doses for the drug selected. Postblock patient monitoring should continue for at least 20 minutes. Accidental widespread neuraxial block has been reported after intraoperative intrathoracic block by the surgeon.[16] Injection under direct vision by the surgeon at a medial location may result in local anesthetic placement into a dural cuff or into the nerve itself, with resultant occurrence of total spinal anesthesia (Table 99–2).

REFERENCES

1. Moore DC, Bridenbaugh LD: Intercostal nerve block in 4,333 patients: Indications, techniques, and complications. Anesth Analg 41:1, 1962.
2. Moore DC: Intercostal nerve block for postoperative somatic pain following surgery of the thorax and upper abdomen. Br J Anaesth 47:184, 1975.
3. Nunn JF, Slavin C: Posterior intercostal nerve block for pain relief after cholecystectomy. Br J Anaesth 52:253, 1980.
4. Bunting P, McGeachie JF: Intercostal nerve blockade producing analgesia after appendectomy. Br J Anaesth 61:169, 1988.
5. Jakobson S, Fridriksson H, Hedenstrom H, et al: Effects of intercostal nerve blocks on pulmonary mechanics in healthy men. Acta Anaesthesiol Scand 24:482, 1980.
6. Faust RJ, Nauss LA: Post-thoracotomy intercostal block: Comparison of its effects on pulmonary function with those of intramuscular meperidine. Anesth Analg 55:542, 1976.
7. Engberg G: Respiratory performance after upper abdominal surgery: A comparison of pain relief with intercostal block and centrally acting analgesics. Acta Anaesthesiol Scand 29:427, 1985.
8. Engberg G, Wiklund L: Pulmonary complications after upper abdominal surgery: Their prevention with intercostal blocks. Acta Anaesthesiol Scand 32:1, 1988.
9. Raj PP, Rai U, Rawal N: Techniques of regional anesthesia in adults. In Raj PP (ed): Clinical Practice of Regional Anesthesia. New York, Churchill Livingstone, 1991, p 271.
10. Hardy PA: Anatomical variation in the position of the proximal intercostal nerve. Br J Anaesth 61:338, 1988.
11. Thompson GE: Intercostal nerve block. In Waldman SD, Winnie AP (eds): Interventional Pain Management. Philadelphia, WB Saunders, 1996, p 311.

TABLE 99–2. COMPLICATIONS OF INTERCOSTAL BLOCK

Pneumothorax
Local anesthetic toxicity
Total spinal anesthesia

12. Moore DC: Intercostal nerve block: Spread of India ink injected into the subcostal groove. Br J Anaesth 53:325, 1981.
13. Kopacz DJ: Regional anesthesia of the trunk. *In* Brown DL (ed): Regional Anesthesia and Analgesia. Philadelphia, WB Saunders, 1996, p 292.
14. Thompson GE, Moore DC: Celiac plexus, intercostal, and minor peripheral blockade. *In* Cousins MJ, Bridenbaugh PO (eds): Neu-
15. Moore DC, Bridenbaugh LD: Pneumothorax: Its incidence following intercostal block. JAMA 182:1005, 1962.
16. Benumof JL, Semenza J: Total spinal anesthesia following intrathoracic intercostal nerve blocks. Anesthesiology 43:124, 1975.
ral Blockade in Clinical Anesthesia and Management of Pain, ed 2. Philadelphia, JB Lippincott, 1988, p 503.

Chapter 100

Paravertebral Somatic Nerve Block

Sam Page, M.D.

Blockade of the paravertebral space offers an alternative regional anesthetic to intercostal and epidural blockade. Patients with chronic pain who require diagnostic or therapeutic nerve blocks and patients who undergo operative procedures of the chest and upper abdomen may benefit. The utility of this procedure is controversial, largely due to concern for pneumothorax and the wide variation of the anatomy of the paravertebral space.

ANATOMY

The thoracic paravertebral space is a narrow, triangular space lateral to the vertebral column. It is bounded posteriorly by the superior costotransverse ligament, anteriorly by the parietal pleura, and superiorly and inferiorly by the heads and necks of adjoining ribs. The base is formed by the posterolateral aspect of the body of the vertebra and the intervertebral foramina, which communicates with the epidural space. Laterally, it communicates with the intercostal space. The paravertebral space contains the sympathetic chain, rami communicantes, and dorsal and ventral roots of the spinal nerve. Local anesthetic injection provides sensory, motor, and sympathetic blockade.

Because the paravertebral space is continuous with the surrounding spaces, injection of local anesthetic can provide anesthesia to several dermatomes through the following means (Fig. 100–1):

Lateral diffusion into the intercostal space
Superior or inferior spread into adjacent paravertebral space
Medial diffusion into the epidural space
A combination of these

If unilateral blockade is maintained, anesthesia and sympathetic blockade are unilateral, and the risk of hypotension is significantly reduced. After injection of 5 mL of contrast into the paravertebral space, the contrast medium will be confined to the paravertebral space about 20% of the time. Epidural and intercostal spread will occur in about 70% and 10% of cases, respectively. A wide range of sensory losses may be seen. This inconsistency in the spread of the solution makes the use of diagnostic blocks without fluoroscopic confirmation a controversial endeavor. Depth from the skin to the transverse process varies significantly, depending on the thickness of the subcutaneous fat layer. The distance from the spinous process laterally to the tip of the transverse process ranges from 2 to 4 cm. A negative pressure gradient exists from the paravertebral space to the epidural space.

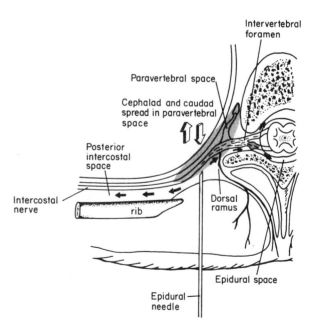

FIGURE 100–1. The paravertebral space is contiguous with surrounding spaces. *Arrows* depict spread of local anesthetic to the intercostal, epidural, and inferior and superior paravertebral spaces. (From Chan VW, Ferrante FM: Continuous thoracic paravertebral block. *In* Ferrante FM, VadeBoncoeur TR (eds): Postoperative Pain Management. New York, Churchill Livingstone, 1993, p 408.)

TECHNIQUE

With the patient in the decubitus or prone position, the back is prepared as for an epidural block placement. Two landmarks are used to enter the paravertebral space at the thoracic level. The inferior portion of the spinous process of the vertebral body corresponding to the desired somatic nerve block is identified. A line is drawn 3 cm laterally, and a point is marked as the needle entry site. This point overlies the transverse process of the vertebral body inferior to the desired paravertebral space.

Local anesthetic infiltration is performed, and in all planes perpendicular to the skin, the same needle is used to seek the transverse process. It is usually 1.5 to 2 cm below the skin, but it may be deeper, depending on the size of the patient. The needle of choice is placed in the same location, and the transverse process is again contacted. The needle is "walked" superiorly until it slips off of the transverse process. A loss-of-resistance technique, using saline or air, is used to identify the paravertebral space as the epidural needle passes through the superior costotransverse ligament. "Walking" off the transverse process superiorly, as opposed to inferiorly, allows entry into the paravertebral space at an angle perpendicular to the superior costotransverse ligament, which allows the best loss-of-resistance technique (Fig. 100–2). The needle will also enter the portion of the paravertebral space that is the deepest, which minimizes the risk of pneumothorax. A needle placed superior to the identified transverse process is immediately inferior to the transverse process of the spinous process that was used as the original landmark.

If a continuous infusion of local anesthetic is planned for postoperative pain, a standard epidural needle is used. After negative aspiration to check for blood, cerebrospinal fluid, and air, a standard epidural catheter is placed 2 to 3 cm into the space.

Another possible variation is placement of a catheter during surgery, when the patient's chest is open. Before closing the thoracotomy incision, an epidural needle can be placed percutaneously into the thorax at the second intercostal space in the midclavicular line. At the level of the third rib, the parietal pleura is opened with a 1 cm incision over the sympathetic nerve trunk. An extrapleural pocket is constructed two spaces above and below the incision. A standard epidural catheter is placed in this pocket and sutured with absorbable suture, and the parietal pleura is closed. Confirmation of correct catheter placement may be done with contrast medium and fluoroscopy. A double-catheter technique (bilateral) has been described for abdominal procedures. Paravertebral blocks, as single injections, have been described for patients having breast surgery. These patients have a higher incidence of nausea and vomiting, which may be significantly less with regional anesthesia.

DOSING

Absorption of local anesthetic from the paravertebral space is difficult to predict. Analgesia has varied from 1 to 10 hours after a single injection. Usually, 15 mL of 0.5% bupivacaine provides analgesia of four dermatomes at the thoracic level. Infusions of 0.25% to 0.5% bupivacaine at 4 to 8 mL/hour have been reported, at an average rate of 0.1 mL/kg/hour. On average, bupivacaine

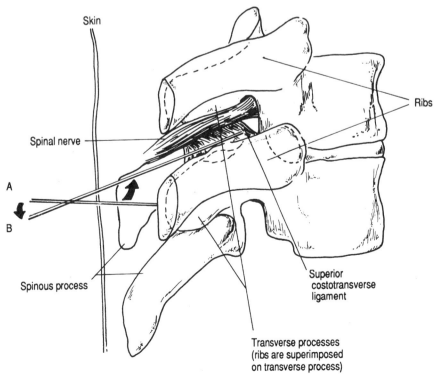

FIGURE 100–2. Direction of the epidural needle. The needle strikes the transverse process and is then angled superiorly to pass through the superior costotransverse ligament. (From Chan VW, Ferrante FM: Continuous thoracic paravertebral block. *In* Ferrante FM, VadeBoncoeur TR (eds): Postoperative Pain Management. New York, Churchill Livingstone, 1993, p 410.)

blood levels are similar to those after epidural bolus injections and continuous infusions, although on an individual basis, larger variations in plasma concentration may be observed from paravertebral local anesthetics.

COMPLICATIONS

The overall failure rate is estimated to be 10%, similar to that for epidural catheter placement. Dural puncture and subarachnoid injection are potential complications. The incidence would likely increase if the needle were directed more medially. This is the widest portion of the paravertebral space, which may minimize the risk of pneumothorax. Pneumothorax is estimated to occur in 0.5% of cases. Vascular injection is thought to occur in about 3% of cases. Hypotension occurs in about 5% of cases, which is much less common than with epidural local anesthetic injection. Urinary retention is infrequent; it was cited to be 10% in one study, as opposed to 60% in patients with epidural analgesia. This is due to the near unilateral block of the paravertebral space. In general, the rate of complications is similar to, if not less than, that seen with placement of epidural catheters.

Continuous paravertebral infusion should remain an option for patients who cannot tolerate the potential respiratory depression of epidural or intravenous opioids, and would have difficulty managing the potential hypotension from epidural local anesthetics. With proper technique, and confirmation by fluoroscopy if necessary, complications can be minimized. As a single-injection technique, paravertebral somatic nerve block remains an alternative to epidural injection and intercostal nerve block for the treatment of chronic pain syndromes.

BIBLIOGRAPHY

Berrisford RG, Sabanathan S, Mearns AJ, et al: Plasma concentrations of bupivacaine and its enantiomers during continuous extrapleural and intracostal nerve block. Br J Anaesth 70:201-204, 1993.

Chan VW, Ferrante FM: Continuous thoracic paravertebral block. *In* Ferrante FM, VadeBoncoeur TR (eds): Postoperative Pain Management. New York, Churchill Livingstone, 1993, p 408.

Lonnqvist PA, MacKenzie J, Soni AK: Paravertebral blockade: Failure rate and complications. Anaesthesia 50:813-815, 1995.

Matthews PJ, Govenden V: Comparison of continuous paravertebral and extradural infusions of bupivacaine for pain relief after thoracotomy. Br J Anaesth 62:204-205, 1989.

Perttunen K, Nilsson E, Heinonen J, et al: Extradural, paravertebral and intercostal nerve blocks for post-thoracotomy pain. Br J Anaesth 75:541-547, 1995.

Purcell-Jones G, Pither CE, Justins DM: Paravertebral somatic nerve block: A clinical, radiographic, and computed tomographic study in chronic pain patients. Anesth Analg 68:32-39, 1989.

Richardson J, Vowden P, Sadanathan S: Bilateral paravertebral analgesia for major abdominal vascular surgery: A preliminary report. Anaesthesia 50:995-998, 1995.

Weltz CR, Greengrass RAA, Lyerly HK: Ambulatory surgical management of breast carcinoma using paravertebral block. Ann Surg 222:19-26, 1995.

Chapter 101

Lumbar Plexus, Femoral, Lateral Femoral Cutaneous, and Obturator Nerve Blocks

Honorio T. Benzon, M.D.

PSOAS COMPARTMENT BLOCK

The lumbar plexus is formed by the ventral rami of the first, second, third, and major part of the fourth lumbar nerves. It is located in the substance of the psoas major muscle in a compartment formed by the bodies of the lumbar vertebrae medially, the psoas major muscle and its fascia anteriorly, and the transverse processes, intertransverse ligaments and muscles, and the quadratus lumborum posteriorly.[1]

At the level between the transverse processes of the fourth and fifth lumbar vertebrae are found the nerves that innervate the upper segment of the lower limb: the femoral, lateral femoral cutaneous, and obturator nerves.

Technique of Chayen and Colleagues

The patient is placed in the lateral decubitus position with the operative limb uppermost and the thighs flexed. A line passing through the iliac crest is made, the insertion site is 3 cm caudal and 5 cm lateral to this intercristal line (Fig. 101–1, small *x*). A 15-cm 22-gauge needle is inserted until it encounters the transverse process of the fifth lumbar vertebra. It is then directed cephalad until it glides off the transverse process, and a 10- or 20-mL syringe is attached it. The needle is advanced slowly, and resistance is felt when the needle

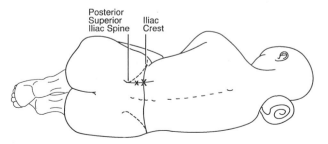

FIGURE 101–1. Psoas compartment block of Chayen and co-workers *(small x)* and lumbar plexus block of Winnie and co-workers *(large X)*. Please see text for details of technique.

enters the quadratus lumborum. This resistance is lost when the tip of the needle enters the psoas compartment, usually at a depth of 12 cm. Paresthesia may be elicited or a nerve stimulator may be used. After a negative aspiration, 30 mL of the local anesthetic is injected.

Chayen and co-workers[1] have had a 90% success rate with their technique. Although they listed the type of surgical procedures in which the block was used, they did not evaluate the quality of blockade of the different areas in the thigh that were innervated by the femoral, lateral femoral cutaneous, and obturator nerves.

Lumbar Plexus Block of Winnie and Colleagues

Winnie and co-workers[2] modified the psoas compartment block of Chayen and others. In this technique, the patient's position is the same as that in the psoas compartment block. A line is drawn across the superior borders of the iliac crests, and a second line is drawn parallel to the spinous processes, passing through the posterior superior iliac spine. The site of needle insertion is at the point at which the paraspinous line crosses the intercristal line (see Fig. 101–1, large *X*). A 3½ in., 22-gauge needle is inserted perpendicular to the skin, in a slightly mesial (medial) direction. The needle is directed slightly caudal if the transverse process is encountered. After paresthesia is elicited, at approximately 5 to 6 cm from the skin, 40 mL of local anesthetic is injected.

The posterior superior iliac spine is 4.5 to 5.5 cm lateral to the spinous process, the same distance from the spine (5 cm) at which the needle is inserted in the procedure of Chayen and co-workers. The difference between the two techniques is that in the technique of Winnie and associates, the need is inserted 3 cm cephalad to the insertion of in the technique of Chayen and others.

Winnie and co-workers theorized that the injection is made into the interfascial space between the quadratus lumborum and psoas major muscles, and, with cephalad and caudal spread of the local anesthetic, both the lumbar and sacral plexuses are blocked.

Comparison of the Lumbar Plexus Block Techniques of Winnie and Chayen

Chayen and others reported the need to combine the psoas compartment block with sciatic nerve block to provide complete anesthesia of the lower extremity. Winnie and co-workers stated that both the lumbar and sacral plexuses are blocked with their technique. Parkinson and associates[3] investigated the extent of blockade with the psoas compartment block and the combined lumbosacral plexus block of Winnie and co-workers. They found that both approaches were effective in blocking the femoral, obturator, and lateral femoral cutaneous nerves. In addition, the nerves to the psoas muscle were reliably blocked. In some patients, there was partial blockade of the nerves receiving contributions from the lumbosacral trunk (L4–5). However, complete blockade of any nerve with a component from S1, S2, or S3 was not achieved.

Cadaver Dissections of the Lumbar Plexus and Clinical Implications

Farny and associates,[4] using cadaver dissections, demonstrated that at the level of L4–5 vertebrae (the site of needle insertion for lumbar plexus block), the lumbar plexus is within the substance of the psoas major muscle rather than between this muscle and the quadratus lumborum. This finding emphasizes the unreliability of the loss-of-resistance technique that Chayen and others advocated, and that the use of a nerve stimulator is more reliable. Farny and colleagues noted that the femoral nerve lies between the lateral femoral cutaneous nerve and the obturator nerve. Although the femoral and the lateral femoral cutaneous nerves were in the same fascial plane (inside a thin fascia at the level of the junction of the posterior third and the anterior two-thirds of the muscle), the obturator nerve was within its own muscular fold in a plane close to the other two nerves. The variability in the anatomy of the obturator nerve may explain the different success rates of obturator nerve blockade with the three-in-one block.

Farny and co-workers[4] found that insertion of the needle more than 6.41 ± 1.61 cm lateral to the midline may miss the psoas muscle, and insertion deeper than 11.6 ± 3 cm may lead to retroperitoneal injection. They noted that the distance from the skin to the femoral nerve was 9.01 ± 2.43 cm. The short distance from the internal border of the psoas muscle to the median sagittal plane, 2.73 ± 0.64 cm, may explain the occurrence of bilateral blockade.[5,6] Whether the bilateral blockade is due to epidural or subarachnoid blockade is not completely known.

COMBINED LUMBAR PLEXUS BLOCK AND SCIATIC NERVE BLOCK

Combined lumbar plexus and sciatic nerve block has been performed in patients undergoing lower extremity surgery, using the lumbar plexus block of Winnie and others and the classic posterior approach to the sciatic nerve block.[6] There was complete sensory blockade of the femoral, lateral femoral cutaneous, obturator, and sciatic nerves within 13 ± 8.7 minutes. A total of 60 mL of local anesthetic was used: 35 mL was injected in the lumbar plexus block and 25 mL in the sciatic nerve block when the operation was at or above the knee. For procedures below the knee, 25 mL was injected at the lumbar plexus and 35 mL in the sciatic nerve (the reverse proportion was utilized). It was surprising that the serum concentrations of lidocaine were within safe limits, given the high dose of lidocaine that was used.[6]

FEMORAL NERVE BLOCK

The femoral nerve lies in a groove between the psoas major muscle and the iliac muscle while entering the thigh deep to the inguinal ligament. At the inguinal ligament, it lies anterior to the iliopsoas muscle and lateral to the femoral artery. The femoral nerve divides into anterior (superficial) and posterior (deep) branches. The anterior branch provides cutaneous innervation to the skin overlying the anterior surface of the thigh and provides motor innervation to the sartorius muscle. The posterior branch provides innervation to the quadriceps muscle and the knee joint and gives rise to the saphenous nerve.[7]

Technique

The needle is inserted 1 to 2 cm inferior to the inguinal ligament, lateral to the femoral artery, and advanced in a lateral and posterior direction (Fig. 101–2).

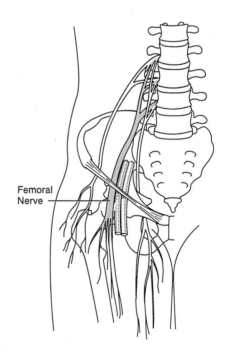

Femoral Nerve

FIGURE 101–2. Femoral nerve block. The needle is inserted 1 to 2 cm inferior to the inguinal ligament and lateral to the femoral artery.

A "pop" is felt when the needle penetrates the fascia lata and iliac fascia. Stimulation of the nerve with a nerve stimulator results in contraction of the quadriceps femoris muscle. Ten to 15 mL of the local anesthetic is adequate to block the femoral nerve.

Perioperative Applications

Femoral nerve block is used, in conjunction with the lateral femoral cutaneous nerve block, to provide anesthesia for malignant hyperthermia biopsy. (The three-in-one block is probably just as effective as the combined femoral and lateral femoral cutaneous nerve block.) Combined femoral and genitofemoral nerve block was found to be comparable to spinal anesthesia for patients who underwent long saphenous vein stripping surgery.[8] Recovery was faster and incidences of back pain and complications were lower in the femoral-genitofemoral nerve block group.

Femoral nerve block has been found to be effective in providing analgesia in patients with fracture of the shaft of the femur, with complete relief and abolition of muscle spasm within a few minutes.[9] It has been used to provide anesthesia for insertion of percutaneous screws in the surgical treatment of subcapital fracture of the femur, although skin infiltration had to be made in the areas innervated by the lateral femoral cutaneous nerve.[10] As a supplement to general anesthesia in patients undergoing anterior cruciate ligament reconstruction, femoral nerve block has been found to reduce the opioid requirements by 80% in the recovery room and by 40% the first postoperative day.[11] Preoperative blockade was more effective than when performed after the surgery.[11] Continuous femoral nerve block has been utilized for postoperative analgesia after a knee operation in a patient with cystic fibrosis.[12]

THREE-IN-ONE BLOCK

The technique of three-in-one block was introduced by Winnie and co-workers in 1973, wherein the femoral, lateral femoral cutaneous, and obturator nerves are blocked with one injection. In this technique, the insertion point is the same as for the femoral nerve block (see Fig. 101-2) with the needle oriented in a slightly cephalad direction. After needle placement, digital pressure is applied distal to the needle entry site, and 30 mL of local anesthetic is injected.[13]

Extent of Blockade

Winnie and associates found a 98.6% success rate (69 of 70 patients) with this technique so long as 20 mL or more of local anesthetic was injected.[13] Other investigators found inconsistent blockade of the obturator nerve. Parkinson and others, using 0.5 mL/kg of body weight of local anesthetic, found no evidence of obturator nerve block with this technique.[3] In his clinical experience, Spillane found evidence of obturator nerve blockade in 4 out of more than 300 patients.[14] Lang and others found that the incidences of femoral, lateral femoral cutaneous, and obturator nerve block were 81%, 96%, and 4%, respectively.[15] Using compound muscle action potential (CMAP) of the obturator nerve as a parameter, Atanassof and co-workers found that the CMAP amplitude decreased by 88.8% ± 21% with direct obturator nerve blockade. In contrast, depression of the CMAP amplitude with the three-in-one technique was 7.4% ± 19%.[16] Finally, Ritter injected 40 mL of dye into the area of the femoral nerve in cadavers and found that the dye always stained the femoral nerve and usually stained the lateral femoral cutaneous nerve, but it did not stain the obturator nerve.[17] He concluded that there was no evidence of a femoral nerve sheath capable of carrying the dye into the area of the lumbar plexus.

Perioperative Applications

Continuous infusions of local anesthetic through a catheter placed in the area of the femoral nerve have been used postoperatively. After an open knee operation, the continuous three-in-one block technique was found to be as effective as epidural morphine and with a significantly lower incidence of nausea, vomiting, pruritus, and urinary retention.[18] Following arthroscopic knee surgery, continuous three-in-one block resulted in significantly lower visual analogue pain scores compared to those with intra-articular bupivacaine or intra-articular morphine.[19]

LATERAL FEMORAL CUTANEOUS NERVE BLOCK

The lateral femoral cutaneous nerve (L2–3) emerges along the lateral border of the psoas muscle caudal to the ilioinguinal nerve. It courses obliquely across the iliac muscle, deep to the iliac fascia, and enters the thigh by passing posterior to the inguinal ligament, medial to the anterior superior iliac spine. It has an anterior and a posterior branch. The anterior branch provides cutaneous innervation to the anterolateral aspect of the thigh while the posterior branch courses backward to supply the skin on the lateral aspect of the thigh from below the greater trochanter of the femur to the middle of the thigh.[20]

Technique

The patient is in a supine position and the anterior superior iliac spine is palpated. The needle is inserted 1 to 2 cm medial and 1 to 2 cm inferior to the anterior superior iliac spine and advanced deep to the fascia lata (Fig. 101-3). Ten to 15 mL of local anesthetic is injected in a fanwise manner, depositing the local anesthetic above and below the fascia.

The nerve can also be blocked by directing the needle in a lateral and cephalad direction to strike the iliac bone, inferior and medial to the anterior superior iliac spine. Ten milliliters of local anesthetic is injected in a fanwise manner.

Blockade of the lateral femoral cutaneous nerve was

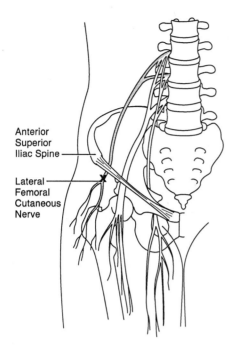

FIGURE 101–3. Lateral femoral cutaneous nerve block. The needle is inserted 2 cm medial and 2 cm inferior to the anterior superior iliac spine.

found to be more effective with the aid of a nerve stimulator compared to the classic technique (100% vs. 40%).[21] Paresthesia to the lateral aspect of the knee with 0.6 mA stimulus intensity was the end point.

Comments

The local anesthetic may spread beneath the iliac fascia, and the femoral nerve may be unintentionally blocked. Lateral femoral cutaneous nerve block is used in the treatment of meralgia paresthetica. Relief of pain in the presence of a good block signifies involvement of the nerve at or distal to its exit, whereas the absence of pain relief may mean involvement of the nerve proximal to the iliac spine, along its course, from the iliac gutter (ovarian and colon problems) to the L2 and L3 vertebral areas. Lateral femoral cutaneous nerve block is utilized, in conjunction with femoral nerve block, to provide analgesia for malignant hyperthermia (MH) biopsies.

OBTURATOR NERVE BLOCK

The obturator nerve, formed by the ventral branches of the anterior primary rami of L2, L3, and L4, emerges from the medial border of the psoas muscle at the brim of the pelvis. It courses inferiorly and anteriorly along the lateral wall of the pelvis to the obturator foramen, where it enters the thigh. It divides into the anterior and posterior branches as it passes through the obturator canal. The anterior branch sends cutaneous branches to the medial aspect of the thigh in addition to supplying the hip joint and the anterior adductor muscles. The

posterior branch supplies the deep adductor muscles and sends a branch to the knee joint.

Technique

The patient is supine and the leg placed in slight abduction. The site of needle insertion is 1 to 2 cm inferior and 1 to 2 cm lateral to the pubic tubercle. After contacting the horizontal ramus of the pubic bone, the needle is redirected in a lateral and superior direction until paresthesia is elicited (Fig. 101–4). Adduction of the hip is elicited when the nerve is stimulated with a nerve stimulator. Ten milliliters of local anesthetic is injected.

An alternative approach has been described by Wassef.[22] In this technique, a mark is made on the skin 1 to 2 cm medial to the femoral artery and immediately below the inguinal ligament. The adductor longus tendon is identified near its insertion at the pubis and the needle is inserted behind the tendon and directed laterally toward the skin mark. The needle is advanced until paresthesia is accomplished or adductor muscle contraction is elicited with the nerve stimulator.

Perioperative Applications

Obturator nerve block is used in the treatment of adductor muscle spasm seen after a cerebrovascular accident, spinal cord injury, or multiple sclerosis. It has been reported to be an adjunct to spinal anesthesia (the obturator nerve may not be blocked in spinal anesthesia),[23] or general anesthesia without neuromuscular blockade, in patients who undergo transurethral resection of urinary bladder tumors.[24] In these procedures,

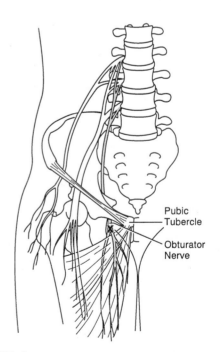

FIGURE 101–4. Obturator nerve block. The site of needle insertion is 1 to 2 cm inferior and 1 to 2 cm lateral to the pubic tubercle. The needle is redirected in a lateral and superior direction after the horizontal ramus of the pubic bone is contacted.

the obturator nerve block may prevent bladder perforation, bleeding, or incomplete resection by preventing inadvertent thigh adductor muscle contractions.[23,24]

REFERENCES

1. Chayen D, Nathan H, Chayen M: The psoas compartment block. Anesthesiology 45:95, 1976.
2. Winnie AP, Ramamurthy S, Durrani Z, et al: Plexus blocks for lower extremity surgery: New answers to old problems. Anesthesiol Rev 1:11, 1974.
3. Parkinson SK, Mueller JB, Little DO, et al: Extent of blockade with various approaches to the lumbar plexus. Anesth Analg 68:243, 1989.
4. Farny J, Drolet P, Girard M: Anatomy of the posterior approach to the lumbar plexus block. Can J Anaesth 41:480, 1994.
5. Dalens B, Tanguy A, Vanneuville G: Lumbar plexus block in children: A comparison of two procedures in 50 patients. Anesth Analg 67:750, 1988.
6. Farny J, Girard M, Drolet P: Posterior approach to the lumbar plexus combined with a sciatic nerve block using lidocaine. Can J Anaesth 41:486, 1994.
7. Rogers JN, Ramamurthy S: Lower extremity blocks. *In* Brown DL (ed): Regional Anesthesia and Analgesia. Philadelphia, WB Saunders, 1996, p 279.
8. Vloka JD, Hadzic A, Mulcare R, et al: Femoral and genitofemoral nerve blocks versus spinal anesthesia for outpatients undergoing long saphenous vein stripping surgery. Anesth Analg 84:749, 1997.
9. Berry FR: Analgesia in patients with fractured shaft of the femur. Anaesthesia 32:576, 1977.
10. Howard CB, Mackie IG, Fairclough J, et al: Femoral neck surgery using a local anesthetic technique. Anaesthesia 38:993, 1983.
11. Ringrose NH, Cross MJ: Femoral nerve block in knee joint surgery. Am J Sports Med 12:398, 1984.
12. Rosenblatt RM: Continuous femoral nerve anesthesia for lower extremity surgery. Anesth Analg 59:631, 1980.
13. Winnie AP, Ramamurthy S, Durrani Z: The inguinal paravascular technique of lumbar plexus anesthesia: The three-in-one block. Anesth Analg 52:989, 1973.
14. Spillane WF: Three-in-1 blocks and continuous 3-in-1 blocks. Reg Anesth 17:175, 1992.
15. Lang SA, Yip RW, Chang PC, et al: The femoral 3-in-1 block revisited. J Clin Anesth 5:292, 1993.
16. Atanassof PG, Branko BM, Brull SJ, et al: Electromyographic comparison of obturator nerve block to three-in-one block. Anesth Analg 81:529, 1995.
17. Ritter JW: Femoral nerve sheath for inguinal paravascular lumbar plexus block is not found in human cadavers. J Clin Anesth 7:470, 1995.
18. Schultz P, Anker-Moller E, Dahl JB, et al: Postoperative pain treatment after open knee surgery: Continuous lumbar plexus block with bupivacaine versus epidural morphine. Reg Anesth 16:34, 1991.
19. De Andres, Bellver J, Barrera L, et al: A comparative study of analgesia after knee surgery with intraarticular bupivacaine, intraarticular morphine, and lumbar plexus block. Anesth Analg 787:727, 1993.
20. Bridenbaugh PO, Wedel DJ: The lower extremity somatic blockade. *In* Cousins MJ, Bridenbaugh PO (eds): Neural Blockade in Clinical Anesthesia and Management of Pain. Philadelphia, Lippincott-Raven, 1998, p 384.
21. Shannon J, Lang SA, Yip RW, et al: Lateral femoral cutaneous nerve block revisited: A nerve stimulator technique. Reg Anesth 20:100, 1995.
22. Wassef MR: Interadductor approach to obturator nerve blockade for spastic conditions of adductor thigh muscles. Reg Anesth 18:13, 1993.
23. Atanassoff PG, Weiss BM, Horst A, et al: Electroneurographic study on the obturator nerve. Anesthesiology 81:A1043, 1994.
24. Atanassoff PG, Weiss BM, Brull SJ, et al: Compound motor action potential recording distinguishes differential onset of motor block of the obturator nerve in response to etidocaine or bupivacaine. Anesth Analg 82:317, 1996.

Chapter 102

Sciatic Nerve Block

Robert E. Molloy, M.D.

Spinal and epidural anesthesia are the most widely utilized forms of regional anesthesia. They provide very reliable anesthesia for lower extremity surgery. They may produce undesirable cardiovascular effects secondary to sympathetic blockade. Although surgical anesthesia is predictable, prolonged postoperative analgesia is less reliable, particularly for outpatients. Sensory block does not persist without associated motor and sympathetic blockade, which may prevent early postoperative ambulation. Lower extremity plexus anesthesia is not as easy to perform and as effective as brachial plexus block.[1] The innervation of the lower extremity includes widely separated peripheral nerves arising from the lumbar and sacral plexuses. They cannot be blocked in one location unless an intraspinal level of injection is selected. However, it has recently become more desirable to provide ambulatory patients with effective anesthesia, rapid and simple recovery, persistent postoperative analgesia, early ambulation with the assist of crutches and braces as needed, and efforts to prevent severe postoperative pain. Lower extremity nerve blocks have become more attractive to the extent that they can meet these objectives.[2] Popliteal sciatic nerve block may be well suited for this purpose. More classic, proximal approaches may play a role in prolonged postoperative analgesia after major knee surgery for inpatients and in cases in which neither intraspinal nor general anesthesia is a good choice.

Sciatic nerve block produces anesthesia of the leg and foot, except for the medial surface, which requires saphenous or femoral nerve block (see Fig. 104-1). The sciatic nerve is the largest peripheral nerve in the body, being almost 2 cm wide and 1 cm thick.[3] It originates from both the lumbar and sacral plexuses. The lumbosacral trunk (L4-5) joins branches of three sacral roots (S1-3) to form the sciatic nerve (Fig. 102-1). The sciatic nerve actually consists of two separate major nerves: the tibial and common peroneal nerves. The sciatic nerve leaves the pelvis passing through the sciatic foramen. It passes deep to the piriformis muscle, and then it passes between the ischial tuberosity and the greater trochanter of the femur. It becomes superficial beyond the gluteus maximus muscle, and it courses down the posterior thigh.[1] It divides into the separate peroneal and tibial nerves before it reaches the popliteal fossa. The sciatic nerve provides sensory innervation to the posterior thigh and most of the leg and foot.[2] It also provides motor innervation of the hamstring muscles and the plantar and dorsiflexor muscles of the ankle and foot. Regional block of the sciatic nerve is usually performed at the sciatic notch or between the greater trochanter and the ischial tuberosity.[2]

CLINICAL APPLICATION OF SCIATIC BLOCK

Sciatic nerve block provides surgical anesthesia and postoperative analgesia for procedures on the foot and the distal leg. Combined with femoral nerve block, it provides anesthesia for the entire leg below the knee. It may allow for prolonged anesthesia with a single injection, limited sympathetic block, no loss of bladder and bowel control, and avoidance of the positioning requirements and complications of central neuraxial block. This can be a painful procedure unless adequate sedation is provided. Sciatic block may be difficult to perform, but use of a peripheral nerve stimulator allows for good results without the necessity of producing painful paresthesia.[4]

Technique

Classic Posterior Approach

This technique blocks the sciatic nerve at the greater sciatic notch. The posterior femoral cutaneous and pudendal nerves are blocked with this approach.[5] The patient is placed in the lateral position with the side to be blocked rotated slightly forward. The uppermost hip and knee are both flexed to near 90 degrees. Two landmarks are identified: the greater trochanter and the posterior superior iliac spine. A line is drawn to connect these points, coinciding with the upper border of the

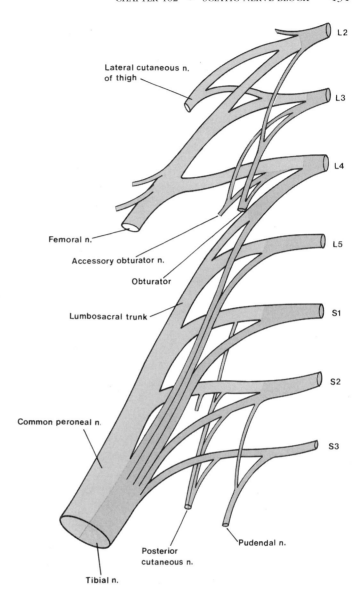

FIGURE 102–1. Anatomy of the lumbosacral plexus, demonstrating formation of the sciatic nerve. (From Macrae WA: Lower limb blocks. *In* Wildsmith JAW, Armitage EN (eds): Principles and Practice of Regional Anesthesia, ed 2. Edinburgh, Churchill Livingstone, 1993, p 189.)

piriformis muscle. It is then bisected, and a perpendicular line is drawn inferiorly from the midpoint of the first line. A third line is drawn from the greater trochanter to the sacral hiatus. The second and third lines intersect over the site of needle insertion. A 22-gauge, 10- to 12.5-cm needle is inserted perpendicular to the skin and advanced until contact with bone or a paresthesia occurs, often at a depth of 6 to 8 cm. If periosteum is contacted, the needle is redirected laterally or medially until paresthesia is elicited. If the needle initially passes into the sciatic notch, it is redirected in a cephalad orientation until bone is contacted, which helps to determine the depth at which paresthesia or a motor response should be sought. The careful injection of 20 to 30 mL of local anesthetic is made after confirming negative aspiration and the absence of painful paresthesia with the initial injection (Fig. 102–2).

The peripheral nerve stimulator is an ideal adjunct to this block. It has been shown to improve the success rate of sciatic block in awake patients and in patients receiving general anesthesia.[4] An insulated needle is connected to the nerve stimulator via the electrode with negative polarity. The nerve is initially approached with 2.0 to 3.0 mA of current, and injection is delayed until a distal motor response is produced with 0.5 mA.

"Supine" Lithotomy Approach

Sciatic nerve block may be performed more distally, between two landmarks: the ischial tuberosity and the greater trochanter. This may be performed with the patient in the supine position, with the extremity to be blocked supported in a position of hip and knee flexion. This avoids rotation of the patient from the supine position. And with this technique, the sciatic nerve remains relatively more superficial than with the lateral and anterior approaches.[6, 7] However, positioning of the leg may prove painful with a traumatized lower extremity. A line is drawn to connect the ischial tuberosity and greater trochanter, and a 22-gauge, 10- to 12.5-cm needle is inserted at the midpoint of this line, perpendicular to the skin. Confirmation of needle placement and local

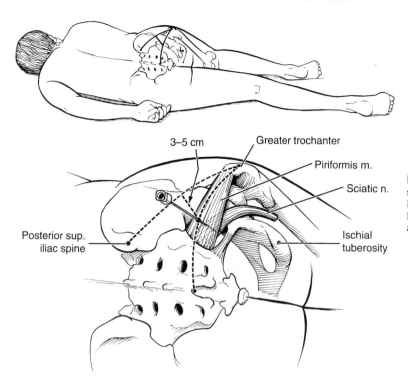

FIGURE 102–2. Patient position and landmarks for classic posterior approach to sciatic nerve block. (From Rogers TN, Ramamurthy S: Lower extremity blocks. *In* Brown DL (ed): Regional Anesthesia and Analgesia. Philadelphia, WB Saunders, 1996, p 279.)

anesthetic injection are similar to the classic sciatic block technique. Essentially the same procedure may be performed with the patient in the prone or lateral position, but no particular advantage seems to recommend these approaches.

Lateral Approach

The lateral and anterior approaches to sciatic block are applied with the patient left undisturbed in the supine position. The lateral approach[8, 9] blocks the sciatic nerve in a plane posterior to the quadratus femoris muscle. The needle is inserted and aimed at the posterior border of the femur, 3 cm distal to the lateral prominence of the greater trochanter. The 22-gauge, 15-cm needle contacts the periosteum and is redirected posteriorly to reach the nerve at a depth of 8 to 12 cm. Good results are obtained when a nerve stimulator is used to produce a distal tibial or peroneal motor response rather than a lateral hamstring or gluteal muscle response.

Anterior Approach

This technique[10, 11] resembles the lateral approach. Both are performed without moving the supine patient who may have leg trauma; but they require deep needle placement, to a depth nearly double that of the classic posterior approach. A line is drawn between the anterior superior iliac spine and the pubic tubercle, and it is trisected. A perpendicular line is drawn inferiorly from the junction of the middle and medial third of the initial line. A third line is drawn parallel to the first, beginning at the greater trochanter and intersecting the second line at the point of needle insertion. The 22-gauge, 15-cm needle strikes the periosteum near the lesser trochanter, and it is redirected medially to seek the sciatic nerve at a depth of 4.5 to 6 cm beyond the femoral surface. A nerve stimulator is again recommended, but a loss-of-resistance technique has been used successfully in children.[11] The anterior approach had been noted to be the most difficult of three approaches when utilized in pediatric patients[12] (Table 102–1).

SIDE EFFECTS AND COMPLICATIONS

Sciatic block can be a prolonged, painful procedure. Hematoma formation, vasodilation, and neural injury may occur. It is essential to take measures to avoid intraneural injection and excessive needle trauma to the sciatic nerve. Analgesia will be inadequate for major knee surgery unless the femoral, obturator, and lateral

TABLE 102–1. APPROACHES TO PROXIMAL SCIATIC NERVE BLOCK

Approach	Position	Needle Depth	Advantages and Disadvantages
Classic posterior	Lateral Sims' position	Moderate	Easiest to perform; patient positioning may be painful
Supine posterior	Supine lithotomy	Moderate	No need to turn patient; leg elevation may be painful
Lateral	Supine position	Double	Position undisturbed; block more difficult
Anterior	Supine position	Double	Position undisturbed; block more difficult

femoral cutaneous nerves are also blocked, individually or by an effective lumbar plexus block procedure. Alternately, heavy sedation or light general anesthesia may be used intraoperatively to supplement combined femoral and sciatic nerve blocks, leading to a quick recovery with excellent postoperative analgesia. Sciatic nerve block is not an "easy" block, and it has a definite failure rate, which may be increased by its very infrequent performance. However, the experienced regional anesthesiologist should be able to perform it carefully and successfully following a quick review of the anatomy and the block technique.

REFERENCES

1. Bridenbaugh PO: The lower extremity: Somatic blockade. *In* Cousins MJ, Bridenbaugh PO (eds): Neural Blockade in Clinical Anesthesia and Management of Pain, ed 2. Philadelphia, JB Lippincott, 1988, p 417.
2. Rogers TN, Ramamurthy S: Lower extremity blocks. *In* Brown DL (ed): Regional Anesthesia and Analgesia. Philadelphia, WB Saunders, 1996, p 279.
3. Wedel DJ: Nerve blocks. *In* Miller RD (ed): Anesthesia, ed 4. New York, Churchill Livingstone, 1994, p 1535.
4. Smith BE, Allison A: Use of a low-power nerve stimulator during sciatic nerve block. Anaesthesia 42:296–298, 1987.
5. Labat G: Regional Anesthesia: Its Techniques and Clinical Applications. Philadelphia, WB Saunders, 1922.
6. Winnie AP, Ramamurthy S, Durrani Z, et al: Plexus blocks for lower extremity surgery: New answers to old problems. Anesthesiol Rev 1:11, 1975.
7. Raj PP, Parks RI, Watson TD, et al: New single-position supine approach to sciatic-femoral nerve block. Anesth Analg 54:489, 1975.
8. Ichiyanagi K: Sciatic nerve block: Lateral approach with the patient supine. Anesthesiology 20:601, 1959.
9. Guardini R, Waldron BA, Wallace WA: Sciatic nerve block: A new lateral approach. Acta Anaesthesiol Scand 29:515, 1985.
10. Beck GP: Anterior approach to sciatic nerve block. Anesthesiology 24:222, 1963.
11. McNicol LR: Anterior approach to sciatic nerve block in children: Loss of resistance or nerve stimulator for identifying the neurovascular compartment. Anesth Analg 66:1199, 1987.
12. Dalens B, Tanguy A, Vanneuville G: Sciatic nerve blocks in children: Comparison of the posterior, anterior, and lateral approaches in 180 pediatric patients. Anesth Analg 70:131, 1990.
13. Macrae WA: Lower limb blocks. *In* Wildsmith JAW, Armitage EN (eds): Principles and Practice of Regional Anaesthesia, ed 2. Edinburgh, Churchill Livingstone, 1993, p 189.

Chapter 103

Sciatic Nerve Block in the Popliteal Fossa

Honorio T. Benzon, M.D.

ANATOMY

The popliteal fossa is a triangular space bounded by the semitendinosus and semimembranosus muscles medially, the biceps femoris muscle laterally, and by the two heads of the gastrocnemius muscle inferiorly. The popliteal vessels are located medial to the sciatic nerve. Although the sciatic nerve is usually one nerve, the tibial and common peroneal nerves can be visualized within the sciatic nerve. Occasionally, the tibial and common peroneal nerves are two separate nerves as soon as they descend from the sacrosciatic foramen, the tibial nerve medially and the common peroneal nerve laterally. The sciatic nerve divides into its tibial and common peroneal branches at the apex of the popliteal fossa, between 4 and 13 cm above the popliteal crease (Fig. 103–1).[1] The tibial nerve immediately gives off the sural nerve and, at the level just above the sole of the foot, gives off the medial calcaneal nerve. The tibial nerve then continues as the posterior tibial nerve, which terminates into the medial plantar and lateral plantar nerves. The common peroneal nerve gives off a sural communicating branch and, once it is below the head of the fibula, divides into the deep peroneal and superficial peroneal nerves. Although the major

branches of the sciatic nerve have muscular branches, the sural nerve has no motor function.

INDICATIONS

Popliteal nerve blocks are indicated for blockade of the foot, either for anesthesia for surgery of the foot or for diagnostic and/or therapeutic blockade for pain management. The block is especially useful when ankle blocks are contraindicated because of the presence of swelling or infection in the ankle. In contrast to ankle blocks, in which up to four injections may be given, only one injection is utilized in popliteal nerve block.

TECHNIQUE

Posterior Approach

The patient is prone and the popliteal fossa is aseptically prepared and draped. The site of needle insertion is 5 to 7 cm above the popliteal crease and 1 cm lateral to a line that bisects the superior part of the fossa. The needle is inserted at a 45 degree angle to the skin and inserted to a depth of 2 to 5 cm until paresthesia is

FIGURE 103–1. Anatomy of the popliteal fossa and technique of sciatic nerve blockade. (Please see text for the technique of nerve blockade.) (From Benzon HT, Kim C, Benzon HP, et al: Correlation between evoked motor response of the sciatic nerve and sensory blockade. Anesthesiology 87:547, 1997.)

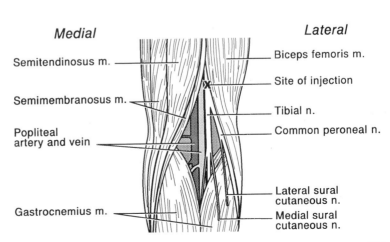

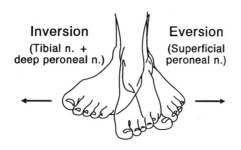

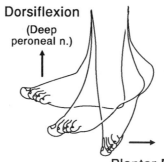

FIGURE 103–2. Elicited motor response of the foot in response to stimulation of the major branches of the sciatic nerve. The nerve responsible for each elicited motor response is indicated; note that the superficial peroneal nerve assists in the elicitation of plantar flexion.

obtained or a motor response is elicited with a nerve stimulator.[1-3] The stimulating current of the nerve stimulator is initially set between 1 and 2 mA, and the needle is advanced until the desired motor response is visible. The needle is further advanced, slowly, until the elicited motor response is maximum. The stimulus intensity is decreased, and visible motor response is elicited with the smallest possible current. The needle is considered close to the nerve when the stimulating current is less than 1 mA, preferably between 0.3 and 0.8 mA. The proximity of the insulated needle to the nerve is confirmed when an injection of 1 or 2 mL of local anesthetic results in an immediate cessation of the elicited motor response.[4] Although several motor responses can be elicited, including eversion, inversion, dorsiflexion, or plantar flexion, elicited inversion or combined inversion–plantar flexion is the preferred response.[1] Thirty to 40 mL of 1% lidocaine is adequate to block the sciatic nerve.

Sciatic nerve block at the popliteal fossa may result in patchy sensory blockade of the foot. This is probably secondary to the considerable size of the sciatic nerve (between 0.9 and 1.5 cm), the variable level at which the sciatic nerve divides into the tibial and common peroneal nerves, the thickness of its epineurium, and the presence of fat in the popliteal fossa.[1] When a nerve stimulator is used, elicited inversion of the foot or combined inversion–plantar flexion is recommended. This is because inversion of the foot is brought about by muscles supplied by both the tibial and deep peroneal nerves, or the sciatic nerve itself is stimulated with inversion. Injection of the local anesthetic after elicited eversion, plantar flexion, or dorsiflexion may result in patchy blockade because these foot movements result from action of the muscles supplied by the major branches of the sciatic nerve, and not the sciatic nerve itself (Fig. 103-2).[1] Complete sensory blockade is also attained when the local anesthetic is injected after elicitation of two foot movements[5]: one injection after stimulation of the tibial nerve (plantar flexion) and the other after stimulation of either the deep peroneal nerve (dorsiflexion) or the superficial peroneal nerve (eversion).

Lateral Approach

Vloka and colleagues described the lateral approach to sciatic nerve block in the popliteal fossa.[6] In this approach, the patient is in the supine position with the legs extended at the knee joint. The long axis of the foot is positioned at a 90 degree angle to the table. A 10-cm-long 21-gauge insulated needle, attached to a nerve stimulator, is inserted in a horizontal plane 7 cm cephalad to the lateral femoral epicondyle, in the groove between the biceps femoris and the vastus lateralis muscles. The needle is advanced until the shaft of the femoral bone is contacted. The needle is then withdrawn and redirected posteriorly at a 30 degree angle to the horizontal plane. With the nerve stimulator stimulus intensity set between 0.8 and 1.5 mA at 1 Hz, the needle is slowly advanced until plantar flexion or dorsiflexion of the foot is elicited. If the nerve is not identified during the first attempt, then the needle is redirected anteriorly or posteriorly 5 to 10 degrees relative to the plane of the initial attempt. Forty milliliters of local anesthetic is injected.

Comparison of the posterior and lateral approaches showed the two approaches to be equally effective.[7] More attempts were necessary to localize the nerve in the lateral approach. Stimulation of the common peroneal nerve was more frequent with the lateral approach, whereas the tibial nerve was more easily identified in the posterior approach. These findings are not surprising as the common peroneal nerve is located laterally in relation to the tibial nerve.

REFERENCES

1. Benzon HT, Kim C, Benzon HP, et al: Correlation between evoked motor response of the sciatic nerve and sensory blockade. Anesthesiology 87:547, 1997.
2. Rorie DK, Byer DE, Nelson DO, et al: Assesment of block of the sciatic nerve in the popliteal fossa. Anesth Analg 59:371, 1980.
3. Singelyn FJ, Gouverneur JA, Gribomont BF: Popliteal sciatic nerve block aided by a nerve stimulator: A reliable technique for foot and ankle surgery. Reg Anesth 16:178–281, 1991.
4. Sims JK: A modification of landmarks for infraclavicular approach to brachial plexus block. Anesth Analg 56:554, 1977.
5. Bailey SL, Parkinson SK, Little WL, et al: Sciatic nerve block: A comparison of single versus double injection technique. Reg Anesth 19:9, 1994.
6. Vloka JD, Hadžić A, Kitain E, et al: Anatomic considerations for sciatic nerve block in the popliteal fossa through the lateral approach. Reg Anesth 21:414, 1996.
7. Hadžić A, Vloka JD: A comparison of the posterior versus lateral approaches to the block of the sciatic nerve in the popliteal fossa. Anesthesiology 88:1480, 1998.

Chapter 104

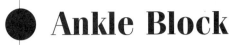

Ankle Block

Robert E. Molloy, M.D.

Ankle block can provide anesthesia for most surgery performed on the foot and toes. Good results have been reported for procedures such as excision of an interdigital neuroma, bunionectomy, amputations of the great toe or of the midfoot and toes for peripheral vascular disease, metatarsal osteotomy, incision and drainage, and debridement procedures.[1, 2] The advantages of ankle block include simplicity and ease of technique, extremely high success rates, lack of significant complications, analgesia without motor block of the foot, ability to ambulate early, and good patient acceptance. There are particular advantages for efficient ambulatory surgery as well as for limiting anesthetic administration with high-risk vascular patients. Disadvantages include the need for multiple painful injections and for repositioning of the patient's foot and ankle during the block. Analgesia for tourniquet application is not provided, but use of a distal leg or ankle tourniquet has been well tolerated by most patients. Patient acceptance is dependent on provision of adequate intravenous sedation and analgesia for the brief period of injections around the ankle. An attempt to limit the number of percutaneous punctures can also be made.

ANATOMY

Ankle blocks interrupt transmission in five nerves at the level of the upper border of the malleoli. The five nerves are the posterior tibial, deep peroneal, saphenous, superficial peroneal, and sural nerves (Table 104–1). The saphenous nerve is the terminal sensory branch of the femoral nerve, whereas the other four nerves arise from the sciatic nerve. The superficial and deep peroneal nerves are derived from the common peroneal nerve, whereas the posterior tibial nerve arises from the tibial nerve. The sural nerve is connected to branches of both the peroneal and tibial nerves. The saphenous, superficial peroneal, and sural nerves are blocked by subcutaneous infiltration. The deep peroneal and posterior tibial nerves are blocked deep to the extensor and flexor retinacula, respectively. Additional anatomic detail is considered with the description of each nerve block (Figs. 104–1 and 104–2).[3]

TECHNIQUE

Ankle blocks are performed with short 25- to 22-gauge needles. Intermediate concentration local anesthetic solutions are injected for surgical anesthesia (e.g., 1.0% to 1.5% lidocaine or mepivacaine). Bupivacaine or ropivacaine may be used to provide prolonged postoperative analgesia.[4] Epinephrine is not added to the local anesthetic solution to prevent unwanted distal vasoconstriction and ischemia. The multiple injections required can be painful, and patient comfort usually requires appropriate intravenous medication prior to blockade.

TABLE 104–1. TECHNIQUE FOR NERVE BLOCKS AT THE ANKLE

Nerve Blocked	Source of Nerve	Area of Anesthesia	Depth of Injection
Saphenous nerve	Femoral nerve (L2–4)	Medial surface of foot	Superficial, subcutaneous
Superficial peroneal nerve	Common peroneal nerve (L4–S2)	Dorsal surface of foot and toes, except space between 1st and 2nd toes	Superficial, subcutaneous
Sural nerve	Branches from tibial and peroneal nerves	Lateral surface of heel, foot, and 5th toe	Superficial, subcutaneous
Posterior tibial nerve	Tibial nerve (L4–S3)	Plantar surface of foot and toes	Subfascial, deep to flexor retinaculum
Deep peroneal nerve	Common peroneal nerve (L4–S2)	Dorsal surface of foot, between great and 2nd toes	Subfascial, deep to extensor retinaculum

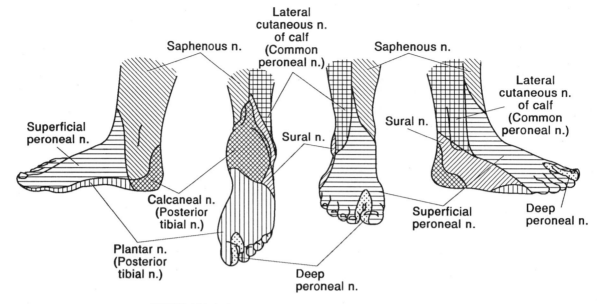

FIGURE 104–1. Cutaneous innervation of the distal lower extremity.

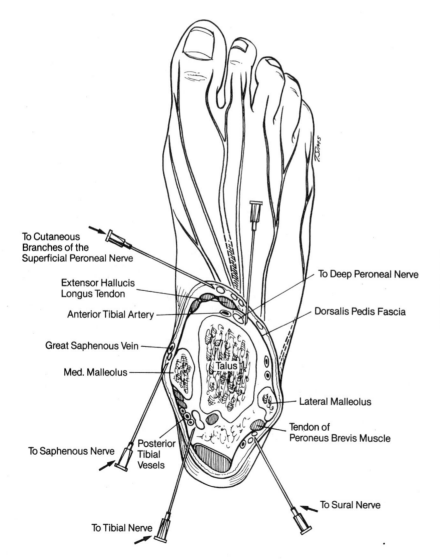

FIGURE 104–2. Transverse section through the ankle demonstrating the anatomy and technique of ankle block. (From Raj PP, Pai U, Rawal N: Techniques of regional anesthesia in adults. *In* Raj PP (ed): Clinical Practice of Regional Anesthesia. New York, Churchill Livingstone, 1991, p 271.)

Posterior Tibial Nerve

The posterior tibial nerve divides into medial and lateral plantar nerves and supplies the plantar surface of the foot and toes. Blockade of this nerve is the most critical technical component of the ankle block. It is most easily performed in the prone position, but supine and lateral positions can be used. The nerve lies posterior and medial to the posterior tibial artery, between the medial malleolus and the Achilles tendon, which are the landmarks for needle insertion. At the level of the upper border of the malleolus, it lies deep to the flexor retinaculum. The classic block is performed at this level, with the needle inserted toward the artery and advanced so that it passes through the flexor retinaculum. The end point for injection may be one of the following: plantar paresthesia, perivascular injection after blood aspiration, or diffuse infiltration from the tibial periosteum back to the retinaculum. The volume injected is 5 mL for the first two end points and 10 mL for the infiltration technique.[5] This nerve may be blocked with greater ease at the midtarsal level, as reported by Sharrock and co-workers.[6] The posterior tibial artery is palpated in a more superficial position where it passes below the medial malleolus. Three to 5 mL of local anesthetic is injected deep to the fascia on either side of the artery. For patients with no palpable arterial pulse, 3 to 5 mL of local anesthetic may be injected immediately posterior and inferior to the sustentaculum tali, a bony ridge below the medial malleolus. This subcalcaneal approach, described by Wassef,[7] utilizes a bony landmark and a superficial nerve location to improve success rate (Fig. 104–3).

Sural Nerve

The sural nerve is formed by branches of the tibial and peroneal nerves. It supplies sensory innervation to the lateral heel, foot, and fifth toe. The nerve is blocked where it passes subcutaneously between the Achilles tendon and the lateral malleolus. With the patient in the same position as for posterior tibial nerve block, the sural nerve is blocked by subcutaneous infiltration from the Achilles tendon to the lateral malleolus at the level of the upper malleolar border. The volume of local anesthetic required varies from 3 to 5 mL.

Deep Peroneal Nerve

The deep peroneal, superficial peroneal, and saphenous nerves may be blocked through a single needle insertion site, with the patient's ankle supported in a supine position.

The deep peroneal nerve (anterior tibial nerve) courses down the leg anterior to the interosseous membrane, and it passes between the malleoli deep to the extensor retinaculum and on to the dorsum of the foot. It supplies sensory innervation to adjacent areas of the great and second toes. At the upper level of the malleoli, it lies between the tendons of tibialis anterior and extensor hallucis longus, just lateral to the anterior tibial (dorsalis pedis) artery. At this site, the 25-gauge needle is inserted between the two tendons, identified by dorsiflexing first the ankle and then the great toe. After the needle passes through the extensor retinaculum, 3 to 5 mL of local anesthetic is injected. A midtarsal variation of this block, described by Sharrock and colleagues,[6] injects the same volume of drug on either side of the dorsalis pedis artery below the extensor retinaculum. At the midtarsal level, the dorsalis pedis artery and the deep peroneal nerve lie lateral to the extensor hallucis longus tendon.

Superficial Peroneal Nerve

The superficial peroneal nerve runs subcutaneously on the anterior surface of the distal leg. It supplies sensory innervation to the dorsum of the foot and toes except for the opposing surfaces of the first two toes. This nerve is blocked by a subcutaneous infiltration of 5 mL of local anesthetic from the deep peroneal nerve injection site laterally toward the upper border of the lateral malleolus.

Saphenous Nerve

The saphenous nerve, derived from the femoral nerve, travels subcutaneously along the leg from the medial aspect of the knee to the medial malleolus along with the great saphenous vein. It supplies sensory innervation to the anteromedial leg and medial foot, stopping before reaching the great toe. A subcutaneous infiltration of local anesthetic from the deep peroneal nerve injection site medially to the medial malleolus will block the saphenous nerve. An anterior subcutaneous ring of local anesthetic is thereby deposited between the two malleoli.

REFERENCES

1. Bridenbaugh PO: The lower extremity: Somatic blockade. *In* Cousins MJ, Bridenbaugh PO (eds): Neural Blockade in Clinical Anesthesia and Management of Pain, ed 2. Philadelphia, JB Lippincott, 1988, p 417.
2. Rogers JN, Ramamurthy S: Lower extremity blocks. *In* Brown DL

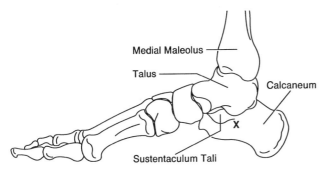

FIGURE 104–3. Subcalcaneal approach to posterior tibial nerve block, identifying the bony landmarks and the point of needle entry at X. (Modified from Wassef MR: Posterior tibial nerve block: A new approach using the bony landmark of the sustentaculum tali. Anaesthesia 46:841, 1991.)

Medial Maleolus

Talus

Calcaneum

X

Sustentaculum Tali

(ed): Regional Anesthesia and Analgesia. Philadelphia, WB Saunders, 1996, p 279.

3. Raj PP, Pai U, Rawal N: Techniques of regional anesthesia in adults. *In* Raj PP (ed): Clinical Practice of Regional Anesthesia. New York, Churchill Livingstone, 1991, p 271.

4. Mineo R, Sharrock NE: Venous levels of lidocaine and bupivacaine after midtarsal ankle block. Reg Anesth 17:47, 1992.

5. Wedel DJ: Nerve blocks. *In* Miller RD (ed): Anesthesia, ed 4. New York, Churchill Livingstone, 1994, p 1535.

6. Sharrock NE, Waller JF, Fierro LE: Midtarsal block for surgery of the forefoot. Br J Anaesth 58:37, 1986.

7. Wassef MR: Posterior tibial nerve block: A new approach using the bony landmark of the sustentaculum tali. Anaesthesia 46:841, 1991.

Chapter 105

Stellate Ganglion Block

Raghavender Thunga, M.D.

ANATOMY

The stellate ganglion, also called the cervicothoracic ganglion, is the fusion of the most inferior cervical and the first thoracic sympathetic ganglia. It is located at the inferior margin of the head of the first rib, immediately lateral to the longus colli muscle and posterior to the vertebral artery. In some older texts its location has been inaccurately displayed at sites more cephalad, perhaps guided by dissection studies that did not account for the downward traction of the lung in living anatomy.[1] At the level of injection (C6–7) the prevertebral fascia extends from the anterior tubercle of C6 and covers the anterior scalene muscle laterally and the longus colli muscle medially. The cervical trunk at this level lies within the superficial layers of this fascia (Fig. 105-1).

The vertebral artery lies anterior to the C7 transverse process, but then enters a foramen (foramen transversaria) to ascend posterior to the anterior tubercle of C6 (Chassaignac's tubercle). In a small percentage of patients, however, the vertebral artery passes anterior to the C6 anterior tubercle. The carotid artery usually lies anterior to the sympathetic chain at the level of injection (C6–7) and is usually retracted laterally during the injection.

INDICATIONS

I. Diagnosis and treatment of autonomic dysfunction
  A. Vascular insufficiency in the upper extremity
    1. Traumatic or embolic vascular occlusion or impaired circulation
    2. Postembolectomy vasospasm
    3. Raynaud's disease
    4. Arteriopathies (scleroderma)
    5. Frostbite
    6. Occlusive vascular disease

  B. Ventricular arrhythmias due to "sympathetic imbalance" on left side
  C. Hyperhidrosis
II. Painful syndromes
  A. Complex regional pain syndrome type I (RSD) and II (causalgia)
  B. Neuropathic states (herpes zoster, postherpetic neuralgia)

TECHNIQUES

Paratracheal (Anterior) Technique[2, 3]

With the patient lying supine, the head is slightly extended and lifted forward perhaps with a pillow or blanket roll (see Fig. 105-1). By asking the patient to keep the mouth slightly open, the neck muscles are kept relaxed. After sterile preparation, the anterior tubercle of C6 is straddled with the index and middle fingers of the nondominant hand. The carotid artery and sternocleidomastoid muscle are retracted laterally in some cases to appreciate the anterior tubercle. Gentle pressure should be directed downward to position the tubercle as superficial as possible relative to the skin.

A 25- or 22-gauge, 1½ in. short-bevel needle connected to a 10-mL syringe is advanced perpendicular to the horizontal plane with the dominant hand until the anterior tubercle of C6 is encountered. Some practitioners interpose a short extension tubing between the needle and the syringe and have an assistant aspirate while the practitioner advances the needle. The needle is then withdrawn about 1 to 2 mm and fixed with the nondominant hand. The syringe is aspirated. Some practitioners will aspirate after turning the needle in 90-degree increments to seek blood return in four quadrants. Even if the needle is in a blood vessel, however, aspiration with 25- or 22-gauge needle may be negative.

A volume as small as 1 mL, if directly injected into the vertebral artery, will produce convulsions. Following the test dose (0.5 to 1 mL), increments of 3 mL are

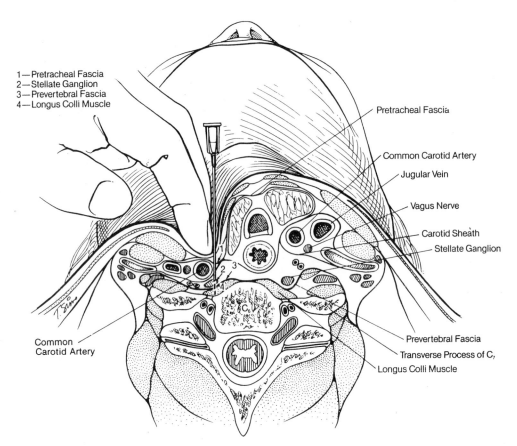

1—Pretracheal Fascia
2—Stellate Ganglion
3—Prevertebral Fascia
4—Longus Colli Muscle

Pretracheal Fascia

Common Carotid Artery

Jugular Vein

Vagus Nerve

Carotid Sheath

Stellate Ganglion

Common
Carotid Artery

Prevertebral Fascia

Transverse Process of C7

Longus Colli Muscle

FIGURE 105–1. Cross-sectional anatomy and technique of paratracheal approach to stellate ganglion block at the level of C6. (From Raj PP: Chronic pain. *In* Raj PP (ed): Clinical Practice of Regional Anesthesia. New York, Churchill Livingstone, 1991, p 489.)

given, up to a total volume of 10 to 12 mL. The patient is advised not to talk during the injection, as even slight movement may alter needle position. Also, between incremental injections, reconfirmation of contact with bone is prudent to ensure that no alteration occurs in the position of the needle. The head of the patient's bed can be raised after injection, presumably allowing the solution to travel caudally toward the stellate ganglion.

The injection should meet little resistance if the needle is properly positioned. If injection is difficult, the needle may be embedded in the periosteum, requiring slight withdrawal. If injection is moderately difficult, the needle may still be positioned within the prevertebral muscle. If the patient complains of extreme radiating pain during injection, the needle may be located intraneurally, requiring slight withdrawal or repositioning.

C7 Approach[1]

In this approach, the needle is placed below the level of the cricoid cartilage, presumably at the C7 level. Because there is no anterior tubercle at C7, the first bony contact is the transverse process of C7. As a result, injection may be made directly into the compartment containing the brachial plexus, which may result in a less selective sympathetic block. The risk of entering the vertebral artery is also increased. These risks may

outweigh the advantage of injecting closer to the stellate ganglion with this approach.

Computed Tomography-Guided (T1) Approach[4]

This technique allows a very accurate method for deposition of solution at the stellate ganglion. With computed tomographic (CT) guidance, the stellate ganglion can be visualized just lateral to the longus colli muscle at the level of the first rib. A needle can then be inserted to contact the first rib near this site, and confirmation with injection of contrast material can be made. No data are available to justify routine use of a CT-guided approach, which is expensive in terms of both cost and time.

MONITORING SYMPATHETIC BLOCK

With successful blockade of the stellate ganglion, the patient may notice increased warmth, decreased moisture, and, in cases of "sympathetically mediated" pain, decreased pain.

Quantitative measurements of decreased sympathetic innervation of the extremity include changes in sweating (abolition of sweating or of the sympathogalvanic response) and vasodilation (increase in skin temperature).[3] A distinctive rise in temperature should be evident on the injected side that approximates, but rarely reaches, core temperature. A successful block will raise the temperature to at least 34°C. Simply noting an increase in temperature compared to that of the contralateral side is not sufficient.

SIDE EFFECTS AND COMPLICATIONS[5]

1. Blockade of the recurrent laryngeal nerve. The patient complains of hoarseness or a lump-in-the-throat sensation. The patient should be kept NPO (nothing by mouth) until the hoarseness resolves.

2. Blockade of cervical sympathetic nerves. Horner's syndrome (ptosis, miosis, and enophthalmos) occurs with blockade of cervical sympathetic nerves. The patient may have anhidrosis, flushing of skin and conjunctiva, and ipsilateral nasal stuffiness (due to engorgement of nasal mucosa).

3. Brachial plexus blockade.

4. Phrenic nerve blockade.

Complications

1. Pneumothorax

2. Subarachnoid or epidural block (if the needle is located near the dural sheath)

3. Injection into the vertebral artery (convulsion and immediate loss of consciousness)

4. Trauma to the thoracic duct (left side)

5. Esophageal puncture (with medial angulation of the needle)

6. Osteitis (infection in the transverse process)

Full resuscitative equipment should always be available when performing this block. Most practitioners avoid bilateral blocks because of the added risk of a bilateral recurrent laryngeal nerve blockade, phrenic nerve blockade, or pneumothorax.

REFERENCES

1. Hogan QH: Stellate ganglion. *In* Hahn MB, McQuillan PM, Sheplock GJ (eds): Regional Anesthesia: An Atlas of Anatomy and Techniques. St Louis, Mosby–Year Book, 1996, p 169.
2. Raj PP: Chronic pain. *In* Raj PP (ed): Clinical Practice of Regional Anesthesia. New York, Churchill Livingstone, 1991, p 489.
3. Lofstrom B, Cousins MJ: Sympathetic neural blockade of upper and lower extremity. *In* Cousins MJ, Bridenbaugh PO (eds): Neural Blockade, ed 2. Philadelphia, JB Lippincott, 1988, p 461.
4. Erickson SJ, Hogan QH: CT-guided injection of the stellate ganglion: Description of technique and efficacy of sympathetic blockade. Radiology 188:707, 1993.
5. Abram SA, Hogan QH: Complications of nerve blocks. *In* Benumof JL, Saidman LJ (eds): Anesthesia and Perioperative Complications. St Louis, Mosby–Year Book, 1992, p 52.

Chapter 106

Lumbar Paravertebral Sympathetic Block

Honorio T. Benzon, M.D.

ANATOMY

The sympathetic chain lies along the anterolateral surface of the lumbar vertebral bodies, the psoas muscle and fascia separating the sympathetic nerves from the somatic nerves. The lumbar sympathetic chain contains preganglionic and postganglionic fibers to the pelvis and lower extremities. The location of the sympathetic ganglia on the vertebrae at the level of the second and third lumbar vertebral bodies, from which the sympathetic innervation of the lower extremities primarily originates, was studied in cadavers. The ganglia were most frequently found at the level of the lower third of the second lumbar vertebra, at the L2-3 interspace, and at the upper third of the third lumbar vertebra.[1] Therefore, the best site for placement of the tip of the needle is at the anterolateral surface of the lower third of the second vertebral body or the upper third of the third vertebral body.[1] The segmental artery and vein pass along the midportion of the lumbar vertebral body in a tunnel under the dense fascia. Solutions injected at the midvertebral level may pass posteriorly in this tunnel to the epidural space. Crossover of the sympathetic fibers has been described.

INDICATIONS

Lumbar sympathetic blocks are indicated for determination of the sympathetic component of pain in a patient with acute or chronic pain, as prognostic or therapeutic blocks in patients with sympathetically mediated pain, for the improvement of blood flow in patients with vascular insufficiency of the lower extremities, and for the management of neuralgic pain associated with peripheral nerve injuries such as those caused by trauma or limb amputation. It is rarely used for the relief of pelvic pain.

TECHNIQUE

The patient is placed prone with a pillow beneath the lower abdomen and hips to reduce lumbar lordosis.

Although blind insertion of the needle can be done, radiologic confirmation is needed because of variability of the body habitus, uncertainty of the vertebral level of insertion, and position of the needle tip. The earlier techniques involved injections at the L2, L3, and L4 vertebrae. More recent techniques employ a single needle.[2,3] In the technique of Hatangdi and Boas,[3] the midline is marked and the tip of the 12th rib is palpated on the side to be injected. The site of insertion of the needle is 2 to 3 cm below and medial to the tip of the 12th rib, opposite the body of L3 (Fig. 106-1). A 5- to 7-inch, 22-gauge needle is inserted 8 to 10 cm from the midline at an angle of 30 to 45 degrees, lateral to the spinous process, to reach the anterolateral aspect of the vertebra. Correct placement of the needle is confirmed by the injection of 2 to 3 mL of nonionic contrast medium, with a linear spread of the dye along the anterolateral aspect of the vertebral bodies (Fig. 106-2). Fifteen to 20 mL of local anesthetic is then injected. Some authors first identify the psoas muscle by injecting 0.5 to 1 mL of dye, visualizing the "psoas stripe," and then advancing the needle until it is anterior to the psoas muscle.[4] For neurolytic blocks, a two-needle tech-

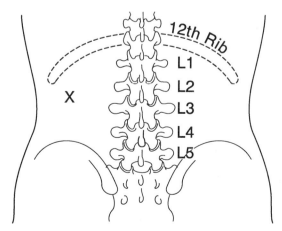

FIGURE 106-1. Single-needle technique of lumbar sympathetic blockade.[3] *X* is the site of the needle insertion.

nique is recommended, with one needle at L2 and the other at L3.[3] The injection of 2 to 4 mL of 6% phenol at each site allows better control of the spread of the neurolytic agent, in comparison with an injection of 6 to 10 mL of phenol at one site. Some investigators recommend confirmation of correct needle placement, by demonstration of a temperature increase after injection of a small volume of local anesthetic, before the phenol is injected. One milliliter of air or local anesthetic is injected before the needle is removed to prevent depositing the neurolytic solution on the somatic nerves during removal of the needle. The patient is kept on the side for 15 to 30 minutes to prevent the phenol from spreading laterally toward the genitofemoral nerve or posteriorly between the slips of origin of the psoas major muscle and along the fibrous tunnel occupied by the rami communicantes, toward the somatic nerve roots.[5] The patient is then turned supine and instructed not to raise the head for at least 1 hour.

The preferred site of insertion of the needle by some investigators is 10 cm.[6] Insertion of the needle closer to the midline takes the needle path close to the somatic nerve roots and lateral to the sympathetic chain. The more lateral the insertion of the needle, the closer is the tip of the needle to the sympathetic chain. There is also less risk of piercing the roots of the lumbar plexus or encountering the transverse process.

Complications of lumbar paravertebral sympathetic blockade include bleeding from puncture of the lumbar vessels or the aorta, hematuria, infection, orthostatic hypotension, perforation of the abdominal viscera, transient backache and stiffness, epidural or subarachnoid blockade, lumbar plexus blockade, and segmental nerve injury. There is a 5% to 40% incidence of postblock neuralgia, but this is usually of limited duration. The genitofemoral nerve passes below L3, so injection at L4 is not advisable.

CONFIRMATORY TESTS OF SYMPATHETIC BLOCKADE

For a discussion of tests of sympathetic blockade, please refer to Chapter 107.

RADIOFREQUENCY LUMBAR SYMPATHOLYSIS

Rocco[7] described the use of radiofrequency (RF) sympathectomy to relieve sympathetically maintained pain (i.e., complex regional pain syndrome type I). The site of RF sympatholysis was slightly cephalad to the middle of the L3 vertebra; contrast material was injected to confirm the correct placement of the needle. Reproduction of the pain, induced dysesthesia, spread of the dye, rapidity of temperature rise in the legs, and increase in the pulse amplitude were useful guides to appropriate

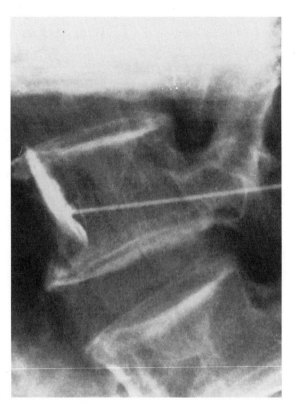

FIGURE 106–2. Linear spread of the dye along the anterolateral aspect of the vertebral body.

placement of the needle tip. The needle tip was heated to 80°C and the temperature was maintained for 90 seconds. Of the 20 patients who had RF sympatholysis, 5 continued to be pain free 5 months to 3 years after the last RF procedure; 15 had temporary relief or no relief at all. Rocco[7] concluded that despite the early sympathetic blockade, as confirmed by a warm foot, long-lasting relief with RF sympatholysis was difficult to obtain.

REFERENCES

1. Umeda S, Arai T, Hatano Y, et al: Cadaver anatomic analysis of the best site for chemical lumbar sympathectomy. Anesth Analg 66:643, 1987.
2. Brown EM, Kunjappan V: Single-needle lateral approach for lumbar sympathetic block. Anesth Analg 4:725, 1975.
3. Hatangdi VS, Boas RA: Lumbar sympathectomy: A single-needle technique. Br J Anaesth 57:285, 1985.
4. Sprague RS, Ramamurthy S: Identification of the anterior psoas sheath as a landmark for lumbar sympathetic block. Reg Anesth 15:253, 1990.
5. Lofstrom JB, Lloyd JW, Cousins MJ: Sympathetic blockade of the upper and lower extremity. *In* Cousins MJ, Bridenbaugh PO (eds): Neural blockade in clinical anesthesia and management of pain. Philadelphia, JB Lippincott, 1980, p 374.
6. Cherry DA, Rao DM: Lumbar sympathetic and coeliac plexus blocks: An anatomical study in cadavers. Br J Anaesth 54:1037, 1982.
7. Rocco AG: Radiofrequency lumbar sympatholysis: The evolution of a technique for managing sympathetically maintained pain. Reg Anesth 20:3, 1995.

Chapter 107

Signs of Sympathetic Blockade: Correlation With Pain Relief

Honorio T. Benzon, M.D.

MONITORING THE ADEQUACY OF SYMPATHETIC BLOCKADE

Signs of successful cervical sympathetic blockade include Horner's syndrome, increased hand temperature, 50% or greater increase in skin blood flow, increased skin resistance, and abolished sympathogalvanic response (SGR).[1, 2] Measurement of skin blood flow and skin resistance usually are not performed clinically. Horner's syndrome signifies cephalic sympathetic blockade but does not imply sympathetic denervation of the arm.[3]

Increase in skin temperature is the most commonly used clinical sign of sympathetic blockade. Different investigators have considered different increases in skin temperature as signifying *effective* sympathetic blockade. After a stellate ganglion block, Carron and Litwiller[4] required a rise of at least 1.5°C in skin temperature to indicate a successful block, whereas other investigators found average increases of 3.8°C and 7.5°C.[5, 6] A mean increase of 3°C was noted after a lumbar paravertebral sympathetic block.[7] Hogan and colleagues[3] recommended that the ipsilateral temperature increase should exceed that of the contralateral side to indicate successful sympathetic blockade. Stevens and associates[8] found that a temperature increase that is 2°C higher than in the contralateral extremity signified *complete* sympathetic blockade in *most* patients.

The magnitude of temperature increases after *complete* sympathetic blockade depend on the baseline values; greater increases are noted in patients with lower preblock temperatures[1] (Fig. 107-1). With vasodilation, the skin temperature approximates core body temperature. Since the upper limit of skin temperature in the fingers and toes is 35 to 36°C,[9] patients other than those with organic peripheral vascular disease can approach 35 to 36°C as a limit of complete sympathetic blockade.[1] Patients with second- or third-stage complex regional pain syndrome (CRPS, or reflex sympathetic dystrophy) whose baseline skin temperatures are low because of vasoconstriction have large increases after complete sympathetic blockade. A patient with first-stage CRPS, who has vasodilation of the involved extremity, can not be expected to have a large temperature increase.

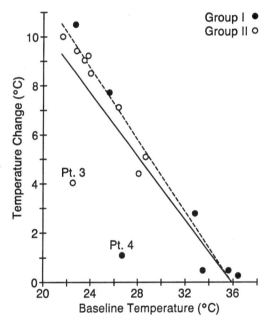

FIGURE 107–1. Temperature changes from baseline values after complete sympathetic block. Group I patients have RSD, whereas group II patients have no RSD. (From Benzon HT, Avram MJ: Temperature increases after complete sympathetic blockade. Reg Anesth 11:27, 1986.)

Abolition of sweating and abolition of the SGR are the standard tests of complete sympathetic blockade.[10-12] The older starch-iodine test is messy and cumbersome, whereas the newer sweat tests, the cobalt blue and the Ninhydrin sweat tests, are easier to perform. Benzon and coworkers[12] modified the preparation of the two sweat tests. For the cobalt blue filter paper 0.5M $CoCl_2$ in 70% ethanol is used. For the Ninhydrin filter paper 2% Ninhydrin in 70% ethanol with 1 mL of 4M acetate buffer (pH 5.5) per 100 mL solution is used. Seventy percent ethanol is used because it dries rapidly and does not require heating of the filter paper. The solution of choice (cobalt blue or Ninhydrin) is applied evenly on a Whatman no. 1 filter paper at 2 mL/100 cm². The papers are dried at room temperature and stored in a desiccator. The sweat tests are performed in

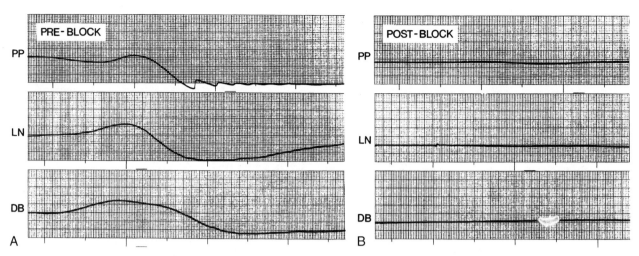

FIGURE 107–2. Sympathogalvanic responses (SGRs) to pin-prick (PP), loud noise (LN), and deep breath (DB). The SGRs were completely abolished after the sympathetic block.

the following manner: the patients' fingers or toes are wiped dry, and the cobalt blue- or Ninhydrin-impregnated filter paper is taped to them. A transparent tape is used so that the changes caused by sweating can be seen. Sweating is signified by a change in color of the cobalt blue filter paper from blue to pink or by the appearance of purple dots in the Ninhydrin filter paper. These sweat tests are not commercially available.

The SGR can be recorded on an ordinary electrocardiogram (ECG) machine. The right arm and left arm leads are placed on the dorsum and palm of the hand (or dorsum and sole of the foot); the other leads are placed on the contralateral extremity, and the lead selector switch is turned to lead I. The stimulus can be a deep breath, a pin-prick, or a loud noise. The response consists of an upward or downward deflection of the ECG tracing, either monophasic or biphasic. Partial sympathetic blockade reduces the response, and complete blockade abolishes it (i.e., the tracing is a straight line) (Fig. 107–2). The SGR has several shortcomings, including marked variation in the responses of patients to the different stimuli and difficulty in obtaining a satisfactory recording under clinical conditions. Also, there is rapid habituation to the stimulus used. In the absence of a sympathetic block, the patient may not have an SGR after several SGR recordings.

The two sweat tests are more reliable than the SGR in predicting complete sympathetic blockade.[12] The sensitivity of the sweat tests and the SGR were found to be 90%. The specificity of the SGR was 56%, compared to 100% for the sweat tests; their accuracies were 74% and 95%, respectively.[12] Because these tests are rarely used clinically, temperature increases to 35 or 36°C can be considered as signifying complete sympathetic blockade.

Relief of pain does not imply complete sympathetic blockade, because patients with chronic pain may exhibit complete pain relief after partial sympathetic blockade. Partial pain relief, on the other hand, signifies one of two things. The patient's pain may be a result of causes other than CRPS (e.g., combined somatic sensory pain and sympathetically mediated pain, combined sympathetically mediated pain and central pain), or the sympathetic

blockade may be partial. A sign of complete sympathetic blockade is necessary in these instances. It is also valuable after surgical or chemical sympathectomy to demonstrate complete sympathetic interruption and to correlate recurrence of pain with sympathetic recovery.[13]

REFERENCES

1. Benzon HT, Avram MJ: Temperature increases after complete sympathetic blockade. Reg Anesth 11:27, 1986.
2. Malmqvist EL, Bengstsson M, Sorensen J: Efficacy of stellate ganglion block: A clinical study with bupivacaine. Reg Anesth 17:340, 1992.
3. Hogan QH, Taylor ML, Goldstein M, et al: Success rates in producing sympathetic blockade by paratracheal injection. Clin J Pain 10:139, 1994.
4. Carron H, Litwiller R: Stellate ganglion block. Anesth Analg 54;567, 1975.
5. Ready LB, Kozody R, Barsa JE, et al: Side-port needles for stellate ganglion block. Reg Anesth 7:160, 1982.
6. Erickson SJ, Hogan QH: CT-guided injection of the stellate ganglion: Description of technique and efficacy of sympathetic blockade. Radiology 188:707, 1993.
7. Hatangdi VS, Boas RA: Lumbar sympathectomy: A single-needle technique. Br J Anaesth 57:285, 1985.
8. Stevens RA, Stotz A, Tzu-Cheg K, et al: The relative increase in skin temperature after stellate ganglion block is predictive of a complete sympathectomy of the hand. Reg Anesth 23:266, 1998.
9. Coller FA, Maddock WG: The differentiation of spastic from organic vascular occlusion by the skin temperature response to high environmental temperature. Ann Surg 96:719, 1932.
10. Lewis LW: Evaluation of sympathetic activity following chemical or surgical sympathectomy. Anesth Analg 34:334-345, 1955.
11. Dhuner KG, Edshage S, Wihelm A: Ninhydrin test an objective method for testing local anaesthetic drugs. Acta Anaesthesiol Scand 4:189, 1960.
12. Benzon HT, Cheng SC, Avram MJ, et al: Sign of complete sympathetic blockade: Sweat test or sympathogalvanic response? Anesth Analg 64:415, 1985.
13. Benzon HT: Importance of documenting complete sympathetic denervation after sympathectomy. Anesth Analg 74:599, 1992.

FURTHER READING

Hogan QH, Abram SE: Neural blockade for diagnosis and prognosis: A review. Anesthesiology 86: 216, 1997.

Chapter 108

Epidural Hematoma

James C. Crews, M.D.

Bleeding into the epidural space, with hematoma formation causing spinal cord compression, is potentially the most serious hemorrhagic complication associated with regional anesthetic or analgesic techniques. Because of the speed at which bleeding into the epidural space can cause significant cord compression and ischemia, early diagnosis and immediate treatment of this complication are essential to prevent permanent spinal cord injury and paraplegia. Spinal epidural hematoma is a rare entity. The total number of reported cases of spinal epidural hematoma exceeded 350 since the late 1950s; the majority of these cases were reported as spontaneous epidural hematoma with no history of trauma or medical procedures.[1] In a review of 199 cases of spontaneous spinal epidural hematoma, Groen and Ponssen[2] reported that, although 25% of these patients had some type of coagulopathy (drug-induced, acquired, or congenital), 103 patients had no relevant medical history.[2] The occurrence of spontaneous epidural hematoma has been reported in patients of all ages, with a slight male predominance. The location of spontaneous epidural hematoma is usually at the lower thoracic level after the fourth decade; before that age, a thoracolumbar location is the exception.

ETIOLOGY OF EPIDURAL HEMATOMA AND NERVE INJURY

The etiologic mechanisms associated with epidural bleeding and hematoma formation that produces symptomatic neurologic injury are in many cases unclear. The majority of cases are thought to be the result of a rupture or trauma to the posterior internal vertebral (epidural) venous plexus.[2] Although this thin-walled, valveless venous plexus is susceptible to injury or spontaneous rupture, the speed and extent to which venous bleeding may cause neurologic injury is limited by the relatively low pressure of this system and the tamponade effect produced by the hydrostatic transdural pressure resulting from the column of the cerebrospinal fluid. Changes in the relative pressures between the

dura and the venous bleed, especially in cases where coagulation is impaired, may produce vascular stasis, tissue congestion, and extrinsic tissue compression of spinal roots or spinal cord tissue, leading to neurologic injury.

Arterial injury (free arteries run along the nerve roots accompanied by the venous plexus) may rapidly produce significant extrinsic neural compression and neurologic injury. Some authors believe that rapidly developing, clinically significant spinal epidural hematomas are more likely to be associated with arterial bleeding than with venous bleeding.[1] Epidural vascular malformations have also been postulated as being responsible for some cases of spinal epidural hematoma.

INCIDENCE OF EPIDURAL HEMATOMA ASSOCIATED WITH CENTRAL NEURAL BLOCKADE

Based on reviews of large series published in the literature, the reported incidence of spinal epidural hematoma associated with central neuraxial blockade (CNB) procedures is estimated at approximately 1 in 190,000 for epidural anesthesia[3] and 1 in 220,000 for subarachnoid block.[4] In a comprehensive review of reported cases of spinal epidural hematomas between 1906 and 1994, 61 published cases of an epidural and/or subdural hematoma involving either an epidural or a subarachnoid block technique were found.[5] The use of anticoagulant medications or the presence of a clotting disorder was reported in 68% of these cases. The procedure was reported as being difficult or traumatic, bloody, and/or with multiple punctures in significant numbers of these cases (25%, 25%, and 20%, respectively). In 87%, one or more of the aforementioned conditions (clotting disorder or technical difficulties) was present. Although 60% of these cases were published after 1980, it is unclear whether this represents an increased frequency of epidural hematomas, an increased use of spinal or epidural analgesia and/or anticoagulant medications, better reporting of anesthesia-related complications, or some combination of these factors.

Another significant factor noted in this review was that the risk of epidural hematoma is most closely associated with placement or removal of the epidural catheter, since bleeding was noted to occur at this time in more than half of the reported cases. From this review it is demonstrated that the presence of a coagulation disorder or a technically difficult procedure (or both) is a critical factor in the most cases of spinal epidural hematoma.

ANTICOAGULANT THERAPY AND CENTRAL NEURAL BLOCKADE

Ruff and Dougherty[6] reported 7 spinal hematomas after 342 diagnostic lumbar punctures followed by intravenous heparinization. It was their conclusion that initiation of heparin therapy within 1 hour of lumbar puncture, traumatic procedures, and concomitant aspirin therapy were significant risk factors in the development of spinal bleeding complications.

Despite the association of epidural hematoma and impaired coagulation status in the cases discussed, the relative safety of CNB techniques in patients receiving various anticoagulants has been reported in several large series including more than 30,000 patients. Several studies reported the relative safety of the use of these techniques in patients undergoing cardiac bypass or peripheral vascular surgical procedures requiring therapeutic heparinization.[6-11] This relative safety seems to be dependent on the variables of strict patient selection, atraumatic technique of epidural or subarachnoid block, willingness to postpone surgery for 24 hours while maintaining rigorous neurologic surveillance of the patient if a traumatic procedure (bleeding) is encountered, delay in the administration of heparin for 60 to 120 minutes after the CNB procedure, and close monitoring of clotting times and maintenance of heparin therapy within a narrow therapeutic window throughout the perioperative period.

Horlocker and colleagues[12] reported the relative safety of maintaining continuous postoperative epidural analgesia in patients receiving low-dose warfarin therapy as prophylaxis for deep venous thrombosis after total knee arthroplasty. No patients in this study had evidence of epidural hematoma, but in most patients the anticoagulant effect of this low dose of warfarin in the postoperative period was not exhibited during the typical duration of postoperative analgesia (38 ± 15 hours).

Several large case series have reported the relative safety of CNB including continuous postoperative epidural analgesia in patients receiving low-dose unfractionated heparin (UH) or low-molecular-weight heparin (LMWH).[13-15] The risk of postoperative pulmonary thromboembolism probably exceeds the risk of spinal hemorrhagic complications with the combination of CNB and low-dose heparin therapy in postoperative patients. Clinical guidelines increasing the safety of these techniques in patients receiving perioperative UH therapy include atraumatic regional anesthetic technique and avoiding initiation of CNB or removal of an epidural catheter within 4 hours of the last dose. For patients receiving LMWH therapy, it is recommended that the dose be administered 10 to 12 hours before performance of a CNB procedure or removal of an indwelling epidural catheter and then withheld for at least 1 to 2 hours after performance of the procedure.

The relative safety of perioperative aspirin or nonsteroidal anti-inflammatory drugs with respect to the risk of epidural hematoma is well accepted.[16-18] The greatest risk associated with these drugs with respect to perioperative spinal hemorrhagic complications relates to their ability to potentiate the anticoagulant effects of heparin or warfarin therapy.

CLINICAL PRESENTATION AND DIAGNOSIS

The symptoms of acute epidural hematoma may include sudden sharp back pain or radicular pain, muscle weakness, sensory deficit, or urinary retention. In some patients the diagnosis may be suspected because of a sensory or motor deficit that lasts beyond the anticipated duration of a regional anesthetic. These initial symptoms may progress to paraplegia within 12 to 18 hours. The diagnosis of epidural hematoma is made by magnetic resonance imaging of the spine. The only treatment for acute compressive epidural hematoma is emergency decompressive laminectomy and hematoma evacuation. Neurologic outcome depends on several factors, including (1) the speed at which the hematoma develops, (2) the severity of the preoperative neurologic deficit, (3) the size and location of the hematoma, and, most importantly, (4) the time span between hematoma formation and surgical decompression.[19, 20] Because of the rapidity at which progressive paraplegia and permanent neurologic injury occur with epidural hematoma, neurologic outcome is enhanced if surgical decompression is performed within 8 hours of the development of paraplegia.

CLINICAL CONSIDERATIONS

Many surgical patients who can benefit from regional anesthetic techniques including subarachnoid or epidural block, spinal opioid administration, or continuous epidural infusion for postoperative pain also have disorders of coagulation or may require anticoagulant therapy as prophylaxis for development of deep venous thrombosis and pulmonary thromboembolism. Therefore, it is essential that considerations for the use of these anesthetic and analgesic techniques be individualized on a patient-by-patient basis. The following clinical considerations are based on large-series case studies, literature reviews, and clinical practice.

In patients with preoperative coagulopathy and those receiving therapeutic anticoagulation with heparin or warfarin, coagulation status should be normalized before performance of a CNB technique. If bleeding occurs in association with performance of a CNB technique before a surgical procedure requiring therapeutic heparinization, consideration should be given to postponing and rescheduling the procedure and performing it with a potentially less traumatic technique (subarachnoid block) or with general anesthesia. Therapeutic heparinization should be delayed for at least 60 minutes after the initiation of CNB procedures. Coagulation indices should be monitored closely throughout the period of therapeutic anticoagulation with maintenance of the activated partial thromboplastin time in the range of less than 1.5 to 2.0 times normal.

In patients receiving perioperative low-dose UH or LMWH, performance of CNB procedures or removal of epidural catheters should be performed near the end of the dosing interval and subsequent doses should be withheld after the procedure for at least 30 minutes for UH or 1 to 2 hours for LMWH. Patients receiving concomitant aspirin, nonsteroidal anti-inflammatory drugs, or other antiplatelet drug therapy must be monitored more closely and with a higher index of suspicion for bleeding complications because of the risk for potentiation of the anticoagulant effects of heparin or warfarin therapy by these drugs.

In the immediate postoperative period, patients must be observed closely for the appropriate return of neurologic function after CNB, regardless of whether they have received or will receive perioperative anticoagulant therapy. Regression of segmental sensory level to pin-prick is not adequate for ensuring return of postoperative neurologic function. Patients must be observed until evidence of return of sensory and motor function in the lumbosacral segments has been documented. For patients receiving continuous postoperative epidural analgesia, any recurrence or persistence of dense sensory or motor deficit should be monitored closely and allowed to regress before reinstitution or continuation of the infusion.

Bleeding into the closed epidural space, with hematoma formation causing spinal cord compression, is clearly a risk associated with central regional anesthetic or analgesic techniques, especially in patients with coagulation disorders and in those requiring perioperative anticoagulant therapy. However, with an appropriate understanding of the pharmacologic properties of the anticoagulant medications, adherence to strict patient selection criteria, individual patient analysis of associated risk-benefit ratios, atraumatic procedural techniques, observation of time intervals between anticoagulant administration and procedures or catheter removal, and continuous awareness of the potential for development of serious hemorrhagic complications in the perioperative period, the safety of these beneficial anesthetic and analgesic techniques may be optimized.

REFERENCES

1. Rainov NG, Heidecke V, Burkert WL: Spinal epidural hematoma: Report of a case and review of the literature. Neurosurg Rev 18:53, 1995.
2. Groen RJM, Ponssen H: The spontaneous spinal epidural hematoma: A study of the etiology. J Neurol Sci 98:121, 1990.
3. Wulf H: Epidural anaesthesia and spinal haematoma. Can J Anaesth 43:1260, 1996.
4. Tryba M: Epidural regional anesthesia and low molecular weight heparin: Pro [German]. Anasth Intensivmed Notfallmed Schmerzther 28:179, 1993.
5. Vandermeulen EP, Aken V, Vermylen J: Anticoagulants and spinal-epidural anesthesia. Anesth Analg 79:1165, 1994.
6. Ruff RL, Dougherty JH: Complications of lumbar puncture followed by anticoagulation. Stroke 12:879-881, 1981.
7. Mathews ET, Abrams LD: Intrathecal morphine in open heart surgery. Lancet 2:543, 1980.
8. El Baz N, Goldin M: Continuous epidural infusion of morphine for pain relief after cardiac operations. J Thorac Cardiovasc Surg 93:878-883, 1987.
9. Rao TL, El-Etr AA: Anticoagulation following placement of epidural and subarachnoid catheters: An evaluation of neurologic sequelae. Anesthesiology 55:618-620, 1981.
10. Ellison N, Jobes DR, Schwartz AJ: Implications of anticoagulant therapy. Int Anesthesiol Clin 20:121-135, 1982.
11. Odoom JA, Sih IL: Epidural analgesia and anticoagulatant therapy: Experience with one thousand cases of continuous epidurals. Anaesthesia 38:254-259, 1983.
12. Horlocker TT, Wedel DJ, Schlichting JL: Postoperative epidural analgesia and oral anticoagulant therapy. Anesth Analg 79:89-93, 1994.
13. Schwander D, Bachmann F: Heparin and spinal or epidural anaesthesia: Clinical decision making [French]. Ann Fr Anaesth Reanim 10:284-296, 1991.
14. Bergqvist D, Landblad B, Matzsch T: Low molecular weight heparin for thromboprophylaxis and epidural/spinal anaesthesia: Is there a risk? Acta Anaesthesiol Scand 36:605-609, 1992.
15. Bergqvist D: Review of clinical trials of low molecular weight heparins. Eur J Surg 158:67-78, 1992.
16. Benzon HT, Brunner EA, Vaisrub N: Bleeding time and nerve blocks after aspirin. Reg Anesth 9:86-89, 1984.
17. Horlocker TT, Wedel DJ, Offord KP: Does preoperative antiplatelet therapy increase the risk of hemorrhagic complications associated with regional anesthesia? Anesth Analg 70:631-634, 1990.
18. Horlocker TT, Wedel DJ, Schroeder DR, et al: Preoperative antiplatelet therapy does not increase the risk of spinal hematoma associated with regional anesthesia. Anesth Analg 80:303-309, 1995.
19. McQuarrie IG: Recovery from paraplegia caused by spontaneous spinal epidural hematoma. Neurology 28:224-228, 1978.
20. Foo D, Rossier AB: Preoperative neurological status in predicting surgical outcome of spinal epidural hematomas. Surg Neurol 15:389-401, 1981.

FURTHER READING

Rauck RL: The anticoagulated patient. Reg Anesth 21:51-56, 1996.

Chapter 109

Epidural Abscess

James C. Crews, M.D.

Infection leading to abscess formation in the spinal epidural space is among the most serious of the potential complications associated with epidural anesthesia or analgesia. Without early diagnosis and appropriate treatment, epidural abscess can progress to produce severe and permanent neurologic sequelae including paralysis and death. Spinal epidural abscess occurs rarely, with a reported frequency of 0.2 to 1.2 cases per 10,000 hospital admissions. The most common location for a spinal epidural abscess is in the posterior thoracic or lumbar epidural space. In a review of 39 cases of spinal epidural abscess at Massachusetts General Hospital during the period 1947 to 1974, only 1 case was associated with epidural anesthesia or analgesia.[1] More frequently, spinal epidural abscess is associated with complications of degenerative disease of the spine, laminectomy procedures, diabetes mellitus, or cancer. This chapter reviews spinal epidural abscess from the perspective of a potentially serious complication of epidural anesthesia and analgesia.

INCIDENCE OF EPIDURAL ABSCESS ASSOCIATED WITH EPIDURAL ANESTHESIA AND ANALGESIA

The incidence of occurrence of epidural abscess associated with perioperative epidural anesthesia for surgery, based on reports in the literature, is estimated to be less than 0.01%. Based on an analysis of 5241 patients receiving postoperative epidural analgesia for a few to several days postoperatively, the incidence of infection was low, with an overall incidence of local infection (skin insertion site or catheter) of between 0.6% and 1.6%.[2, 3] In these series, no perioperative spinal space infections were reported. A series of 75 patients receiving postoperative care in an intensive care unit revealed a 36% incidence of local inflammation, a 12% incidence of local infection, a 5.3% incidence of epidural catheter-related infection, and no spinal space infections.[4] However, isolated cases of epidural abscess in patients receiving postoperative epidural analgesia have been reported.

In an analysis of 517 parturients who received epidural analgesia for labor and delivery and were subsequently found to have evidence of chorioamnionitis on the basis of examination of the placenta, there was no evidence of epidural or spinal abscess in any patient despite a high percentage of patients with fever, leukocytosis, and lack of antibiotic therapy before placement of the epidural catheter. Of the 146 patients for whom blood culture results were reported, 13 cultures were positive.[5] For patients receiving long-term epidural analgesia for chronic or cancer-related pain, the rate of epidural abscess is approximately 0.6 per 1000 days of treatment, despite an overall catheter site infection rate of 5% to 15% (1 to 6 infections per 1000 days of treatment).[6, 7] Considering the relatively long duration of catheter implantation and the health status of patients requiring long-term epidural analgesia, the incidence of serious infection in this high-risk patient population is surprisingly low.

MICROBIOLOGY AND PATHOPHYSIOLOGY OF EPIDURAL ABSCESS

Potential patient-related risk factors for epidural abscess include immunocompromised states (e.g., diabetes mellitus, cancer, intravenous drug abuse, steroid therapy) and local or systemic infection producing local contamination or bacteremia. The potential mechanisms for epidural space infection associated with epidural anesthesia and analgesia include (1) direct inoculation during epidural needle or catheter placement; (2) invasion by way of the epidural needle and catheter track; (3) contamination of the injectate; and (4) hematogenous spread from a distant focus of infection. The microbial organisms most commonly associated with epidural infection and abscess are *Staphylococcus epidermidis, Staphylococcus aureus, Streptococcus* spp., *Pseudomo-*

nas aeruginosa, and *Escherichia coli.* Staphylococci are associated with approximately 60% of cases of epidural abscess.

Based on observations of the most frequently isolated organisms associated with epidural catheter-related infection and epidural abscess, contamination by skin flora represents a potential source of infection. Several studies have demonstrated significant numbers of residual skin flora organisms despite the careful application of various surgical skin preparation solutions. One study reported significantly better antimicrobial potency against staphylococci after skin disinfection with a solution of 0.5% chlorhexidine in 80% ethanol than after 10% povidone-iodine.[8] Meticulous sterile technique from the beginning of skin preparation until the sterile dressing is applied over the epidural insertion site is essential to minimize the risks of epidural catheter–related infection.

An epidural abscess causes progressive neurologic injury predominantly by compression of the spinal cord and nerve roots within the closed space of the vertebral canal.[9] Spinal cord tissue is extremely vulnerable to extrinsic compression. Spinal cord compression produces primarily changes in the white matter, including vacuolization, loss of myelin, and axonal swelling, resulting in progressive, potentially permanent loss of neural function.

CLINICAL PRESENTATION AND DIAGNOSIS

In a 1947 review of 20 patients with spinal epidural infections, Heusner described the four classic clinical phases of an epidural abscess: initial back pain, followed by root pain, muscle and sphincter weakness, and finally paralysis.[10] The back pain and spinal tenderness usually bring a patient to the attention of a physician within 24 hours. Root pain radiating from the site of spinal tenderness may begin by the second or third day. Fever and leukocytosis usually are present by this time. Changes in deep tendon reflexes may be helpful for diagnosis of the anatomic level of the compression-depression of lower extremity reflexes if the compression overlies the cauda equina and of accentuation if the compression overlies the spinal cord. If undiagnosed and untreated, the advanced clinical phases of the disease include progressive motor weakness, ascending hypesthesia, impairment of bowel and bladder function, and finally paralysis.

Epidural abscess should be considered in the differential diagnosis for any patient presenting with symptoms of back pain and fever. Other considerations may include meningitis, spinal subdural abscess, acute transverse myelopathy, vertebral disc space disease, vertebral osteomyelitis, vascular lesions, and spinal cord tumor. Local spine tenderness in association with back pain and fever suggests the possibility of an epidural space process. Despite the relative rarity of spinal epidural abscess, the complications are so serious that prompt diagnosis and treatment are of paramount importance.

Immediate surgical intervention is associated with the best chance of recovery of neurologic function.

In cases of acute epidural abscess associated with epidural catheters, the reported duration of catheter maintenance has ranged from 24 hours to 4 days, with abscess symptoms occurring between 24 hours and 14 days after catheter insertion. In a patient with a history of recent epidural catheterization or with a temporary epidural catheter in place, the symptoms of back pain and fever should initially be addressed by careful physical examination, including a neurologic examination, percussion of the vertebral spines, and examination of the epidural site. Local erythema, tenderness, and drainage at the epidural catheter insertion site are suggestive of epidural catheter–related infection. Any drainage at the epidural skin site should be sent for Gram staining and culture; the skin site should then be disinfected, the epidural catheter carefully removed, and the catheter tip sent for culture. If local vertebral pain or tenderness is present, prompt cerebrospinal fluid examination should be considered and a magnetic resonance imaging (MRI) scan should be performed. In a patient with evidence of neurologic impairment, *immediate* MRI scanning and a neurosurgical consultation should be obtained. Prompt surgical laminectomy, decompression, and drainage, in addition to appropriate antibiotic therapy, should be implemented as indicated.

In patients with permanently implanted and subcutaneously tunneled epidural catheters, local erythema and drainage at the catheter exit site without vertebral pain or tenderness, signs of systemic infection, or neurologic impairment has been treated successfully with local exit-site care including topical disinfectants and antibiotics. However, patients with suspected deep track or epidural space infection without neurologic impairment should be evaluated by MRI and treated with catheter removal and culture and systemic antibiotics. For patients with MRI evidence of epidural space infection, a neurosurgical and infectious diseases consultation should be considered. Patients with neurologic signs should immediately be evaluated by MRI, and a neurosurgical consultation and antibiotic therapy should be instituted as outlined previously.

Epidural abscess has been reported in a few cases after epidural steroid injection. Patients should be informed of the potential for local immunosuppressive effects, the possibility of infectious complications after epidural steroid injection, and the need to seek medical attention early if any new or otherwise unexplained symptoms develop after the procedure.

SPECIAL CLINICAL SITUATIONS

Several common clinical situations deserve special consideration with respect to clinical management of epidural anesthesia or analgesia in patients with fever, bacteremia, or depressed immune status. Infectious complications of epidural anesthesia and analgesia occur rarely. However, the potential morbidity associated with these complications requires that the physician maintain a high index of suspicion for their development, especially in patients with depressed immune status. An ongoing assessment of the risk of infection vs. the analgesic benefit of epidural placement or maintenance must ultimately be made on an individual case basis.

Fever in the perioperative or peripartum period is not an uncommon occurrence and does not contraindicate the placement or maintenance of an epidural catheter for short-term anesthetic or analgesic management in immunocompetent patients. Patients with fever (including those suspected of having transient bacteremia) should be evaluated for potential sources of infection (e.g., pulmonary, urinary tract, surgical wound) and observed for any signs of erythema or tenderness at the catheter insertion site, spinal tenderness, signs of meningeal irritation, or changes in neurologic status. In postoperative patients with bacteremia, one may consider the removal and replacement of the potentially hematogenously contaminated catheter with a new catheter after administration of appropriate antibiotic therapy for the suspected pathogen. This practice would naturally be based on the anticipated benefit of the continuation of epidural analgesia vs. other analgesic modalities.

Patients who are immunocompromised or who are receiving long-term steroid therapy require an even higher level of suspicion with respect to the development of infectious complications. These patients may benefit greatly from the use of epidural anesthetic and analgesic techniques, especially in the intraoperative and early postoperative periods. It is my practice to selectively use epidural anesthesia and analgesia in these patients, with adherence to strict aseptic technique, close postoperative observation, and a duration of catheter maintenance of approximately 24 to 48 hours.

As with any invasive procedure, the decision to place or maintain an epidural catheter in any given patient must be based on an understanding of the risks of the procedure and the potential benefits for the individual patient. Physicians and other health care personnel caring for patients receiving epidural anesthesia and analgesia must understand the risks and the signs and symptoms of epidural catheter–related infections and epidural abscesses as a feature of their ongoing observation and management. With these principles in mind and maintenance of an appropriate index of suspicion, the risk and associated morbidity of epidural abscess can be reduced.

REFERENCES

1. Baker AS, Ojemann RG, Swartz MN, et al: Spinal epidural abscess. N Engl J Med 293:463, 1975.
2. de Leon-Casasola OA, Parker M, Lema MJ, et al: Postoperative epidural bupivacaine-morphine therapy. Anesthesiology 81:368, 1994.
3. Scott DA, Beilby DSN, McClymont C: Postoperative analgesia using epidural infusions of fentanyl with bupivacaine. Anesthesiology 66:729, 1995.
4. Darchy B, Forceville X, Bavoux E, et al: Clinical and bacteriologic survey of epidural analgesia in patients in the intensive care unit. Anesthesiology 85:988, 1996.
5. Goodman EJ, DeHorta E, Taguiam JM: Safety of spinal and epidural anesthesia in parturients with chorioamnionitis. Reg Anesth 21:436, 1996.
6. de Jong PC, Kansen PJ: A comparison of epidural catheters with or without subcutaneous injection ports for treatment of cancer pain. Anesth Analg 78:94, 1994.
7. Du Pen SL, Peterson DG, Williams A, et al: Infection during chronic epidural catheterization: Diagnosis and treatment. Anesthesiology 73:905, 1990.
8. Sato S, Sakuragi T, Dan K: Human skin flora as a potential source of epidural abscess. Anesthesiology 85:1276, 1996.
9. Feldenzer JA, McKeever PE, Schaberg DR, et al: Experimental spinal epidural abscess: A pathophysiological model in the rabbit. Neurosurgery 20:859, 1987.
10. Heusner AP: Nontuberculous spinal epidural infections. N Engl J Med 239:845, 1948.

FURTHER READING

Danner RL, Hartman BJ: Update of spinal epidural abscess: 35 cases and review of the literature. Rev Infect Dis 9:265, 1987.
Dawson P, Rosenfeld JV, Murphy MA, et al: Epidural abscess associated with postoperative epidural analgesia. Anaesth Intensive Care 19:569, 1991.
Holt HM, Andersen SS, Andersen O, et al: Infections following epidural catheterization. J Hosp Infect 30:253, 1995.
Strafford MA, Wilder RT, Berde CB: The risk of infection from epidural analgesia in children: A review of 1620 cases. Anesth Analg 80:234, 1995.
Wood CE, Goresky GV, Klassen KA, et al: Complications of continuous epidural infusions for postoperative analgesia in children. Can J Anaesth 41:613, 1994.

Chapter 110

Unintentional Subdural Injections

Cynthia A. Wong, M.D.

Epidural anesthesia complicated by total spinal anesthesia, after negative aspiration for cerebrospinal fluid (CSF), was first described in three case reports by de-Saram in 1956.[1] It was listed as a complication of epidural anesthesia ("massive epidural") by Dawkins in 1969.[2] Boys and Norman reported the first case of unintentional subdural placement of an epidural catheter for labor analgesia[3] and were the first to suggest that so-called massive epidurals were the result of subdural injection of local anesthetic. Since then, there have been multiple case reports of radiographically confirmed subdural injections of local anesthetics resulting in unusual blocks, or high- or total spinal anesthesia or analgesia. Therefore, anesthesiologists performing epidural anesthesia or analgesia should be aware that unintentional subdural injection can occur and contribute to morbidity.

Subdural injection can also occur during attempted subarachnoid anesthesia[4] or the subarachnoid injection of contrast material during myelography.[5]

ANATOMY OF THE SUBDURAL SPACE

The subdural space has classically been defined as a potential space between the dura and arachnoid membranes, containing a small amount of serous fluid.[6] Recently, this concept has been questioned.[7] Newer information suggests that the subdural space is not a true space. It is not lined by mesothelial cells and a basement membrane, as are other body spaces. In contrast, a specialized layer of fibroblasts with no extracellular collagen and few cell junctions lines the inner dura. This layer is structurally weak compared with the external dura. It opposes an arachnoid layer composed of larger cells with many tight junctions, which acts as the major barrier against movement of substances, including drugs, across the dura. Haines and associates[7] reviewed the literature, which suggests that the subdural space is created by traumatic shearing between the weak inner dural cell layer and the outer arachnoid layer. The ability

to perform spinaloscopy of the extra-arachnoid subdural space suggests that this shearing is easy to accomplish.[8]

The subdural space does exist pathologically. The spinal subdural space connects with the intracranial space and ends at the lower border of the S2 vertebral body, where the filum terminale becomes closely invested by dura.[6] Injected contrast material collects in larger volumes in the lateral and dorsal aspects of the space.[9] Along the dorsal nerve roots, the dura fuses with the epineurium distal to the ganglion, whereas, the arachnoid ends proximal to the ganglion.[6] In contrast, along the ventral nerve roots, the dura and arachnoid fuse together with the epineurium. This may explain the larger dorsal space and the propensity of subdural blocks to exhibit a greater sensory than motor component (see later).

INCIDENCE AND CHARACTERISTICS OF A SUBDURAL BLOCK

The incidence of subdural injection through a Tuohy needle was 0.82% in a retrospective chart review of epidural steroid injections.[10] Dawkins described the incidence of "massive epidural" as 0.1%.[2] The risk of unintentional subdural injection is most likely increased in patients with previous back surgery.[10] Intentional subdural injections have been described.[11] The technique involves identifying the epidural space and then rotating the needle 180 degrees with gentle pressure. Therefore, needle rotation may increase the incidence of subdural injection.

The incidence of unintentional subdural placement of an epidural catheter is not known.

The characteristics of the subdural injection of local anesthetic can best be described as atypical. The onset may be 5 to 30 minutes after injection.[10] This is in contrast to the unintentional injection of local anesthetic into the subarachnoid space, when symptoms, including total spinal anesthesia, occur within 1 to 2 minutes. Because of the prolonged onset time, a normal test dose will not rule out the subdural placement of a needle or catheter.

The presentation of a subdural block probably depends on the concentration and volume of local anesthetic injected, whether the injection is entirely into the subdural space or also into the epidural space, and perhaps on the position of the patient. Usually, the sensory level is significantly higher than expected, based on the volume of injected local anesthetic. Total spinal anesthesia can occur.[1] Even if local anesthetic spread is limited to the spinal subdural space, block of the trigeminal nerve can occur.[12] (The spinal tract of the trigeminal nerve extends down to C2.[6]) Sacral spread is usually limited. Motor block may be more profound than expected,[10] although usually the sensory block is more extensive than the motor block, and the motor block can be patchy. This may be explained by the fact that the dorsal subdural space, where the sensory nerve roots are located, is larger. Occasionally, blocks may be unilateral.[12] Hypotension can be profound but is usually much easier to treat than the hypotension associated with unintentional subarachnoid injection.[10] Again, this may be explained by the fact that sympathetic nerve fibers travel with the ventral (motor) nerve roots, which tend to be less blocked.

SUMMARY OF CASE REPORTS

Case reports have described a variety of circumstances in which unintentional injection of the subdural space has occurred. For the purposes of this review, only the most recent case reports are referenced.

There are several case reports of multiorifice epidural catheters placed with the tip and distal orifices located in the subdural space and the proximal orifices located in the epidural space, resulting in a combined epidural/subdural block.[13] A functioning epidural catheter can migrate into subdural space.[14] In an attempt to salvage an epidural catheter unintentionally placed in the subarachnoid space, the catheter was pulled back into the subdural space, and a subdural block resulted.[15] In another case, a subarachnoid catheter was placed after unintentional dural puncture. Despite the ability to withdraw CSF, injection of local anesthetic through the catheter resulted in no neuraxial block. Radiologic examination demonstrated that the catheter tip was located in a pool of CSF in the subdural space.[16]

Although unintentional subdural injection is most often associated with attempted epidural anesthesia or analgesia, it can occur with other nerve blocks. A lumbar sympathetic block complicated by unilateral sensory block and Horner's syndrome may have been secondary to the subdural injection of local anesthetic.[17, 18] Subdural injection during attempted retrobulbar block can result in sudden respiratory arrest.[19] Unintentional subdural injection can also complicate stellate ganglion blocks,[20] interscalene brachial plexus blocks,[21] and attempted placement of a caudal catheter.[22]

The subdural injection of air during attempted identification of the epidural space using the loss-of-resistance-to-air technique has been described in several case reports.[23] The headaches occurred immediately after injection and were not postural.

Finally, after unintentional placement of subdural catheters, opioids have been injected into the subdural space for both chronic[24] and acute[25] pain control. Opioid doses less than the normal epidural dose resulted in analgesia lasting longer than single-shot opioid epidural analgesia.

MANAGEMENT OF UNINTENTIONAL SUBDURAL INJECTION

Management of the side effects of unintentional subdural catheter placement includes support of circulation and respiration should a high spinal anesthetic develop.

Several authors have reported successfully maintaining recognized subdural catheters, using infusions with smaller drug volumes.[24, 26] However, McMenemin and associates[27] reported that the computed tomography examination of a patient who had received an unintentional subdural injection showed a space-occupying lesion that displaced the spinal cord anteriorly. They suggest that this mass in the subdural space could exert pressure on the nerve roots or spinal cord or cause compression of spinal vessels and may be an explanation for rare permanent neurologic damage after epidural anesthesia. Hilgenhurst and coworkers[28] reported permanent neurologic injury after infusion of meperidine through a subdural catheter. A computed tomographic scan documented fluid in the subdural space and altered subarachnoid anatomy. Several authors have documented the subarachnoid[29] and epidural[30] migration of subdural catheters. Therefore, in light of the possibility of unrecognized subarachnoid migration of a subdural catheter and the unpredictable and varied block that results from the injection of local anesthetics and opioids into the subdural space, it seems prudent to replace an unintentional subdural catheter whenever possible.

SUMMARY

Unintentional subdural injection via a needle or catheter can occur during attempted epidural anesthesia or analgesia, as well as during other nerve blocks adjacent to the central nervous system. A normal test dose may not rule out subdural injection, as the onset of the block can be delayed. The clinical presentation of the block resulting from the subdural injection of local anesthetics is atypical and varied, depending on the site of injection, concentration and volume of anesthetic injection, and perhaps the position of the patient.

REFERENCES

1. deSaram M: Accidental total spinal anesthesia. Anaesthesia 11:77, 1956.
2. Dawkins CJM: An analysis of the complications of extradural and caudal block. Anaesthesia 24:554, 1969.

3. Boys JE, Norman PF: Accidental subdural analgesia: A case report, possible clinical implications and relevance to "massive extradurals." Br J Anaesth 47:1111, 1975.

4. Sechzer PH: Subdural space in spinal anesthesia. Anesthesiology 24:869, 1963.

5. Dake MD, Dillon WP, Dorwart RH: CT of extraarachnoid metrizamide instillation. Am J Roentgen 147:583, 1986.

6. Romanes GJ: Cunningham's Manual of Practical Anatomy. Oxford, England, Oxford University Press, 1986.

7. Haines DE, Harkey HL, al-Mefty O: The "subdural" space: A new look at an outdated concept. Neurosurgery 32:111, 1993.

8. Blomberg RG: The lumbar subdural extraarachnoid space of humans: An anatomical study using spinaloscopy in autopsy cases. Anesth Analg 66:177, 1987.

9. Shapiro R: Myelography. Chicago, Year Book Medical Publishers, 1986.

10. Lubenow T, Keh-Wong E, Kristof K, et al: Inadvertent subdural injection: A complication of an epidural block. Anesth Analg 67:175, 1988.

11. Mehta M, Maher R: Injection into the extra-arachnoid subdural space. Anaesthesia 32:760, 1977.

12. Manchanda VN, Murad SH, Shilyansky G, et al: Unusual clinical course of accidental subdural local anesthetic injection. Anesth Analg 62:1124, 1983.

13. Sala-Blanch X, Martinez-Palli G, Agusti-Lasus M, et al: Misplacement of multihole epidural catheters—a report of two cases. Anaesthesia 51:386, 1996.

14. Abouleish E, Goldstein M: Migration of an extradural catheter into the subdural space. A case report. Br J Anaesth 58:1194, 1986.

15. Stevens RA, Stanton-Hicks MD: Subdural injection of local anesthetic: A complication of epidural anesthesia. Anesthesiology 63:323, 1985.

16. van der Maaten JM, van Kleef JW: Failure of anaesthesia after accidental subdural catheter placement. Acta Anaesthesiol Scand 36:707, 1992.

17. Willis MH, Korbon GA, Arasi R: Horner's syndrome resulting from a lumbar sympathetic block. Anesthesiology 68:613, 1988.

18. Sugar RG: A new complication due to the lumbar sympathetic block [letter]? Anesthesiology 69:803, 1988.

19. Drysdale DB: Experimental subdural retrobulbar injection of anesthetic. Ann Ophthalmol 16:716, 1984.

20. Bruyns T, Devulder J, Vermeulen H, et al: Possible inadvertent subdural block following attempted stellate ganglion blockade. Anaesthesia 46:747, 1991.

21. Tetzlaff JE, Yoon HJ, Dilger J, et al: Subdural anesthesia as a complication of an interscalene brachial plexus block [case report]. Reg Anesth 19:357, 1994.

22. Calder TM, Harris AP: Subdural block during attempted caudal epidural analgesia for labor. Anesthesiology 76:316, 1992.

23. Hogan QH, Haddox JD: Headache from intracranial air after a lumbar epidural injection: subarachnoid or subdural? Reg Anesth 17:303, 1992.

24. Brown G, Atkinson GL, Standiford SB: Subdural administration of opioids. Anesthesiology 71:611, 1989.

25. Chadwick HS, Bernards CM, Kovarik DW, et al: Subdural injection of morphine for analgesia following cesarean section: A report of three cases. Anesthesiology 77:590, 1992.

26. Collier CB, Gatt SP, Lockley SM: A continuous subdural block. Br J Anaesth 70:462, 1993.

27. McMenemin IM, Sissons GR, Brownridge P: Accidental subdural catheterization: Radiological evidence of a possible mechanism for spinal cord damage. Br J Anaesth 69:417, 1992.

28. Hilgenhurst G, Sukiennik AW, Anderson ML, et al: Paraplegia after continuous subdural meperidine infusion. Anesthesiology 80:462, 1994.

29. Foster PN, Stickle BR, Griffiths JO: Variable presentation of subdural block [letter]. Anaesthesia 50:178, 1995.

30. Ralph CJ, Williams MP: Subdural or epidural? Confirmation with magnetic resonance imaging. Anaesthesia 51:175, 1996.

Chapter 111

Cauda Equina Syndrome After Continuous Spinal Anesthesia

Tom C. Krejcie, M.D.

There have been a total of 11 reported cases of cauda equina syndrome following continuous spinal anesthesia.[1-3] The syndrome results from a dysfunction of the various components of the cauda equina's roots. It comprises a tetrad of symptoms including low back pain, saddle anesthesia, bowel and bladder sphincter dysfunction, and, possibly, chronic paraplegia. The structures of the conus medullaris and the cauda equina are prone to injury from a variety of causes, including drug (local anesthetic) toxicity and direct trauma. Whereas this chapter deals with cauda equina syndrome as it relates to spinal anesthesia, all of the many causative factors have to be considered if the onset of symptoms is temporally related to the performance of spinal anesthesia, be it a single-injection technique or a continuous technique requiring placement of a subarachnoid catheter. Table 111–1 contains the various etiologies for this class of neuropathies.

PERTINENT ANATOMY

The cauda equina (horse's tail) begins immediately below the conus medullaris of the spinal cord at the level of the third lumbar vertebra at birth and, through growth and development, is located below the first lumbar vertebra in adults. It includes both lumbar and sacral spinal roots. The cauda equina results from the spinal cord being shorter than the vertebral column, with the incongruity between vertebral level and spinal roots being greatest at the caudal terminus. This arrangement results in the roots forming the cauda equina being in close proximity to one another and therefore being more susceptible to combined injury, as well as traversing a relatively long distance within the subarachnoid space before reaching and exiting their respective neural foramina. The cauda equina roots provide motor and sensory innervation of most of the lower extremities, pelvic floor, and the sphincters. The nerves also provide afferent and efferent autonomic activity to these nerve areas and, as such, are responsible for bowel and bladder function. The cauda equina and other spinal nerve roots are surrounded by a root sheath, rather than the more substantial perineurium that covers nerves distal to the subarachnoid angle. The physical differences in this component of the blood-nerve barrier may be exaggerated in sacral roots, making them more susceptible to neurotoxic injury. Although subarachnoid-administered local anesthetics act on superficial layers of the spinal cord, their primary site of action is on the nerve fibers.

The vascular supply to these nerves is very complex and highly variable between individuals. The major consequence of these varied vascular arrangements is that the area is prone to ischemic injury. Blood supply to the conus medullaris and the cauda equina is from the anterior and paired posterior spinal arteries, branches of the vertebral arteries, and from various radicular arteries with a unilateral (usually left-sided) predominance. The major anterior radicular artery supplying this area with a higher, usually thoracic, origin is the artery of the lumbar enlargement, also known as the arteria radicularis magna or the artery of Adamkiewicz.

LOCAL ANESTHETIC NEUROTOXICITY

Based on multiple studies of diverse local anesthetic agents, it is clear that local anesthetics, per se, are toxic to nerves. Ready and colleagues[4] have demonstrated the potential neurotoxicity of 5% lidocaine in dextrose. In a review of the physiologic mechanisms by which local anesthetics may cause nerve injury, Kalichman[5] concluded that the toxic *potential* of the local anesthetics *is not* correlated with pH or osmolality of the solution or the presence or absence of additives (sodium bisulfite, sodium metabisulfite, or methylparaben). There is no evidence that ester- or amide-linked local anesthetics have a greater potential for causing nerve injury. Toxicity does depend on local anesthetic concentration, *not* total dose, and the relative potency for nerve injury with four different local anesthetic agents is the same as their relative potency for producing nerve conduction block. It is interesting to note that lidocaine and tetra-

TABLE 111-1. CAUSES OF CAUDA EQUINA SYNDROME

A. Compressive etiologies
  1. Intramedullary, extramedullary-intradural, epidural tumors
  2. Epidural hematomas and abscesses
  3. Herniated lumbosacral disks
  4. Spinal stenosis
B. Noncompressive etiologies
  1. Spinal arachnoiditis
    a. Drug toxicity
    b. Surgical intervention
    c. Idiopathic
  2. Infectious etiologies
    a. Bacterial
    b. Viral
       i. Genital herpes virus
      ii. Cytomegalovirus
     iii. Varicella-zoster
  3. Inflammatory
  4. Ischemic insults
  5. Large vessel compression (i.e., anterior spinal artery syndrome)
  6. Microscopic (drug toxicity)

caine are the most water soluble of the local anesthetics and, as such, can be prepared for clinical administration in relatively high concentrations. The concentration-dependent effect of anesthetics causes, in moderate doses, endoneural edema that resolves without sequelae, but high concentrations are associated, initially, with greater volumes of edema and subsequent, primary ischemic injury to Schwann cells. Local anesthetics can reduce nerve blood flow, and it may be through this mechanism that injury occurs.[5] Diseases affecting the caliber of the microvasculature or stretching the nerve by flexing the back or hip may reduce the margin of safety and predispose the tissue to neuropathologic changes when vasoconstrictive drugs (local anesthetics) are administered; moderate levels of nerve ischemia cause demyelination, but severe ischemia causes axonal injury. The damage results from ischemia of or a direct neurotoxic effect to the neurons or glia. Ischemia is a common cause of neurologic deficits ranging from transient dysfunction to permanent paralysis.

MECHANICAL AND TECHNICAL PROBLEMS

The continuous spinal anesthesia tray as originally supplied by the Kendall Healthcare Corporation contained a 28-gauge microbore catheter that was threaded through a conventional 22-gauge Quincke bevel spinal needle. Unlike an epidural needle, the microbore catheter would exit the end of the spinal needle in a straight coaxial direction without a directional bias. The catheter, when threaded, would have a propensity to travel initially in a cephalad direction only because of the angle used when placing the spinal needle into the subarachnoid space. However, once the catheter leaves the spinal needle its subsequent course is affected by the subarachnoid structures. In a nice demonstration by Möllmann and associates,[6] the disposition of a microbore catheter was followed using a 2-mm endoscope

(spinaloscopy) inserted from the caudal end of a freshly prepared cadaveric human spinal column (T12-S1). From their observations, they concluded that the direction taken by the spinal catheter could not be controlled, nor could the final position of the catheter tip be predicted if the catheter was inserted more than 2 cm past the end of the needle. Using a paramedian approach in placing the spinal needle did not help in this matter, nor did rotating the bevel of the needle. There was no apparent trauma to spinal nerves by either placement of the spinal needle or catheter due to the mobility of these structures within the spinal canal. It is possible that the catheter may lean against a single nerve and over time cause mechanical damage. This does not, however, explain the multilevel injury exhibited by most patients. These findings support the report of Chan and Smyth,[7] who demonstrated radiographically the caudad position and restricted sacral block in a patient. The likelihood that a catheter would be positioned in the sacral terminus is further quantitated by a radiographic evaluation by Standl and Beck.[8] In their report, they found that 16% of the 28-gauge catheters placed into the subarachnoid space were directed caudally. Rigler and Drasner,[9] using a model of the subarachnoid space, have demonstrated pooling of highly concentrated hyperbaric lidocaine when a 28-gauge is directed caudally and that the pooling is independent of the speed with which the local anesthetic is injected.

TRANSIENT RADICULAR IRRITATION

Transient radicular irritation (TRI) is thought to be the cause of the vague sensations that a patient may relate if carefully questioned in the period following the normal clinical resolution of a spinal anesthetic. I have included TRI in this chapter on cauda equina syndrome because it may represent a subset of the same "toxic" phenomenon or be one point in a spectrum of disease. For reasons that are not clear, this syndrome appears to be occurring with increasing frequency. It consists of aching pain and/or dysesthesias in a dermatomal distribution over the buttocks and radiating to both dorsolateral sides of the thighs and calves. The pain seems to be worse at night and is relieved when the patient stands up and walks around. Nonsteroidal anti-inflammatory agents provide incomplete analgesia.

In the case report of Schneider and co-workers,[10] the authors presented four cases of TRI of 88 patients receiving 5% hyperbaric lidocaine for similar surgical procedures performed in the lithotomy position. During this same time period, 120 patients received a bupivacaine spinal anesthetic with no apparent sequelae. In their report, the authors noted that the L5 and S1 spinal nerves lie in the most dorsal position in the spinal canal. They hypothesized that in the supine position, the sensory fibers of these nerves are most exposed to a hyperbaric local anesthetic solution pooling in this area. Furthermore, placing a patient into the lithotomy position is generally linked to a reduction of the physiologic lordosis of the lumbar spine and induces stretching of the cauda equina. Stretching of nerves may decrease their perfusion and increase their vulnerability to a local anesthetic. In a prospective study, Pollock and associates[11] compared 5% hyperbaric lidocaine (with 0.2 mg epinephrine) to either 2% isobaric lidocaine or 0.75% bupivacaine and surveyed the incidence of TRI. Sixteen percent of patients receiving either 5% lidocaine with epinephrine (8 of 51) or 2% lidocaine (8 of 51) complained of symptoms consistent with TRI. None of the patients given a bupivacaine spinal had similar complaints. The incidence of back pain without radiation (non-TRI back pain) was also highest in the 5% lidocaine group, compared with 2% lidocaine or bupivacaine (20% vs. 6% vs. 8%, respectively).

The significance of TRI, which spontaneously resolves over a maximum of 4 days, is that lidocaine, when administered in the subarachnoid space, can produce a "toxic" effect, although at this time, without demonstrating a persistent deficit, the clinical significance of this syndrome remains unclear.

CONCLUSIONS

Following the flurry of case reports and the subsequent withdrawal of microbore catheters from the North American market, a symposium on continuous spinal anesthesia was held in August 1993. The manuscripts that resulted from this comprehensive meeting have been published.[12] After reviewing the literature on cauda equina syndrome as it relates to continuous spinal anesthesia and my own clinical experience with the technique and this particular complication,[1] several conclusions may be drawn.

Our initial case report on cauda equina syndrome after continuous spinal anesthesia has often been misquoted. This syndrome is not limited to, but rather is dominated by, microbore catheters and 5% hyperbaric lidocaine. This may be because of the commercial availability of the combination of a microbore catheter and 5% hyperbaric lidocaine and the resurgence of continuous spinal anesthesia or because of the fact that this combination of drug and technique unveiled a previously unappreciated local anesthetic toxicity. Three of the four cases we reported involved the 28-gauge microcatheter threaded through a conventional 22-gauge Quincke spinal needle and an initial dose of 5% lidocaine with 7.5% dextrose exceeding 100 mg. The fourth case involved placing a 20-gauge catheter threaded through an 18-gauge modified Tuohy epidural needle (epidural anesthetic kit) into the subarachnoid space, after which 28 mg of 0.5% tetracaine with 5% dextrose was incrementally administered to obtain adequate lower extremity anesthesia. In all four cases, more than one ampule of the local anesthetic solution was administered to obtain the *initial* surgical anesthetic. In no case was evidence of sacral anesthesia evaluated in the supine patient. The other seven reported cases of cauda equina syndrome occurred after the patient received a continuous spinal anesthetic with 5% hyperbaric lidocaine administered through a microbore catheter.

The most consistent explanation for this sequela is the inhomogeneous distribution of the local anesthetic resulting in an anesthetic concentration undiluted by cerebral spinal fluid resulting in local anesthetic toxicity. The initial administration of more than 100 mg of 5% hyperbaric lidocaine becomes a necessary but not sufficient requirement for a cauda equina syndrome to ensue. It is a necessary requirement because there is no case report of cauda equina syndrome when less than 100 mg of lidocaine was given. The minimum dose requirement is not sufficient because there is evidence in the literature that initial doses of lidocaine exceeding 100 mg have been given without subsequent evidence of a cauda equina syndrome. Obviously there are other factors that alter the disposition or toxicity of the spinal lidocaine.

The microbore spinal catheter increases the likelihood of local anesthetic toxicity by (1) providing the route for repeated injections of a short-duration local anesthetic (5% hyperbaric "spinal" lidocaine); (2) slowing injection of the local anesthetic and thus inhibiting mixing within the cerebrospinal fluid; and (3) its possibly greater potential for caudal positioning permits the local anesthetic to be deposited in the confined area of the sacral terminus. These conclusions are consistent with those concerns expressed by deJong in his editorial, "Last round for a heavyweight?"[13] In this editorial, he summarized the then-current literature surrounding the use of 5% lidocaine in 7.5% dextrose, including the 11 reported cases of cauda equina syndrome as well as the earliest report of TRI. Although deJong advised against using spinal lidocaine, Carpenter recommended its continued use until a "safer" short-acting alternative becomes available.[14] Douglas also recommended the continued use of spinal lidocaine but with adherence to the following guidelines: informed consent by the patient, cephalad direction of the spinal needle opening, and rapid lidocaine injection.[15]

REFERENCES

1. Rigler ML, Drasner K, Krejcie TC, et al: Cauda equina syndrome after continuous spinal anesthesia. Anesth Analg 72:275–281, 1991.
2. Schell RM, Brauer FS, Cole DJ, et al: Persistent sacral nerve root deficits after continuous spinal anaesthesia. Can J Anaesth 38:908–911, 1991.
3. Ross BK, Coda B, Heath CH: Local anesthetic distribution in a spinal model: A possible mechanism of neurologic injury after continuous spinal anesthesia. Reg Anesth 17:69–77, 1992.
4. Ready LB, Plumer MH, Haschke RH, et al: Neurotoxicity of intrathecal local anesthetics in rabbits. Anesthesiology 63:364–370, 1985.
5. Kalichman MW: Physiologic mechanisms by which local anesthetics may cause injury to nerve and spinal cord. Reg Anesth 18:448–452, 1993.
6. Möllmann M, Holst D, Lübbesmeyer H, et al: Continuous spinal anesthesia: Mechanical and technical problems of catheter placement. Reg Anesth 18:469–472, 1993.
7. Chan VWS, Smyth RJ: Radiographic examination of catheter position in restricted sacral block after continuous spinal anesthesia. Anesth Analg 75:449–452, 1992.
8. Standl T, Beck H: Radiological examination of the intrathecal position of microcatheters in continuous spinal anaesthesia. Br J Anaesth 71:803–806, 1993.
9. Rigler ML, Drasner K: Distribution of catheter-injected local anes-

thetic in a model of the subarachnoid space. Anesthesiology 75:684–692, 1991.

10. Schneider M, Ettlin T, Kaufmann M, et al: Transient neurologic toxicity after hyperbaric subarachnoid anesthesia with 5% lidocaine. Anesth Analg 76:1154–1157, 1993.

11. Pollock JE, Neal JM, Stephenson CA, et al: Prospective study of the incidence of transient radicular irritation in patients undergoing spinal anesthesia. Anesthesiology 84:1361–1367, 1996.

12. Scientific publications ASRA continuous spinal anesthesia symposium. Reg Anesth 18:1993.

13. deJong RH: Last round for a "heavyweight?" Anesth Analg 78:3–4, 1994.

14. Carpenter RL: Hyperbaric lidocaine spinal anesthesia: Do we need an alternative? Anesth Analg 81:1125, 1995.

15. Douglas MJ: Neurotoxicity of lidocaine—does it exist? Can J Anaesth 42:181, 1995.

Chapter 112

Back Pain After Epidural Chloroprocaine Injection

Cynthia A. Wong, M.D.

HISTORY

In the 1980s, reports appeared in the literature documenting adhesive arachnoiditis after the inadvertent subarachnoid injection of 2-chloroprocaine preparations containing sodium bisulfite, an antioxidant additive. In October 1987, Astra Pharmaceuticals (Astra USA, Inc., Westborough, Mass) changed the formulation of 2% and 3% Nesacaine (2-chloroprocaine), eliminating the sodium bisulfite and replacing it with the chelating agent disodium ethylenediaminetetraacetic acid (EDTA, 0.111 mg/mL) (Nesacaine-MPF).

Beginning in April 1988, Fibuch and Opper documented severe lower back pain in 8 of 20 patients after resolution of epidural 2-chloroprocaine anesthesia using the new formulation.[1] The pain was described as intense, localized to the lower back, and associated, in some patients, with palpable muscle spasm and localized tenderness. Possible mechanisms included the unlikely possibility of local muscle trauma due to technical difficulties administering the epidural anesthetic, direct nerve damage, or local anesthetic induced myotoxicity. A more likely etiology was muscle spasm secondary to local hypocalcemia. Disodium EDTA actively chelates calcium. Diffusion of Nesacaine-MPF through vertebral foramina into the lumbar muscles might lead to localized hypocalcemia. Ackerman[2] suggested that the symptoms might be associated with skin, subcutaneous, and intramuscular injection of Nesacaine and local irritation caused by the low pH of the formulation.

Meanwhile, Astra Pharmaceuticals was contacted by other anesthesiologists reporting the same observation, and in December 1988, the company wrote a "Dear Doctor" letter alerting anesthesiologists to this phenomena and suggesting that back pain was associated with larger volumes (>20 to 25 mL) of Nesacaine-MPF and the use of the same local anesthesia for skin and needle tract local anesthesia infiltration.

PRELIMINARY STUDIES

In 1989, Levy and colleagues[3] studied 54 patients who were randomly assigned to receive epidural anes-

thesia with 3% Nesacaine-MPF with or without epinephrine or 2% lidocaine with or without epinephrine. Lidocaine was used for local infiltration. Their results confirmed a higher incidence of moderate and severe lower back pain in patients receiving Nesacaine-MPF compared with lidocaine. The exact mechanism remained unclear. However, in support of the localized hypocalcemia theory, Dirkes[4] reported the dramatic resolution of back pain in one patient after the intravenous administration of calcium chloride.

Subsequently, two studies in volunteers,[5, 6] designed to study physiologic effects of epidural anesthesia, provided the researchers with the opportunity to document Nesacaine-MPF associated back pain in a prospective manner. Hynson and colleagues[5] reported severe, spasmodic back pain in four of five volunteers receiving Nesacaine-MPF but no severe back pain in 14 remaining volunteers who received epidural lidocaine or saline injections. Large volumes (>30 mL) of all three solutions were injected, suggesting that the back pain was indeed related to the epidural injection of Nesacaine-MPF, not to large volumes of local anesthetic solutions. Similarly, back pain developed in 10 of 10 volunteers who received large doses of Nesacaine-MPF in three separate injections over a 7-hour period.[6] There was a significant upward increase in Visual Analog Pain scores as the volume of local anesthetic injected increased. In both studies, the pain was not associated with paraspinous muscle spasm, nor was it relieved with a change in position, massage, or the local application of heat. Several volunteers (all medically sophisticated) localized the pain to deep back muscles (psoas or quadratus lumborum).[6]

DEFINITIVE EVIDENCE

Stevens and colleagues[7] studied 100 patients scheduled for outpatient knee arthroscopies. Patients were randomly assigned to one of five groups: (1) 2% lidocaine (initial dose, 30 mL), (2) 3% 2-chloroprocaine with EDTA (initial dose, 15 mL), (3) 3% 2-chloroprocaine with EDTA (initial dose, 30 mL), (4) 3% 2-chloroprocaine without EDTA (initial dose, 30 mL), and (5) 3% 2-chloroprocaine with EDTA, pH adjusted to 7.27 (initial dose, 30 mL). Epinephrine 1:200,000 was freshly added to all the local anesthetic solutions, and 1% lidocaine was used for local skin and needle tract infiltration. A blinded investigator evaluated knee and back pain after the resolution of the epidural anesthesia. Patients in group 2 received a mean of 21 mL local anesthesia; patients in the other groups received means of 40 to 43 mL of local anesthesia. Type II back pain (described as a deep, aching, burning pain in the lumbar region) occurred in 50% of group 3 patients compared with 10% of group 2 and 4, 25% of group 5, and 5% of group 1 patients. The authors concluded that the presence of disodium EDTA and total injected volume of local anesthesia were important factors contributing to postepidural anesthesia back pain. Increasing the pH of the solution lessened the severity but did not eliminate the incidence of back pain. Limiting the dose of 2-chloroprocaine with EDTA to less than 25 mL resulted in a similar low incidence of back pain to that after epidural lidocaine.

SUMMARY

2-Chloroprocaine with disodium EDTA should be limited to doses of less than 25 mL to avoid postanesthesia back pain. If higher volumes or repeat doses are anticipated, then a different local anesthetic should be chosen.

In December 1996, Astra released a new formulation of 2% and 3% 2-chloroprocaine (Nesacaine-MPF 2% and 3%) that contains no preservative (no disodium EDTA and no methylparaben). Nesacaine 1% and 2% (Astra USA, Inc.) contains both disodium EDTA (0.111 mg/mL) and methylparaben.

REFERENCES

1. Fibuch EE, Opper SE: Back pain following epidurally administered Nesacaine-MPF. Anesth Analg 69:113, 1989.
2. Ackerman WE: Back pain after epidural Nesacaine-MPF [letter]. Anesth Analg 70:224, 1990.
3. Levy L, Randel GI, Pandit SK: Does chloroprocaine (Nesacaine MPF) for epidural anesthesia increase the incidence of backache [letter]? Anesthesiology 71:476, 1989.
4. Dirkes WE Jr: Treatment of nesacaine-MPF–induced back pain with calcium chloride [letter]. Anesth Analg 70:461, 1990.
5. Hynson JM, Sessler DI, Glosten B: Back pain in volunteers after epidural anesthesia with chloroprocaine. Anesth Analg 72:253, 1991.
6. Stevens RA, Chester WL, Artuso JD, et al: Back pain after epidural anesthesia with chloroprocaine in volunteers: Preliminary report. Reg Anesth 16:199, 1991.
7. Stevens RA, Urmey WF, Urquhart BL, et al: Back pain after epidural anesthesia with chloroprocaine. Anesthesiology 78:492, 1993.

Chapter 113

Transient Radiculitis After Subarachnoid Lidocaine Injection

Cynthia A. Wong, M.D.

HISTORY

Subarachnoid lidocaine for spinal anesthesia has been used for nearly half a century. Phillips and associates[1] prospectively evaluated 5% hyperbaric lidocaine in the 1960s in 10,440 patients and reported an excellent safety profile. Fewer than 0.5% of the patients had post-anesthesia peripheral nerve symptoms.

In 1991, two small series of case reports were published describing cauda equina syndrome after continuous spinal anesthesia with microcatheters.[2, 3] Five of the six patients received 5% hyperbaric lidocaine; one patient received hyperbaric tetracaine. A study of 5% hyperbaric lidocaine distribution after injection through a microcatheter into a spinal canal model implicated high (toxic) local cerebrospinal fluid drug concentrations as a possible etiology for the reported nerve damage.[4] Microcatheters were subsequently withdrawn from the market.

Soon thereafter, Schneider and colleagues[5] reported four patients who experienced transient radicular irritation after completely recovering from spinal anesthesia with 5% hyperbaric lidocaine. The anesthetics were administered uneventfully through 24- to 25-gauge pencil-point needles. One to 20 hours after complete recovery from the anesthetic, the patients complained of pain, radiating from the lower back to the dorsolateral thighs and calves. Subsequently, Snyder and colleagues[6] documented five similar cases, Sjöström and Bläss,[7] one case, and Pinczower and co-workers,[8] nine cases. Case reports have continued to be published,[9] including three cases using isobaric 2% lidocaine.[10]

The pain described by the patients is aching or cramping, worse at night, may improve with ambulation and treatment with nonsteroidal anti-inflammatory drugs, and lasts several days.[5, 8] The neurologic examination reveals normal results.

PROSPECTIVE STUDIES

Hampl and colleagues[11] prospectively studied 270 patients undergoing spinal anesthesia with either hyperbaric lidocaine or bupivacaine. Patients were not randomized. Forty-four of 120 patients (37%) receiving lidocaine complained of transient radicular pain, and only 1 of 150 patients receiving bupivacaine had complaints. The groups were similar, except that duration of surgery was shorter in the lidocaine group and all patients in the lidocaine group were in the lithotomy position, compared with 62% in the bupivacaine group.

In another prospective, nonrandomized study of 600 patients undergoing spinal anesthesia, the incidence of transient radicular pain was 10% after 5% hyperbaric lidocaine and 0% after hyperbaric and isobaric bupivacaine.[12] In a third prospective study of 54 patients, the incidence of transient radicular pain after 5% hyperbaric lidocaine was 24%.[13]

Pollock and associates[14] prospectively randomized patients undergoing inguinal hernia repair and knee arthroscopy to receive subarachnoid 5% hyperbaric lidocaine with epinephrine, 2% isobaric lidocaine without epinephrine, or 0.75% hyperbaric bupivacaine without epinephrine. There was a 16% incidence of transient radicular irritation in patients receiving both concentrations of lidocaine, compared with 0% in the bupivacaine group. The incidence was significantly higher in the knee arthroscopy patients compared with the inguinal hernia patients. Needle type was not controlled.

Other studies also have compared different concentrations of lidocaine. In a study designed to compare the sensory and motor block characteristics of 5% and 1.5% lidocaine with dextrose and 1.5% lidocaine without dextrose,[15] volunteers reported transient radicular pain after spinal anesthesia with all three solutions of lidocaine. Hampl and co-workers[16] randomized 54 patients to receive 5% lidocaine with 7.5% or 2.7% dextrose, or 0.5% bupivacaine with 8.5% dextrose. Thirty percent to 33% of the lidocaine patients, but none of the bupivacaine patients, complained of transient radicular symptoms. Finally, Hampl and colleagues[17] randomized 50 patients to receive either 5% or 2% hyperbaric lidocaine. Thirty-two percent of the 5% lidocaine group and 40% of the 2% lidocaine group experienced transient radicular pain.

POSSIBLE FACTORS CONTRIBUTING TO TRANSIENT RADICULAR IRRITATION

It is interesting that lidocaine for subarachnoid anesthesia has been used for nearly 50 years, but transient radicular irritation has been reported only recently. Several mechanisms contributing to transient radicular irritation after spinal anesthesia have been suggested, although none has been proven to cause the syndrome or even to be associated with it. Several editorials have addressed the issue.[18-20] Suggested mechanisms or associated factors include local anesthetic neurotoxicity,[18-20] maldistribution of local anesthetic in the subarachnoid space after injection through pencil-point needles (used much more frequently now than in the past),[20] hyperosmolarity of the anesthetic solution,[19] operative position of the patient,[19, 20] and early ambulation.[20]

ANIMAL STUDIES OF LOCAL ANESTHETIC TOXICITY TO NERVES

Animal studies on peripheral nerves,[21] isolated nerve tissue,[22, 23] and intact subarachnoid anesthesia models[24, 25] have consistently demonstrated that high concentrations of local anesthetics are toxic to nerves. In desheathed bullfrog sciatic nerves, lidocaine caused progressive nonreversible loss of impulse activity with increasing concentration, beginning with 1% lidocaine.[23] In the same model, 5% lidocaine with and without 7.5% dextrose caused irreversible conduction blockade, whereas 7.5% dextrose alone had little residual conduction blockade.[22] Tetracaine 0.5% also caused irreversible blockade, whereas lidocaine 1.5% and bupivacaine 0.75% caused less.

In a rabbit model of subarachnoid anesthesia, concentrations of lidocaine and tetracaine slightly greater than those used clinically in humans produced dose-related neural injury, whereas 2-chloroprocaine and bupivacaine did not.[24] In a rat model, tail-flick latency 4 to 6 days after subarachnoid infusion was significantly prolonged after infusion of 5% hyperbaric lidocaine, compared with bupivacaine, tetracaine, and saline.[25] In the same model, 5% lidocaine infusion with and without glucose produced similar neurologic impairment.[26]

MALDISTRIBUTION OF LOCAL ANESTHETIC WITH PENCIL-POINT NEEDLES

Beardsley and colleagues[27] used an in vitro model of the spinal canal to address the issue of local anesthetic maldistribution after injection through pencil-point needles. They found that slow injection (2 mL in 60 seconds) through 25- and 27-gauge pencil-point needles, with the opening directed sacrally, resulted in higher local dye concentrations, compared with rapid injections (2 mL in 10 seconds) through the same needles,

through a 25-gauge Quincke needle and through needles with the opening directed cephalad.

CONCLUSIONS

Transient radicular irritation after spinal anesthesia appears to be a real entity with an unknown etiology. Studies have definitively shown that it is associated with lidocaine anesthesia in all clinically used concentrations (1.5% to 5%), with and without dextrose. Although the pain appears radicular in distribution, there is no evidence to support a neurologic origin for it.[19] The pain appears hours after the complete resolution of the neuraxial blockade and likely has a different mechanism than that responsible for permanent neurologic injury (e.g., cauda equina syndrome associated with microcatheters).[19] Pencil-point needles are now in vogue, but the syndrome is also common after spinal anesthesia with beveled needles.[7, 8, 13, 14, 28] Patient position may play a role,[29] but again, the syndrome has been described in all positions, and this has not been studied in a rigorous fashion.

The morbidity associated with the syndrome is low. No permanent neurologic sequelae have been reported, although one study documented an average verbal rating pain score (scale 1 to 10) of 6.2.[29] Astra USA mailed a "Dear Doctor" letter in 1995 and changed the package insert for its 5% hyperbaric spinal lidocaine. It suggested diluting 5% lidocaine with an equal volume of cerebrospinal fluid or saline, a maximum dose of 100 mg, replacement of the needle if spread of sensory blockade is inadequate and an additional dose is necessary, and use of spinal needles that allow aspiration of cerebrospinal fluid before and after anesthetic administration. Whether any of these suggestions would contribute to a decreased incidence of transient radicular irritation is unclear.

Experts differ on the issue of whether 5% lidocaine should continue to be used in clinical practice. deJong[18] advises against using it, Douglas[20] advises using it with appropriate precautions (informed consent of the patient, cephalad needle opening, rapid injection), and Carpenter[19] plans to continue using it until a safer, short-acting alternative is available.

REFERENCES

1. Phillips OC, Ebner H, Nelson AT, et al: Neurologic complications following spinal anesthesia with lidocaine: A prospective review of 10,440 cases. Anesthesiology 30:284, 1969.
2. Rigler ML, Drasner K, Krejcie TC, et al: Cauda equina syndrome after continuous spinal anesthesia. Anesth Analg 72:275, 1991.
3. Schell RM, Brauer FS, Cole DJ, et al: Persistent sacral nerve root deficits after continuous spinal anaesthesia. Can J Anaesth 38:908, 1991.
4. Ross BK, Coda B, Heath CH: Local anesthetic distribution in a spinal model: A possible mechanism of neurologic injury after continuous spinal anesthesia. Reg Anesth 17:69, 1992.
5. Schneider M, Ettlin T, Kaufmann M, et al: Transient neurologic toxicity after hyperbaric subarachnoid anesthesia with 5% lidocaine. Anesth Analg 76:1154, 1993.
6. Snyder R, Hui G, Flugstad P, et al: More cases of possible neuro-

logic toxicity associated with single subarachnoid injections of 5% hyperbaric lidocaine [letter]. Anesth Analg 78:411, 1994.

7. Sjöstrom S, Bläss J: Severe pain in both legs after spinal anaesthesia with hyperbaric 5% lignocaine solution. Anaesthesia 49:700, 1994.

8. Pinczower GR, Chadwick HS, Woodland R, et al: Bilateral leg pain following lidocaine spinal anaesthesia. Can J Anaesth 42:217, 1995.

9. Cozanitis DA: Leg pains after spinal anaesthesia [letter]. Can J Anaesth 42:657, 1995.

10. Hampl KF, Schneider MC, Bont A, et al: Transient radicular irritation after single subarachnoid injection of isobaric 2% lignocaine for spinal anaesthesia. Anaesthesia 51:178, 1996.

11. Hampl KF, Schneider MC, Ummenhofer W, et al: Transient neurologic symptoms after spinal anesthesia. Anesth Analg 81:1148, 1995.

12. Tarkkila P, Huhtala J, Tuominen M: Transient radicular irritation after spinal anaesthesia with hyperbaric 5% lignocaine. Br J Anaesth 74:328, 1995.

13. Salmela L, Aromaa U, Cozanitis DA: Leg and back pain after spinal anaesthesia involving hyperbaric 5% lignocaine. Anaesthesia 51:391, 1996.

14. Pollock JE, Neal JM, Stephenson CA, et al: Prospective study of the incidence of transient radicular irritation in patients undergoing spinal anesthesia. Anesthesiology 84:1361, 1996.

15. Liu S, Pollock JE, Mulroy MF, et al: Comparison of 5% with dextrose, 1.5% with dextrose, and 1.5% dextrose-free lidocaine solutions for spinal anesthesia in human volunteers. Anesth Analg 81:697, 1995.

16. Hampl KF, Schneider MC, Thorin D, et al: Hyperosmolarity does not contribute to transient radicular irritation after spinal anesthesia with hyperbaric 5% lidocaine. Reg Anesth 20:363, 1995.

17. Hampl KF, Schneider MC, Pargger H, et al: A similar incidence of transient neurologic symptoms after spinal anesthesia with 2% and 5% lidocaine. Anesth Analg 83:1051, 1996.

18. de Jong RH: Last round for a "heavyweight" [editorial]? Anesth Analg 78:3, 1994.

19. Carpenter RL: Hyperbaric lidocaine spinal anesthesia: do we need an alternative [editorial]? Anesth Analg 81:1125, 1995.

20. Douglas MJ: Neurotoxicity of lidocaine—does it exist [editorial]? Can J Anaesth 42:181, 1995.

21. Kalichman MW, Moorhouse DF, Powell HC, et al: Relative neural toxicity of local anesthetics. J Neuropathol Exp Neurol 52:234, 1993.

22. Lambert LA, Lambert DH, Strichartz GR: Irreversible conduction block in isolated nerve by high concentrations of local anesthetics. Anesthesiology 80:1082, 1994.

23. Bainton CR, Strichartz GR: Concentration dependence of lidocaine-induced irreversible conduction loss in frog nerve. Anesthesiology 81:657, 1994.

24. Ready LB, Plumer MH, Haschke RH, et al: Neurotoxicity of intrathecal local anesthetics in rabbits. Anesthesiology 63:364, 1985.

25. Drasner K, Sakura S, Chan VW, et al: Persistent sacral sensory deficit induced by intrathecal local anesthetic infusion in the rat. Anesthesiology 80:847, 1994.

26. Sakura S, Chan VW, Ciriales R, et al: The addition of 7.5% glucose does not alter the neurotoxicity of 5% lidocaine administered intrathecally in the rat. Anesthesiology 82:236, 1995.

27. Beardsley D, Holman S, Gantt R, et al: Transient neurologic deficit after spinal anesthesia: Local anesthetic maldistribution with pencil point needles? Anesth Analg 81:314, 1995.

28. Hampl KF, Schneider MC: Transient neurologic symptoms after spinal anesthesia [letter]. Anesth Analg 83:437, 1996.

29. Pollock JE, Mulroy MF, Stephenson C: Spinal anesthetics and the incidence of transient radicular irritation [abstract]. Anesthesiology 81:A1029, 1994.

● I n d e x